PUBLIC HEALTH

James M. Shultz, PhD, MS, is a population health scientist and associate professor, Department of Public Health Sciences, University of Miami Miller School of Medicine, and Member, Sylvester Comprehensive Cancer Center. He is the Director of P3H: Protect & Promote Population Health *in Complex Crises*. With a strong focus on medically high-risk patients, the mission of P3H is to optimize health by safeguarding populations from cascading crises and extreme events. He also directs the Center for Disaster and Extreme Event Preparedness (DEEP Center), well known for training in the field of disaster behavioral health and mental health and psychosocial support. He is currently conducting research and publishing on themes of population health science, safeguarding medically high-risk patients, disaster public and behavioral health, climate change impacts on population health, and complex and compounding disaster risks and resilience. Dr Shultz holds a PhD in behavioral epidemiology and a master of science degree in health behavior research from the University of Minnesota.

Lisa M. Sullivan, PhD, MA, is associate dean for education, professor, and former chair of biostatistics at Boston University School of Public Health. She is engaged in a wide range of research endeavors including the Framingham Heart study and is an award-winning educator. She is currently chairing the Association for Schools and Programs of Public Health's Framing the Future: Education for Public Health 2030 initiative.

Sandro Galea, MD, DrPH, a physician, epidemiologist, and author, is dean and Robert A. Knox Professor at Boston University School of Public Health. He is former chair of the board of the Association of Schools and Programs of Public Health and past president of the Society for Epidemiologic Research and of the Interdisciplinary Association for Population Health Science.

SECOND EDITION

PUBLIC HEALTH

An Introduction to the Science and Practice of Population Health

James M. Shultz, PhD, MS

Lisa M. Sullivan, PhD, MA

Sandro Galea, MD, DrPH

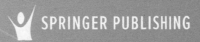

First Springer Publishing edition 2020 (978-0-8261-7753-7).

Springer Publishing Company, LLC
www.springerpub.com
connect.springerpub.com

Senior Acquisitions Editor: David D'Addona
Senior Director, Content Development: Taylor Ball
Production Editor: Joseph Stubenrauch
Compositor: S4Carlisle Publishing Services

ISBN: 978-0-8261-8042-1
ebook ISBN: 978-0-8261-8043-8
DOI: 10.1891/9780826180438

SUPPLEMENTS:

 A robust set of instructor resources designed to supplement this text is located at **http://connect.springerpub.com/content/book/978-0-8261-8043-8.** Qualifying instructors may request access by emailing **textbook@springerpub.com.**

LMS Common Cartridge With All Instructor Resources ISBN: 978-0-8261-8041-4
Instructor Manual ISBN: 978-0-8261-8044-5
Instructor Test Bank ISBN: 978-0-8261-8048-3
Instructor PowerPoints ISBN: 978-0-8261-8045-2
Instructor Syllabus ISBN: 978-0-8261-8047-6
Podcast Transcript ISBN: 978-0-8261-8046-9

23 24 25 26 / 5 4 3 2 1

The author and the publisher of this Work have made every effort to use sources believed to be reliable to provide information that is accurate and compatible with the standards generally accepted at the time of publication. Because medical science is continually advancing, our knowledge base continues to expand. Therefore, as new information becomes available, changes in procedures become necessary. We recommend that the reader always consult current research and specific institutional policies before performing any clinical procedure or delivering any medication. The author and publisher shall not be liable for any special, consequential, or exemplary damages resulting, in whole or in part, from the readers' use of, or reliance on, the information contained in this book. The publisher has no responsibility for the persistence or accuracy of URLs for external or third-party internet websites referred to in this publication and does not guarantee that any content on such websites is, or will remain, accurate or appropriate.

Library of Congress Cataloging-in-Publication Data

Names: Shultz, James M., 1950- author. | Sullivan, Lisa M. (Lisa Marie),
  1961- author. | Galea, Sandro, author.
Title: Public health: an introduction to the science and practice of
  population health / James M. Shultz, Lisa M. Sullivan, Sandro Galea.
Identifiers: LCCN 2023025615 (print) | LCCN 2023025616 (ebook) | ISBN
  9780826180421 (paperback) | ISBN 9780826180438 (ebook) | ISBN
  9780826180445 (Instructor's manual) | ISBN 9780826180483 (Instructor's
  test book) | ISBN 9780826180452 (Instructor's PowerPoints)
Subjects: MESH: Public Health Practice | Population Health | Public Health
  | Socioeconomic Factors
Classification: LCC RA425 (print) | LCC RA425 (ebook) | NLM WA 100 | DDC
  362.1–dc23/eng/20230721
LC record available at https://lccn.loc.gov/2023025615
LC ebook record available at https://lccn.loc.gov/2023025616

Contact sales@springerpub.com to receive discount rates on bulk purchases.

Printed in the United States of America by Hatteras, Inc.

This book is dedicated to Rosemary Park—and Sebastian, Luca, Theo, and Evangeline—Schiumo; Mariel Kim—and Nolan and Lucy—Crouser; and Dr. Zelde Espinel (JS); family, friends, and colleagues (LS); and Isabel Tess Galea, Oliver Luke Galea, and Dr. Margaret Kruk (SG).

CONTENTS

SECTION IV: THE METHODS OF PUBLIC HEALTH

PREFACE

We all care about our health. We all want to be healthy individuals and want our children, parents, partners, and friends to be healthy. Public health aspires to create a world where we can all live our healthiest possible life, to realize our full human potential. This book aims to serve as an introduction to public health for anyone who is interested in this ideal.

Public Health: An Introduction to the Science and Practice of Population Health is designed to introduce the reader to the fundamentals that they will need either to build a career in public health, or simply to know enough about public health to inform a career in other sectors. The second edition builds on the first edition, incorporating feedback from readers, and evolving in the aftermath of the COVID-19 pandemic that has transformed public health and adding a series of new and timely case studies.

The name of the book is meant to illustrate our bringing together of science and practice. Population health science helps us understand how health is generated in populations. Population health science is the foundation of public health practice that takes that understanding and makes populations healthier. Therefore, this book serves as an introduction to the science of population health, leading directly to the practice of public health.

The book starts from one fundamental premise: our health is generated throughout our lives and by the world around us—by where we live, where we work, and who we interact with on a daily basis. Once we understand that, we can then understand the work of public health through the study of two types of factors. First are the influences of our behaviors: our interactions with our family, friends, and communities; the places where we live; and the policies and norms that shape all that we do. This is called the social ecological perspective. Second are the forces that affect our health as we experience them throughout our life, from infancy to old age. This is called the life course perspective.

A note about one notable change in this edition. In the first edition of *Public Health* we referred to the framework that guides our thinking as the eco-social model. On reflection, and upon receiving feedback from readers, we recognize that the eco-social model is best reserved for a more specific theoretical framework. Our intention was always to use a term to broadly conceptualize the relations among personal and environmental factors that shape health, without reliance on any specific theoretical model. As such, in the second edition we use the term social ecological to capture these relations.

This book is organized such that the reader is introduced to these factors in sequence, learning first about the influences across social ecological levels, and then about how health is generated throughout the life course. This serves to organize the student's thinking and also guide the student in learning how we can design interventions at each of these levels that can improve our health and the health of others.

Bookending our discussions of the social ecological and life course perspectives is a discussion of the foundational concepts of public health, including the central roles of prevention, health equity, quantitative methods, how we have to think of population health as a complex system to guide intervention, and how those interventions must engage communities to be effective. The book includes access to podcasts that illustrate the key points of each chapter.

We recognize that our approach in this book is different than that taken by most other textbooks of public health. Our hope here is that an approach grounded in social ecological and life course perspectives can uniquely introduce the student to the science and practice of public health, and provide the instructor with a framework that can organize a rich body of material efficiently. Our goal ultimately is to help prepare the next generation of population health scientists and public health practitioners. If this book can be part of that effort, it shall have achieved its purpose.

Thank you for joining us on this journey.

James M. Shultz, Lisa M. Sullivan, Sandro Galea

Qualified instructors may obtain access to supplementary material (Instructor's Manual, PowerPoints, Test Bank, Case Study podcast transcripts, and Syllabus) by emailing textbook@springerpub.com.

ACKNOWLEDGMENTS

This book would not have been possible without the help of many. A formal thank you goes to Dr. Salma Abdalla who coauthored several chapters and lent a critical eye to many sections in the first edition, and to Haradeen Dhillon who provided extensive editorial assistance, careful review and updating of important data sources throughout the second edition. Thank you to Eric DelGizzo for fine-tooth-comb help with final copy-editing. Parisa Varanloo worked tirelessly on the figures and diagrams that illustrate the book throughout. Thanks to Nick Gooler who recorded and updated the podcasts associated with the book to add color and depth to the book's content. We are grateful to the editorial team at Springer who shepherded this project from start to finish, particularly David D'Addona and Taylor Ball, and to Joseph Stubenrauch who guided the production of the book. Colleagues, far too many to name, have shaped our thinking about the science of population health and the practice of public health. None of us would be here without their help, and this book would be infinitely poorer without their generous engagement with us throughout our lives. We are indebted to all of them. And finally, we are grateful to all our students who over the years have taught us how to teach public health and many who provided ideas, input, and thoughts about our teaching that ultimately shaped this book. This book would not have been possible without them. Thank you.

CASE STUDY PODCASTS

The authors of *Public Health: An Introduction to the Science and Practice of Population Health* have recorded a set of podcasts to illustrate the key points of each chapter. These podcasts are narrated by graduate students of public health and feature case studies pertinent to the chapter themes, most of which appear in the chapter text. It is our intention that they pique students' interests and inspire discussion both inside and outside of the classroom. Access the podcasts by following this link to Springer Publishing Company Connect™: https://connect.springerpub.com/content/book/978-0-8261-8043-8

ABBREVIATIONS AND COMMON DEFINITIONS

ABBREVIATIONS

AAA: Agricultural Adjustment Act

AACAP: American Academy of Child and Adolescent Psychiatry

ABM: agent-based model

ACA: Affordable Care Act

ACE: adverse childhood experience

ACL: Administration for Community Living

ADHD: attention deficit hyperactivity disorder

ADLs: activities of daily living

AHA: American Heart Association

AI/AN: American Indian/Alaska Native

AMA: American Medical Association

ANHB: Alaska Native Health Board

AoA: Administration of Aging

APHA: American Public Health Association

ATF: Bureau of Alcohol, Tobacco, Firearms and Explosives

ASPH: Association of Schools of Public Health

ASPPH: Association of Schools and Programs of Public Health

ASPR: Assistant Secretary for Preparedness and Response

BMI: body mass index

BNI: basic needs insecurities

BP: blood pressure

CBT: cognitive behavioral therapy

CDC: Centers for Disease Control and Prevention

CEPH: Council on Education for Public Health

CHA: community health assessment

CIA: Central Intelligence Agency

CIHR: Canadian Institutes of Health Research

CLRD: chronic lower respiratory disease

CMS: Center for Medicare and Medicaid Services

CMV: cytomegalovirus

CO$_2$: carbon dioxide

COP: Conference of the Parties

COPD: chronic obstructive pulmonary disease

CVD: cardiovascular disease

DALY: disability-adjusted life year

DBP: diastolic blood pressure

DCM: depression care management

DEEP: Disaster and Extreme Event Preparedness

DFA: Dementia Friendly America

DHEW: Department of Health, Education, and Welfare

DM: diabetes mellitus

EBP: Evidence-Based Practice

ED: emergency department

EMS: emergency medical services

EPA: Environmental Protection Agency

ESKD: end-stage kidney disease

EUA: emergency use authorization

EVALI: e-cigarette, or vaping, product use-associated lung injury

EVD: Ebola Virus Disease

FAS: fetal alcohol syndrome

FASD: fetal alcohol spectrum disorder

FDA: Food and Drug Administration

FEMA: Federal Emergency Management Agency

FHA: Federal Housing Administration

FoMO: fear of missing out

FPL: federal poverty level

GBD: global burden of disease (Global Burden of Diseases, Injuries, and Risk Factors Study)

GDP: gross domestic product

GIS: geographic information system

GM: General Motors

GPEI: Global Polio Eradication Initiative

GRIDS: gay-related immunodeficiency syndrome

HALE: health-adjusted life expectancy

HBM: Health Belief Model

HCV: Hepatitis C Virus

HDL: high-density lipoprotein

HHS: U.S. Department of Health and Human Services

HIA: health impact assessment

HiAP: Health in All Policies

HIPAA: Health Insurance Portability and Accountability Act

HPV: human papillomavirus

HSV: herpes simplex virus

HUD: Department of Housing and Urban Development

ICD-11: 11th Revision of the *International Statistical Classification of Diseases and Related Health Problems*

ICDS: India's Integrated Child Development Services

ICP: Inclusive Communities Project

IDMC: Internal Displacement Monitoring Centre

IDP: internally displaced person

IHD: Ischemic Heart Disease

IHS: Indian Health Service

IMR: infant mortality rate

INGOs: International Nongovernmental Organizations

IPV: intimate partner violence

IRR: Incident Rate Ratio

K2A: Knowledge to Action

LDL: low-density lipoprotein

LE: life expectancy

LGB: lesbian, gay, bisexual

LHD: local health department

LHI: Leading Health Indicator

LIA: Lead Industries Association

LMIC: low- to middle-income country

LRC: Linkage to, Retention in, Re-engagement in HIV Care

LTOT: long-term oxygen therapy

MADD: Mothers Against Drunk Driving

MBSR: Mindfulness-Based Stress Reduction

MBTA: Massachusetts Bay Transportation Authority

MedVP: medically vulnerable patient

MHS: U.S. Marine Hospital Service

MIDAS: Models of Infectious Disease Agent Study

MMWR: Morbidity and Mortality Weekly Report

MPH: Master of Public Health

MSM: men who have sex with men

NAHIC: National Adolescent and Young Adult Health Information Center

NAPA: National Alzheimer's Project Act

NCD: noncommunicable disease

NCI: National Cancer Institute

NGO: nongovernmental organization

NIH: National Institutes of Health

NIMH: National Institute of Mental Health

NPA: National Partnership for Action

NPR: National Public Radio

NSDUH: National Survey on Drug Use and Health

NSSI: nonsuicidal self-injury

ODD: oppositional defiant disorder

ODPHP: Office of Disease Prevention and Health Promotion

OEM: Office of Emergency Management

OPR: opioid pain relievers

OSHA: Occupational Safety and Health Administration

PAHO: Pan-American Health Organization

PPE: Personal Protective Equipment

PrEP: pre-exposure prophylaxtics

PSA: prostate specific antigen

PTSD: posttraumatic stress disorder

QALY: quality-adjusted life year

QOL: quality of life

QOLS: Quality of Life Scale

REACH: Racial and Ethnic Approaches to Community Health

RR: risk ratio *or* relative risk

RWJF: Robert Wood Johnson Foundation

SAMHSA: Substance Abuse and Mental Health Services Administration

SBP: systolic blood pressure

SDG: Sustainable Development Goal

SDI: Sociodemographic Index

SDOH: social determinants of health

SDWA: Safe Drinking Water Act

SES: socioeconomic status

SIDS: sudden infant death syndrome

SITB: self-injurious thoughts and behaviors

SNAP: Supplemental Nutrition Assistance Program

STI: sexually transmitted infections

SUL: Shelter Unit Leader

TANF: Temporary Assistance for Needy Families

TDHCA: Texas Department of Housing and Community Affairs

T1D: type 1 diabetes

T2D: type 2 diabetes

UHC: universal health coverage

UN: United Nations

UNAIDS: United Nations Programme on HIV and AIDS

UNFPA: United Nations Population Fund

UNHCR: United Nations High Commissioner for Refugees

UNICEF: United Nations International Children's Emergency Fund

UNODC: United Nations Office on Drugs and Crime

UNRWA: United Nations Relief and Works Agency for Palestine Refugees in the Near East

USAID: U.S. Agency for International Development

USDA: United States Department of Agriculture

USDHEW: U.S. Department of Health, Education, and Welfare

USDHHS: U.S. Department of Health and Human Services

USPHS: U.S. Public Health Service

USPSTF: U.S. Preventive Services Task Force

VMT: vehicle miles traveled

VOAD: voluntary organizations active in disasters

VOC: variant of concern

WFP: World Food Programme

WHA: World Health Assembly

WHO: World Health Organization

WIC: Special Supplemental Nutrition Program for Women, Infants and Children

WISEWOMAN: Well-Integrated Screening and Evaluation for Women Across the Nation

WTO: World Trade Organization

YLD: years lived with disability

YLLs: years of life lost

YRBS: Youth Risk Behavior Survey

YRBSS: Youth Risk Behavior Surveillance System

COMMON DEFINITIONS

Age-standardized death rates: rates of death applied to a standard age distribution to allow for fair comparison

Biostatistics: the study of understanding variability in potential causes and outcomes in order to infer associations and relationships among them

Communicable disease: a disease that is passed from an infected person (a person who harbors an infectious agent, such as a bacteria or virus) to a previously noninfected person

Dose-response: an upward stairstep relationship between exposure and outcome

Efficiency: a term often used in economics to describe the maximization of the total economic output of a system

Epidemiology: the study of the distribution and determinants of disease

Incidence: the number of new cases of specific disease conditions

Life course perspective: a perspective stating that our health is produced throughout our life, through the perinatal period, infancy, and childhood (before birth through age 14); adolescence and young adulthood (ages 15–24); adulthood (ages 25–64); and older adulthood (ages 65 and older)

Meta-analysis: a type of statistical analysis that pools data from multiple smaller studies on a particular topic to build more precise estimates of association

Population health science: the study of the conditions that shape distributions of health within and across populations, and the mechanisms through which these conditions manifest as the health of individuals

Prevalence: the number of existing cases of specific disease conditions

Primary prevention: actions that keep people from becoming ill or injured in the first place

Secondary prevention: actions aimed to reduce the impact of a disease or injury in the earliest stages of occurrence

Social ecological perspective: a perspective explaining that our health is produced through a variety of levels starting from the individual and extending to an individual's family members and friends, their neighborhoods, their cities, and their countries

Tertiary prevention: actions that reduce the impact of an ongoing injury or disease once an individual has been diagnosed and treated for clinical disease

SPRINGER PUBLISHING CONNECT™ RESOURCES

 A robust set of instructor resources designed to supplement this text is located at **http://connect.springerpub.com/content/book/978-0-8261-8043-8**. Qualifying instructors may request access by emailing **textbook@springerpub.com**.

Instructor Resources

- LMS Common Cartridge With All Instructor Resources
- Instructor Manual
  - Active Learning Exercises for Instructors
- Instructor Test Bank
  - Multiple-Choice Questions with Answers/Rationales
- Instructor PowerPoints
- Instructor Syllabus

Student Resources

- Case Study Podcasts
- Podcast Transcripts

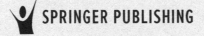

Visit https://connect.springerpub.com/ and look for the "**Show Supplementary**" button on the **book homepage**.

INTRODUCTION

1

THE ORIGINS OF PUBLIC HEALTH

OVERVIEW: PUBLIC HEALTH, POPULATION HEALTH, AND POPULATION HEALTH SCIENCE: KEY DISTINCTIONS

Humans have long recognized the need to develop systems that can create healthy populations. The roots of organized public health extend back millennia.[1] Roman aqueducts were built, in part, to accommodate the need of growing cities to have clean water that was not contaminated by urban effluent. Jump forward to the mid-19th century where modern public health as we know it emerged principally from western European countries, particularly England, France, and Germany. Spurred by industrialization and the need to create healthier cities, the first formal health departments were established. Organized public health soon became one of the most important advances in human history, leading to a period of a worldwide unprecedented increase in life span with the average life expectancy jumping from around 40 years in the mid-1800s to around 80 years in many high-income countries in the present day.

Those starting on a journey in public health build upon this legacy. This chapter aims to give the reader the foundations that can create a path for a lifetime of study or work in public health. To set those foundations, we first (a) explain core terms that underlie what we cover in this book, (b) describe the evolution of public health departments and methods of research and practice in 19th-century Europe, (c) discuss the evolution of public health practice in the United States in the 20th century, (d) outline the current organization of public health practice in the United States, including the Centers for Disease Control and Prevention (CDC) and local state and municipal health departments, (e) discuss the organization of public health globally with particular reference to the World Health Organization (WHO), and (f) describe the evolution of academic schools of public health as the academic soul of public health.

POPULATION

Public health, being about populations, requires that students actively think in terms of population health. Although population thinking is essential to public health science and practice, it is not an intuitive way of thinking. More often than not, our attention gravitates to a particular important individual: the person at the center of our "selfies." Population thinking necessarily moves us beyond ourselves to considering more than one individual. This certainly includes other individuals with whom we are closely connected and groups of individuals of which we are a part. Extending beyond our own social networks, such thinking has us consider many other groups in which we have no obvious membership or deep connection.

So, what is a population? Two properties are necessary to describe a population.[2] First, a population requires more than one individual. Second, these individuals share one or more common characteristics.

> **Two properties are necessary to describe a population:**
> **First, a population requires more than one individual.**
> **Second, these individuals share one or more common characteristics.**

So really, a population of interest could be as small as two persons or as encompassing as the citizenry of the entire planet. By way of example, at the expansive extreme of this continuum, while the world was suffering the ravages of World War I one century ago, pandemic influenza was circling the globe.[3] The death toll from this deadly outbreak was estimated in the range of 50 to 100 million at a time when the global population was about 1.5 billion people and everyone was susceptible.

Quite often, we define a population as people in a particular place. Places have discernible geopolitical boundaries; we can talk about the population of a city, region, or country. A population may be further defined by a set of commonalities, one or more characteristics shared by members of the population. For example, we may have a population of employees in a particular workplace, or a population of people who have common hobbies or experiences. Either way, the study of public health rests on understanding the population we are concerned with so that we can improve the health of that population. Now, with a population lens in mind, we can start thinking about health.

HEALTH

What do we mean by health? The classic definition comes from the Constitution of the WHO, defining health as a state of complete physical, mental, and social well-being and not merely the absence of disease or infirmity.[4] Through this definition, dating from 1948, the WHO described the enjoyment of the highest attainable standard of health as a fundamental right of every human being. Further, the WHO indicated that this is a right that should be accorded to all world citizens irrespective of race, economic or social condition, religion, or political belief. The WHO also noted that achieving health for all peoples is fundamental to the attainment of peace and security. To this day, the WHO Constitution continues to read like an enlightened call to arms more than seven decades after it was written. Importantly, this conception of health makes it clear that health is not just about the absence of disease. That means we are not interested only in giving people medicines to make them healthy after they get sick. Rather, we want to keep people healthy to begin with so that they can go about their business, living their lives. In this way of thinking, health is not an end—it is a means. It is a human right, one we should all have, so that we can choose to live our life as we wish to live it.

PUBLIC HEALTH AND POPULATION HEALTH SCIENCE

Now, with this in mind, what do we mean by public health?

There are many definitions of public health that we can lean on. The CDC Foundation notes that public health is the science of protecting and improving the health of families and communities through the promotion of healthy lifestyles, research for disease and injury prevention, and detection and control of infectious diseases.[5]

The American Public Health Association (APHA), the primary membership organization for public health professionals in the United States, considers the role of public health to be the promotion and protection of the health of people and the communities where they live, learn, work, and play.[6]

These definitions have not changed much over time. In 1920, Dr. Charles-Edward Amory Winslow, who established the Department of Public Health inside the Yale School of Medicine, described public health as the science and art of preventing disease, prolonging life, and promoting health through the organized efforts and informed choices of society, public and private organizations, communities, and individuals.[7]

The common theme in all these definitions is that public health is about collective effort, work done by groups of us, aiming to create the conditions that can keep us all healthy. This definition informs how we approach this book.

Importantly, we consider public health to be grounded in the science of population health. Population health science is the study of the conditions that shape distributions of health within and across populations, and the mechanisms through which these conditions manifest as the health of individuals.[2] Population health science provides us with the science and tells us what we need to know to understand what it is that causes health, so that then, in public health, we can intervene to make populations better.

> **Population health science provides us with the science and tells us what we need to know to understand what it is that causes health, so that then, in public health, we can intervene to make populations better.**

Therefore, this book is about public health practice and population health science. Throughout this book, we aim to explore how population health is produced, and what it is that public health does, or can do, to make populations healthier.

THE HISTORY OF PUBLIC HEALTH

THE EARLY DAYS OF PUBLIC HEALTH

Human habitation on this planet did not start out with populations as we think of them today. Human societies of *Homo erectus*, dating from 1.8 million years ago, and *Homo sapiens*, dating from 200,000 years ago, employed hunting and gathering as their predominant subsistence strategies. The survival of early humans depended on mobility in search of water and sustenance. At the most basic level, a primary indicator of health was staying alive. The average life expectancy was just over 20 years. Pockets of early humans regularly died out.

> **Health and public health today are strongly shaped by how our primeval physiologies interact with our present-day lifestyles.**

Our nomadic forebears established the baseline for what constitutes health today. Our human physiology developed and functioned optimally for this hunter–gatherer lifestyle. Health and public health today are strongly shaped by how our primeval physiologies interact with our present-day lifestyles.

The subsistence tasks of hunter–gatherer life were all-consuming. One of the initial economies that came from the clustering of humans into small bands was the development of the technology of the hunt. Even with the sporadic successful hunt, the bulk of the human diet still consisted of naturally occurring foods including fruits, berries, nuts, seeds, tubers, and primitive grains. Humans remained nomadic, propelled by the imperative to seek and find available food and fresh water sources in their environment.

The hunter–gatherer diet was rich in foods of plant origin, high in fiber, and low in fat, saturated fat, sodium, and calories. Daily, periodically strenuous physical activity was a mainstay of all subsistence activities. Hunter–gatherers needed to live close to sources of clean water, generally the same sources on which their plant-based diet depended. The constant mobility that defined hunter–gatherer life minimized the need to develop systems for sanitation. Although parasitic and communicable infectious diseases posed major threats to the health and longevity of hunter–gatherers, cardiovascular diseases and colon and lung cancers were virtually unknown.

Only in recent millennia (the most recent 7,000–8,000 years) have humans shifted toward settling in place and forming agriculture-based communities. For this to take place required the emergence of staple grains, like the fertile bread wheat, and the refinement of skills for cultivating and harvesting crops. The upside was the relative stability of the groups, now putting down roots and remaining in one locale. This was balanced against the downside that reliance on one primary grain led to widespread nutritional deficiencies and starvation following poor growing seasons. This was the epoch when populations, and by extension, population health, became meaningful.

The impetus for public health comes from humans living together in populations. As populations form and settle, two of the most basic survival concerns are ensuring a safe water supply and disposing of wastes; these remain central to public health today. The act of populating and residing in an area, and the ability to sustain that population, requires that water be brought in and wastes be shipped out or otherwise neutralized. This requires organization—collective action to promote health, or, in other words, public health. The construction of conduits for bringing water to human settlements dates back thousands of years. Excavations in the Indus Valley and the Punjab reveal primitive bathrooms, drains, and covered sewers.[1] A hemisphere away, the Incas constructed elaborate baths and sewage systems.

In the Middle Ages, as European cities grew, several outbreaks of bubonic plague, caused by *Yersinia pestis* (*Y. pestis*), illustrated the challenges occasioned by city living not accompanied by public health efforts to ensure health.[8] *Y. pestis* resides in the intestines of fleas whose bites transmit the bacterium to rats. Rat populations thrived in the cities, harboring the disease and ensuring the survival of the bacterium. Fleas also fed on humans, who were merely incidental hosts, infecting them as they ingested a blood meal. Once an individual was infected, the bacteria replicated in the lymph nodes and spread to other tissues, producing a severe febrile illness with delirium and headache. Sixty percent of infected individuals died. Originating in Asia, bubonic plague epidemics surged throughout the entirety of Europe from the mid-1300s through the late 1700s.

Two public health tools emerged from the plague years in Europe in the Middle Ages to help cope with these epidemics: quarantine and isolation. As the scourge of bubonic plague, the Black Death, was ransacking Europe, quarantine measures were imposed on ships, passengers, and their cargo that had been potentially exposed to the disease.[8] Ships were forced to anchor off port for a period of 40 days (in Italian, *quaranta giorni*, the origin of the term "quarantine") to ensure that the disease was not on board or had run its course. The parallel process for

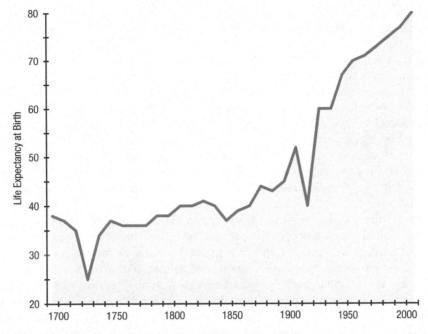

FIGURE 1.1 Life expectancy at birth in England and Wales, 1700 to 2005.
Source: Data from Roser M, Ortiz-Ospina E, Ritchie H. Life Expectancy. 2019. https://ourworldindata.org/life-expectancy

restricting entry and movement of possibly infected persons traveling over land was the erection of a cordon sanitaire. This was a physical barrier that could not be crossed without permission. The use of this practice continued up to the early 20th century.

Fast forward to the mid-1800s and we come to mid-19th-century London, where Edwin Chadwick advocated for improving living conditions in order to improve health. Chadwick argued, correctly, that improved health would increase productivity and reduce social costs. The tie-in to public health was his proposal to improve systems for providing clean water and removing wastes and toxic substances. In this manner, the emerging field of public health found acceptability because it aligned with the economic priorities of the government. Public health actions to improve living conditions contributed to advancing life expectancy. Average life expectancy had hovered around 35 to 40 years throughout the 1700s and the first half of the 1800s in England and Wales (**Figure 1.1**). The latter half of the 1800s saw a quantum gain of almost 10 years in life expectancy.

One of the most practical aspects of this movement was the passage of the Public Health Act of 1848.[9] The act created and operationalized the General Board of Health in London. In turn, the General Board directed the creation of local health boards that were charged with remedying environmental threats to health in their localities. This set the model for much of what is modern public health practice to this day.

THE EVOLUTION OF PUBLIC HEALTH IN THE UNITED STATES

Several events that are relevant to public health in the United States date back to the late 1700s when Congress established the U.S. Marine Hospital Service (MHS) to deal with the health problems of sick and disabled seamen. MHS created a network of hospitals in port cities to provide care for seamen, who were regarded as a critical asset for the new nation. MHS was the predecessor of the U.S. Public Health Service (USPHS). The city of Boston played a central role as the site of the first marine hospital, and the city created the first board of health and the first health department in the United States. None other than the legendary Bostonian, Paul Revere, was the nation's first health officer.

It was a Massachusetts legislator, Lemuel Shattuck, who developed the first system for record-ing vital statistics—births, deaths, and marriages—in the United States, one that became an exam-ple for emulation by other states. Shattuck's contributions were substantial. He cross-tabulated mortality data by age, sex, occupation, socioeconomic level, and location. Further, he extended the use of health data to the recording of immunizations, smoking status, and alcohol abuse. Shattuck was also the architect of a public health survey for use throughout Massachusetts that was published in the *New England Journal of Medicine*, along with a consolidated set of 50 recommendations.

The 20th century was the era when the science and practice of public health truly came into its own in the United States. Key events in the timeline include the official naming of the USPHS in 1912. The USPHS was charged with investigating a range of human diseases. Prominent concerns at that time were tuberculosis, malaria, and leprosy. Within the purview of the USPHS were such mainstays of public health as safeguarding water supplies, sanitation, and sewage dis-posal. National disease reporting was initiated in 1925. As one safeguard for the nation's health, legislation passed in 1938 created the Food and Drug Administration (FDA), a key public health agency, responsible for ensuring the safety of the U.S. food supply and the efficacy of drugs and medical devices, and for promoting innovations that lead to new drugs and devices that are safer, more effective, and more affordable for all.

In 1946, the Communicable Disease Center (CDC) was launched as a new program within the USPHS, with approximately 400 employees who were mostly engineers and epidemiologists with experience working on malaria control in the southern states. The program occupied a small space in Atlanta, Georgia, and the goal of the newly formed CDC was to expand its focus to all communicable diseases. Within 2 years, the CDC began a disease-surveillance program which effectively changed the practice of public health. One of its first notable accomplishments was the eradication of malaria from the United States. This set the stage for evidence-based public health practice.

Over the coming decade, the CDC expanded in size and scope. The CDC created the Epi-demic Intelligence Service (EIS), comprised of trained epidemiologists, who investigated hun-dreds of outbreaks related to communicable diseases, and environmental and biological hazards. The CDC created and expanded systems to gather data to monitor health and established a Bu-reau of Health Education with curricula for educators to use across the educational continuum. In 1970, while retaining the CDC acronym, the Communicable Disease Center was renamed the Center for Disease Control. In 1981, Center (singular) was changed to Centers (plural). In 1992, the phrase "and Prevention" was appended, but the CDC acronym was left unchanged: Centers for Disease Control and Prevention (CDC). The CDC is guided by the following mission statement:

> *CDC works 24/7 to protect America from health, safety and security threats, both foreign and in the U.S. Whether diseases start at home or abroad, are chronic or acute, curable or preventable, human error or deliberate attack, CDC fights disease and supports communities and citizens to do the same.*
>
> *CDC increases the health security of our nation. As the nation's health protection agency, CDC saves lives and protects people from health threats. To accomplish our mission, CDC conducts critical science and provides health information that protects our nation against expensive and dangerous health threats, and responds when these arise.*[10]

TABLE 1.1   Three Core Functions of Public Health and 10 Essential Public Health Services

CORE FUNCTIONS			ESSENTIAL SERVICES
1	**Assessment**	1	Assess and monitor population health
		2	Investigate, diagnose, and address health hazards and root causes
2	**Policy development**	3	Communicate effectively to inform and educate
		4	Strengthen, support, and mobilize communities and partnerships
		5	Create, champion, and implement policies, plans, and laws
		6	Utilize legal and regulatory actions
3	**Assurance**	7	Enable equitable access
		8	Build a diverse and skilled workforce
		9	Improve and innovate through evaluation, research, and quality improvement
		10	Build and maintain a strong organizational infrastructure for public health

Source: Adapted from Centers for Disease Control and Prevention. Public health system and the 10 essential public health services. n.d. https://www.cdc.gov/publichealthgateway/publichealthservices/essentialhealthservices.html

In 1988, the Institute of Medicine issued a report entitled "The Future of Public Health," and in it, articulated three core functions of public health: assessment, policy development, and assurance.[11] Assessment involves collecting and analyzing data to monitor health outcomes and to identify emerging health issues that need attention. Policy development involves recommendations for interventions, programs, and policies to address health problems that have been identified. Assurance involves enforcement of policies, allocation of resources to support programs and interventions, and evaluation of how well these interventions, programs, and policies are working to promote health. In 1994, a Core Public Health Functions Steering Committee was organized with representation from the CDC and other U.S. public health agencies to develop specific functions and activities within each core function. Ten essential public health services were articulated that to this day provide a framework for nearly every public health activity (**Table 1.1**).

THE U.S. PUBLIC HEALTH SYSTEM

The public health system in the United States is organized across federal, state, municipal, and local health authorities. Other public health services are delivered by nongovernmental agencies and community programs.

THE U.S. FEDERAL PUBLIC HEALTH SYSTEM

Administratively, the U.S. federal public health system resides under the executive branch of government, principally centered within the U.S. Department of Health and Human Services (HHS). Health-related functions are also performed by the departments of Defense, Veterans Affairs, Homeland Security, and Labor, and the Social Security Administration.

The stated mission of the HHS is to enhance and protect the health and well-being of all Americans.[12] HHS seeks to achieve this mission in several ways. Not only does HHS deliver a range of health and human services, the department also actively promotes advances in public health and medical research and carries out aspects of health policy. The Office of the Secretary includes a complement of administrative officers.[13] Among these are the Assistant Secretary of Health who oversees the office of the U.S. Surgeon General.[14] After the terrorist attacks of September 11, 2001, public health preparedness became a priority public health issue and a new office was created to house the Assistant Secretary for Preparedness and Response (ASPR).[15] This purview of this office was expanded in 2022, retaining the ASPR acronym while modifying the name of the entity to Administration for Strategic Preparedness and Response.

Perhaps most well known to the general public are the CDC,[16] the National Institutes of Health (NIH),[17] and the FDA.[18] The Center for Medicare and Medicaid Services (CMS) is rarely mentioned by name but its component programs, Medicare and Medicaid, are broadly known.[19] CMS performs one of the most essential functions of HHS, administering the major federal healthcare funding programs for older adults (Medicare); and for low-income families, pregnant women, people of all ages with disabilities, and people who need long-term care (Medicaid). Another division, the Substance Abuse and Mental Health Services Administration (SAMHSA), supports substance abuse treatment and prevention programs.[20] The HHS is also charged with providing healthcare to American Indians/Alaska Natives residing on government lands through the Indian Health Services.[21]

STATE, MUNICIPAL, AND LOCAL HEALTH AUTHORITIES

Much of the direct delivery of public health services to individual recipients occurs at state, county, city, and municipality levels. Correspondingly, the majority of government public health professionals work in state, county, and local health departments close to their places of residence. CDC is a resource to local health officials and operations. CDC provides technical guidance, consultations, toolkits, data, and assistance connecting local health officials with others outside of specific jurisdictions who may be experiencing similar issues or who have particular expertise that might be useful.

Apart from the practicality of bringing services directly to the people, this structure aligns with the tradition, since the founding of the nation, of vesting significant governing power in the states. In the case of public health, where needs reach down to the community, the family unit, and the individual, the provision of public health programs and services is shared among state and local levels. The specific division of labor and the delegation of duties between state and local levels differ across states.

GLOBAL PUBLIC HEALTH

On an international level, the WHO is the body charged with protecting and promoting health and preventing disease on a global scale. Moreover, public health services are also delivered by national and international nongovernmental agencies and community programs around the globe.

THE WORLD HEALTH ORGANIZATION

The WHO is part of the United Nations (UN) system.[22] The WHO is the organization most directly involved in global health. Many other UN agencies also participate in functions that bear directly on the health of populations. As examples, UN entities focus on women's health (UN Women),[23] HIV/AIDS (United Nations Programme on HIV and AIDS [UNAIDS]),[24] drug abuse (United Nations Office on Drugs and Crime [UNODC]),[25] refugee health (United Nations High Commissioner for Refugees [UNHCR] and United Nations Relief and Works Agency for Palestine Refugees in the Near East [UNRWA]),[26,27] children's health (United Nations International Children's Emergency Fund [UNICEF]),[28] and famine prevention/intervention through the World Food Programme (WFP),[29] among other entities.

Established in 1948 and headquartered in Geneva, Switzerland, the WHO has six regional offices and 150 country offices. The Pan-American Health Organization (PAHO),[30] based in Washington, DC, is the WHO regional office for the entire Western Hemisphere, the "Americas."

The WHO addresses health needs that may be brought forward by any of the 193 UN member states (as of 2022). The organization has 7,000 staff members worldwide, and more than 700 institutions support the WHO's work.

GLOBAL NONGOVERNMENTAL ORGANIZATIONS AND CIVIL SOCIETY

Many thousands of national and international nongovernmental organizations (NGOs) focus their activities on some aspect of public health. Name a major disease, and there will be an organization advocating for prevention and effective treatment of that medical condition. Consider cancer. Well known is the American Cancer Society.[31] There are counterpart cancer organizations beginning with the names of dozens of other nations (e.g., Dutch Cancer Society, Saudi Cancer Society).[32,33] Many organizations have a focus on a specific cancer. In the United States, Susan G. Komen for the Cure is well known for fundraising for breast cancer using community walks and running events to garner community participation.[34] The most common and major cancers (lung, breast, colorectal) have organizations; so too do little-known cancers. (The Acoustic Neuroma Association is the first listed on the alphabetical index of more than 300 cancer organizations.)[35]

In parallel, other prominent diseases are represented by associations that seek funding for research and offer support to persons living with the disease and their family members. Diseases that are the leading causes of death in the United States are represented by such organizations as the American Heart Association,[36] the American Cancer Society[30], the American Lung Association,[37] the American Diabetes Association,[38] and the Alzheimer's Association.[39] The recent appearance of COVID-19 as a new entry among the leading causes of disease and death has given rise to new organizations including the Long-COVID Alliance.

There are associations for surviving family members who have lost a loved one to drunk driving (Mothers Against Drunk Driving),[40] gun violence (The Sandy Hook Promise),[41] and suicide (Alliance of Hope).[42]

There are health professional organizations for public health (APHA)[43] and for most every type of health and medical professional. Some professional organizations represent a broad occupational category (American Medical Association)[44] while others represent a specific specialty (American Psychiatric Association)[45] or even subspecialty (Academy of Consultation-Liaison Psychiatry).[46]

By way of example, disasters, humanitarian emergencies, and public health crises bring together governmental and nongovernmental entities to assist populations in need. ReliefWeb serves as an international online hub and information resource, helping to coordinate humanitarian assistance for specific disaster events.[47] ReliefWeb lists more than 3,000 organizations that may be active in disasters. Well known among NGOs and international nongovernmental organizations (INGOs) are the American Red Cross,[48] International Federation of Red Cross and Red Crescent Societies,[49] CARE,[50] Caritas,[51] and Doctors Without Borders (Médecins Sans Frontières).[52] Large numbers of religiously affiliated NGOs also operate in this space (e.g., Catholic Charities USA, Episcopal Relief and Development, Lutheran World Relief, and Mennonite Central Committee).[53-56]

THE EVOLUTION OF ACADEMIC SCHOOLS OF PUBLIC HEALTH IN THE UNITED STATES

THE EARLY ORIGINS OF ACADEMIC PUBLIC HEALTH

Academic schools of public health date back to the time of the Great Influenza.[57] Years of planning went into the creation of health education that was distinct from the traditional medical school curriculum. In 1916, just prior to the onset of the global influenza pandemic, the Johns Hopkins University School of Hygiene and Public Health became the first school of public health, endowed by the Rockefeller Foundation. Early schools of public health were private institutions that were populated almost exclusively by professionals with medical degrees. Not surprisingly, the education focused on infectious diseases. In the early decades, the prioritized enrollment of physicians, coupled with the failure to include field training, did not succeed in producing a cadre of graduates who could assume roles as public health officers and sanitarians.

Impetus for expanding public health education was provided by the Social Security Act of 1935. The act increased funding for the USPHS and upgraded qualifications for federally funded health personnel that translated, in most states, into a requirement of at least 1 year of graduate education. This increase in public health positions created demand for public health credentials that triggered state universities to open new schools. By 1936, graduate public health training was offered in 10 institutions: Johns Hopkins, Harvard, Columbia, Michigan, University of California at Berkeley, Massachusetts Institute of Technology, Minnesota, Pennsylvania, Wayne State, and Yale. During the 1930s, there was a proliferation of 1-year graduates who received a Master of Public Health (MPH) degree with a strong emphasis on applied field training.

The expansion of public health training continued during the Second World War to prepare physicians, nurses, and sanitarians with skills to deal with tropical and parasitic diseases, sexually transmitted infections, and sanitation in the theaters of war. Training was also provided to impart industrial hygiene skills to ensure the health of workers in the domestic industries that supported the war effort. This boom in public health training was accompanied by the formation of the Association of Schools of Public Health (ASPH) in 1941 and the establishment of the Council on Education for Public Health (CEPH) of the APHA, adding rigor and standardization to public health curricula.

Some of the earliest insights from population health scholarship that informed public health were studies that elucidated the causal relationship between cigarette smoking and rising lung cancer rates, published by Doll and Hill in 1948. In the same year, the Framingham Heart Study was launched. This research continues more than 70 years later as one of the most consequential studies that connects a series of lifestyle risk factors to the onset, progression, and mortality associated with cardiovascular and other noncommunicable diseases (NCDs).

In 1953, President Eisenhower created the U.S. Department of Health, Education, and Welfare (DHEW). The year 1970 expanded the breadth of the public health agenda, marking the inception of both the Occupational Safety and Health Administration (OSHA) and the Environmental Protection Agency (EPA). In 1979, reorganization of the executive branch separated health and education into separate departments. Public health functions resided within the renamed and reorganized HHS.

POST–WORLD WAR II AND ACADEMIC PUBLIC HEALTH TODAY

The focus on preparing public health practitioners through applied courses and fieldwork took a downturn after the war when university funding for public health faculty shifted toward an imperative for these professionals to compete for research grant support. Foundation support for public health education dwindled. Schools of public health found themselves at a disadvantage when competing with medical schools for NIH funding and other research support. Community-focused field training educational programs vanished. Nationwide, enrollment in graduate public health education decreased by half by the mid-1950s.

Later that decade, an emergency infusion of federal funding partially revived public health education. In 1958, the First National Conference on Public Health Training was held. The introduction of major national social programs of the 1960s—Medicare and Medicaid—once again increased the demand for public health education, this time focusing on healthcare delivery. The 1960s and 1970s saw a revitalization of graduate public health training as schools of public health received direct funding for training along with an enhanced ability to compete for research grants.

However, in 1973, just as the number of graduate public health degrees awarded annually was approaching 5,000, President Nixon attempted to eliminate all federal funding for schools of public health and for research training grants. Fortunately, funding was not terminated and in 1976, the Milbank Memorial Fund published a detailed public health roadmap report, *Higher Education for Public Health*, that proposed a three-tiered structure for public health education.[58] This included the preparation of public health leaders; created specialist public health training for nurses, health educators, and environmental health professionals; and added an undergraduate training component to graduate entry-level personnel. The report defined core disciplines within public health and recommended a role for the schools as regional resources to educational institutions in the area of public health research. It also highlighted engagement of schools in local community health services and renewed emphasis on public health practice.

There are currently 68 schools of public health and 139 programs in public health that are accredited by the CEPH. These programs are distributed across 47 states and eight countries.

Today, the public health ecosystem includes schools of public health, official governmental bodies charged with promoting health, NGOs, and a range of international bodies, all aspiring to create the conditions for states of complete physical and mental well-being for as many people as possible.

WHAT ARE THE MAJOR PUBLIC HEALTH ACHIEVEMENTS OVER THE 20TH CENTURY AND MORE RECENTLY IN THE UNITED STATES?

Public health has transformed healthy life and catapulted life expectancy forward within the past 125 years. During the 20th century, life expectancy in the United States increased by 30 years. The CDC credits 25 years of this unprecedented jump in life expectancy to 10 great public health achievements during the 20th century, 1900–1999.[59] Here is the list:

Ten Great Public Health Achievements—United States, 1900–1999[58]:

- Control of infectious diseases
- Decline in deaths from coronary heart disease and stroke
- Family planning
- Fluoridation of drinking water
- Healthier mothers and babies
- Motor vehicle safety
- Recognition of tobacco use as a health hazard
- Safer and healthier foods
- Safer workplaces
- Vaccination

We select a subset of these achievements for further discussion.

VACCINATION AND CONTROL OF INFECTIOUS DISEASES— TWO CLOSELY INTERRELATED ACHIEVEMENTS

Vaccination was a major contributor to the control of infectious diseases in past decades. Smallpox was declared eradicated in 1979. Smallpox, a disease that produced illness exclusively in humans, transformed the course of history over centuries. European explorers unknowingly introduced smallpox to the Americas, decimating populations of First Nations peoples who were immunologically naïve to the disease.[60] Poliomyelitis was banished from the Western Hemisphere during the 20th century. The spread of measles, diphtheria, rubella, and tetanus became well controlled through childhood vaccination.

Beyond vaccine-preventable diseases, water purification and improved sanitation—fundamental pillars of public health—successfully decreased the disease burden of major killers like typhoid and cholera. The introduction of antimicrobial therapies diminished the spread of tuberculosis and some sexually transmitted infections.

HEALTHIER MOTHERS AND BABIES, FAMILY PLANNING, AND FOOD SAFETY

The health and survival of mothers and their children benefitted from improved hygiene and better nutrition. Expanded access to healthcare, advances in medical procedures, antibiotic medications, and the introduction of prenatal and neonatal care also improved the well-being of mothers and babies. Collectively, these developments translated into a startling 90% decline in the infant mortality rate and a 99% decrease in the maternal mortality rate over the 20th century. Related to the realm of maternal and child health, the 1900s also ushered in the era of family planning. The availability of preconception counseling and contraceptive options paved the way for smaller families. Planned pregnancies and prenatal care combined to lower rates of fetal, infant, and maternal deaths.

The United States made strides to improve the safety of foods and the purity of the water supply. The introduction of safer and healthier foods had the complementary effects of decreasing food contamination and improving the nutritional content of foods. The ability to supplement vital micronutrients and to fortify foods led to the virtual elimination of nutritional deficiency diseases in childhood. As examples, in the United States, diseases such as rickets, pellagra, and goiter have vanished.

WATER FLUORIDATION

In the mid-20th century, the United States began to fluoridate the drinking water, reaching more than half the population by the end of the century. This public health action benefits people across the socioeconomic spectrum. As a result of this simple low-cost action, rates of tooth decay in children and tooth loss in adults were reduced by more than half.

SAFER WORKPLACES

During the 20th century, major reductions were achieved in rates of work-related injuries and deaths in the mining, construction, and manufacturing sectors. Toxic and disease-producing exposures to hazardous materials, poisons, dusts, fumes, and carcinogens in work settings have been monitored and significantly controlled. Worksite risk reduction occurred through combinations of regulations, installation of safety equipment, workforce training, use of personal protective equipment, attentive worker supervision, and when necessary, litigation.

MOTOR VEHICLE SAFETY

The introduction of the automobile and motorized transportation early in the 20th century redefined mobility and simultaneously created new patterns of unintentional injury. In the United States, unintentional injury is the leading cause of death for people aged 1 to 44 years. For multiple decades prior to the opiate epidemic, motor vehicle crash deaths were the principal cause of death from unintentional injury—and now rank second, following "unintentional poisonings" (drug overdose deaths).

There are multiple pathways available for successfully mitigating motor vehicle crash trauma and death (**Figure 1.2**). These include training motorists and passengers on every-time use of seat belts, child safety seats, and motorcycle helmets. Safety technology rapidly evolved. Carmakers began to design vehicles with rigid passenger cages surrounded by deformable extremities. In a crash, the passenger compartment would remain intact while the bumpers and the motor or trunk compartments would collapse and absorb the impact. A similar mind-set went into the design of the passenger compartment, replacing metals with softer, cushioned plastics to reduce trauma during a collision.

The national highway system continuously upgrades the quality of roadways; improves highway lighting; and introduces new signals, signage, and safeguards to make motoring safer. Onboard navigation systems and smart technologies are being used to alert drivers to dangerous situations and to diminish distractions. Laws have been passed to keep drivers in their lanes and driving within specified speed limits. Significant penalties are set for risky human behaviors including driving while under the influence of substances or while texting or using other electronics. New sensor technologies increasingly allow vehicles to sense—and avoid—road hazards such as side-impact collisions and rear-end collisions when vehicles in front decelerate quickly. Sensors can detect persons or objects passing behind the vehicle and rapidly apply the brakes. The evolving technology of self-driving vehicles holds considerable future promise for decreasing collision risks.

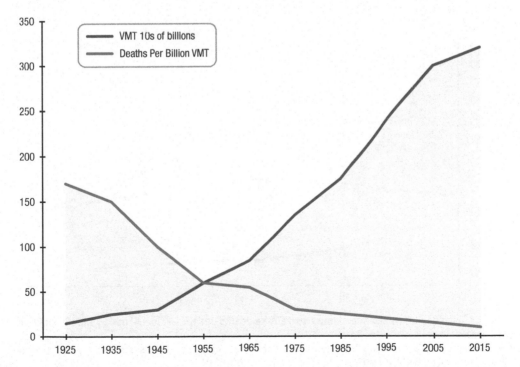

FIGURE 1.2 VMT and deaths per billion VMT, United States, 1925 to 2015. VMT, vehicle miles traveled.
Source: Data from Bratland D. US traffic deaths per VMT, VMT, per capita, and total annual deaths. 2018. https:// commons.wikimedia.org/wiki/File:US_traffic_deaths_per_VMT,_VMT,_per_capita,_and_total_annual_deaths.png

DECLINE IN DEATHS FROM CORONARY HEART DISEASE AND STROKE

While rates of communicable diseases were declining, the number of cases of NCDs was increasing. Most notably, heart disease rates rose steadily during the first half of the 20th century. With the successful identification of modifiable lifestyle-related risk factors that were associated with heart disease, programs were devised for risk factor modification at both the individual and population levels. A combination of decreased saturated fat intake in the habitual diet; improved detection, treatment, and control of high blood pressure; and smoking cessation contributed to steady, long-term declines in both stroke and ischemic heart disease mortality rates beginning in the 1960s and continuing for more than 50 years. By the 2010s, heart disease death rates were only slightly higher than cancer death rates for men and actually lower than cancer death rates for women. The downward trends in heart disease and stroke present a visible contrast to the relatively unchanging cancer death rates from the late 1970s onward (**Figure 1.3**).

RECOGNITION OF TOBACCO USE AS A HEALTH HAZARD

The widespread adoption of the cigarette smoking habit was a 20th-century phenomenon. Shrewd marketing coupled with the addictive properties of nicotine led to a surge in smoking rates, first for men and later for women throughout the first half of the 1900s (**Figure 1.4**). Although by the late 20th century, cigarette smoking was described as the chief preventable cause of death in the United States, public recognition that tobacco posed a grave health hazard was slow to develop. One of the reasons is the 20-year time lag between rising smoking rates and rising deaths from smoking-related diseases. This is due, in part, to the fact that it takes a matter of decades, on average, for a regular smoking habit to produce fatal cancer, respiratory disease, or cardiovascular disease.

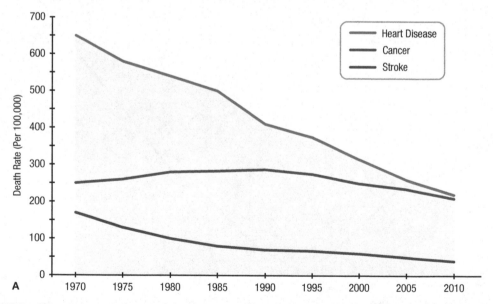

FIGURE 1.3 Trends in heart disease, cancer, and stroke deaths per 100,000 for (A) males and (B) females, United States, 1970 to 2010.
Source: Data from Ma J, Ward EM, Siegel RL, Jemal A. Temporal trends in mortality in the United States, 1969–2013. Original Investigation. *JAMA.* 2015;314(16):1731-1739. doi:10.1001/jama.2015.12319

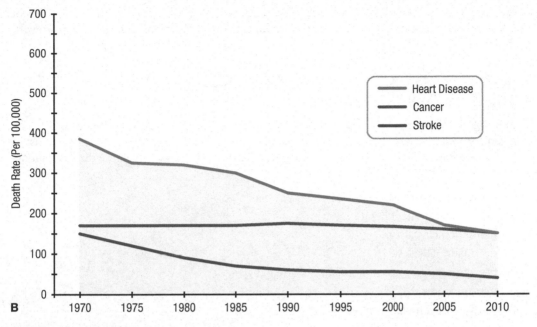

B

FIGURE 1.3 (*continued*)

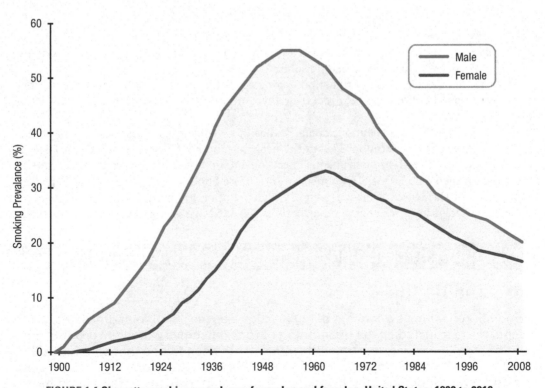

FIGURE 1.4 Cigarette smoking prevalence for males and females, United States, 1900 to 2010.

Following the release of the landmark 1964 Surgeon General's Report on the health risks of smoking, there was an abrupt drop in numbers of smokers, followed by a long-term downward trend in tobacco use.[61]

PUBLIC HEALTH ACHIEVEMENTS CONTINUING INTO THE 21ST CENTURY

Taken together, these public health achievements throughout the 1900s continue to produce favorable trends that have extended into the 21st century. The CDC presented an updated list of major public health achievements for the first decade of the 2000s.[62] Seven are direct offshoots of the original list for the 20th century:

- cardiovascular disease prevention
- maternal and infant health
- motor vehicle safety
- occupational safety
- prevention and control of infectious diseases
- tobacco control
- vaccine-preventable diseases

Three new achievements were introduced into the roster:

- cancer prevention
- childhood lead poisoning prevention
- improved public health preparedness and response

The new additions include public health preparedness that became a priority following the September 11, 2001, terrorist attacks. The other two new achievements are in the areas of prevention of cancer and childhood lead poisoning.

The interconnection and coordination among academic, public health, governmental, and nongovernmental entities will be a recurring theme as we explore the science and practice of population health.

Now we explore the concept of population health thinking using a case study example that describes how early misperceptions about risk behaviors for the transmission of HIV/AIDS—and the populations affected—had detrimental effects on disease control and proved to be highly stigmatizing for men who have sex with men (MSM). (Case Study 1.1; you can access the podcast accompanying Case Study 1.1 by following this link to Springer Publishing Company Connect™: http://connect.springerpub.com/content/book/978-0-8261-8043-8/part/part01/chapter/ch01).

 CASE STUDY 1.1: POPULATION HEALTH THINKING (HIV/AIDS)

POPULATION HEALTH

Population health, as a concept of health, signifies the health outcomes of a group of individuals, including the distribution of such outcomes within the group.[63] Population health science, in turn, is the study of the conditions that shape distributions of health within and across populations, and of the mechanisms through which these conditions manifest as the health of individuals.[64] Population health science provides the quantitative scaffolding for public health and the allied field of preventive medicine.

(continued)

POPULATION HEALTH THINKING

One of the most important skills in public health is being able to think in terms of populations. This skill, if applied effectively, can be life-changing and life-saving. This skill is critical to be able to differentiate the relationship between individual and population health.[65] Here is an illustration of why it is important to develop this facility using the example of what was once an emerging infectious disease outbreak that expanded to global pandemic proportions. The initial cases were reported as a case series report of a mysterious and perplexing illness with an unusual presentation.

In the early 1980s, information based on several early cases of a new disease led to major misconceptions about the true population dynamics of the outbreak. These misconceptions continue to this day as the disease has grown into a pandemic. We begin a case report of an individual who was among the first to be diagnosed.

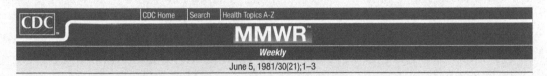

CDC	CDC Home	Search	Health Topics A-Z

MMWR™
Weekly
June 5, 1981/30(21);1–3

Persons using assistive technology might not be able to fully access information in this file. For assistance, please send e-mail to: mmwrg@cdc.gov. Type 508 Accommodation and the title of the report in the subject line of e-mail.

Epidemiologic Notes and Reports

Pneumocystis Pneumonia — Los Angeles

In the period October 1980-May 1981, 5 young men, all active homosexuals, were treated for biopsy-confirmed *Pneumocystis carinii* pneumonia at 3 different hospitals in Los Angeles, California. Two of the patients died. All 5 patients had laboratory-confirmed previous or current cytomegalovirus (CMV) infection and candidal mucosal infection. Case reports of these patients follow.

Patient 1: A previously healthy 33-year-old man developed *P. carinii* pneumonia and oral mucosal candidiasis in March 1981 after a 2-month history of fever associated with elevated liver enzymes, leukopenia, and CMV viruria. The serum complement-fixation CMV titer in October 1980 was 256; in May 1981 it was 32.* The patient's condition deteriorated despite courses of treatment with trimethoprim-sulfamethoxazole (TMP/SMX), pentamidine, and acyclovir. He died May 3, and postmortem examination showed residual *P. carinii* and CMV pneumonia, but no evidence of neoplasia.

Patient 2: A previously healthy 30-year-old man developed *P. carinii* pneumonia in April 1981 after a 5-month history of fever each day and of elevated liver-function tests, CMV viruria, and documented seroconversion to CMV, i.e., an acute-phase titer of 16 and a convalescent-phase titer of 28* in anticomplement immunofluorescence tests. Other features of his illness included leukopenia and mucosal candidiasis. His pneumonia responded to a course of intravenous TMP/SMX, but, as of the latest reports, he continues to have a fever each day.

Patient 3: A 30-year-old man was well until January 1981 when he developed esophageal and oral candidiasis that responded to Amphotericin B treatment. He was hospitalized in February 1981 for *P. carinii* pneumonia that responded to TMP/SMX. His esophageal candidiasis recurred after the pneumonia was diagnosed, and he was again given Amphotericin B. The CMV complement-fixation titer in March 1981 was 8. Material from an esophageal biopsy was positive for CMV.

Patient 4: A 29-year-old man developed *P. carinii* pneumonia in February 1981. He had had Hodgkins disease 3 years earlier, but had been successfully treated with radiation therapy alone. He did not improve after being given intravenous TMP/SMX and corticosteroids and died in March. Postmortem examination showed no evidence of Hodgkins disease, but *P. carinii* and CMV were found in lung tissue.

Patient 5: A previously healthy 36-year-old man with clinically diagnosed CMV infection in September 1980 was seen in April 1981 because of a 4-month history of fever, dyspnea, and cough. On admission he was found to have *P. carinii* pneumonia, oral candidiasis, and CMV retinitis. A complement-fixation CMV titer in April 1981 was 128. The patient has been treated with 2 short courses of TMP/SMX that have been limited because of a sulfa-induced neutropenia. He is being treated for candidiasis with topical nystatin.

(continued)

The following case report of a single patient was published in the *Morbidity and Mortality Weekly Report* (*MMWR*).[66]

Patient: A previously healthy 33-year-old man developed Pneumocystis carinii *pneumonia and oral mucosal candidiasis in March after a 2-month history of fever associated with elevated liver enzymes, leukopenia, and CMV viruria. The serum complement-fixation CMV titer in October was 256; in May it was 32. The patient's condition deteriorated despite courses of treatment with trimethoprim-sulfamethoxazole (TMP/SMX), pentamidine, and acyclovir. He died May 3, and postmortem examination showed residual* P. carinii *and CMV pneumonia, but no evidence of neoplasia.*

Actually, this description of a novel patient presentation was the first listed among a total of five similar reports that were compiled into a case series published on June 5, 1981, describing a medical curiosity.

Here is what was known:

- All five case patients were previously healthy young adult men, ages 29 to 36 years.
- All five cases were patients of one Los Angeles internist.
- All cases were white.
- All cases were male.
- All cases were gay (MSM).
- All reported having multiple sexual partners.
- All cases had multiple, simultaneous, diverse opportunistic diseases (parasitic, fungal, viral):
  o All cases had biopsy-confirmed *P. carinii* pneumonia—a parasitic disease.
  o All cases had oral mucosal candidiasis ("oral thrush")—a fungal infection.
  o All cases had laboratory-confirmed cytomegalovirus infection of the brain—a viral disease.
- All died.

Despite the similarities:

- The five patients did not know each other.
- These patients did not have any known sexual contacts in common.

Based on a small number of individual cases, what were some hunches at the time that were circulated rampantly?

Certainly, the commonalities among the cases would lead to speculation that this was

- a white, gay male disease;
- a disease that ransacks the immune system;
- a disease that allows multiple types of infections to spread simultaneously and unchecked; and
- a disease that kills.

Indeed, the spectre of a white, gay male disease was all over the news. The illness was variously described as "the gay plague," or gay cancer, or even as gay-related immunodeficiency syndrome (GRIDS).[67]

(continued)

Within the first year, it became known that this yet-unnamed disease could also be transmitted through contaminated blood and blood products, setting off an alarm worldwide. This was likely to be a viral disease and there was potential for anyone to become infected. Within the early months, Miami, Florida, became an epicenter for multiple modes of transmission. It was in Miami that the first case was diagnosed in a person with hemophilia. Some of the first cases in Haitian nationals and injection drug users were also first identified in southern Florida. Internally, some investigators referred to this strange ailment with the shorthand mnemonic, "4H disease." While clever, this was in fact an extremely stigmatizing and pejorative expression that signified four population subgroups thought to be at higher risk for the disease: homosexuals, hemophiliacs, Haitians, and heroin-users.[68]

It took 13 months following the publication of the case series for this disease to be officially named:

Acquired immunodeficiency syndrome: AIDS. Four more years would elapse before the virus was isolated and given a consensus name, human immunodeficiency virus: HIV. Sometimes, both names are combined and the disease is referred to as HIV/AIDS.

The early consensus conceptualization that this was a white, gay male disease was highly stigmatizing and discriminatory. It was also wrong. Seen through the lens of population health thinking on a global scale, HIV/AIDS is a pandemic that affects men and women of all races and has multiple modes of sexual and drug-use-associated transmission.

On a global scale, by the numbers:

- HIV/AIDS is currently more prevalent in non-Whites than Whites.
- Heterosexual contact—not male-to-male sex—is the primary mode of HIV/AIDS virus transmission.
- There are slightly more women than men living with HIV/AIDS. Among HIV/AIDS cases worldwide, 52% are women.[69]

Therefore, numerically, HIV/AIDS cases globally are

- not predominantly white,
- not primarily gay, and
- not primarily male.

The initial speculations, based on a few individual cases, suggesting that this strange disease—that would later be named HIV/AIDS—could be described as a white, gay male disease, were inaccurate on all counts.

Failing to apply a population health lens has real-world, life-and-death consequences.

In the case of HIV/AIDS, these were the consequences:

- discrimination and stigma against gay men and other persons living with HIV
- delays in funding and providing care
- disease cases that could have been prevented by timely action
- death due to discrimination, delays, and preventable disease transmission

Consider population health thinking to be an essential skill.

SUMMARY

Public health focuses on the health of populations. Public health has been relevant since the time when early humans transitioned to living as populations in communal settings. Public health issues that immediately came to prominence were providing the population with clean water and adequate nutrition while disposing of wastes. Existential challenges were posed by population encounters with common communicable diseases that caused high rates of infant and early childhood mortality, punctuated by periodic plagues that swept broad geographic regions and decimated communities.

The 20th century was remarkable based on public health achievements that collectively accounted for a more than 25-year surge in average life expectancy. Particularly notable was the successful conquest of infectious diseases, coupled with the development and widespread distribution of vaccines; these advances had the effect of markedly decreasing childhood disease and death, and dramatically increasing life expectancy.

Two mass-produced and effectively marketed human inventions, the tobacco cigarette and the automobile, introduced entirely new patterns of illness and injury. Fortunately, public health interventions have been instrumental in diminishing the population burdens of smoking-attributable diseases and motor vehicle accidents.

Lifestyles changed markedly (and continue to do so), propelling NCDs, notably cardiovascular diseases and cancers, to the forefront. The recognition of disease risk factors led to public health interventions that have successfully decreased the population impact of disability and early death from lifestyle-related diseases. Nevertheless, in the early 21st century, the escalating prominence of NCDs poses an ongoing challenge, and some disease trends such as obesity are visibly worsening. However, the unanticipated and globe-changing appearance of the COVID-19 pandemic thrust communicable diseases back into the forefront as leading causes of disease and death worldwide.

Public health, powered by population health science, continues to make strides toward achieving disease prevention and health promotion. Concurrently, humans continue to demonstrate their capacity to both generate health threats (climate change is the most obvious and compelling at this moment) and create innovative solutions. Health-enhancing endeavors are aided by the structure of the public health system, ranging from municipal health departments to state, federal, and global governmental institutions and nongovernmental programs and policies.

End-of-Chapter Resources

Access additional case study podcasts online at http://connect.springerpub.com/ content/book/978-0-8261-8043-8/

DISCUSSION QUESTIONS

1. Considering the list of the top 10 public health achievements for the 20th century, and again for 2001 to 2010, make your predictions for the top 10 achievements that will be on the list for 2011 to 2022 and future decades.
2. With each new era, populations encounter—and sometimes create—major threats to population health. Discuss the likely population health implications of current trends in climate change.

3. As some learners contemplate a future career in public health itself, or in public health–informed professions, discuss your preferences for working in public health at the municipal, state, federal, and international levels.

A robust set of instructor resources designed to supplement this text is located at **http://connect.springerpub.com/content/book/978-0-8261-8043-8**. Qualifying instructors may request access by emailing **textbook@springerpub.com**.

REFERENCES

1. Rosen G. *A History of Public Health*. 2nd ed. Johns Hopkins University Press; 2015.
2. Keyes KM, Galea S. *Population Health Science*. Oxford University Press; 2016. https://global.oup.com/academic/product/population-health-science-9780190459376?cc=us&lang=en&
3. Barry JM. *The Great Influenza: The Story of the Deadliest Pandemic in History*. Penguin Books, Ltd; 2004.
4. World Health Organization. *Constitution of WHO: principles*. https://www.who.int/about/governance/constitution
5. CDC Foundation. *What is public health?* https://www.cdcfoundation.org/what-public-health
6. American Public Health Association. *What is public health?* https://www.apha.org/what-is-public-health
7. Winslow CE. The untilled fields of public health. *Science*. 1920;51(1306):23-33. doi:10.1126/science.51.1306.23
8. Frith J. The history of plague—part 1. The three great pandemics. *J Mil Veterans Health*. 2012;20(2):11-16. https://jmvh.org/article/the-history-of-plague-part-1-the-three-great-pandemics
9. UK Parliament. *The 1848 public health act*. https://www.parliament.uk/about/living-heritage/transformingsociety/towncountry/towns/tyne-and-wear-case-study/about-the-group/public-administration/the-1848-public-health-act
10. Centers for Disease Control and Prevention. *Mission, role and pledge*. Published February 25, 2022. https://www.cdc.gov/about/organization/mission.htm
11. Institute of Medicine. *The Future of Public Health*. National Academies Press; 1988.
12. U.S. Department of Health & Human Services. *About HHS*. https://www.hhs.gov/about/index.html
13. U.S. Department of Health & Human Services. *HHS secretary*. Published 2019. https://www.hhs.gov/about/leadership/secretary/index.html
14. U.S. Department of Health & Human Services. *Office of the Surgeon General*. https://www.surgeongeneral.gov
15. Public Health Emergency. *HHS Office of the Assistant Secretary for preparedness and response*. Published 2019. https://www.phe.gov/ABOUT/ASPR/Pages/default.aspx
16. Centers for Disease Control and Prevention. https://www.cdc.gov
17. National Institutes of Health. https://www.nih.gov
18. U.S. Food and Drug Administration. https://www.fda.gov
19. The U.S. Centers for Medicare & Medicaid Services. https://www.cms.gov
20. Substance Abuse and Mental Health Services Administration. https://www.samhsa.gov
21. Indian Health Service (IHS). https://www.ihs.gov
22. World Health Organization. https://www.who.int
23. UN Women. http://www.unwomen.org/en
24. UNAIDS. http://www.unaids.org/en
25. United Nations Office on Drugs and Crime. http://www.unodc.org
26. UNHCR: The UN Refugee Agency. https://www.unhcr.org
27. UNRWA. United Nations Relief and Works Agency for Palestine refugees. https://www.unrwa.org
28. UNICEF for every child. https://www.unicef.org
29. World Food Programme. https://www1.wfp.org
30. Pan American Health Organization. https://www.paho.org/hq/index.php?lang=en
31. American Cancer Society. https://www.cancer.org
32. Dutch Cancer Society. https://www.kwf.nl/english/Pages/The-organisation.aspx
33. Saudi Cancer Society. http://saudicancer.org
34. Susan G. Komen Breast Cancer Foundation. https://ww5.komen.org
35. Acoustic Neuroma Association. https://www.anausa.org
36. American Heart Association. https://www.heart.org
37. American Lung Association. https://www.lung.org
38. American Diabetes Association. http://www.diabetes.org

39. Alzheimer's Foundation of America. https://alzfdn.org
40. Mothers Against Drunk Driving. https://www.madd.org
41. Sandy Hook Promise. https://www.sandyhookpromise.org
42. Alliance of Hope. *Hope after suicide.* https://allianceofhope.org
43. American Public Health Association. https://www.apha.org
44. American Medical Association. https://www.ama-assn.org
45. American Psychiatric Association. https://www.psychiatry.org
46. Academy of Consultation-Liaison Psychiatry. https://www.clpsychiatry.org
47. Reliefweb. *Informing humanitarians worldwide.* https://reliefweb.int
48. American Red Cross. https://www.redcross.org
49. International Federation of Red Cross and Red Crescent Societies. https://media.ifrc.org/ifrc
50. CARE. https://www.care.org
51. Caritas. https://www.caritas.org
52. Doctors without Borders (Médecins Sans Frontières) International. https://www.msf.org
53. Catholic Charities USA. https://www.catholiccharitiesusa.org
54. Episcopal Relief & Development. https://www.episcopalrelief.org
55. Lutheran World Relief. https://lwr.org
56. Mennonite Central Committee. https://mcc.org
57. Committee on Educating Public Health Professionals for the 21st Century. History and current status of public health education in the United States. In: Gebbie K, Rosenstock L, Hernandez LM, eds. *Who Will Keep the Public Healthy?* National Academies Press; 2003:41-60. https://www.nap.edu/read/10542/chapter/5
58. Sheps CG. *Higher Education for Public Health: A Report of the Milbank Memorial Fund Commission.* Milbank Memorial Fund; 1976.
59. Centers for Disease Control and Prevention. Ten great public health achievements—United States, 1900–1999. *MMWR Morb Mortal Wkly Rep.* 1999;*48*(12):241-243. https://www.cdc.gov/mmwr/preview/mmwrhtml/00056796.htm
60. McNeill WH. *Plagues and Peoples.* Anchor Books; 1976.
61. Surgeon General's Advisory Committee on Smoking and Health. *Smoking and Health: Report of the Advisory Committee to the Surgeon General of the Public Health Service.* Public Health Service Publication No. 1103. Office of the Surgeon General; 1964. https://profiles.nlm.nih.gov/ps/retrieve/ResourceMetadata/NNBBMQ
62. Centers for Disease Control and Prevention. *CDC identifies 10 public health achievements of first decade of 21st century.* Published May 19, 2011. https://www.cdc.gov/media/releases/2011/p0519_publichealthachievements.html
63. Kindig D, Stoddart G. What is population health? *Am J Public Health.* 2003;*93*(3):380-383. doi:10.2105/ajph.93.3.380
64. Keyes KM, Galea S. *Population Health Science.* Oxford University Press; 2016.
65. Arah OA. On the relationship between individual and population health. *Med Health Care Philos.* 2009;*12*(3):235-244. doi:10.1007/s11019-008-9173-8
66. Centers for Disease Control and Prevention. Pneumocystis pneumonia—Los Angeles. *MMWR Morb Mortal Wkly Rep.* 1981;*30*(21):1-3.
67. Gander K. *The terror and prejudice of the 1980s AIDs crisis remembered by a gay man who lived through it. The Independent.* Published January 6, 2017. https://www.independent.co.uk/life-style/love-sex/aids-crisis-1980-eighties-remember-gay-man-hiv-positive-funerals-partners-disease-michael-penn-a7511671.html
68. Cohen J. The Caribbean. *Science.* 2006;*313*(5786):470. doi:10.1126/science.313.5786.470a
69. UN Women. *Facts and figures: HIV and AIDS.* Updated July 2018. https://www.unwomen.org/en/what-we-do/hiv-and-aids/facts-and-figures

2

UNDERSTANDING THE GLOBAL BURDEN OF DISEASE AND DISABILITY

LEARNING OBJECTIVES

- Define disease and disability.
- Introduce the Global Burden of Disease and disability-adjusted life years (DALYs).
- Distinguish and give examples of communicable and noncommunicable diseases.
- Identify the leading causes of death and disability in the United States and globally.

OVERVIEW: WHAT IS DISEASE AND DISABILITY?

As introduced in Chapter 1, "The Origins of Public Health," health is a state of physical and mental well-being that is much more than the absence of disease. In contrast, disease is a deviation from normal structure or function characterized by specific signs that may be directly observable or detectable using available screening measures. Illness usually describes a set of symptoms such as pain, distress, or fatigue that often accompanies disease. The causes of disease are many and varied and may include harmful exposures, infection, or degeneration. Health professionals and their healthcare systems are engaged in disease detection, control, and treatment. While the optimal outcome would be to effectively manage illness and cure disease, the reality is that disease compromises the health of many, leading to disability and untimely mortality.

This chapter aims to provide the student with an understanding of the Global Burden of Disease by exploring population patterns of disease and disability. We (a) contrast the concepts of health and disease; (b) introduce the Global Burden of Disease; (c) discuss disability and the universal measure of DALYs; (d) present current data on leading causes of death and disability in the United States and worldwide; (e) distinguish and compare death and disability for communicable diseases, noncommunicable diseases, and injuries; and (f) describe the relationship of mortality to life expectancy.

CONTRASTING HEALTH AND DISEASE

WHAT DOES IT MEAN TO BE HEALTHY?

Chapter 1 introduced the World Health Organization (WHO) definition of health as a state of complete physical, mental, and social well-being and not merely the absence of disease or infirmity.[1] Health encompasses multiple dimensions of physical and mental well-being. Individual and population health are influenced by many factors. Health-promoting behaviors include engaging in physical activity, eating nutritious foods, getting enough sleep, managing stress, successfully completing important tasks at work and at home, engaging in mutually supportive social relationships, practicing good hygiene, and getting preventive care. These behaviors are supported by having an environment that is conducive to health, including having access to neighborhood parks and opportunities for recreation, working in safe workplaces, and benefitting from policies and laws that protect and produce health.

WHAT IS DISEASE AND HOW DO WE CLASSIFY DISEASE?

Disease signals that something is amiss and the body is not fully healthy. This creates an opportunity for a disorder to be detected, diagnosed, named, and classified. International systems have been developed for systematic disease categorization. In 2018, the WHO released its landmark 11th Revision of the *International Statistical Classification of Diseases and Related Health Problems* (ICD-11).[2] The WHO aims for ICD-11 to map the human condition from birth to death: any injury or disease we encounter in life—and anything we might die of—is coded.[3] Diseases are listed numerically with numbers pertaining to larger disease categories such as neoplasms (cancers), diseases of the circulatory system, diseases of the respiratory system, and mental/behavioral/neurodevelopmental disorders.

Each new edition of the ICD codes is years in the making because defining diseases and disorders is a complex process and classifications change over time. A disorder is a disturbance or disruption of normal functioning, even if there may not be a sufficient burden of symptoms to diagnose a specific disease. Disorders that are classified as diseases change with each new ICD edition as diagnostic capabilities improve, understanding of the disease process advances, and the social and economic implications of the disorder are elucidated.

COMMUNICABLE AND NONCOMMUNICABLE DISEASES AND INJURIES

When considering global disease patterns and burdens, diagnosed diseases and disorders are sorted into three large buckets: communicable diseases, noncommunicable diseases (NCDs), and injuries. Communicable diseases, also known as infectious or transmissible diseases, are diseases that are transmitted from an infected person, a person who harbors an infectious agent (such as a bacteria or virus), to a previously noninfected person. The movement of the infectious agent is necessary for causing new infection that may progress to a diagnosable disease.

In contrast, at the most literal level, an NCD, also known as a nontransmissible disease, is defined in the negative—by what it is not. An NCD is not a communicable disease. An NCD is not caused by a contagious or communicable infectious agent. The term "NCD" is now preferred to the less specific, but still popular, term "chronic disease." As we see in later chapters, the term "noncommunicable" is not precisely accurate because these diseases are transmitted between people through social interactions as well. Since the mid-1900s, NCDs have greatly exceeded communicable diseases as the primary causes of death worldwide, even as COVID-19 suddenly emerged on the scene. Among NCDs, diseases of the heart and cancers are especially prominent causes of death and disability worldwide.

Injuries and violence comprise the third major category for classification of diseases. Globally, motor vehicle crashes, leading to injury and death, are the best known example, but this diverse and expansive category also includes drug overdoses (unintentional poisonings), suicide, homicide, and armed conflict.

THE GLOBAL BURDEN OF DISEASE

Understanding the global landscape of disease and disability takes a global scientific enterprise. To tackle the extraordinary complexity of quantifying worldwide patterns, the Institute for Health Metrics and Evaluation at the University of Washington launched the ongoing and continuous Global Burden of Diseases, Injuries, and Risk Factors Study (GBD). The GBD is generally considered to be the gold standard for measuring disease burden worldwide. The GBD engages thousands of researchers distributed across more than 145 countries to examine trends in health indicators.[4]

The GBD is premised on the idea that all world citizens deserve to live a long life in full health. Two different phenomena impede the achievement of this desirable goal. First, some people die early, prematurely, from certain diseases. Second, some people continue to live on, even to advanced years of life, but their quality of life and their life experience are constrained by disability. They are living, but not in "full health."

Part of the impetus for creating the GBD was the realization that favorable trends in mortality patterns could be offset by unfavorable trends in disability. This was precisely the situation before there was COVID-19. Mortality rates were generally decreasing worldwide, and correspondingly, life expectancies were increasing. This favorable trend had continued for decades and was not anticipated to abate. Nevertheless, rates of disability and various forms of impairment were steadily rising. These well-documented increasing rates of disability were partially explained by the fact that as people lived longer, their chances for acquiring a disabling condition increased.

GBD researchers cleverly developed a measure for examining mortality and disability simultaneously. The primary metric used in the GBD, the DALY, compares hundreds of diseases and types of injuries in terms of risks for dying early and/or living with decreased capacity and quality of life due to disability. For each health condition, the GBD quantifies both years of life lost (YLLs) and years lived with disability (YLDs) and adds them together to estimate DALYs. Premature death is measured as YLLs. Living with diminished health and functionality is quantified as YLDs. Summing these together for each health condition, DALYs = YLLs + YLDs.

> **DALYs: disability-adjusted life years**
>
> **One DALY equals one lost year of healthy life.**
>
> **For each disease or medical condition, DALYs are made up of two components:**
>
>   1. **Dying early—premature death—is measured as YLLs.**
>   2. **Living with decreased capacity and quality of life due to disability is measured as YLDs.**
>
> **These two pieces are added together to get DALYs:**
>
> **DALYs = YLLs + YLDs**

One DALY equals one lost year of healthy life. Of course, dying early is counted as a complete loss of potential life. However, living with disability can range from partial to near total in terms of impact on living healthfully. YLDs are expressed as fractions. For example, an individual with mild chronic lower respiratory disease may be initially estimated to be living at 50% capacity—0.5 DALY for the year. Later, as disease and disability progress, the final year of life might be estimated at 0.75 DALY or higher.

A DALY is described as a universal metric that compares and contrasts health conditions across populations across time. The GBD uses DALYs to estimate the years of healthy life lost by type of health condition and by risk factor on multiple levels: country, region, and worldwide. One aim of the GBD is to equip decision makers with the necessary evidence to confront health issues that detract from healthy life. A related aim is to carefully allocate resources, professional talent, and funding to the cause of improving health by intervening on the major risk factors.

The already daunting challenges faced by GBD researchers were suddenly amplified with the appearance of COVID-19 in 2020. The pandemic added a deadly and debilitating disease to the panoply of disorders that were already harming and killing individuals—and populations. Moreover, COVID-19 interacted with a broad swath of prevalent diseases and medical conditions, both communicable diseases and NCDs, to worsen the prognosis for millions of patients living with these other diseases who became ill with COVID-19 while also hobbling the healthcare systems that treated them, triggering patterns of excess mortality—from many causes—around the globe.

DISABILITY-ADJUSTED LIFE YEARS

Pre-COVID, in 2019, what were the subcategories of disease or injury contributing the highest percentages of DALYs to the GBD? NCDs, illustrated in blue in **Figure 2.1**, predominated with cardiovascular diseases and cancers as the top two conditions generating DALYs. Prominent NCDs also included musculoskeletal disorders, mental disorders, and diabetes and kidney diseases. Neonatal conditions were third in rank order. The combination of respiratory infections (e.g. influenza) and tuberculosis—communicable diseases—were in fourth place (Figure 2.1). Unintentional injuries—other than transport injuries—were the leading cause of DALYs among multiple forms of injury and violence. COVID-19 is expected to both appear high in the ranks once GBD data are updated and also boost the numbers of DALYs from other causes.

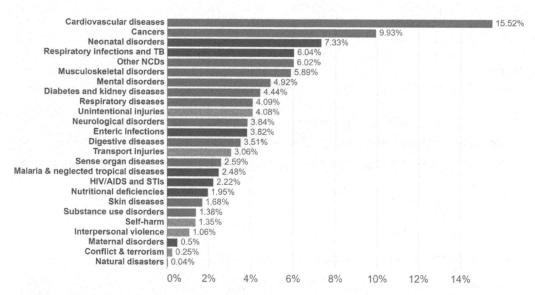

FIGURE 2.1 Global share of total disease burden, 2019. Total disease burden, measured in disability-adjusted life years (DALYs) by subcategory of disease or injury. DALYs measure the total burden of disease—both from years of life lost due to premature death and years lived with a disability. One DALY equals one lost year of healthy life.
Note: Noncommunicable diseases are shown in blue; communicable, maternal, neonatal, and nutritional diseases in red; injuries in gray.
Source: IHME, Global Burden of Disease 2019. https://ourworldindata.org/burden-of-disease

Remember that the YLD measure focuses on disability rather than death. When examining the leading causes of YLDs globally for 2019, we see a strong preponderance of musculoskeletal and sensory disorders and mental health conditions. In rank order for 2019, the top 10 conditions contributing YLDs were low back pain, depressive disorders, headache pain, hearing loss, other musculoskeletal disorders, diabetes mellitus, gynecologic diseases, anxiety disorders, dietary iron deficiency, and oral disorders.

Major causes of DALYs shift over time. For example, NCDs contribute to DALYs directly because premature deaths from NCDs get tallied as YLLs. NCDs also contribute to DALYs through increasing YLDs. NCDs are lifestyle-related diseases with risk factors that cluster and worsen, leading to more days of disability. Also, prior to death, many NCDs produce significant nonfatal episodes of illness and injury (e.g. heart attacks, strokes, falls leading to fractures) that are severely disabling. So before NCDs contribute to YLLs from premature death, they contribute to YLDs in a major way through years of suboptimal living with a disability chronologically across the life course of many individuals.

Leading Risk Factors for DALYs Worldwide

GBD researchers have examined and rank-ordered the primary risk factors that contribute to DALYs worldwide. It seems expectable that some of the most potent risk factors are lifestyle behaviors (e.g. smoking, high salt diet) or the physiological measures that reflect a high-risk lifestyle (e.g. high blood pressure, high blood sugar, high cholesterol; **Figure 2.2**). However, perhaps surprisingly, among the highest ranking factors are such environmental risks as air pollution, particulate matter pollution, unsafe water source, and unsafe sanitation.

LEADING CAUSES OF DEATH IN THE UNITED STATES

Between 1900 and the early decades of the 2000s, the number of U.S. deaths per 1,000 citizens per year dropped by half. The top 10 causes of death in the United States transformed in

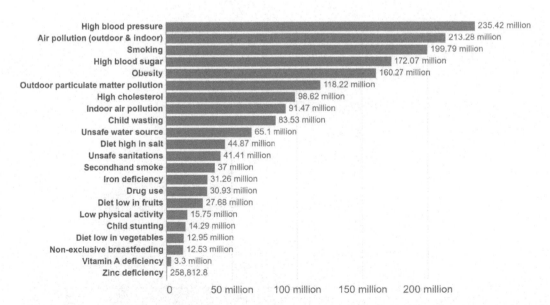

FIGURE 2.2 Global disease burden by risk factor, 2019. Disease burden is measured as disability-adjusted life years (DALYs). One DALY is the equivalent of losing one year in good health because of either premature mortality or disability. One DALY represents one lost year of healthy life.
Source: IHME, Global Burden of Disease 2019. https://ourworldindata.org/burden-of-disease

a remarkable fashion (**Figure 2.3**).[5,6] In the year 1900, four infectious diseases—pneumonia/influenza, tuberculosis, gastrointestinal infections, and diphtheria—were all ranked among the top 10. These infectious diseases collectively accounted for more deaths per 1,000 U.S. citizens in 1900 than the full top 10 list in 2016 summed together. In contrast, in 2016, NCDs accounted for seven of the top 10 causes of death with heart disease and cancer each accounting for about one-quarter of all deaths. Only a single infectious disease cause of death appeared among the top 10 in 2016 (pneumonia and influenza).

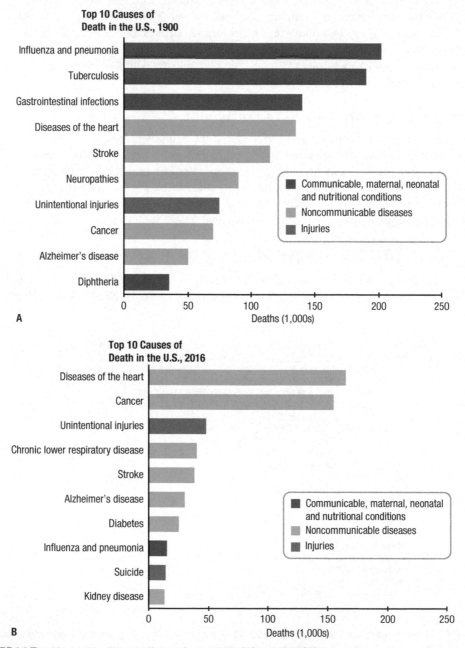

FIGURE 2.3 Top 10 causes of death, United States, 1900 (A) and 2016 (B).
Source: Data from Jones DS, Podolsky SH, Greene JA. The burden of disease and the changing task of medicine. *N Engl J Med.* 2012;366(25):2333-2338. doi:10.1056/NEJMp1113569; Heron M. National vital statistics reports, deaths: leading causes for 2016. 2016. https://www.cdc.gov/nchs/data/nvsr/nvsr67/nvsr67_06.pdf

Then came COVID-19 in 2020. By 2021, the leading causes of death in the United States now included COVID-19 in third place, accounting for more than 400,000 deaths (**Figure 2.4**). Heart disease and cancer remained in the top two slots. Yet, even with the introduction of COVID-19, the number of NCDs actually increased to eight of the top 10. COVID-19 was the sole infectious disease with influenza dropping out of the top 10. A far more dramatic finding was how COVID-19 had contributed to excess mortality across a wide range of other causes of death, most particularly prominent NCDs (**Figure 2.5**). These patterns merit further exploration as COVID-19 equilibrates and produces a lower and more predictable number of annual deaths that will nevertheless remain in the top 10 causes of death for the foreseeable future.

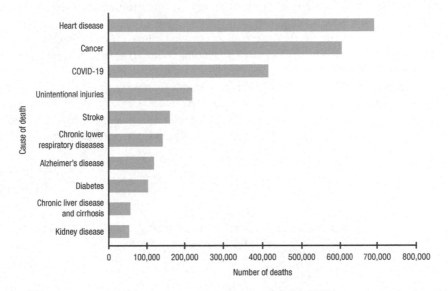

FIGURE 2.4 Provisional number of leading underlying causes of death, 2021.
Source: Ahmad FB, Cisewski JA, Anderson RN. Provisional mortality data – United States, 2021. *MMWR Morb Mortal Wkly Rep.* 2022;71(17):597-600. doi:10.15585/mmwr.mm7117e1

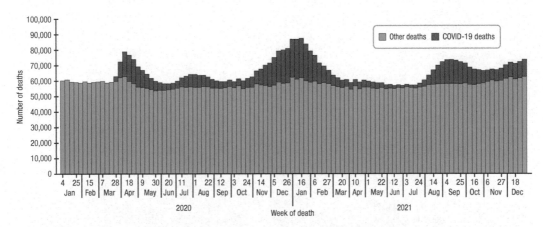

FIGURE 2.5 National Vital Statistics System provisional data for 2021 are incomplete. Data from December 2021 are less complete because of reporting lags. Data for 2020 are final. These data exclude deaths that occurred in the United States among residents of U.S. territories and foreign countries; number of COVID-19 deaths (deaths with confirmed or presumed COVID-19, coded to *International Classification of Diseases, Tenth Revision* code U07.1 as an underlying or contributing cause of death), by week of death, 2020–2021.
Source: Ahmad FB, Cisewski JA, Anderson RN. Provisional mortality data – United States, 2021. *MMWR Morb Mortal Wkly Rep.* 2022;71(17):597-600. doi:10.15585/mmwr.mm7117e1

LEADING CAUSES OF DEATH GLOBALLY

According to the GBD database for 2019, cardiovascular diseases, including ischemic heart disease and stroke, topped the list of leading causes of death globally, followed by cancers, respiratory diseases, digestive diseases, and lower respiratory infections (primarily pneumonia and influenza; **Figure 2.6**). When data are updated to include COVID-19, pandemic deaths will rank in the top five causes of death, at least for the years 2020 and 2021.

When comparing the leading causes of death globally for 1990 and 2019, it is notable that NCDs are more numerous and higher ranking in 2019. Examining global mortality patterns in greater detail, when countries are classified and divided into the four World Bank income categories (low, lower-middle, upper-middle, and high income), trends and distinctions become readily apparent (**Figure 2.7**).[7]

Here is a series of observations that you can confirm for yourself. First, communicable disease causes of death are particularly concentrated in low-income countries where six of 10 causes of death are infectious diseases. At the other extreme, for high-income countries, only a single infectious disease, lower respiratory infections—primarily influenza and pneumonia—appears among the top 10.

Second, not unexpectedly, in the high-income countries, NCD causes of death predominate and account for nine of 10 leading causes of death. At the opposite pole, for low-income countries, only three of the 10 top causes are NCDs: ischemic heart disease, stroke, and cirrhosis of the liver.

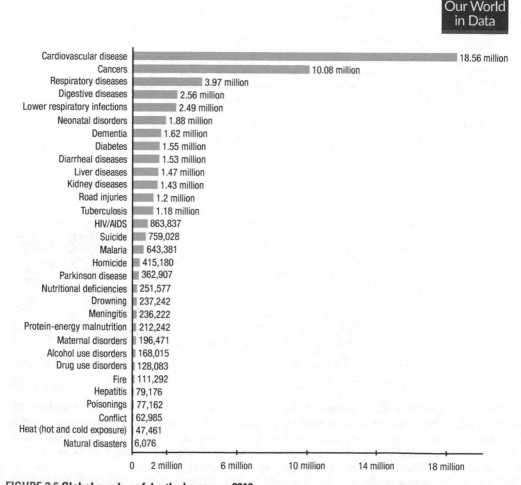

FIGURE 2.6 Global number of deaths by cause, 2019.
Source: IHME, Global Burden of Disease 2019. https://ourworldindata.org/burden-of-disease

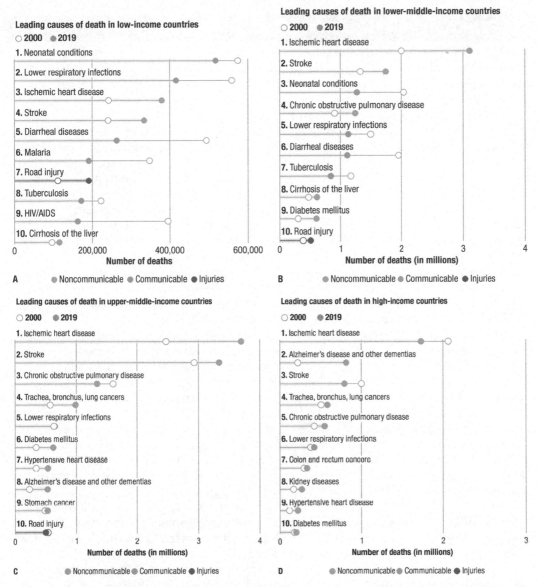

FIGURE 2.7 Top 10 global causes of death by World Bank income category, 2019. (A) Low income; (B) lower-middle income; (C) upper-middle income; and (D) high income.
Note: World Bank 2020 income classification.
Source: Reproduced with permission from the World Health Organization. The top 10 causes of death. 2020. https://www
.who.int/news-room/fact-sheets/detail/the-top-10-causes-of-death\

Third, as one observed commonality, cardiovascular diseases—the combination of heart disease and stroke—are the leading causes of death in lower-middle, upper-middle, and high-income countries. In each of these three income categories, ischemic heart disease ranks first. Stroke ranks second in both lower-middle and upper-middle countries and third in high-income nations. Now contrast this with low-income countries where ischemic heart disease ranks third and stroke is in fourth place.

Fourth, it is useful to ask, how different are these specific causes of death across income categories? The answer is very different. In fact, only three causes of death share the top 10 in both low-income and high-income countries. These three are ischemic heart disease, stroke, and lower respiratory infections. (Case Study 2.1; you can access the podcast accompanying Case Study 2.1 by following this link to Springer Publishing Company Connect™: http://connect .springerpub.com/content/book/978-0-8261-8043-8/part/part01/chapter/ch02).

CASE STUDY 2.1: FALLING LIFE EXPECTANCY IN THE UNITED STATES

Tracking patterns of health and disease in a population informs our future policies and practices, providing actionable guidance to collectively better the health of the public. Life expectancy is one key indicator of a nation's health status. Each nation computes life expectancy, a vital statistic that is current and readily available, allowing easy comparisons across countries.

Life expectancy in the United States soared by an astonishing 30 years during the 1900s, an accomplishment that cannot be replicated, given the limitations of human physiology.[9] At the turn of the millennium, the U.S. Centers for Disease Control and Prevention proudly ballyhooed how 10 Great Public Health Achievements accounted for 25 years of the 30-year gain. Prominent among these achievements was the successful conquest of communicable diseases through a combination of vaccination and basic public health measures that assured population-wide access to clean water and sanitation and healthier foods.[10] This was coupled with advances in the prevention and treatment of cardiovascular diseases, control of tobacco consumption, ongoing enhancements in motor vehicle and workplace safety, and improvements in maternal and child health.[10] This 30-year increase in life expectancy within one century is breathtaking across the course of human history. This is certainly cause for celebration, optimism, and expected future gains. Right?

Not so fast. First, dating from the 1980s, U.S. life expectancies have fallen below those of comparable countries. The gap has been growing for more than 40 years. Although U.S. life expectancy increased during most years through 2014, these gains did not keep pace with "peer" nations. Second, since 2014, the United States has experienced a plateauing and some reversal of U.S. life expectancy gains, rather than a continued ascent. U.S. life expectancy has dropped. Several factors have been at play.

Starting in 2014, overall U.S. life expectancy actually dipped slightly due to the opiate epidemic.[11] Overdose deaths rose steadily over multiple years, exceeding 107,000 deaths in 2021. Declining life expectancy in the United States contrasted with the ongoing upward trajectory for peer nations that were not experiencing widespread opiate abuse and rising overdose deaths.

Then, starting in 2020, U.S. life expectancy took a sharp hit during the first years of the COVID-19 pandemic. Life expectancy declined globally during 2020, the pandemic's pre-vaccine year. Yet, U.S. COVID-19 mortality rates fared much worse than peer nations, creating a disproportionate drop in life expectancy.[12]

A graphic prepared by the Health System Tracker (**Figure 2.8**), a collaboration between Peterson Center for Health Care and the Kaiser Family Foundation, is rich in comparative detail.

First, we observe the steady upward trajectory of life expectancy for the United States and comparable peer countries that actually extended throughout much of the 20th century. This graphic "picks up the story" in 1980 when U.S. life expectancy was already below the overall average of peer nations by about two years, but not the lowest of the group.

Second, we see that for 40 years—4 decades—through 2019, the upward slope of U.S. gains in life expectancy was lower than for peer countries. Already starting with a lower life expectancy than the average of comparable countries in 1980, over this 40-year span, U.S. life expectancy dropped farther away from the average of this select group of high-income nations through 2019.

Third, for the 5 years, 2015 to 2019, the departure from peer countries became more pronounced as drug overdose deaths proliferated in the United States, amplified by the appearance of synthetic opiates, most notably fentanyl, and also a diversion to using heroin as a cheaper alternative drug.

(continued)

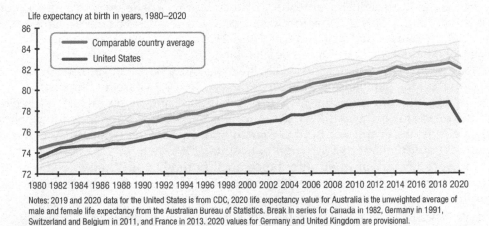

Life expectancy improved for the United States and most comparable countries in 2019 but decreased in 2020 due to COVID-19.

Life expectancy at birth in years, 1980–2020

Notes: 2019 and 2020 data for the United States is from CDC, 2020 life expectancy value for Australia is the unweighted average of male and female life expectancy from the Australian Bureau of Statistics. Break in series for Canada in 1982, Germany in 1991, Switzerland and Belgium in 2011, and France in 2013. 2020 values for Germany and United Kingdom are provisional.

FIGURE 2.8 Life expectancy comparing the United States to comparable countries, 1980–2020. DALYs, disability-adjusted life years; SDI, sociodemographic index.
Source: Data from Health System Tracker – Ortaliza J, Ramirez G, Satheeskumar V, Amin K. How does U.S. life expectancy compare to other countries? Kaiser Family Foundation Health System Tracker. https://www.healthsystemtracker .org/chart-collection/u-s-life-expectancy-compare-countries/#Life%20expectancy%20at%20birth%20in%20years,%20 1980-2020%C2%A0

Heroin and other street drugs were often laced with fentanyl, adding to the steeply rising burden of deaths classified as "unintentional poisonings." During this period, U.S. mortality patterns from unintentional injuries were transformed. Following decades when motor vehicle crash deaths predominated as the primary form of what the public describes as "accidental deaths", suddenly drug overdose deaths—"unintentional poisonings"—jumped into first place.

Fourth, the steep downturn in life expectancy between 2019 and 2020 is largely attributable to the COVID-19 pandemic, yet here again, the downward inflection for the United States is sharper than for comparable nations.

Taken together, this graphic presents a stark picture of diminished U.S. life expectancy, both absolutely and relatively, when displayed alongside the experience of peer countries.

These startling mortality dynamics call out for further exploration and explanation. Prior to the appearance of COVID-19, the dip in life expectancy from the all-time high of 78.9 years in 2014 had been largely made up, with a value of 78.8 years in 2019. Encouragingly, the United States seemed poised to advance onward to higher life expectancy once again.

That was not to be. COVID-19 caused a global downturn in life expectancy during 2020.[12] Yet despite superior healthcare capabilities and vastly larger per capita healthcare expenditures, the United States experienced more severe COVID-19 mortality and a deeper dive in the U.S. life expectancy indicator than did almost all peer countries.

When COVID-19 arrived, the average life expectancy for peer nations was almost 4 years higher than for the United States (82.6 years versus 78.8 years in 2019).[13] At year-end 2020, the average peer nation life expectancy had shed 0.5 years, dropping to 82.1 years.[14] In contrast, U.S. life expectancy plummeted 1.8 years to just 77.0 years, expanding the gap between U.S. life expectancy and the average for comparable countries to over 5 years!

(*continued*)

COVID-19 was so deadly that pandemic fatalities immediately inserted themselves into the leading causes of death for the United States. In 2020, the first year of the pandemic, COVID-19 instantly became the third leading cause of death with about 350,000 deaths recorded.[15] Only deaths from diseases of the heart and cancers claimed more lives. U.S. life expectancy dropped again in 2021, a year that saw an estimated 475,000 COVID-19 deaths.[16] Indeed, excess deaths due to COVID-19 and other causes in 2020 and 2021 led to an overall decline in U.S. life expectancy between 2019 and 2021 of 2.7 years for the total population, 3.1 years for males, and 2.3 years for females.

Resulting U.S. life expectancy by the end of 2021 had fallen to 76.1 years overall, 73.2 years for men, and 79.1 years for women, revealing a sprawling gender gap of almost six years! For both U.S. men and women, life expectancy at birth is the lowest among nations with high per capita GDPs.[14]

A powerful driver of lower life expectancy in the United States relates to the extraordinary disparities in mortality rates and life expectancy by race/ethnicity. Overall, increases in excess deaths during the first 2 pandemic years, 2020 and 2021, led to decreases in life expectancy at birth of 7.1 years for non-Hispanic American Indian/Alaska Native (AI/AN) males, 5.8 years for non-Hispanic AI/AN females, 4.7 years for Hispanic males, 4.6 years for non-Hispanic Black males, 3.4 years for Hispanic females, 3.3 years for non-Hispanic Black females, 2.6 years for non-Hispanic White males, 2.3 years for non-Hispanic Asian males, 2.1 years for non-Hispanic White females, and 1.8 years for non-Hispanic Asian females.

In summary, despite the extraordinary 30-year gain in life expectancy during the 1900s, the United States failed to keep pace with comparable high-income countries, falling progressively behind peer nations over a 40-year period, from the 1980s forward. Then, the double whammy of the opiate epidemic followed immediately by the COVID-19 pandemic dropped U.S. life expectancy sharply, giving back a portion of the gains achieved in the previous century and careening far below comparable countries.

SUMMARY

Health is a complex construct, encompassing physical and mental well-being, and is not simply the absence of disease. Diseases are diagnosed, based on specific criteria, and these diagnoses can also be complicated. Diseases are classified as communicable (also known as infectious or transmissible) or noncommunicable (also called chronic). Communicable diseases are often of shorter duration as compared to noncommunicable diseases. Communicable diseases are passed from one infected person to another, while noncommunicable diseases are often caused by lifestyle factors or environmental or social conditions and are the leading causes of death worldwide.

The leading causes of disability and death have changed over time and will likely continue to change. As of March 2022, COVID-19 was responsible for more than 6.2 million deaths worldwide, and that number continues to climb. A little over 1 year into the COVID-19 pandemic, global cases of major depressive disorder spiked up 27.6%.[8] The full consequences of COVID-19, particularly on mental health, have yet to be realized.

End-of-Chapter Resources

 Access additional case study podcasts online at http://connect.springerpub.com/ content/book/978-0-8261-8043-8/

DISCUSSION QUESTIONS

1. Given the changing patterns of COVID-19, where does COVID-19 currently rank among the leading causes of death in the United States?

2. Among deaths from unintentional injuries, drug overdose deaths (listed as unintional poisonings) have outnumbered motor vehicle crash deaths during the second decade of the 2000s. What have been the trends over the most recent 2 years and where do unintentional injury deaths currently rank in U.S. leading causes of death?

3. What has been the impact of long COVID-19 on U.S. patterns of disability and DALYs?

A robust set of instructor resources designed to supplement this text is located at **http://connect.springerpub.com/content/book/978-0-8261-8043-8**. Qualifying instructors may request access by emailing **textbook@springerpub.com**.

REFERENCES

1. World Health Organization. *Constitution of WHO: principles.* https://www.who.int/about/governance/constitution

2. World Health Organization. *WHO's new International Classification of Diseases comes into effect.* https://www.who.int/news/item/11-02-2022-who-s-new-international-classification-of-diseases-(icd-11)-comes-into-effect

3. World Health Organization. *ICD-11: classifying disease to map the way we live and die.* Published June 18, 2018. https://www.who.int/news-room/spotlight/international-classification-of-diseases

4. Institute for Health Metrics and Evaluation. *Global burden of disease (GBD).* http://www.healthdata.org/gbd

5. Jones DS, Podolsky SH, Greene JA. The burden of disease and the changing task of medicine. *N Engl J Med.* 2012;366(25):2333-2338. doi:10.1056/NEJMp1113569

6. Heron M. Deaths: leading causes for 2016. *Natl Vital Stat Rep.* 2018;67(6):1-77. https://www.cdc.gov/nchs/data/nvsr/nvsr67/nvsr67_06.pdf

7. The World Bank. *World Bank country and lending groups.* https://datahelpdesk.worldbank.org/knowledgebase/articles/906519-world-bank-country-and-lending-groups

8. Santomauro DF, Mantilla Herrera AM, Shadid J, et al. Global prevalence and burden of depressive and anxiety disorders in 204 countries and territories in 2020 due to the COVID-19 pandemic. *Lancet.* 2021;398(10312):1700-1712. https://doi.org/10.1016/s0140-6736(21)02143-7

9. Roser M, Ortiz-Ospina E, Ritchie H. *Life expectancy.* Our World in Data. Published 2013. https://ourworldindata.org/life-expectancy

10. Centers for Disease Control and Prevention. *Ten great public health achievements–United States, 1900-1999.* https://www.cdc.gov/mmwr/preview/mmwrhtml/00056796.htm

11. Stein R. *Life expectancy drops again as opioid deaths surge in U.S.* NPR. Published December 21, 2017. https://www.npr.org/sections/health-shots/2017/12/21/572080314/life-expectancy-drops-again-as-opioid-deaths-surge-in-u-s

12. Aburto JM, Schöley J, Kashnitsky I, et al. Quantifying impacts of the COVID-19 pandemic through life-expectancy losses: a population-level study of 29 countries. *Int J Epidemiol.* 2022;51(1):63-74. https://doi.org/10.1093/ije/dyab207

13. Woolf SH, Masters RK, Aron LY. Effect of the covid-19 pandemic in 2020 on life expectancy across populations in the USA and other high income countries: simulations of provisional mortality data. *BMJ.* 2021;373:n1343. https://doi.org/10.1136/bmj.n1343

14. Ortaliza J, Ramirez G, Satheeskumar V, Amin K. *How does U.S. life expectancy compare to other countries?.* Health System Tracker. Published September 28, 2021. https://www.healthsystemtracker.org/chart-collection/u-s-life-expectancy-compare-countries/

15. Centers for Disease Control and Prevention. *2020 final death statistics: COVID-19 as an underlying cause of death vs. contributing cause.* Published January 7, 2022. https://www.cdc.gov/nchs/pressroom/podcasts/2022/20220107/20220107.htm

16. Donovan, D. *U.S. officially surpasses 1 million COVID-19 deaths.* Johns Hopkins Coronavirus Resource Center. Published May 17, 2022. https://coronavirus.jhu.edu/from-our-experts/u-s-officially-surpasses-1-million-covid-19-deaths

3

AT THE HEART OF PUBLIC HEALTH: PREVENTION

Salma M. Abdalla also contributed to this chapter

LEARNING OBJECTIVES

- Explain the concept of prevention as a core principle for public health.
- Distinguish primordial, primary, secondary, and tertiary disease prevention.
- Explain the science of screening and provide examples of how screening is applied.
- Discuss the principles of disease prevention and health promotion in public health interventions, locally, nationally, and globally.

OVERVIEW: CORE PRINCIPLE OF PUBLIC HEALTH: PREVENTION

There are two core principles we consider central to the work of public health, prevention (this chapter) and health equity (see Chapter 4, "At the Heart of Public Health: Social Determinants of Health and Health Equity"). Regarding the core principle of prevention, public health is concerned with creating the healthiest possible populations. As such, public health is about the creation of the conditions that are conducive to keeping us all healthy for as long as possible. With prevention in mind, public health is different from clinical medicine. Clinical medicine is concerned with treating us once we are sick, restoring us to health when possible, and slowing the progression of disease and disability. Public health tries to ensure that we do not get sick to begin with. Importantly, public health is about the health of all of us. This has implications for how public health does its work and how anyone in public health engages with the profession.

With prevention as a guiding principle, in this chapter we (a) discuss the principles of primordial, primary, secondary, and tertiary disease prevention; (b) introduce the concept of screening, including when to screen and when not to screen; and (c) apply the notions of prevention to various populations, with local, national, and global examples.

PREVENTION: CREATING THE HEALTHIEST POSSIBLE LIFE

PREVENTING DISEASE

One century ago, in 1920, Charles-Edward A. Winslow defined public health as "the science and art of preventing disease, prolonging life, and promoting physical health and efficiency through organized community efforts for the sanitation of the environment, the control of community infections, the education of the individual in principles of personal hygiene, the organization of medical and nursing service for the early diagnosis and preventive treatment of disease, and the development of the social machinery which will ensure to every individual in the community a standard of living adequate for the maintenance of health, so organizing these benefits as to enable each citizen to realize his birthright of health and longevity."[1] This definition, which puts prevention at the heart of public health, has stood the test of time and remains broadly applicable today.

Disease prevention is one of the cornerstones of public health. Prominent among the great public health achievements of the 20th century[2] are prevention activities (e.g., vaccination and control of communicable diseases) that are central to the practice of public health. Investing in disease prevention is one of the most cost-effective and commonsense approaches to improve health. Prevention spares people from developing avertable illnesses in the first place, thereby setting off a cascade of beneficial outcomes including reduced healthcare costs, improved productivity, and enhanced quality of life.

CASE STUDY 3.1: AMERICAN INDIAN / ALASKA NATIVE LEADERSHIP IN COVID-19 VACCINATION

At the front end of the COVID-19 pandemic, the American Indian/Alaska Native (AI/AN) population in the United States experienced disproportionately high rates of COVID-19 infection, hospitalization, and death[3] in the context of ongoing structural inequalities and discrimination.[4,5] Yet, when vaccines became available in early 2021, offering the option to significantly reduce COVID-19 transmission and disease risks, it was the non-Hispanic AI/AN population that rapidly achieved the highest first dose and second dose vaccination rates in the nation.[6,7] According to the Centers for Disease Control and Prevention (CDC), which publishes available vaccination data according to race and ethnic group, non-Hispanic AI/ANs led the United States in rates of first-dose and full vaccination through late 2021.[6] Furthermore, state- and county-level data confirmed these high vaccination rates for AI/AN populations.[7]

These stunning achievements in vaccination rates, playing against a backdrop of long-standing health inequities, reflect unique aspects of the diverse AI/AN cultures that allowed greater autonomy and agency in the selection of population protection strategies. Approaches to COVID-19 vaccination were able to build upon prior successes in adapting community mitigation strategies for the unique needs of AI/AN tribes during the 2020 prevaccine era.

The focus of this case study, COVID-19 vaccination for AI/AN communities, advances our conversation regarding two themes at the heart of public health, prevention—COVID-19 vaccines dramatically lower rates of severe COVID-19 disease, hospitalization, and mortality—and health equity, noting the extraordinary disease burden of COVID-19 for AI/AN peoples. Here we primarily describe AI/AN vaccination in a manner that illuminates the workings of societal and structural levels of the COVID-19 response, including federal agencies and tribal governments, in carrying out timely and effective vaccination campaigns that created ripple effects down to the levels of communities, social networks, families, and individuals.

As background, 9.7 million people, representing 2.9% of the United States population, identify as AI/AN. This includes those who specify solely AI/AN identity

(*continued*)

and a larger number who identify as AI/AN in combination with other races. The diversity of AI/AN tribes and nations is notable, with some residing on reservations and others dwelling in urban Indian enclaves. AI/AN lands are sovereign territories, covering 100 million acres, including 44 million acres in Alaska. The Indian Health Service (IHS), a federal agency within the Department of Health and Human Services, serves just over one-quarter (2.6 million) of those who identify as AI/AN, including many of the 574 federally recognized AI/AN tribes distributed across Alaska and 34 of the 48 contiguous states.

Early on, immediately upon approval of emergency use authorization (EUA) for the Pfizer and Moderna mRNA vaccines, the IHS received sizable allocations. Using its established and fully operational national distribution system, IHS was able to rapidly ship allotments of vaccines throughout an extensive network of "receiving facilities" located in all IHS areas. Receiving facilities were frequently colocated at tribal health programs on reservations and accessible sites specified by urban Indian organizations. Concurrently, the Alaska Native Health Board (ANHB), the statewide entity representing Alaska's 229 federally recognized tribes and villages, adopted an alternative strategy. ANHB developed a partnership with Alaska state government to procure and distribute COVID-19 vaccines.

These strategies, tailored for timely and efficient vaccine distribution, propelled AI/AN populations into the forefront early in the 2021 vaccine era. This was simultaneously reflected in how quickly AI/AN vaccination rates surged into the lead among race/ethnic groups.

While nimble distribution systems provided the logistics for getting vaccines to AI/AN communities, the high rate of vaccine uptake observed among AI/ANs was buoyed by much more profound influences. The sovereignty of AI/AN nations played a decisive role in allowing these communities to self-direct their own COVID-19 vaccination campaigns. Sovereignty gave AI/AN tribes and nations considerable power to define their own destinies relative to COVID-19. Essentially, the COVID-19 response within tribal communities—for mitigating transmission risks, promoting vaccination and forestalling vaccine resistance—can be visualized as an ecosystem of healthcare and information services involving cooperation among AI/AN governments, tribal health systems, and allied community-based organizations.

As examples of the autonomy of tribal decision-making, in the earliest months of the pandemic's prevaccine era, AI/AN communities implemented such stalwart outbreak investigation and control measures as case identification, case isolation, contact tracing, and quarantine for identified contacts in adherence with CDC protocols. AI/AN nations improvised strategies for safely treating COVID-19 patients within their communities, making use of trained patient transport teams, food delivery teams during times of lockdown, and enforcement using their own patrols.

Social media channels were used to maintain tribal continuity and connectedness. During times of COVID-19 lockdown, the use of social media—which had been previously instrumental for social interaction and support during the long winter seasons—was amplified in importance. Social media provided opportunities to enhance such mainstays as storytelling, talking circles, and educational programs and to expand into the realm of public health engagement, providing updates on effective strategies for surviving COVID-19.

Once vaccines became available, AI/AN communities distinguished themselves in several ways.

(*continued*)

First, the pandemic's quantifiably unequal impact on AI/AN nations became a potent motivator for concerted activity on vaccination. Cumulatively, throughout the first 2 full years of the pandemic, non-Hispanic AI/AN populations experienced COVID-19 case rates at 1.5 times the baseline comparison group of non-Hispanic Whites; COVID-19 hospitalizations at 3.2 times the baseline; and COVID-19 deaths at 2.2 times the baseline. The COVID-19 case rate ratio for non-Hispanic AI/ANs was higher than for non-Hispanic Blacks/African Americans, or for non-Hispanic Asians, and identical to the rate ratio for Hispanics. For both COVID-19 hospitalizations and deaths, the rate ratios were higher for non-Hispanic AI/ANs than for any other race/ethnic category. COVID-19 was quite literally decimating AI/AN nations.

Second, health messaging was a key to raising vaccine coverage rates in AI/AN communities. A poll that included 2,000 AI/AN respondents documented the favorability of health messaging that presented COVID-19 vaccination for AI/AN communities as a means for combatting a pandemic that had caused such disproportionate suffering.[8] The power—and the rationale—of messaging that portrayed vaccination as a way to fight back was strongly grounded on the COVID-19 surveillance findings.

Third, COVID's concentrated impact on older adults threatened the health and life of AI/AN tribal elders and, by extension, posed an existential dilemma for tribal culture and viability.[6] One of the earliest findings from CDC pandemic surveillance data was the exponential rise in COVID-19 mortality rates with age. Beyond the name itself, tribal "elders" tend to be older members of their communities. Therefore, AI/AN governments and tribal leaders, supported by community-based organizations, prioritized vaccination for community members whose roles are instrumental for preserving the AI/AN way of life. According to Foxworth and colleagues (2021), among tribal members who were placed first in line for vaccination—both to optimize their own health and to role model the act of safely receiving the COVID-19 vaccine—were "tribal elders, council members, knowledge keepers, Indigenous-language speakers, and tribal health providers."[6] The same poll that included 2,000 AI/AN respondents identified strong support for protecting tribal elders through first-in-line vaccination and taking steps to preserve the integrity of AI/AN culture and heritage.[8]

Fourth, tribal leadership had the discretion to determine vaccination priorities, particularly in early 2021 when vaccine supplies were not adequate to cover the entire U.S. population. Some AI/AN nations opted to make vaccines available to younger members of their tribes sooner than happened in neighboring non-AI/AN communities.

Fifth, AI/AN communities were able to use their own venues for drive-through and outdoor vaccination events. Among the tribal facilities that could be repurposed as vaccination sites were schools, casinos, urban Indian community centers, parks, and lodges.

Sixth, tribes had the ability to incentivize vaccination in several ways. Some communities provided direct cash payments to community members who could provide proof of vaccination. Other incentives were tied to tribal ceremonial seasons that are so central to the AI/AN way of life (e.g., Lenten and Easter season for the Pascua Yaqui Tribe, summer feast days for Pueblo communities, and the Hanbleceya ceremony for the Crow Creek Sioux Tribe). While some ceremonies were canceled due to concerns about transmission during COVID-19 surges, a

(continued)

number of AI/AN communities went forward with these sacred events; however, only community members who could provide proof of vaccination were permitted to attend.

Ongoing research is likely to enrich our understanding of contributors to high rates of vaccine uptake among AI/AN communities. These are multitiered actions that incorporate the novel aspects of tribal governance. Some prominent lessons learned during 2021, the first year of vaccine availability, have been concisely summarized by Foxworth et al.[6]

> First, having the autonomy to establish their own policies and priorities was instrumental for AI/AN communities to proactively vaccinate their populations.
>
> Second, communities benefited from creating innovative, inclusive approaches to increase vaccination uptake, which included tailoring outreach and messaging strategies to their individual cultures.
>
> Third, although the IHS, state governments, and the federal government facilitated timely vaccine delivery and distribution to tribal communities, they should enhance their collaborations with tribes to address the underlying inequities that have made AI/ANs especially vulnerable to COVID-19.

MAINTAINING HEALTH AS LONG AS POSSIBLE

Prevention has played a major role in elevating life expectancy to the levels we experience today. Early humans, dwelling on the planet 25,000 to 40,000 years ago, survived, on average, only 20 to 30 years.[9,10] During the intervening 25,000 years, global life expectancy gains crept upward almost imperceptibly, hovering in the mid-30s by the year 1900.[10] It was only during the 20th century that the human species witnessed an exponential rise in life expectancy. Throughout the 1900s, average life expectancy surged upward by more than 30 years in high-income countries, including the United States. Most of this startling increase came from preventing infant and early life mortality. Prevention held the key. This phenomenon is not expected to be repeated. Going forward, additional gains in life expectancy are likely to be much more limited.[11,12]

The dramatic improvement in average life expectancy can be attributed, in large part, to accelerating economic growth, effective control of infectious diseases, and improved sanitation. These three factors collectively contributed to better living conditions, improved nutrition, and the development and widespread use of vaccines and antimicrobials to prevent and combat communicable diseases.[13]

The dramatic improvement in global average life expectancy can be attributed, in large part, to accelerating economic growth, effective control of infectious diseases, and improved sanitation.

PREVENTION BASICS: TYPES OF PREVENTION

Prevention is a core population health concept. Prevention describes actions that ward off or forestall the occurrence of disease in populations.[14] The notion of prevention expands to include a range of possibilities. The ideal preventive intervention would aim to achieve disease eradication, to effectively banish disease. During the 20th century, this occurred globally with smallpox and across much of the planet with poliomyelitis. Prevention activities may also be directed toward buffering the severity of the population impact of disease. When disease occurrence cannot be prevented outright, preventive measures can still be applied to dampen and slow the progression of disease, disability, and death.

Prevention science has been conceived in terms of levels using "primary," "secondary," and "tertiary" prevention terminology. As an alternative, prevention science professionals sometimes prefer to describe three levels of preventive interventions using the terms "universal," "selective," and "indicated" prevention. Both sets of terms are useful for understanding how prevention strategies are focused and applied at various points along a continuum as disease develops and interacts with a population. In this chapter, we examine the different levels, highlighting the primary, secondary, and tertiary nomenclature.

PRIMARY DISEASE PREVENTION

Primary prevention refers to actions that keep people from becoming ill or injured in the first place. These strategies prevent disease. Primary prevention actions are core elements of public health and health promotion: immunizing the population against infectious diseases, ensuring safe water supplies and sanitation, improving the nutritional status of the population, decreasing or eliminating hazardous exposures, and diminishing health-compromising behaviors.[15]

In the realm of chronic disease (noncommunicable disease) prevention, some investigators insert primordial prevention as an approach that precedes primary prevention.[16] Primordial prevention aims to completely prevent the expression of a risk factor. Quite straightforwardly, primordial prevention of hypertension uses strategies that keep blood pressures in a normal range from early childhood forward, thereby preventing the occurrence of blood pressure elevations that signify hypertension. Primordial prevention activities take place far "upstream," applying systems-level interventions to diminish the appearance of risk factors, like hypertension or obesity, at the population level (**Figure 3.1**).[17] When successful, primordial/primary prevention lowers disease incidence (the proportion of people developing new-onset disease).

Let us play out the scenario of a population or a society—let us call it Primaria—that subscribes wholly and successfully to the precepts of primordial and primary prevention. Over time, what

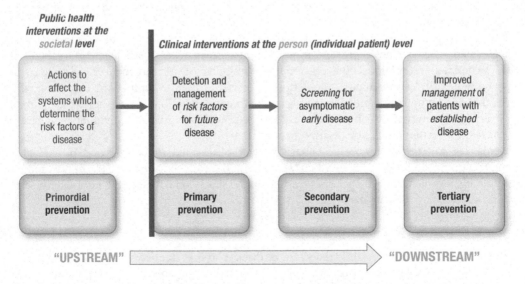

FIGURE 3.1 Disease prevention intervention strategies: primordial, primary, secondary, and tertiary.
Source: Frank JW. Prevention and control strategies for non-communicable disease: Goldberger, Pellagra and Rose revisited. *Epidemiologia.* 2022;3(2):191-198. https://doi.org/10.3390/epidemiologia3020015

does our Primarian society look like in terms of the production of health and disease? The answer is very healthy. The hallmark of Primaria is robust population health. Primaria is composed of persons whose mothers received prenatal care, who were breastfed as infants, and who were vaccinated on schedule. Primarians observe a healthy diet lifelong (high in vegetables, fruits, whole grains, and fiber; low in red meats, high-fat dairy products, soft drinks, and processed foods), and maintain a daily physical activity regimen that includes regular periods of movement throughout the day as well as bouts of cardiovascular and resistance training throughout the week. Primarians as a population do not use nicotine products or other addictive substances in any form with the possible exception of moderate caffeine intake and minimal or no alcohol consumption. They are every-time users of seat belts who do not drive and text and who observe traffic laws while driving. They maintain a schedule of regular preventive medical visits and educate themselves on new developments in the realm of healthy lifestyles. They are environmentally conscious, minimize their carbon footprint, and advocate for programs and policies that promote the public's health—and social justice—at levels ranging from local to planetary. Primarians live long, healthy lives.

Primaria, of course, does not exist. There are no cultures that come close to universal adoption of primordial and primary prevention principles. However, for the sake of illustrating primary prevention, it is interesting to contemplate how healthy such a society could be. Optimal health and minimal disease: all good, right? Perhaps not quite; there are powerful countervailing human tendencies as we will see at the next, more realistic, level of prevention.

SECONDARY DISEASE PREVENTION

Secondary prevention aims to reduce the impact of a disease or injury in the earliest stages of occurrence. Secondary prevention focuses on detecting and treating subclinical (i.e., not yet outwardly recognizable or detectable) diseases or injuries as soon as possible.

By achieving early detection, secondary prevention holds promise for halting and reversing the disease course, and possibly restoring persons to full health. Assuming that effective treatments or lifestyle interventions are available, these individuals are likely to return to disease-free living. Therefore, secondary prevention can reduce the numbers of persons currently living with disease, especially among the ranks of those with minor or outwardly undetectable disease. When successful, secondary prevention lowers disease prevalence (the proportion of persons currently living with disease).

Secondary prevention most notably features the broad application of screening to detect elevated risks or early signs and symptoms of disease. The World Health Organization (WHO) defines screening as "the presumptive identification of unrecognized disease in an apparently healthy, asymptomatic population by means of tests, examinations or other procedures that can be applied rapidly and easily to the target population."[18] In other words, screening is a process through which tests are used to determine whether an individual likely has or will develop a certain disease or health outcome.

Screening for risk factors, risk behaviors, and observable functional and physiological changes is premised on the concept of early detection. Early detection creates the opportunity to apply timely intervention, which ideally translates to disease control, minimizing disability, and, hopefully, restoring full health.

More on Screening

The objective of screening is early detection of disease so that treatments can be implemented as early as possible, when they are often most effective.[19] Common screening tests used include Pap smear for cervical cancer, prostate specific antigen (PSA) blood measurements for prostate cancer, colonoscopy for colon cancer, mammography for breast cancer, and cholesterol measurements for cardiovascular disease. Screening tests do not diagnose disease, but rather, identify persons at highest risk for disease who then undergo further evaluation and testing to diagnose disease if it is present.

Some screening tests work very well in that they very accurately differentiate persons most likely to have and not have disease. There are key performance measures that summarize how well a screening test works: sensitivity, specificity, false positive fraction, and false negative fraction.

- The sensitivity of a screening test is its ability to correctly identify a person with disease, or the percentage of persons with disease who screen positive.

- The specificity of a screening test is its ability to correctly identify a person without disease, or the percentage of persons without disease who screen negative.

- The false positive fraction of a screening test is an error, measured as the percentage of persons without disease who screen positive.

- The false negative fraction of a screening test is also an error, measured as the percentage of persons with disease who screen negative.

A perfect screening test has 100% sensitivity and specificity, and 0% false positive and false negative fractions. Unfortunately, performance measures like these are usually unattainable. A screening test might, for example, have a sensitivity of 80%, a specificity of 90%, a false positive fraction of 10%, and a false negative fraction of 20%. Is this a good screening test? The answer is, it depends. It depends on what we are screening for and the implications of errors. On the surface, we might feel that these performance measures are quite good. Suppose, for example, that these are the performance characteristics for a new low-cost, rapid test to screen for COVID-19 in asymptomatic persons. A sensitivity of 80% means that 80% of persons truly infected with COVID-19 screen positive. This is helpful to these people who can self-isolate to prevent the spread of infection. But, what of the other 20%? The other 20% are false negatives. These are people truly infected with COVID-19, but they screen negative. They might feel falsely reassured that they do not have COVID-19 and venture out to the grocery store or meet friends for dinner, potentially infecting others. A specificity of 90% means that 90% of persons free of COVID-19 screen negative. This means that there is a 10% false positive fraction, or 10% of people free of COVID-19 screen positive. These people might immediately isolate, unnecessarily, so as not to spread infection. When evaluating performance characteristics of any screening test, it is important to think through the implications of errors to determine what levels of performance would be acceptable and useful.

Some screening tests are designed to identify issues that might be addressed to prevent disease, for example, the use of endoscopy to locate and remove intestinal polyps that may later develop into cancer.[20] Other screening tests, such as mammography for breast cancer, are screening tests for disease diagnoses. There are benefits and risks associated with screening tests that must be considered when deciding if screening is appropriate for a particular circumstance. Screening for preventive measures, like removing intestinal polyps, might be controversial as not all persons with polyps would develop cancer. Other screening tests might carry specific risks. For example, x-ray imaging exams introduce exposure to radiation, a risk factor for cancer.[21] So how do we approach these complex challenges to determine appropriate uses for screening?

A rule of thumb is using screening tools where the benefits outweigh the risks. The WHO established the following criteria to determine the suitability of a screening test:

1. "Screening should be done only for diseases with serious consequences, so that screening tests could potentially have clear benefits to people's health.
2. The test must be reliable enough, and not harmful in itself.
3. There must be an effective treatment for the disease when detected at an early stage—and there has to be scientific proof that that treatment is more effective when started before symptoms arise.
4. Factual information should be made available to the public to help people decide for themselves whether or not to have a screening test."[22]

Performance characteristics of the screening test are also of concern. We might decide, for example, that a screening test is not appropriate because it has low specificity and a high false positive fraction. Recall, specificity measures a screening test's ability to produce a negative result in people free of the disease of interest. Screening tests with a higher false positive fraction—patients who are actually well but erroneously screen positive on the test—can create unnecessary stress, and lead to unnecessary diagnostic procedures before the false result is ruled out. Inaccurate screening introduces further risks and costs.

When a cure or a life-extending treatment is available, the optimal triad of early detection, early diagnosis, and early treatment can occur. Conversely, early detection of the presence of an incurable disease, with no available treatments to prolong survival, results in persons who screen positive living with the awareness of their untreatable terminal condition for a longer period.

Overdiagnosis describes the situation where screening tends to detect less consequential disease cases that are unlikely to progress, become clinically significant, or pose a threat to life.[23] As a classic instance of overdiagnosis, conducting repetitive cancer screenings is especially likely to detect slower growing, less aggressive cancers (**Figure 3.2**). In contrast, faster growing, aggressive cancers are often missed during screening and not diagnosed until symptom onset leads to diagnosis in a clinical setting.

As we continue to explore levels of prevention, let us consider what a society that makes extensive use of population screening for disease would look like. How are health and disease produced in a population that prizes and prioritizes secondary prevention in the form of screening, a population we will call Secondaria?

Residents of Secondaria, like much of the real world, do not consistently observe the principles of primary prevention when they make their behavioral choices. In fact, there is considerable experimentation among population members with a range of risk behaviors. Some members of this population even engage avidly in thrill-seeking, risk-taking, mood-altering, highly experiential activities that activate the brain's positive reinforcement and pleasure pathways. Many Secondarians participate in hazardous risk behaviors, and their

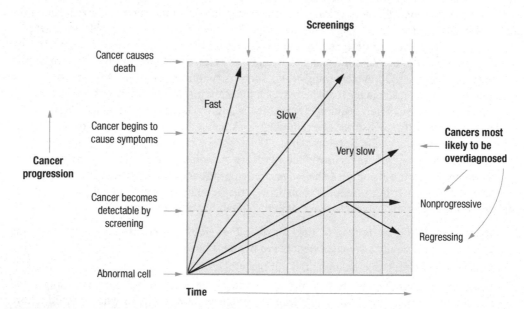

FIGURE 3.2 Cancer heterogeneity and multiple screenings drive overdiagnosis.
Source: Carter SM, Barratt A. What is overdiagnosis and why should we take it seriously in cancer screening? *Public Health Res Practice.* 2017;27(3):2731722. https://doi.org/10.17061/phrp2731722

lifestyles and exposures over time lead to physiological changes and subclinical disease states that can be detected on screening.

Secondarians do not come close to Primarians in terms of attaining optimal levels of health for all, and they have shorter life expectancies. What does distinguish Secondarians, however, is their widespread reliance on screening tests. Screenings are conducted in community, school, and worksite settings as well as in physician practices and medical clinics. Secondarians screen extensively for noncommunicable disease (NCD) risk factors such as elevated blood pressure, blood glucose and blood lipid levels, and liver function. Primary care providers determine each patient's risk profile (e.g., diet, activity, overweight, smoking, drinking, seat-belt use, or sun exposure). Providers counsel Secondarians on lifestyle modification options and prescribe medications to treat physiological risk factors detected by screening, such as elevated blood pressure. Follow-up appointments focus on progress in achieving reductions in identified lifestyle risks and improving follow-up screening test results. Through the conscientious application of screening tests and medical follow-up, Secondarians are able to live with awareness of their risks and make modest adjustments to their lifestyles to decrease risk, increase their disability-free life span, and extend their life span compared to persons who do not receive regular screenings and make lifestyle adjustments based on screening results.

TERTIARY DISEASE PREVENTION

Tertiary prevention refers to actions that reduce the impact of an ongoing injury or disease once an individual has been diagnosed and treated for clinical disease. At this stage, the interaction of the individual's physiological makeup, coupled with lifestyle risks and environmental exposures, has resulted in clinically diagnosable disease. What remains for tertiary prevention is to manage existing disease in a manner that improves a population member's ability to function, enhances quality of life, and maximizes the patient's remaining life span or length of survival.[15] Rehabilitation is the central theme of tertiary disease prevention. Examples of tertiary disease prevention include cardiac rehabilitation programs for people who survive a heart attack and interventions to promote weight loss in persons who develop type 2 diabetes.

As we continue to explore levels of prevention, let us consider what a society, Tertiaria, that focuses on management of existing diseases would look like. How are health and disease produced in a population that prioritizes tertiary prevention?

> **Examples of tertiary disease prevention include cardiac rehabilitation programs for people who survive a heart attack and interventions to promote weight loss in persons who develop type 2 diabetes.**

Residents of Tertiaria do not consistently observe the principles of primary and secondary prevention when they make their behavioral choices. This population experiments with a range of risk behaviors that lead to diseases, and screening services are not widely adopted.

Tertiarians fall far behind Primarians and Secondarians in terms of their levels of health and well-being—and their life expectancies are substantially reduced. What does distinguish Tertiarians, however, is a robust rehabilitation system for those already diagnosed with disease. Providers counsel Tertiarians on lifestyle modification options and prescribe medications to manage their conditions, improve their quality of life, and extend their years of survivorship—albeit after disease has occurred. Follow-up appointments focus on managing signs of disease progression. Through conscientious participation in rehabilitation and medical follow-up, Tertiarians are able to live with and manage their diseases and modify their degree of disability.

LEVERAGING PREVENTION: UPSTREAM VERSUS DOWNSTREAM APPROACHES

A useful concept when distinguishing public health from clinical medical approaches to the production of health and disease is that of upstream versus downstream strategies.

Primordial prevention and primary prevention actions operate upstream, producing health by intervening to prevent the occurrence of the risk factor (primordial prevention) or the adoption of risk-elevating behaviors (primary prevention). In the best case, some individuals will engage in almost no risk-elevating behaviors throughout life, and physiological health and function will remain intact throughout most of the life span. Primary prevention exerts the greatest leverage in terms of setting the individual on track for a long, risk-free, disease-free life course (**Figure 3.3**). Disease, when it occurs, happens rarely and mostly during a compressed period late in life.

Secondary prevention strategies operate throughout the lifetime, in essence, in midstream. Substantial proportions of the population develop identifiable risk factors for disease, but screening allows these risk factors to be detected, sometimes eliminated, and often favorably modified through behavior change (e.g., weight loss) or effective pharmacological treatment (e.g., blood

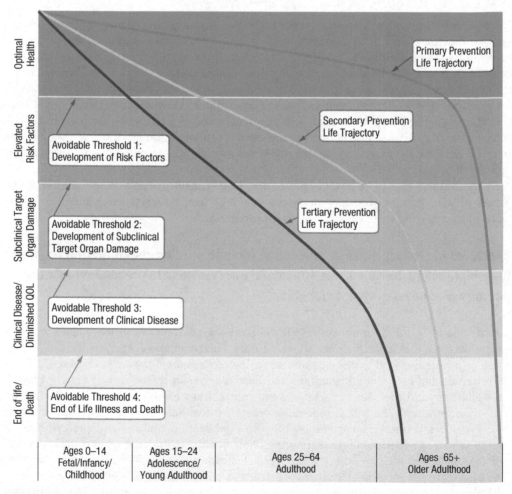

FIGURE 3.3 Primary, secondary, and tertiary prevention in relation to the healthy life course. QOL, quality of life. Artistic credit: Parisa Varanloo.

pressure control involving a combination of antihypertensive medications and lifestyle change). Knowledge of risk coupled with effective strategies to manage risk can avert or slow the progression from very early physiological changes to more significant target organ damage to diagnosable clinical disease. Secondary prevention approaches allow an intermediate degree of leverage to be applied to the restoration and ongoing production of health.

Tertiary prevention is purely a downstream approach. Health has already been compromised. Target organ damage has occurred. Clinical disease has been diagnosed. Symptoms of pain or discomfort, functional impairment, and disability are present and may be worsening. Nevertheless, within a much narrower range of influence at this stage, there is an opportunity to regain stamina, restore function, and live healthier and longer following treatment and rehabilitation.

Prevention strategies differ based on the type of disease. As one example, consider the prevention approaches for type 1 versus type 2 diabetes (Table 3.1). Both forms of diabetes are

TABLE 3.1   Prevention Strategies for Type 1 and Type 2 Diabetes

	PREVENTION STRATEGIES			
	PRIMARY	SECONDARY	TERTIARY	EXPANDED TERTIARY/ "QUATERNARY"
Prevention strategies	• Prevention of disease risk factors • Prevention of disease onset	• Early detection • Early treatment • Restoring health when possible	• Prevention of disease progression through optimal disease control	• Preventing harm from interventions
T1D	• No known primary prevention	• Screening of relatives of patients with T1D • Population screening • Insulin treatment	• Tight glucose control • Frequent self-monitoring • Insulin pump	• Hypoglycemia awareness • Education • Advocacy
T2D	• Community-based healthy lifestyle programs • Physical activity • Nutritious diet • Obesity prevention • Preventive checkups	• Population screening • Routine preventive medicine screening • At-risk population screening • Behavioral/ lifestyle intervention • Diet/exercise prescription • Medications as indicated	• Management of cardiovascular risk factors • Behavioral/ lifestyle intervention • Diet/exercise prescription • Glucose control medications	• Matching level of glucose control to the patient population • Avoidance of overmedication

T1D, type 1 diabetes; T2D, type 2 diabetes.

disorders of glucose (blood sugar) metabolism. Type 1 diabetes is an autoimmune disease in which the pancreas is unable to make insulin in sufficient quantity. In contrast, type 2 diabetes is a lifestyle-related disorder in which the body does not use insulin properly, so prevention approaches focus on health behaviors.

Just for completeness, we present a simplified example of the use of terminology that has been strongly espoused by prevention scientists: universal, selected, and indicated prevention. Table 3.2 presents these terms as they are applied broadly to the prevention of mental health disorders.

TABLE 3.2 Prevention Strategies for Mental Health Disorders

PREVENTION STRATEGIES	TARGET	APPROACH
Universal preventive interventions	General population	Education for populations with no identified risks: • Community- and school-based mental health and substance abuse curricula • Educational resources in multiple media • Public awareness and education campaigns
Selective preventive interventions	Subgroups with biological, psychological, social risk factors	Surveillance and interventions for youth and adults at risk: • Youth exposed to ACEs • Youth experiencing academic problems • Youth who are isolating or lacking healthy friendships
Indicated preventive interventions	High-risk individuals with detectable signs/symptoms of mental/behavioral disorder	High-risk individuals with observable signs/symptoms of mental disorder (do not meet diagnostic criteria): • Programs to teach/reinforce social skills • Teaching coping strategies • Special skills training • Monitoring these individuals—supportive observation
Psychological/psychiatric treatment	Individuals with current diagnosed mental disorder	Persons with diagnosed mental disorder: • Psychotherapy tailored to diagnosis and needs • Evidence-based practices • Medication prescription and careful monitoring for efficacy and side effects

ACEs, adverse childhood experiences.

Source: Data from youth.gov. Mental health: promotion and prevention. https://youth.gov/youth-topics/youth-mental-health/mental-health-promotion-prevention

PREVENTION BASICS: APPLYING NOTIONS OF PREVENTION TO LOCAL, NATIONAL, AND GLOBAL POPULATIONS

Employing the principle of prevention means designing public health interventions and policies that focus on the forces that create health rather than interventions that are concerned with controlling diseases. The notions of prevention can be applied on the local level—local governments generally oversee and implement programs—through providing preventive services widely to the public. National efforts that focus on prevention include national screening and surveillance programs. On a global level, international entities such as the WHO can support countries in developing national prevention protocols that are suitable for local adaptation.

PUBLIC HEALTH VERSUS MEDICAL CARE

Clinical medicine generally aims to restore patients to their earlier "normal" healthy existence, prior to getting sick. When a patient develops symptoms and seeks medical care, the physician's goal is to diagnose the disease, understand the pathology, identify the optimal treatment, and care for that individual patient.[13] In that sense, because curing and caring for the patient are the top priorities for the healthcare system, it is not particularly relevant to medicine how many in the community may experience the same disease.

While clinical medicine is concerned with individuals, public health is concerned with populations. Public health aims to minimize the need for clinical interventions. A public health approach means identifying potential causes or determinants of disease, reducing the risk of exposure to these causes, and thereby reducing the risk of disease through a wide array of interventions ranging from policies that promote health, to altering the social conditions people live in, to individual education and behavior change.

> While clinical medicine is concerned with individuals, public health is concerned with populations.

Improving the health of a population through preventive health measures is in some respects more challenging than delivering healthcare to an individual. Yet, funding for clinical medicine continues to be prioritized over that for public health; for too long, we have been focusing on treatment rather than preventing diseases from occurring in the first place. Using the United States as an example, despite spending more per person on healthcare than other comparable countries,[24] public health remains chronically underfunded. A 2015 report found that combined federal, state, and local public health spending was below prerecession levels.[25] This reflects both the immediacy of concern about clinical health as a common experience, and that public health has not yet been able to make its case robustly enough, two challenges we hope that future students of public health can help overcome.

During the last decades of the 20th century, public health was heavily focused on behavior modification and individual responsibility for health. The 21st century, however, is emerging as the era for population health in which the focus is not only on the individual but the collective health of entire communities and populations. A focus on population health means more recognition and emphasis on social determinants of health (Box 3.1) and on the cultural and built environments that shape the health of a population as a whole (refer to the section in Chapter 4, "At the Heart of Public Health: Social Determinants of Health and Health Equity" focusing on the social determinants of health for more information). Tackling these determinants requires using innovative interventions to improve safety, the environment, housing, schools, transportation, and many other public policy areas that can only be achieved through multidisciplinary approaches.

BOX 3.1 SOCIAL DETERMINANTS OF HEALTH

The WHO defines social determinants of health as "the circumstances in which people are born, grow up, live, work and age, and the systems put in place to deal with illness. These circumstances are in turn shaped by a wider set of forces: economics, social policies, and politics."[28]

To that end, a population health perspective ideally embraces a wide spectrum of approaches that partner not only traditional aspects of public health and clinical medicine but also social interventions such as improving the built environment and providing better access to healthy food (see Chapter 4, "At the Heart of Public Health: Social Determinants of Health and Health Equity").[26]

The main purpose of the prevention principle is to implement interventions designed to prevent specific health problems identified through community concerns or assessment processes initiated by public health professionals. Thus, a prevention-based public health approach works through identifying a health problem, identifying the causes or determinants of the problem, developing and testing interventions to prevent or control these determinants, and then implementing and monitoring these interventions to assess their effectiveness.[27]

SUMMARY

Prevention and health equity have to be at the heart of all we do, informing how we think in public health practice. A public health practice that is rooted in the principle of prevention means working to identify and eliminate risks to maximize the production of health rather than intervening to mitigate and control the consequences of diseases. There are multiple levels of prevention: primordial/primary, secondary, and tertiary. Primordial and primary prevention operate upstream, producing health by intervening to prevent the occurrence of a risk factor or the adoption of risk-elevating behaviors. Secondary prevention efforts, such as screening, operate midstream to avert or slow the progression of disease. Tertiary prevention efforts operate downstream, aiming to slow and reduce the impact of damage once clinical disease has been diagnosed. Employing the principle of prevention means designing public health interventions and policies that transcend the focus on clinical medicine and address the forces that create health rather than interventions that are concerned with controlling diseases.

End-of-Chapter Resources

 Access additional case study podcasts online at http://connect.springerpub.com/ content/book/978-0-8261-8043-8/

DISCUSSION QUESTIONS

1. "Improving the health of a population through preventive health measures is in some respects more challenging than delivering healthcare to an individual." Why would that be? Discuss such challenges for a chosen health problem.

2. Read the "Declaration of Human Rights" and discuss how and why health is linked to the fulfillment of human rights (access the declaration at https://www.un.org/en/about-us/universal-declaration-of-human-rights).

3. Thinking about existing public health services and the overall social and political atmosphere, would it be realistic to propose adopting a primary prevention national strategy in your country? Why? (Explain the existing system to provide public health services in your country.)

A robust set of instructor resources designed to supplement this text is located at http://connect.springerpub.com/content/book/978-0-8261-8043-8. Qualifying instructors may request access by emailing **textbook@springerpub.com**.

REFERENCES

1. Winslow CE. The untilled fields of public health. *Science*. 1920;*51*(1306):23-33. doi:10.1126/science.51.1306.23
2. Centers for Disease Control and Prevention. Ten great public health achievements–United States, 1900–1999. *MMWR Morb Mortal Wkly Rep*. 1999;*48*(12):241-243. https://www.cdc.gov/mmwr/preview/mmwrhtml/00056796.htm
3. Centers for Disease Control and Prevention. *Risk for COVID-19 infection, hospitalization, and death by race/ethnicity*. Published February 1, 2022. https://www.cdc.gov/coronavirus/2019-ncov/covid-data/investigations-discovery/hospitalization-death-by-race-ethnicity.html
4. Yellow Horse AJ, Yang TC, Huyser KR. Structural inequalities established the architecture for COVID-19 pandemic among Native Americans in Arizona: a geographically weighted regression perspective. *J Racial Ethn Health Disparities*. 2022;9(1):165-175. doi:10.1007/s40615-020-00940-2
5. Foxworth R, Evans LE, Sanchez GR, Ellenwood C, Roybal CM. "I hope to hell nothing goes back to the way it was before": COVID-19, marginalization, and native nations. *Perspect Politics*. 2022;*20*(2):439-456. doi:10.1017/S1537592721001031
6. Foxworth R, Redvers N, Moreno MA, Lopez-Carmen VA, Sanchez GR, Shultz JM. COVID-19 vaccination in American Indians and Alaska Natives–lessons from effective community responses. *N Engl J Med*. 2021;*385*(26):2403-2406. doi:10.1056/NEJMp2113296
7. Hill L, Artiga S. *COVID-19 vaccination among American Indian and Alaska Native people*. Kaiser Family Foundation. Published April 9, 2021. https://www.kff.org/racial-equity-and-health-policy/issue-brief/covid-19-vaccination-american-indian-alaska-native-people/
8. Sanchez GR, Foxworth R. *Native Americans and COVID-19 vaccine hesitancy: pathways toward increasing vaccination rates for native communities*. Health Affairs Blog. Published July 29, 2021. https://www.healthaffairs.org/do/10.1377/forefront.20210723.390196/full/
9. Caspari R, Lee SH. Older age becomes common late in human evolution. *Proc Natl Acad Sci USA*. 2004;*101*(30):10895-10900. doi:10.1073/pnas.0402857101
10. Galor O, Moav O. The neolithic origins of contemporary variations in life expectancy. *SSRN Electron J*. 2007:40. doi:10.2139/ssrn.1012650
11. Cave C. *Did ancient people die young?* Sapiens. Published August 17, 2018. https://www.sapiens.org/body/human-lifespan-history
12. Ruggeri A. *Do we really live longer than our ancestors?*. BBC Future. Published October 3, 2018. http://www.bbc.com/future/story/20181002-how-long-did-ancient-people-live-life-span-versus-longevity
13. Fineberg HV. The paradox of disease prevention: celebrated in principle, resisted in practice. *JAMA*. 2013;*310*(1):85-90. doi:10.1001/jama.2013.7518
14. Porta M, ed. *A Dictionary of Epidemiology*. 6th ed. Oxford University Press; 2014.

15. Institute for Work & Health. *Primary, secondary and tertiary prevention.* Published April 2015. https://www
.iwh.on.ca/what-researchers-mean-by/primary-secondary-and-tertiary-prevention

16. Falkner B, Lurbe E. Primordial prevention of high blood pressure in childhood: an opportunity not to be
missed. *Hypertension.* 2020;75(5):1142-1150. doi:10.1161/HYPERTENSIONAHA.119.14059

17. Frank JW. Controlling the obesity pandemic: Geoffrey Rose revisited. *Can J Public Health.* 2022;113(5):736-
742. doi:10.17269/s41997-022-00636-6

18. World Health Organization. *Cancer: screening.* https://www.who.int/cancer/prevention/diagnosis-screening/
screening/en

19. Wilson JMG, Jungner G. *Principles and practice of screening for disease.* World Health Organization. Accessed
January 1, 1968. https://apps.who.int/iris/handle/10665/37650

20. Sweetser S, Smyrk TC, Sinicrope FA. Serrated colon polyps as precursors to colorectal cancer. *Clin
Gastroenterol Hepatol.* 2013;11(7):760-e55. https://doi.org/10.1016/j.cgh.2012.12.004

21. American Cancer Society. *Understanding radiation risk from imaging tests.* https://www.cancer.org/treatment/
understanding-your-diagnosis/tests/understanding-radiation-risk-from-imaging-tests.html

22. Wilson JMG, Jungner G. *Principles and practices of screening for disease.* Geneva, Switzerland: World Health
Organization; 1968. Report No.: Public Health Papers No. 34. Available from: http://whqlibdoc.who.int/php/
WHO_PHP_34.pdf

23. Carter SM, Barratt A. What is overdiagnosis and why should we take it seriously in cancer screening? *Public
Health Res Pract.* 2017;27(3):2731722. https://doi.org/10.17061/phrp2731722

24. Sawyer B, Cox C. *How does health spending in the U.S. compare to other countries?* Peterson-Kaiser Health
System Tracker. 2019. Published December 7, 2018. https://www.healthsystemtracker.org/chart-collection/
health-spending-u-s-compare-countries/#item-relative-size-wealth-u-s-spends-disproportionate-amount-health

25. Levi J, Segal LM, Gougelet R St, Laurent R. *Investing in America's health: a state-by-state look at public health
funding & key health facts 2015.* Trust for America's Health. 2015. https://www.tfah.org/report-details/
investing-in-americas-health-a-state-by-state-look-at-public-health-funding-key-health-facts-1/

26. Centers for Disease Control and Prevention. *Public health system and the 10 essential public health
services.* Published June 26, 2018. https://www.cdc.gov/publichealthgateway/publichealthservices/
essentialhealthservices.html

27. Schneider M-J. *Introduction to Public Health.* Jones and Bartlett; 1999. https://books.google.com/
books?id=OEDhCwAAQBAJ&printsec=frontcover&dq=Introduction+to+Public+Health&hl=en&sa=X-
&ved=0ahUKEwiH5Nfgz5LdAhUPm-AKHaoGDYQQ6AEIKTAA#v=onepage&q=prevention&f=false

28. World Health Organization. *Social determinants of health: key concepts: what are the social "determinants" of
health?* https://www.who.int/news-room/questions-and-answers/item/social-determinants-of-health-key-concepts

4

AT THE HEART OF PUBLIC HEALTH: SOCIAL DETERMINANTS OF HEALTH AND HEALTH EQUITY

Salma M. Abdalla also contributed to this chapter

LEARNING OBJECTIVES

- Explain the differences between health equity and health equality.
- Discuss current patterns of health inequity in the United States.
- Provide examples of global health inequities.
- Describe the role of social determinants of health and how they create health inequities.

OVERVIEW: THE RELATIONSHIP BETWEEN HEALTH INEQUITIES AND THE SOCIAL DETERMINANTS OF HEALTH

Alongside prevention, health equity is the second core principle at the heart of public health. Public health aims to improve the health of whole populations. On the surface, this may sound easy: We aim to improve the health of everyone within a population. Contemplated more thoughtfully, however, this concept poses a fundamental challenge: How do we improve the health of all without having any health left-behinds? Health equity suggests that, within the limits of what is preventable and what is amenable to public health interventions, everyone should have the same health.

Health equity is not the same as health equality. It is not feasible to produce equal health for all. For example, we can reasonably expect that those who are younger may have better health than those who are older. Nevertheless, seeking health equity for all is a worthy goal. Unfortunately, the United States has long been characterized by enormous health equity gaps. As examples, significant health inequities exist and persist between White and African

American/Black populations, and between persons with high versus low socioeconomic positions. Many of these differences are due to differences in the social determinants of health. Social determinants of health are the conditions of our unique environments that shape our daily lives and our health. And because these environments differ so dramatically, these social determinants of health create health inequities.

In this chapter we (a) define and contrast health equity and health inequality, (b) outline historical and current patterns of health inequity in the United States, (c) examine global health inequities, (d) explore the role of social determinants of health in determining health inequities, and (e) analyze the trade-offs that may be inherent in improving overall health and reducing health inequities.

HEALTH EQUITY

HEALTH EQUITY SUGGESTS THAT EVERYONE CAN HAVE THE SAME HEALTH

Although there are several definitions of health equity, each of them revolve around social justice and the principle that all social groups should have a minimum level of health and well-being. In the 1990s, Margaret Whitehead articulated a concise definition that characterized health inequities as unnecessary, avoidable, unfair, and unjust. She wrote, "equity in health implies that ideally everyone should have a fair opportunity to attain their full health potential and, more pragmatically, that no one should be disadvantaged from achieving this potential, if it can be avoided."[1]

Another definition of health equity is the "attainment of the highest level of health for all people. Achieving health equity requires valuing everyone equally with focused and ongoing societal efforts to address avoidable inequalities, historical and contemporary injustices, and the elimination of health and healthcare disparities."[2]

A related term that is often used, health disparities, is defined as "differences that occur by gender, race or ethnicity, education or income, disability, living in rural localities, or sexual orientation."[3] As such, health equity means ensuring that everyone has access to health, and achieving that often requires giving special attention to those who are at the greatest risk of experiencing poor health outcomes based on their social conditions.[4]

HEALTH EQUITY AS A CORE ABIDING PRINCIPLE FOR PUBLIC HEALTH

Health equity underlines a commitment to reduce and eliminate health differences and their determinants and to ensure the attainment of the highest level of health for all people.[4] As one of the core principles of public health, health equity is driven by the values of social justice and human rights. The right to health and the need to address social determinants of health in order to enhance the well-being of a population are recognized as core values by both the World Health Organization (WHO) Constitution and the United Nation's (UN) Universal Declaration of Human Rights. Both documents use the principles of nondiscrimination and equal opportunity to assert health as a human right.[5]

HEALTH EQUITY AND HEALTH EQUALITY

Although they are often used interchangeably, health equity and health equality are not synonymous. The concept of health equity is value-based while health equality is an empirical measure.

Inequality generally refers to any differences between groups. Health inequity, on the other hand, is the product of modifiable systematic inequalities in the distribution of resources, or other processes, between more and less advantaged social groups. In other words, health inequities are avoidable, unnecessary, and unfair.[6]

For example, it is difficult to argue that health inequalities due to biological differences are unjust. We expect that younger individuals are, on average, healthier than older adults. It is, however, a cause for concern from a health equity point of view when we detect nutritional differences between girls and boys, or racial differences in the likelihood of receiving treatment for a specific disease (health inequities).[7]

There are widely circulated depictions that distinguish the terms inequality/equality and inequity/equity. These depictions illustrate a point of unequal (and also inequitable) access to resources, such as healthcare. In a series of 5 panels, **Figure 4.1** illustrates the "reality" of unequal and inequitable access, in contrast to displaying "equality" of the supports provided (that nevertheless do no achieve equity), and "equity" where the supports provided are carefully aportioned to match the needs. Two additional panels illustrate "justice," where all structural barriers are removed and "inclusion" where equality, equity, and justice are joined by opportunities for full participation.

We note that the term "health disparities" is often used in public health. "Disparities" literally means "great differences" and, as such, the problem is more accurately considered as "inequalities." However, the term is often used interchangeably to signify inequities or inequalities. Hence, we prefer to use the terms "inequities" and "inequalities" to be precise about their meaning.

TRADE-OFFS THAT MAY BE INHERENT IN IMPROVING OVERALL HEALTH AND REDUCING HEALTH INEQUITIES

PUBLIC HEALTH AIMS TO IMPROVE THE HEALTH OF WHOLE POPULATIONS

Public health is concerned with improving the health of the entire population. As such, public health interventions traditionally aim to achieve the greatest health gains on a population level, which we call efficiency.[8] Efficiency is a term often used in economics to describe the maximization of the total economic output of a system. Using the efficiency principle to maximize the total health of a population includes minimizing disability-adjusted life years (DALYs) owing to acute and chronic conditions, minimizing quality-adjusted life years (QALYs) for those with disabilities, and extending years of productive life.

AIMING TO IMPROVE THE HEALTH OF EVERYONE WITHIN A POPULATION

Taking an efficiency approach toward the health of a population can also mean that we may forget that individuals within a population are heterogeneous. Populations are composed of individuals who differ by race and ethnicity, gender, socioeconomic status, and many other factors.

There is ample evidence that social factors, including income level, gender, education level, employment status, and race and ethnicity, exert a great influence on how healthy a person is. Using a health equity approach means that people's needs guide the allocation of resources to improve the well-being of individuals within a population. Unfortunately, this allocation strategy can reduce the overall efficiency of an intervention.

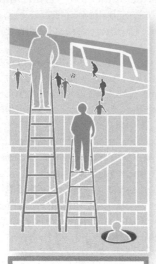

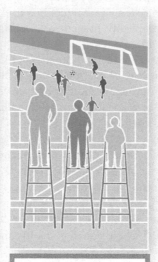

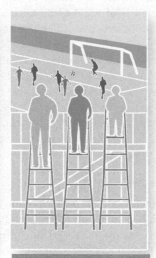

Reality

One gets more than is needed, while the other gets less than is needed. Thus, a huge disparity is created.

Equality

The assumption is that everyone benefits from the same supports. This is considered to be equal treatment.

Equity

Everyone gets the support they need, which produces equity.

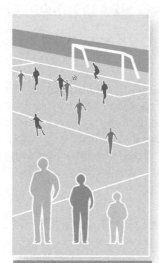

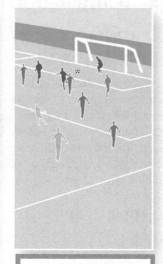

Justice

All three can see the game without supports or accommodations because the cause(s) of the inequity was addressed. The systemic barrier has been removed.

Inclusion

Everyone is included in the game. No one is left on the outside; we didn't only remove the barriers keeping people out, we made sure they were valued and involved.

FIGURE 4.1 What is health equity?
Source: Rodriguez LJ, Mullen J. Addressing vulnerability through the pursuit of health equity. In: Knickman JR, Elbel B, eds. *Jonas & Kovner's Health Care Delivery in the United States.* 13th ed. Springer Publishing Company; 2023:219.

There is ample evidence that social factors, including income level, gender, education level, employment status, and race and ethnicity, exert a great influence on how healthy a person is.

CORE CHALLENGE: HOW DO WE IMPROVE THE HEALTH OF ALL WITHOUT HAVING ANY HEALTH LEFT-BEHINDS?

While public health efforts over the past century have led to significant improvements in many health indicators, these gains have not benefited everyone. Health inequities in a number of health outcomes have increased. Maximizing the overall health of a population is one of the goals of public health. However, as we design and implement interventions to achieve this goal, we can sometimes exacerbate health inequities within a population. The need to make trade-offs between improving the health of the population as a whole and reducing health inequities is not always present when designing and implementing interventions. However, this tension is often present as public health resources are finite.[9] One example of an intervention that improved overall health but did not reduce health inequities is the cervical cancer screening program implemented in both the United States and Canada in the 1990s. Women with higher incomes were more likely to access the intervention and be screened than those from a lower socioeconomic status.[10]

To minimize the need for trade-offs between improving the health of the entire population and addressing health inequities, several countries adopted policy recommendations that coupled overall health improvement with reducing health inequities. Such policies include the United Kingdom's "Tackling Health Inequalities: A Program for Action," the "Integrated Pan-Canadian Healthy Living Strategy," and the Swedish "Health on Equal Terms Public Health Policy."[10]

HEALTH INEQUITIES IN THE UNITED STATES

HEALTH INEQUITIES BY RACE

Racial and ethnic minorities represent more than a third of the U.S. population. The percentage is increasing, and the U.S. Census Bureau projects that by 2044, minority subpopulations combined will together constitute the majority of the American population. Minorities face health inequities in the United States compared to White Americans. As one potent example, for the period 2014 to 2018, age-adjusted breast cancer mortality for Black women was 40% higher than for non-Hispanic White women (27.7 versus 20.0 deaths per 100,000 women), yet the incidence rate for Black women was slightly lower than for White women. Moreover, this finding related to an "emerging racial disparity" dating from the 1980s (see **Figure 4.2**). In fact, prior to 1980, breast cancer mortality was initially lower in Black women.

Moreover, in 2018, African American/Black individuals were 30% more likely than their White counterparts to die prematurely from heart disease and twice as likely to die from a stroke.[11] Another example is obesity. Obesity, which is associated with a number of other chronic conditions, affects minorities disproportionately. Between 2017 and 2018, almost 25.6% of Latinx children and adolescents between the ages of 2 and 19 were obese, the highest proportion among all racial/ethnic groups of the same age in the United States.[12]

Health inequities extend beyond health indicators and disease prevalence to average life expectancy and mortality rates. This has never been more apparent than during the COVID-19 pandemic. COVID-19-specific and overall mortality rates surged globally and very steeply for all races and ethnicities in the United States. As mortality rose, life expectancies declined at highly differential rates worldwide and in the United States. The startling differences in U.S. life

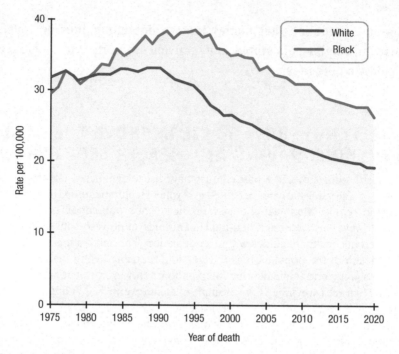

FIGURE 4.2 Trends in breast cancer mortality among Black women and White women in the United States, 1975 through 2020.

expectancies by race/ethnicity are visually apparent in **Figure 4.3** both prior to the pandemic (2019) and during the first 2 years of the pandemic (2020 and 2021). When pandemic-era life expectancy declines are compared directly (**Figure 4.4**), the race/ethnic disparities are clear to see.

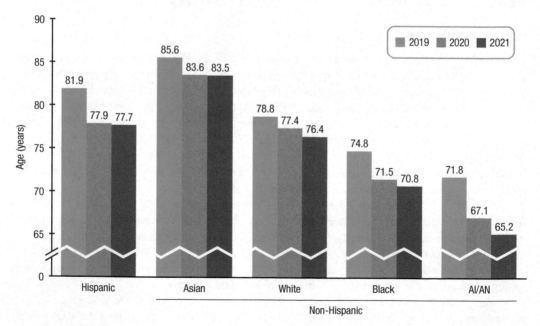

FIGURE 4.3 United States life expectancy at birth, by Hispanic origin and race, 2019 to 2021. AI/AN, American Indian/Alaska Native.
Source: Provisional Life Expectancy Estimates for 2021. NVSS Vital Statistics Rapid Release. Report No. 23. August 2022. https://www.cdc.gov/nchs/data/vsrr/vsrr023.pdf

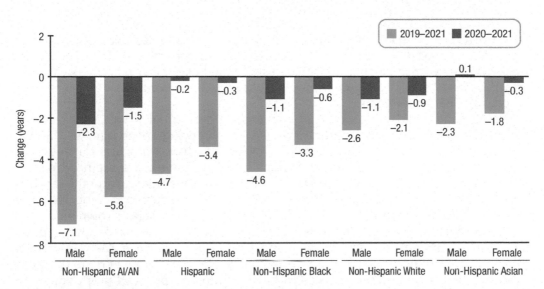

FIGURE 4.4 United States change in life expectancy at birth, by Hispanic origin and race, 2019 to 2021 and 2020 to 2021. AI/AN, American Indian/Alaska Native.
Source: Provisional Life Expectancy Estimates for 2021. NVSS Vital Statistics Rapid Release. Report No. 23. August 2022. https://www.cdc.gov/nchs/data/vsrr/vsrr023.pdf

Further, although the national infant mortality rate had an overall decrease between 2004 and 2021, inequities among a number of racial and ethnic groups persisted over the same period.[13] Native Americans and Alaskan Americans have an infant mortality rate that is 60% higher than their White counterparts. In 2018, African American/Black infants experienced the highest infant mortality rates (10.8 infant deaths per 1,000 live births) while infants born to Asian mothers had the lowest (3.6 infant deaths per 1,000 live births).[14] Ultimately, as illustrated by Case Study 4.1, these health inequalities reflect structural inequities and are the product of forces that have, over time, resulted in poorer health for minority groups in the country.

CASE STUDY 4.1: YOU CAN'T LIVE HERE: GOVERNMENTAL AND CORPORATE REDLINING PRACTICES AND RACIAL SEGREGATION IN AMERICAN CITIES

In 2019, the median wealth of White households in America was $188,200; the median wealth of African American/Black households was $24,100.[15] The health benefits associated with higher income levels have been well established, with lower income individuals experiencing worse health outcomes.[16] Deeper to these discussions is the role of wealth in providing access to a full slate of resources and experiences that together create healthy populations. A look at the history of racial segregation shows how policy decisions can have long-lasting, multigenerational effects on populations.

An African American/Black family's median wealth is estimated to be less than 15% of that of a White family.[15] In 2019, 37% of African American/Black households and 33% of Latinx households had zero or negative wealth compared to 15.5% of White households.[15] Three-in-four (74%) White Americans own a home while fewer than 45% of African American/Black Americans are homeowners. Homes owned by African American/Black Americans tend to be segregated from White

(continued)

neighborhoods. This is not surprising as access to resources accumulates over time. Families pass assets from one generation to the next. African American/Black families whose wealth potential was capped have fewer resources to share with the next generation, creating even larger gaps between White and African Americans/Black Americans.

The National Housing Act of 1934 was passed during the Great Depression to help make housing and mortgages more affordable for American families. The act was created the Federal Housing Administration (FHA) to "encourage improvement in housing standards and conditions [and] to provide a system of mutual mortgage insurance."[17] While the FHA helped to stimulate homeownership and allow families to accumulate wealth, it explicitly limited resources to minorities and segregated neighborhoods. The FHA distributed a set of policies known as redlining. Neighborhoods were color-coded and ranked to identify which neighborhoods should or should not receive mortgage and home loan assistance. Neighborhoods with "inharmonious" racial groups were literally outlined in red, and areas where minorities lived were denied access to federal loans.[18] Approved mortgages and home loans were concentrated in segregated neighborhoods. African Americans/Blacks received only 2% of all federally insured home loans between 1945 and 1959.[19] This systematically discriminatory practice resulted in racial segregation of housing units. Segregated housing limited the wealth accumulation of African American/Black families (they were relegated to poorer neighborhoods) and denied them mortgage and home loan resources available to their White counterparts. Redlining stifled the property value of African American/Black homes and decreased tax revenues. In turn, this limited access to the host of public goods and services provided to neighborhoods, including public schools, health centers, parks, and public transportation. Redlining was finally made illegal by the Fair Housing Act of 1968.

Another example of using housing-related policies to support segregation is the Servicemen's Readjustment Act of 1944. The act, better known as the G.I. Bill, created benefits for returning servicemen, including low interest rates and zero down payment for mortgages for veterans. Of the first 67,000 mortgages insured by the G.I. Bill, fewer than 100 went to non-Whites.[20] These racially motivated, discriminatory practices systematically prevented African Americans/Blacks from accessing the same types and levels of housing as Whites, maintaining deep racial divides that also created health gaps we see today.

Unequal access to housing has a lasting effect that translates to poor health outcomes. People concentrated in lower income neighborhoods (usually predominately inhabited by minorities) have consistently higher mortality rates than those in wealthier ones.[21,22] In addition to the direct effect of housing quality on health, housing segregation affects health through other determinants. For example, majority minority neighborhoods receive less public investment. This results in limited wealth accumulation, limited access to healthy foods, fewer high-quality public schools, and living in neighborhoods with more hazardous environmental exposures.[23] A study of exposures to air toxins showed that African Americans/Blacks consistently experience more exposures to industrial air toxins than Whites and Latinx.[24] Indeed, African American/Black children have almost twice the rate of asthma (22%) compared to their White (12%) and Latinx (14%) counterparts.[25] Higher asthma rates in African American/Black youth relate to the social, structural, and physical disadvantages of living in segregated neighborhoods.[26]

(continued)

Unequal access to housing has a lasting effect that translates to poor health outcomes.

When we look to policies that have shaped the environment we live in, housing policies in the 20th century shed light on racial disparities that exist between Whites and African Americans/Blacks in the United States. Systematic segregation has not only defined the places where African Americans/Blacks and Whites live, it has shaped, for generations, access to goods and services that contribute to health and prosperity.

HEALTH INEQUITIES BY SOCIOECONOMIC POSITION

Another major source for health inequity in the United States is socioeconomic status, whether measured by income, employment status, or educational attainment. Socioeconomic inequities in the United States are sizable and growing. Child health indicators, including infant mortality, follow a socioeconomic gradient that relates to underlying income and educational inequities. Specifically, the most adverse health outcomes for children and adults were observed for the lowest income and lowest educational attainment groups (**Figure 4.5**).[27]

Health inequities go beyond health indicators; average life expectancy increases continuously with higher income in the United States (**Figure 4.6**). For example, a national analysis found that, overall, average life expectancy between the top and bottom 1% of income differed by 15 years for men and 10 years for women between the years 2001 and 2014. Moreover, inequity in average life expectancy has been on the rise; between 2001 and 2014, the top 1% of income earners gained 3 years in life expectancy while those in the bottom 1% showed no gains.[28]

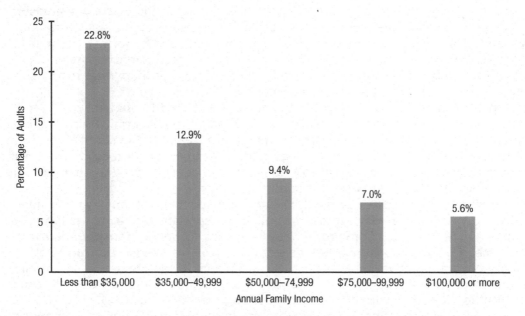

FIGURE 4.5 Poor self-rated health in relation to annual family income category in the United States.
Source: Data from Schiller JS, Lucas JW, Peregoy JA. Summary health statistics for U.S. adults: national health interview survey, 2011. *Vital Health Stat.* 10. 2012;(256): 76-78. https://www.cdc.gov/nchs/data/series/sr_10/sr10_256.pdf

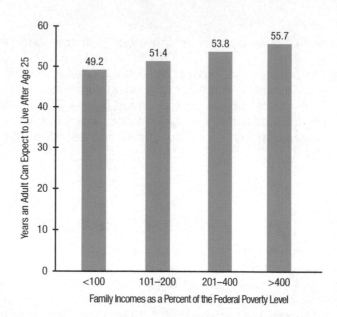

FIGURE 4.6 Life expectancy from age 25 by family income bracket in relation to the FPL. FPL, federal poverty level.
Source: Kincaid E. Residents of one Virginia county live 18 years longer than people just 350 miles away—here's why. *Business Insider.* April 14, 2015. https://www.businessinsider.com/how-income-affects-health-2015-4

CASE STUDY 4.2: GETTING FROM HERE TO THERE WHEN YOU HAVE NO OTHER OPTION: PUBLIC TRANSPORTATION ROUTES, LIKELIHOOD OF STABLE EMPLOYMENT, AND HEALTH

Despite the U.S. government's decision to invest in private vehicles and highways since the 1960s, the use of public transportation in the United States is increasing. In 2019, for example, Americans took 9.9 billion trips on public transportation.[29] Nonetheless, the upsurge in demand is highlighting the need for maintenance of existing public transit and investment in new options.[30] Unfortunately, the demand for public transportation is becoming much higher than what the existing systems were designed to accommodate.[30]

About 10% of the nation's urban bus fleet and 3% of the rail fleet need repair, along with 17% of transportation operating systems, 35% of guideway elements such as tracks, and 37% of transport stations. It is clear that the country needs an infusion of investment in public transportation. Further, for our focus here, investing in public transportation will contribute to the betterment of the health for the American population as we will describe.

Making the case for investment in public transportation to advance the health of the population is easy; access to public transportation directly leads to better healthcare access. Conversely, lack of access to public transportation leads to missed doctor appointments, missed or delayed medication use, and delayed care seeking.[31] Between 10% and 51% of patients in the United States identify transportation as a barrier to healthcare access.[32] Transportation barriers cause 5.8 million Americans to miss or delay seeking medical care anually.[33] Lack of access to public transportation is more common among minorities and persons of

(continued)

low socioeconomic status. In 1997, minority patients in Texas were more likely to forgo cancer treatment owing to transportation barriers when compared with their White counterparts.[34] In 2001, about one-third of those living at or below 125% of the federal poverty level in Cleveland, Ohio, reported that finding transportation to healthcare providers was hard or very hard.[35] In 2013, lack of transportation led to 25% of low-income patients missing or rescheduling their appointments.[32] Families with an income below $50,000 per year were particularly susceptible; about 4 million children from these families missed essential doctor appointments because of transportation barriers each year. Better access to public transportation will translate directly into better access to healthcare and decreased healthcare costs.[36]

The relation between available public transportation and health extends beyond access to healthcare. Transportation influences other health determinants. Access to public transportation is critical for maintaining stable employment and relates directly to income levels. The manner in which a city's public transportation system is structured influences the number of jobs, the size of the labor market, and the income level of its citizens.[37] For example, a recent study in New York City found that people with poor access to public transportation had lower average incomes and higher unemployment rates.[38]

The relation between available public transportation and health extends beyond access to healthcare. Transportation influences other health determinants. Access to public transportation is critical for maintaining stable employment and relates directly to income levels.

On a broader level, the American Public Transportation Association estimates that $1 billion invested in public transportation creates and supports more than 50,000 jobs.[29] In addition to directly affecting employment opportunities, investment in public transportation drives community growth, development, and economic viability. For each dollar invested in public transportation, the economic return is estimated to be $4. Moreover, a $10 million capital investment in public transportation is linked to a $32 million increase in business sales.[29]

Reducing air pollution is perhaps the most beneficial aspect of investing in public transportation. Nearly four in 10 people in the United States live in areas where the air is too dangerous to breathe.[39] Harmful motor vehicle emissions are responsible for between one-quarter and one-half of air pollutants in these areas.[36] However, improved availability and utilization of public transportation can dramatically reduce motor vehicle emissions. On average, public transportation produces, per passenger mile, 95% less carbon monoxide and 45% less carbon dioxide when compared to private vehicles.[40]

Despite the clear advantages of investing in public transportation, most, if not all, public transportation systems in the United States remain underfunded. There is currently a $90 billion backlog in funding needed to restore U.S. transportation systems to the status of "good repair" (i.e., functional to work well), a figure that is estimated to grow to $122 billion by 2032.[30]

It is important to note that the crumbling public transportation system contributes to health inequality in the United States. The people who experience the worst of the public transportation system are those who need it most.[41] Although all Americans may be concerned about improving public transportation, these systems are most essential for those who are the most impoverished.

(continued)

Increasing the use of public transportation in the United States is not only attainable but also crucial to improving the health of the population and reducing inequalities. Approaching public transportation planning through public health and social justice lenses is an intelligent and economically sound investment. Expanding and improving accessibility to public transportation contributes to urban development and access to the job market, reduces air pollution, leads to better access to the healthcare system, and results in better health outcomes, especially for minorities.

HEALTH INEQUITIES BY SEXUAL ORIENTATION

The Centers for Disease Control and Prevention (CDC) supports the Youth Risk Behavior Survey (YRBS), conducted nationwide with U.S. high school students. In 2019, special analyses were conducted to examine a wide range of health risks and health-related behaviors by sexual orientation. The YRBS respondents were predominantly students who self-identified their sexual orientation as heterosexual (straight), accounting for 84.5% of the sample. Around 11% self-identified as lesbian, gay, or bisexual—the LGB subset. The remaining 4.5% self-described as "not sure."

Particularly distinguishing was the comparison between LGB youth and heterosexual youth on a series of items that asked about exposures to interpersonal violence and self-harm. As outlined in **Table 4.1**, LGB youth were more likely to have been exposed to threats, bullying (in person and online), physical assault, dating violence (both physical and sexual), and forced sexual experience compared to their heterosexual student counterparts. Moreover, LGB youth were almost five times more likely to have attempted suicide. These data reveal stark disparities in exposures to violence and self-harm behaviors experienced by high school students who identify as LGB.

TABLE 4.1 Health Inequities in Violence Exposures for LGB Youth: Youth Risk Behavior Survey, 2019

	SEXUAL ORIENTATION		
EXPOSURES TO VIOLENCE	**HETEROSEXUAL (STRAIGHT) 84.5% OF TOTAL (%)**	**LGB 11% OF TOTAL (%)**	**NOT SURE 4.5% OF TOTAL (%)**
Carried a weapon	16.0	18.9	14.7
Threatened or injured by a weapon on school property	5.1	10.0	12.6
Injured in a physical fight	2.5	4.9	8.7
Did not go to school because they felt unsafe	4.6	12.5	10.8

(continued)

TABLE 4.1   Health Inequities in Violence Exposures for LGB Youth: Youth Risk Behavior Survey, 2019 (*continued*)

	SEXUAL ORIENTATION		
EXPOSURES TO VIOLENCE	HETEROSEXUAL (STRAIGHT) 84.5% OF TOTAL (%)	LGB 11% OF TOTAL (%)	NOT SURE 4.5% OF TOTAL (%)
Electronically bullied	14.2	28.0	22.5
Bullied on school property	18.8	34.2	24.9
Physically forced to have sexual intercourse	5.4	17.8	12.6
Experienced physical dating violence	8.3	17.5	24.5
Experienced sexual dating violence	9.1	22.7	23.8
Felt sad or hopeless	26.4	60.4	46.5
Attempted suicide	6.4	23.4	13.7

LGB, lesbian, gay, bisexual.

Source: Data from Centers for Disease Control and Prevention. CDC releases 2019 youth risk behavior survey results. August 20, 2020. https://www.cdc.gov/healthyyouth/data/yrbs/feature/index.htm

HEALTH INEQUITIES GLOBALLY

Health inequities are even more pronounced on a global level. Perhaps most compelling, there is currently a 20-year gap in average national life expectancy at birth between countries. A child born in Japan is expected to live 84 years while a child born in the Central African Republic is expected to live only 54 years, and a child born in Malawi is expected to live only 64 years. In the European Union region, four children out of 1,000 die before the age of 5,[42] while in Chad, the number dramatically increases to 110 children out of 1,000.[43]

Inequities in health outcomes are significant within countries as well. These inequities are rooted in differences in socioeconomic status, race, ethnicity, disability, sexual orientation, and gender. For example, on a global level, children under 5 years of age from poor rural households die at disproportionally higher rates than their counterparts from richer urban areas. Worldwide, a child from the poorest 20% of households is twice as likely to die compared to a child from the richest 20%.

About 150 million people face catastrophic healthcare costs annually. Even if people can afford to pay for healthcare, access to physicians can be a challenge in many countries. Low-income countries have ten-fold fewer doctors than high-income countries. For example, consider the contrast between Myanmar, with four physicians per 10,000 individuals, compared to Norway, with 40 physicians per 10,000 individuals. As another indicator of health inequities, globally, the richest 20% of women are more than 20 times more likely to have a skilled health professional to attend their birth than poor women.[44]

Addressing these inequities requires complex approaches that tackle healthcare system reforms in addition to taking action in multiple sectors that affect social determinants of health, including transportation and educational systems.

THE SOCIAL DETERMINANTS OF HEALTH

THE SOCIAL DETERMINANTS AS A PART OF CONTEMPORARY PUBLIC HEALTH PRACTICE

The social determinants of health (SDOH) represent a propelling force for moving toward equity and justice in public health. The SDOH are predicated on the understanding that economic and social conditions play a leading role in producing health. The SDOH was introduced and promoted by the WHO, which defines SDOH as:

> *The social determinants of health (SDOH) are the non-medical factors that influence health outcomes. They are the conditions in which people are born, grow, work, live, and age, and the wider set of forces and systems shaping the conditions of daily life. These forces and systems include economic policies and systems, development agendas, social norms, social policies, and political systems.*[25]

HISTORY OF THE SOCIAL DETERMINANTS OF HEALTH

The SDOH have come to the forefront in recent decades. However, historically, the philosophical groundwork for the SDOH was laid following the Industrial Revolution when disease and poverty were on the rise.[45] Following the typhus epidemic, German physician, Ruldolf Virchow, stated, "If medicine is to fulfill her great task, then she must enter the political and social life. Do we not always find the diseases of the populace traceable to defects in society?"[45] Although the term SDOH would not be introduced until decades later, key concepts underpinning what would become the SDOH were apparent in the foundational documents that created the UN and the WHO in the 1940s.[46] Social and political factors were acknowledged to contribute centrally and influentially to population health, and were infused into both the classic WHO definition that declares health to be "a state of complete physical, mental, and social well-being and not merely the absence of disease or infirmity" and the clarion call to advocate for health as a fundamental human right.[46] Over the next 75 years, the SDOH would come to prominence as a framework upon which to think about health, fashion evidence-based interventions, and promulgate health policies.

THE SDOH AND HEALTHY PEOPLE 2030

The CDC has embraced the WHO's definition of the SDOH. One major goal-setting initiative for tracking, evaluating, and promoting the health of the nation is Healthy People 2030, based administratively in the CDC's Office of Disease Prevention and Health Promotion (ODPHP). Healthy People 2030's three closely interconnected priority areas are the SDOH, health equity, and health literacy. With each 10-year cycle, Healthy People generates an expansive array of objectives with many tagged specifically to five key domains of the SDOH: healthcare access and quality, education access and quality, social and community context, economic stability, and neighborhood and built environment (**Figure 4.7**).

DOMAINS OF THE SOCIAL DETERMINANTS OF HEALTH

The CDC's Healthy People 2030 initiative defines and intervenes on five domains of the SDOH. We will systematically and sequentially describe each of these five domains. In practice, the nation's most salient and compelling health issues are influenced by multiple social determinants

Social Determinants of Health

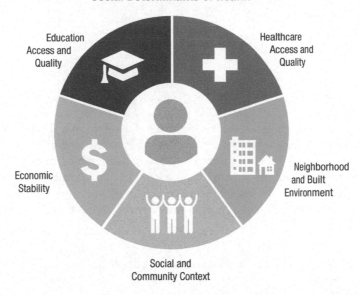

FIGURE 4.7 Domains of the social determinants of health.
Source: U.S. Department of Health and Human Services. Social determinants of health. Social Determinants of Health—Healthy People 2030. August 18, 2020. https://health.gov/healthypeople/priority-areas/social-determinants-health

interacting in synergistic ways. The CDC describes each of these five domains in terms of the "connection" between key elements of the particular domain—and health. The CDC provides an overarching goal for each of the five domains. In practice, the CDC's Healthy People initiative develops, tracks, and monitors multiple objectives each decade that together, collectively, are aimed at achieving, or at least making demonstrable progress toward achieving, the goal for each of the SDOH domains. Here, for each of the five SDOH domains, we present the name, the goal statement, and the CDC "connection" statement that links the domain to attainment of optimal health and well-being, and then we provide some examples.

DOMAIN: HEALTHCARE ACCESS AND QUALITY

Goal Statement

Increase access to comprehensive, high-quality health care services.

Connection Statement

The connection between people's access to and understanding of health services and their own health.

Key Issues Covered by the Domain

- Access to healthcare
- Access to primary care
- Health insurance coverage
- Health literacy

Access to healthcare, primary care, and health insurance, coupled with health literacy, directly affects health and well-being. The linkage of healthcare access to health is the most straightforward and self-evident of the five domains. Therefore, the Healthy People 2030 focus on the domain of healthcare access aims to ensure timely ease of access to healthcare services of excellence—for all people. The flipside here is avoiding the domino-like cascade of impediments to accessing healthcare that many people still encounter. For example, the one in 10 citizens who lack health insurance are unlikely to have a primary care provider or to be able to buy life-sustaining medications. Training capable health professionals to serve marginalized communities is a significant need.

DOMAIN: EDUCATION ACCESS AND QUALITY

Goal Statement

Increase educational opportunities and help children and adolescents do well in school.

Connection Statement

The connection of education to health and well-being.

Key Issues Covered by the Domain

- Graduating from high school
- Enrollment in higher education
- Educational attainment in general language and literacy
- Early childhood education and development

Higher levels of educational attainment produce health and longevity. Therefore, the Healthy People 2030 focus on educational access and quality is on making sure that children and adolescents are assured of having quality education available from young ages forward that can launch them into higher education and open a range of future professional opportunities that education brings. Objectives in this domain also focus on the obverse; diminishing stressors and threats to health and mental health that concentrate in lower-educated communities targeted for marginalization.

DOMAIN: ECONOMIC STABILITY

Goal Statement

Help people earn steady incomes that allow them to meet their health needs.

Connection Statement

The connection between the financial resources people have—income, cost of living, and socioeconomic status—and their health.

Key Issues Covered by the Domain

- Poverty
- Employment
- Food security
- Housing stability

Employment in a satisfying and meaningful profession, the ability to earn a comfortable income, and the capability to generate wealth over the lifetime, coupled with lifelong food security and housing stability are economic benchmarks of a health-producing lifestyle. Therefore, the Healthy People 2030 focus on the domain of economic stability addresses the one in 10 Americans living in poverty along with the entire population that may be buffeted by cyclical or sudden economic downturns and the ongoing shifts in occupational and career opportunities. People must be able to afford healthy food and a safe home and have resources to pay for preventive and therapeutic healthcare. To improve the employment situation and assure a sustaining income for all, consideration must be given to childcare programs that free parent wage-earners to go to work. Careers and income-earning opportunities must be available and inclusive to facilitate income generation for people living with disabilities or medical conditions that require special accommodation. Underpinning the most marginalized, programs that provide support for basic necessities while providing jobs training and opening doors for employment must be prioritized.

DOMAIN: SOCIAL AND COMMUNITY CONTEXT

Goal Statement

Increase social and community support.

Connection Statement

The connection between characteristics of the contexts within which people live, learn, work, and play, and their health and well-being.

Key Issues Covered by the Domain

- Cohesion within a community
- Civic participation
- Discrimination
- Conditions in the workplace
- Incarceration

Social support comes from influential people at each level from household to societal. Most proximate and often most important, particularly during early life, are relationships and interactions with parents, siblings, grandparents, and others in the household. Beyond the immediate home environments, childcare providers and teachers, as well as a broad spectrum of friends—and for those who play sports, teammates—will be central figures during childhood and beyond. Colleagues, coworkers, and community members also provide health-producing social support. Therefore, the Healthy People 2030 focus on social and community context centers on "helping people get the social support they need in the places where they live, work, learn, and play." Besides maximizing healthy sources of social support, Healthy People objectives also tackle the downside of unsafe environments, including the imperative to diminish discrimination, lack of social support at home or in the community, and lack of resources to afford necessities (linking to the economic stability domain). There is a balancing element here in that the positive relationships in various settings, at multiple levels, can buffer and offset some of the deficits in social support.

DOMAIN: NEIGHBORHOOD AND BUILT ENVIRONMENT

Goal Statement

Create neighborhoods and environments that promote health and safety.

Connection Statement

The connection between where a person lives—housing, neighborhood, and environment—and their health and well-being.

Key Issues Covered by the Domain

- Quality of housing
- Access to transportation
- Availability of healthy food
- Air and water quality
- Neighborhood crime and violence

As is examined in Chapter 7, "Families, Social Networks, Neighborhoods, and Cities," our zip code can tell us more about our health and well-being than our genetic code. Connecting to all the other domains, our neighborhoods are major determinants of our economic stability, access to education, access to healthcare, and community levels of social support. Therefore, the Healthy People 2030 focus on the neighborhood and built environment expands on the central importance of place. Specifically, the objectives address the safety, wholesomeness, and salutary qualities of the places where (as mentioned under social and community context) people live, work, learn, and play. Of course, the flipside is the current reality that many neighborhoods and communities are characterized by the reverse cluster of attributes: unsafe dwellings and commercial structures, substandard housing, high rates of violence and crime, contaminated water supplies, pollution and unsafe air, proximity to toxic waste sites, noise pollution, and more. Therefore, the Healthy People 2030 objectives involve interventions and policy changes, ranging from local to state and federal levels to address these overt risks to health and well-being.

THE SOCIAL DETERMINANTS OF HEALTH DOMAINS: OTHER MODELS

While the CDC's Healthy People 2030 provides us with a concise set of the five SDOH domains just discussed, this framework is not universally adopted. Different programs highlight the SDOH and modify the classification of domains to best suit their work and their agendas.

During the COVID-19 pandemic, the Kaiser Family Foundation observed the SDOH closely. Their classification scheme was almost identical to the CDC/Healthy People domains—but food security was singled out for special attention, bringing the total domains to six (**Figure 4.8**).

The National Health Service of Scotland features eight SDOH domains in the work that they do (**Figure 4.9**).

As another example, a large-scale research endeavor is underway to recruit a cohort of one million subjects and gather detailed medical, genetic, and behavioral data at multiple points over time. Here is the description of the All of Us research program: "All of Us is a research

Social Determinants of Health

Economic Stability	Neighborhood and Physical Environment	Education	Food	Community and Social Context	Healthcare System
Employment	Housing	Literacy	Hunger	Social integration	Health coverage
Income	Transportation	Language	Access to healthy options	Support systems	Provider availability
Expenses	Safety	Early childhood education		Community engagement	Provider linguistic and cultural competency
Debt	Parks	Vocational training		Discrimination	
Medical bills	Playgrounds	Higher education		Stress	Quality of care
Support	Walkability				
	Zip code/ geography				

Health Outcomes
Mortality, Morbidity, Life Expectancy, Healthcare Expenditures, Health Status, Functional Limitations

FIGURE 4.8 The Kaiser Family Foundation social determinants of health domains.
Source: Artiga S, Hinton E. Beyond health care: the role of social determinants in promoting health and health equity. Kaiser Family Foundation. Published May 10, 2018. https://www.kff.org/racial-equity-and-health-policy/issue-brief/beyond-health-care-the-role-of-social-determinants-in-promoting-health-and-health-equity/

Social Determinants of Health

The social determinants of health are the conditions in which we are born, we grow and age, and in which we live and work. The factors below impact on our health and well-being.

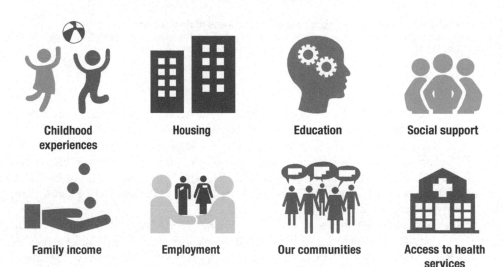

FIGURE 4.9 The National Health Service of Scotland Social Determinants of Health Domains.
Source: Adapted from NHS Health Scotland. https://www.gov.scot/publications/practising-realistic-medicine/pages/9/

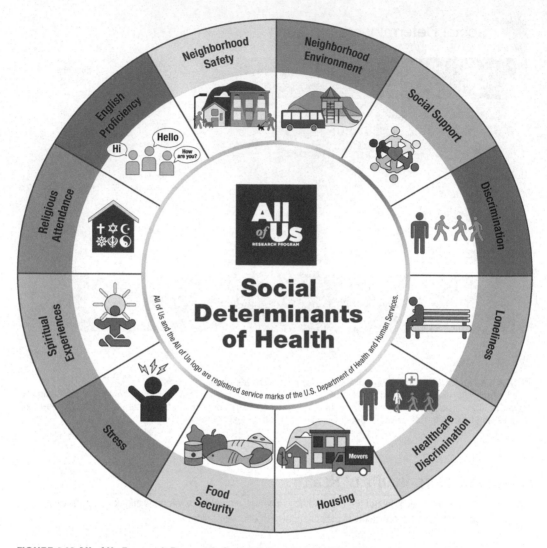

FIGURE 4.10 All of Us Research Program's Social Determinants of Health Domains.
Source: Sayles M. All about the social determinants of health. American Association on Health & Disability. Published May 2, 2022. https://aahd.us/2022/05/all-about-the-social-determinants-of-health/

program from the National Institutes of Health (NIH). It is seeking one million or more people from across the United States. By doing so, it hopes to one day speed up medical research. People who join share information about their health, habits, and what it is like where they live. By looking at patterns, researchers may learn more about what affects people's health."[47] Check out the SDOH graphic used in the All of Us program—with 12 domains illustrated (**Figure 4.10**)! On closer inspection, the 12 topics listed in the SDOH "wheel" used by the All of Us research program closely resemble the "key issues covered" under each of the five CDC/Healthy People domains that were enumerated earlier.

Regardless of the classification and number of domains, the SDOH feature prominently in contemporary public health practice, as articulated for example, in Public Health 3.0: A Call to Action for Public Health to Meet the Challenges of the 21st Century,[48] presented by the U.S. Department of Health and Human Services (HHS). The social determinants are a key force in evolving patterns of population health and disease. They play a role in health behaviors, which are prominent influencers of health outcomes.[49]

THE SOCIAL DETERMINANTS AS DRIVERS OF HEALTH INEQUITIES

It is impossible to examine the SDOH without understanding health inequities and disparities. The SDOH are the very factors that shape health. Differences across populations in the social determinants act as major forces behind observed differences in health. For example, while healthful foods are important for better health outcomes,[50] not everyone can access healthy foods. Not all people can afford healthy and nutritious foods due to their income or employment status, and even if they had the means, such foods may not be available in their neighborhoods. Health and health inequities affect all. Addressing social determinants with a goal of reducing health inequities is important for social justice and improving the health and economic prosperity of the population.[51] Differential exposure to social determinants is often a function of social class, gender, race, ethnicity, language, immigration status, education, occupation, and income.[52]

CORE CHALLENGE: HOW DO WE TARGET PUBLIC HEALTH INTERVENTIONS AROUND THE SOCIAL DETERMINANTS OF HEALTH?

There is no single, overarching determinant of health. The SDOH are a multiplicity. Likewise, there is no single intervention that will be appropriate or effective for any population. To target any issue, we must first assess social needs and circumstances in the population of interest and in ways that are feasible, comfortable, and appropriate.[53] Once evidence-based interventions are established, it is critical to monitor and evaluate them and to make necessary and ongoing adjustments. This iterative process will work to maximize the potential of the intervention. In Chapter 1, "The Origins of Public Health," we outlined the CDC's 10 Essential Public Health Services. In **Table 4.2** we provide examples of how to address the SDOH through each of these 10 Essential Services.[54]

TABLE 4.2 Addressing Social Determinants of Health Through the 10 Essential Public Health Services

ROLES OF PUBLIC HEALTH AGENCY (BASED ON 10 ESSENTIAL PUBLIC HEALTH SERVICES)	EXAMPLES TO ADDRESS THE SDOH THROUGH THE ESSENTIAL PUBLIC HEALTH SERVICES
1. Monitor health status to identify and solve community health problems	Include the SDOH measures as basis for addressing community health problems and inequities Ensure community health assessments (CHA) include the SDOH measures and engage communities and multisectoral partners in CHA efforts
2. Diagnose and investigate health problems and health hazards in the community	Include community-level determinants of health in investigations, as well as policies and practices that involve other sectors to support them. For example • Ensure water sources meet required standards • Ensure brownfield sites identify hazardous waste that might contaminate a community • Address deteriorating housing conditions to prevent lead poisoning and other hazards to health

(continued)

TABLE 4.2   Addressing Social Determinants of Health Through the 10 Essential Public Health Services (*continued*)

ROLES OF PUBLIC HEALTH AGENCY (BASED ON 10 ESSENTIAL PUBLIC HEALTH SERVICES)	EXAMPLES TO ADDRESS THE SDOH THROUGH THE ESSENTIAL PUBLIC HEALTH SERVICES
3. Inform, educate, and empower people about health issues	Ensure outreach and education efforts address social and structural determinants of health inequities Ensure access to culturally and linguistically appropriate approaches to community health (e.g., Racial and Ethnic Approaches to Community Health [REACH]) to help address the SDOH. Approaches should take into account such challenges as structural racism and stigma against immigrants, both of which can decrease likelihood of seeking needed healthcare
4. Mobilize community partnerships and action to identify and solve health problems	Engage and collaborate with community members and non-traditional partners associated with the SDOHs, such as • Housing authorities • Law enforcement • Schools • Community organizations
5. Develop policies and plans that support individual and community health efforts	Leverage evidence-based policies in nonhealth sectors that affect the SDOH and health outcomes, such as • Safe and affordable housing that can reduce risk for asthma, lead poisoning, homelessness • Full-day kindergarten that can reduce adverse health prospects such as teenage pregnancy Develop and implement state/community health improvement plans that include and address the SDOH in collaboration with community partners
6. Enforce laws and regulations that protect health and ensure safety	Develop strategies to ensure enforcement of existing regulations and laws that affect health, such as • Housing and health codes to prevent childhood lead poisoning • Batterer intervention program laws to prevent violence against women and children
7. Link people to needed personal health services and ensure the provision of healthcare when otherwise unavailable	Educate community members about their eligibility for and access to entitlement programs: • Medicaid, including its medical, mental health, and housing benefits • Temporary Assistance for Needy Families (TANF) • Supplemental Nutrition Assistance Program (SNAP) Ensure that essential health benefits and the free preventive services provisions of the Affordable Care Act (ACA) are correctly and equitably implemented

(*continued*)

TABLE 4.2   Addressing Social Determinants of Health Through the 10 Essential Public Health Services (*continued*)

ROLES OF PUBLIC HEALTH AGENCY (BASED ON 10 ESSENTIAL PUBLIC HEALTH SERVICES)	EXAMPLES TO ADDRESS THE SDOH THROUGH THE ESSENTIAL PUBLIC HEALTH SERVICES
8. Assure competent public and personal healthcare workforce	Support staff training and development efforts that help workforce incorporate social determinants of health inequity into their job responsibilities
	Promote hiring of workforce that reflects population being served
9. Evaluate effectiveness, accessibility, and quality of personal and population-based health services	Ensure evaluation and research designs include interventions that address the SDOH inequity
	Use performance management and quality improvement methods to explore and address more effectively the root causes of issues, which often include the SDOH
10. Research for new insights and innovative solutions to health problems	Expand research agendas to include the SDOH and related health outcomes, especially in evaluation of natural experiments where a project is already addressing the SDOH but is not studying health effects (e.g., implementation of the Essentials for Childhood Framework)
	Use community-based participatory research designs
	Apply evidence-based practices (e.g., The Community Guide) to address health inequity and demonstrate improved health outcomes

Source: Centers for Disease Control and Prevention. Ten essential public health services and how they can include addressing social determinants of health inequities. March 18, 2021. https://www.cdc.gov/publichealthgateway/publichealthservices/pdf/ten_essential_services_and_sdoh.pdf

SUMMARY

The SDOH must be centered at the heart of all we do, informing how we think in public health practice to bring about health equity. Our everyday conditions and surroundings profoundly shape our health. The influences of the social determinants on health are inextricable. Embracing health equity as a core principle of public health underlines a commitment to reduce and eliminate health inequities—and their social determinants—to ensure the attainment of the highest level of health for all people. In turn, health equity is powered by the values of social justice and human rights.

By definition, health inequities are different from health inequalities; inequities are avoidable, unnecessary, and unfair health inequalities. While public health efforts over the past century have led to significant improvements in many health indicators (efficiency), some of these interventions have exacerbated health inequities. This tension between efficiency and equity is often present when designing interventions as public health resources are finite. As such, adopting a health equity approach means that public health professionals have an obligation to identify and reduce inequities that may arise from interventions aiming to maximize the health of the entire population.

End-of-Chapter Resources

 Access additional case study podcasts online at http://connect.springerpub.com/ content/book/978-0-8261-8043-8/

DISCUSSION QUESTIONS

1. Living in proximity to fossil fuel production sites where petroleum products are extracted, refined, and processed into petrochemicals elevates risks for various forms of cancer. Considering the populations that are affected, how is this a health equity issue?

2. Climate change is making Atlantic hurricanes stronger and more destructive for populations living along the U.S. Gulf Coast. In terms of damage sustained during hurricane landfall, what social determinants of health distinguish the vulnerability of coastal populations?

3. How might the discontinuation of Affirmative Action protections impact educational disparities in the United States?

 A robust set of instructor resources designed to supplement this text is located at **http://connect.springerpub.com/content/book/978-0-8261-8043-8.** Qualifying instructors may request access by emailing **textbook@springerpub.com.**

REFERENCES

1. Braveman P. Health disparities and health equity: concepts and measurement. *Annu Rev Public Health.* 2006;*27*:167-194. doi:10.1146/annurev.publhealth.27.021405.102103
2. Healthy People 2020. *Disparities.* Published 2014. https://www.healthypeople.gov/2020/about/foundation -health-measures/Disparities#5
3. Braveman PA, Kumanyika S, Fielding J, et al. Health disparities and health equity: the issue is justice. *Am J Public Health.* 2011;*101*(suppl 1):S149-S155. doi:10.2105/AJPH.2010.300062
4. Braveman P. What are health disparities and health equity? We need to be clear. *Public Health Rep.* 2014;*129*(suppl 2):5-8. doi:10.1177/00333549141291S203
5. Sadana R, Blas E. What can public health programs do to improve health equity? *Public Health Rep.* 2013;*128*(suppl 3):12-20. doi:10.1177/00333549131286S303
6. Daniels N, Kennedy B, Kawachi I. Social justice is good for our health. *Boston Review.* July 25, 2000. http:// bostonreview.net/forum/norman-daniels-bruce-kennedy-ichiro-kawachi-justice-good-our-health
7. Braveman P, Gruskin S. Defining equity in health. *J Epidemiol Community Health.* 2003;57:254-258. doi:10.1136/jech.57.4.254
8. Reidpath DD, Olafsdottir AE, Pokhrel S, Allotey P. The fallacy of the equity-efficiency trade off: rethinking the efficient health system. *BMC Public Health.* 2012;*12*(suppl 1):S3. doi:10.1186/1471-2458-12-S1-S3
9. Platt JM, Keyes KM, Galea S. Efficiency or equity? Simulating the impact of high-risk and population intervention strategies for the prevention of disease. *SSM Popul Health.* 2017;3:1-8. doi:10.1016/ j.ssmph .2016.11.002
10. Frohlich KL, Potvin L. Transcending the known in public health practice: the inequality paradox: the population approach and vulnerable populations. *Am J Public Health.* 2008;*98*(2):216-221. doi:10.2105/AJPH .2007.114777
11. U.S. Department of Health and Human Services. *Heart disease and African Americans.* U.S. Department of Health and Human Services–Office of Minority Health. https://minorityhealth.hhs.gov/omh/browse.aspx?lvl=4&lvlid=19
12. Fryar CD, Carroll MD, Afful J. *Prevalence of overweight, obesity, and severe obesity among children and adolescents aged 2–19 years: United States, 1963–1965 through 2017–2018.* NCHS Health E-Stats. 2020.

13. MacroTrends. U.S. infant mortality rate 1950-2022. https://www.macrotrends.net/countries/USA/united-states/infant-mortality-rate

14. Ely DM, Driscoll AK. Infant mortality in the United States, 2018: data from the period linked birth/infant death file—National Center for Health Statistics. *Natl Vital Stat Rep.* 2020;69(7):1-18.

15. Bhutta N, Chang A, Dettling LJ, Hsu JW. *Disparities in wealth by race and ethnicity in the 2019 survey of consumer finances.* FEDS Notes. Board of Governors of the Federal Reserve System. Published September 28, 2020. https://doi.org/10.17016/2380-7172.2797

16. Chetty R, Stepner M, Abraham S, et al. The association between income and life expectancy in the United States, 2001–2014. *JAMA.* 2016;315(16):1750. doi:10.1001/jama.2016.4226

17. Living New Deal. *National housing act (1934).* https://livingnewdeal.org/glossary/national-housing-act-1934

18. Badger E. Redlining: still a thing. *Washington Post.* May 28, 2015. https://www.washingtonpost.com/news/wonk/wp/2015/05/28/evidence-that-banks-still-deny-black-borrowers-just-as-they-did-50-years-ago/?noredirect=on&utm_term=.f934b1366f69

19. Bauman JF, Biles R, Szylvian KM. *From Tenements to the Taylor Homes: In Search of an Urban Housing Policy in Twentieth-Century America.* Pennsylvania State University Press; 2000. http://www.psupress.org/books/titles/0-271-02012-1.html

20. Katznelson I. *When Affirmative Action Was White: An Untold History of Racial Inequality in Twentieth-Century America.* W. W. Norton; 2005. https://books.wwnorton.com/books/detail.aspx?id=8023

21. Farley T, Cohen D. *Prescription for a Healthy Nation: A New Approach to Improving Our Lives by Fixing Our Everyday World.* Beacon Press; 2005.

22. Tavernise S. Black Americans see gains in life expectancy. *The New York Times.* May 8, 2016. https://www.nytimes.com/2016/05/09/health/blacks-see-gains-in-life-expectancy.html

23. Williams DR, Mohammed SA. Discrimination and racial disparities in health: evidence and needed research. *J Behav Med.* 2009;32:20-47. doi:10.1007/s10865-008-9185-0

24. Ard K. Trends in exposure to industrial air toxins for different racial and socioeconomic groups: a spatial and temporal examination of environmental inequality in the U.S. from 1995 to 2004. *Soc Sci Res.* 2015;53:375-390. doi:10.1016/j.ssresearch.2015.06.019

25. World Health Organization. *Social determinants of health.* https://www.who.int/health-topics/social-determinants-of-health#tab=tab_1

26. Brewer M, Kimbro RT, Denney JT, et al. Does neighborhood social and environmental context impact race/ethnic disparities in childhood asthma? *Health Place.* 2017;44:86-93. doi:10.1016/j.healthplace.2017.01.006

27. Braveman PA, Cubbin C, Egerter S, et al. Socioeconomic disparities in health in the United States: what the patterns tell us. *Am J Public Health.* 2010;100(suppl 1):S186-S196. doi:10.2105/AJPH.2009.166082

28. Chetty R, Stepner M, Abraham S, et al. The association between income and life expectancy in the United States, 2001–2014. *JAMA.* 2016;315(16):1750-1766. doi:10.1001/jama.2016.4226

29. American Public Transportation Association. *Public transportation facts.* Published April 26, 2020. https://www.apta.com/news-publications/public-transportation-facts/

30. American Society of Civil Engineers. *2017 Infrastructure Report Card.* Author; 2017:88-92. https://www.infrastructurereportcard.org/wp-content/uploads/2017/01/Transit-Final.pdf

31. eCampus Rural Health Stanford Medicine. *Healthcare disparities & barriers to healthcare.* http://med.stanford.edu/ruralhealth/health-pros/factsheets/disparities-barriers.html

32. Syed ST, Gerber BS, Sharp LK. Traveling towards disease: transportation barriers to health care access. *J Community Health.* 2013;38(5):976-993. doi:10.1007/s10900-013-9681-1

33. University of California Davis, Health. *It's not just transportation, it's health justice for patients.* Published April 6, 2022. https://health.ucdavis.edu/news/headlines/its-not-just-transportation-its-health-justice-for-patients/2022/04

34. Guidry JJ, Aday LA, Zhang D, Winn RJ. Transportation as a barrier to cancer treatment. *Cancer Pract.* 1997;5(6):361-366. http://www.ncbi.nlm.nih.gov/pubmed/9397704

35. Ahmed SM, Lemkau JP, Nealeigh N, Mann B. Barriers to healthcare access in a non-elderly urban poor American population. *Health Soc Care Community.* 2001;9(6):445-453. doi:10.1046/j.1365-2524.2001.00318.x

36. American Public Transportation Association. *Benefits of public transportation.* https://www.apta.com/research-technical-resources/transit-statistics/benefits-of-public-transportation/

37. Bacares CAO. *Do public transport improvements increase employment and income in a city?* ERSA conference paper. European Regional Science Association. 2013. https://ideas.repec.org/p/wiw/wiwrsa/ersa13p1040.html

38. Kurtzleben D. *Bad public transit isn't just inconvenient; it keeps people from jobs.* Vox. Published January 6, 2015. https://www.vox.com/2015/1/6/7494641/public-transit-unemployment-income

39. American Lung Association. *State of the Air Report.* Published 2021. https://www.lung.org/our-initiatives/healthy-air/sota

40. Shapiro RJ, Hassett KA, Arnold FS. *Conserving Energy and Preserving the Environment: The Role of Public Transportation.* American Public Transportation Association; 2002. http://biblioteca.cejamericas.org/handle/2015/1589?show=full

41. White GB. Stranded: how America's failing public transportation increases inequality. *The Atlantic.* May 16, 2015. https://www.theatlantic.com/business/archive/2015/05/stranded-how-americas-failing-public-transportation-increases-inequality/393419

42. World Bank Group. *Mortality rate, under-5 (per 1,000 live births)—European Union.* The World Bank Data. https://data.worldbank.org/indicator/SH.DYN.MORT?locations=EU

43. World Bank Group. *Mortality rate, under-5 (per 1,000 live births)–Chad.* The World Bank Data. https://data.worldbank.org/indicator/SH.DYN.MORT?locations=TD

44. World Health Organization. *World conference on social determinants of health; fact file on health inequities.* Published September 14, 2011.

45. Frank JW, Mustard JF. The determinants of health from a historical perspective. *Daedalus.* 1994;*123*(4):1-19. http://www.jstor.org/stable/20027264

46. Grad FP. The preamble of the constitution of the world health organization. *Bull World Health Organ.* 2002;*80*(12):981-984.

47. National Institute of Health. *All of Us Research Program.* https://www.joinallofus.org

48. DeSalvo KB, Wang YC, Harris A, et al. Public Health 3.0: A Call to Action for Public Health to Meet the Challenges of the 21st Century. *Prev Chronic Dis.* 2017; 14: 170017. doi: http://dx.doi.org/10.5888/pcd14.170017

49. Galea S. *Well: What We Need to Talk About When We Talk About Health.* New York: Oxford University Press; 2019.

50. Angelino D, Godos J, Ghelfi F, et al. Fruit and vegetable consumption and health outcomes: an umbrella review of observational studies. *Int J Food Sci Nutr.* 2019;70(6):652-667. doi:10.1080/09637486.2019.1571021

51. Woodward A, Kawachi I. Why reduce health inequalities? *J Epidemiol Community Health.* 2000;54(12):923-929. doi:10.1136/jech.54.12.923

52. Braveman P, Gottlieb L. The social determinants of health: it's time to consider the causes of the causes. *Public Health Rep.* 2014;*129*(suppl 2):19-31. doi:10.1177/00333549141291S206

53. Abir M, Hammond S, Iovan S, Lantz PM. *Why more evidence is needed on the effectiveness of screening for social needs among high-use patients in acute care settings. Health Affairs.* Accessed May 23, 2019. https://www.healthaffairs.org/do/10.1377/forefront.20190520.243444

54. Centers for Disease Control and Prevention. *10 essential public health services.* Accessed March 18, 2021. https://www.cdc.gov/publichealthgateway/publichealthservices/essentialhealthservices.html

5

WHAT CAUSES THE HEALTH OF POPULATIONS? A SOCIAL ECOLOGICAL AND LIFE COURSE APPROACH

LEARNING OBJECTIVES

- Identify the two frameworks that we apply to explain what causes the health of populations.
- Distinguish the differences between the life course and social ecological perspectives.
- Demonstrate the "level of influence" at which health is produced, from the individual to the global policy level.
- Distinguish critical/sensitive periods, chains of risk, and accumulation of risk in relation to producing health and disease at different life stages.
- Demonstrate the scope and scale of public health interventions by mapping them onto a matrix consisting of the multiple social ecological levels and life course age ranges.

OVERVIEW: HOW DO WE EXPLAIN WHAT CAUSES HEALTH AND DISEASE?

Now that we have introduced the history and structure of public health, we move on to presenting a conceptual structure that can guide us through the rest of the book. To do that, we (a) introduce the social ecological perspective and discuss each "level of influence" at which health is produced from the individual level to the global policy level and (b) introduce the life course perspective and discuss how health is produced at each life stage, starting with the intergenerational stage and moving on to the peripartum period and through to old age.

Explaining what causes health and disease is fundamental to public health. Public health focuses on improving the health of entire populations. To accomplish this, public health builds on the science of population health. In turn, population health science is concerned with understanding the causes of health in populations. Here, we consider two concepts that are central to our understanding of the health of populations.

First, building on previous work, we consider causes of events as those factors necessary for the event to occur when and how it did.[1] The corollary is that causes are necessary conditions as evidenced by the fact that the health-related event of interest would not occur in the absence of these conditions.

Second, we also preferentially apply the phrase, "the production of health." Harkening back to the World Health Organization (WHO) definition, health is not merely the absence of disease. Health can be proactively promoted, potentiated, and as we say, produced.[2]

Causal thinking is therefore a fundamental pillar of population health science. Causation is not directly observed but must be inferred.[1] We intuitively and reflexively understand causation at the individual level and we shall use this as the launch point for expanding our conversation toward examining causation at the population level.

CONCEPTUAL FRAMEWORKS INFORM THE PRODUCTION OF HEALTH IN POPULATIONS

Thinking at the population level is not necessarily intuitive. In order to organize our thinking, we use two frameworks or perspectives to guide us through the rest of the book: the social ecological and life course perspectives.

> **Thinking at the population level is not necessarily intuitive. In order to organize our thinking, we use two frameworks or perspectives to guide us through the rest of the book: the social ecological and life course perspectives.**

The **social ecological perspective** explains that our health is produced through a variety of levels starting from the individual, and then moving outward from the individual to include an individual's family members and friends, their neighborhoods, their cities, and their countries. The social ecological perspective is informed by the thinking of a number of scholars who have advanced our understanding in the field over the past several decades.[3-6] Three chapters are dedicated to describing social ecological levels, respectively, focusing on individual behavior; the "between individuals" level that includes families, networks, neighborhoods, and cities; and countries, policies, and health.

The other organizing framework we use is the **life course perspective**. The life course perspective states, simply enough, that our health is produced throughout our life. The life course perspective is informed by a number of scholars who have advanced our understanding in the field.[7,8] Three chapters are devoted to discussion of the perinatal period, infancy, childhood, and adolescence (before birth through age 24); adulthood (ages 25–64); and older age (ages 65 and older).

When considered together, the social ecological and life course dimensions create a useful matrix for understanding the health of populations. This framework appears across multiple case examples introduced throughout this book. In this chapter, we discuss each perspective in more detail, beginning with the social ecological perspective, followed by the life course perspective. Then we bring the two together in a way that allows us to examine issues of population health concern from both perspectives simultaneously.

THE SOCIAL ECOLOGICAL PERSPECTIVE

The social ecological perspective examines how health is produced at multiple levels. In fact, another term for this perspective is the multilevel approach, acknowledging that we are concerned with different levels that influence health. **Figure 5.1** displays the four levels of the social

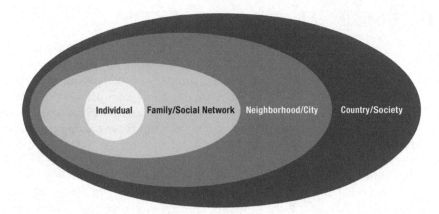

FIGURE 5.1 The multilevel social ecological perspective: social ecological levels illustrated, correspond-ing to levels described in Chapters 6 through 8. Family, social network, neighborhood, and city levels are combined in Chapter 7. Artistic credit: Parisa Varanloo.

ecological dimension that are used for organizing the discussion throughout three chapters: in-dividual behavior (Chapter 6, "Individual Behavior"); family/social network and neighborhood/city (Chapter 7, "Families, Social Networks, Neighborhoods, and Cities"); and country/society (Chapter 8, "Countries, Policies, and Health").

SOCIAL ECOLOGICAL PERSPECTIVE: INDIVIDUAL BEHAVIOR

At the heart of the social ecological framework is the individual. Disease happens in the individ-ual and it is the individual who is healthy. Therefore, we anchor this discussion of health first in ourselves (individuals) and then expand outward to encompass others. By way of illustration, let us consider a high school student who lives somewhere along the U.S. Northeast megalopolis. This adolescent male, age 15, attends the neighborhood public school. He performs adequately but is currently uncertain about his college aspirations (**Figure 5.2**).

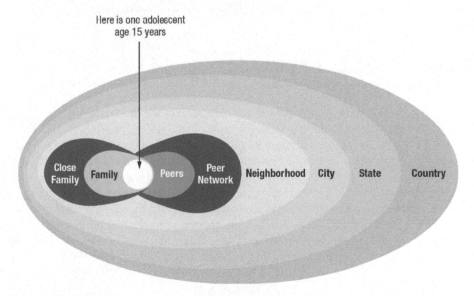

FIGURE 5.2 An illustration of an individual embedded in the social ecological framework. Artistic credit: Parisa Varanloo.

SOCIAL ECOLOGICAL PERSPECTIVE: FAMILY/SOCIAL NETWORKS

Most individuals are intimately embedded within social networks starting with the family or the household. Our student lives at home with both parents and his older sibling who is a senior in high school. Six extended family members, including one set of grandparents (his mother's parents), live nearby in town. He primarily hangs out with a group of five to seven fellow students. All of his friends are from the same neighborhood and live within easy walking distance (they are too young to drive). They visit each other's homes, including in some instances when parental supervision is not available.

Families frequently reside in neighborhoods where children and youth go to the local schools. Residents shop in nearby supermarkets and malls. As noted, our student has a small, tight primary peer group. As context, these peers are enrolled in a large high school with several thousand students. Our adolescent and his peer group take advantage of easy access to local malls where they sometimes play video games or watch newly released films. Many inexpensive but unhealthy fast-food outlets are available inside the mall and in the nearby vicinity. Several members of the group are involved in skateboarding, with sufficient skills to give impromptu demonstrations. They wear minimal protective gear. And the three who avidly participate in skateboarding have already sustained serious injuries, including several fractures, lacerations, and concussions.

SOCIAL ECOLOGICAL PERSPECTIVE: NEIGHBORHOODS/CITIES

Clusters of neighborhoods make up towns and cities that benefit from the efficiencies and economies of shared governance and services. Most of the adult residents of local neighborhoods perform their job duties at workplaces located in the surrounding cities.

Back to our youth and his peer group, access to health and fitness options, as well as potentially health-compromising options such as nonnutritious fast foods and video game arcades, is regulated by city ordinances and local legislation. Local norms, policies, and politics influence the health versus risk seesaw for youth, their families, and social networks.

SOCIAL ECOLOGICAL PERSPECTIVE: COUNTRY/SOCIETY

At a higher level of geopolitical organization, towns, cities, urban metropolitan centers, and rural areas are part of progressively larger entities (e.g., states, provinces) and ultimately nation states. Politics and policies that are formulated at national as well as subnational levels have strong bearing on the health of citizens. Critical issues relevant to population health require coordination on a local, national, regional, continental, or global basis. Although the state and country levels seem distal and far removed from our youth, these are the levels that sponsor, evaluate, and promote evidence-based health education programs for delivery in schools; conduct youth surveys of health behaviors, including patterns of substance use and sexual behaviors; support university-based scientific research on adolescent health behaviors and interventions that work; and regulate the taxation, advertising, and promotion of products that may be harmful to health (e.g., tobacco products, high-sugar content foods, alcohol).

CASE STUDY 5.1: CIGARETTE SMOKING: BACKGROUND AND SOCIAL ECOLOGICAL PERSPECTIVE

BACKGROUND

We illustrate the social ecological and life course perspectives using the example of cigarette smoking, beginning with some historical context. What makes smoking particularly illuminating as an illustration is the fact that the cigarette is a human invention that can be traced from its origin as a mass-produced item. The cigarette is an engineered, paper-wrapped tube containing crushed tobacco leaf and a panoply of other ingredients (up to 7,000!) that the tobacco industry describes as a "nicotine delivery device."

The cigarette is designed for addiction. Unlike earlier forms of smoked tobacco products (pipes, cigars) made from bitter alkaline tobaccos that are too harsh to hold in the lungs, the cigarette, featuring mild burley tobaccos, is designed to allow deep and prolonged inhalation. This allows the smoker to take full advantage of the unique properties of nicotine and also vastly increases the harm inflicted on human physiology that ultimately leads to dozens of diseases and frequently to premature death.

To be clear, the tobacco plant (genus *Nicotiana*) predates human habitation. Cultivation of tobacco by indigenous First Nations peoples in the Americas dates back to 6000 BCE.[9] Tobacco was used for medicinal and ceremonial purposes (usually in the form of pipe tobacco). Christopher Columbus returned to Europe with tobacco following his maiden voyage to the Western Hemisphere in 1492.[9] By the early 1600s, tobacco was grown commercially in the southern colonies to support the proliferation of European markets. A variety of tobacco products competed for consumer preference, including snuff, cigars, pipe tobacco, and self-rolled cigarettes. This was centuries before Big Tobacco coined the term, "nicotine delivery devices."

A major inflection point in the adoption of the smoking habit came as a result of James Albert Bonsack's invention of the cigarette rolling machine, introduced in 1881.[9] Thereafter, cigarettes could be cheaply mass-produced. Still, it took four decades for the cigarette product to gain popularity and accelerate past other forms of tobacco. Around World War I, cigarettes became the dominant tobacco product. Buoyed by effective tobacco marketing, cheap price, and the powerful grip of nicotine addiction, the widespread adoption of the cigarette habit has transformed global patterns of health and disease.[10]

Worldwide, cigarette smoking has been definitively and causally linked to the production of one-third of cancers (most notably lung cancer), chronic respiratory diseases, cardiovascular diseases, cognitive impairment (e.g., Alzheimer's disease), and preventable perinatal deaths. Fully 12% of deaths worldwide, equivalent to more than 5 million deaths per year in persons over the age of 30, are attributable to cigarette smoking.[11] Deaths are concentrated in the Americas and Europe where the tobacco habit has proliferated for more than a century. Considering mortality rates from noncommunicable diseases, tobacco is responsible for 36% of respiratory disease deaths, 22% of cancer deaths, and 10% of cardiovascular disease deaths. Tobacco use is especially notable for causing early death, accounting for 38% of deaths in the age range 30 to 44 years.

(continued)

Remarkably, it took decades to recognize that smoking produces adverse health outcomes. Smoking was socially "cool" in the mid-1900s and heavily marketed.[12] The U.S. government provided cigarettes to soldiers as a benefit, who then introduced their wives to smoking.[13] White-shirted electrical engineers smoked as they tinkered with their warehouse-sized computers. Nurses smoked. Physicians smoked. Cigarette advertising supported medical journals. Best known is the long-running series of "More doctors smoke Camels than any other cigarette" ads.[14]

When U.S. Surgeon General Luther Terry released the trailblazing volume, *Smoking and Health, Report of the Advisory Committee to the Surgeon General of the Public Health Service*, it was 1964.[15] At that time, smoking was a normative behavior for men (52.9% smoked) while 31.5% of women also smoked cigarettes. Almost two decades later, in 1982, more than a century after the automation of cigarette manufacturing, Surgeon General C. Everett Koop declared smoking to be "the chief, single, avoidable cause of death in our society and the most important public health issue of our time."[16]

Given the enormous burden of disease and death associated with cigarette smoking, let us now explore this health risk behavior using the first of the twin dimensions we are introducing in this chapter, the social ecological perspective. The life course perspective is examined in Case Study 5.2.

SOCIAL ECOLOGICAL PERSPECTIVE ON CIGARETTE SMOKING: INDIVIDUAL BEHAVIOR

We can best begin to understand the complex relationship between smoking and health starting at the most familiar level, the level of the self, the individual. At the level of the individual, cigarette smoking is a substance use behavior that has very high addiction potential based on the pharmacologic properties of nicotine acting on the reward circuitry of the brain.[17] With time and practice, each individual smoker develops a repertoire of smoking behaviors. Nicotine is a biphasic drug, capable of producing either stimulant or depressant effects. Therefore, smokers learn to titrate their dose of nicotine with each cigarette smoked. Studies of the "topography" of smoking[18] demonstrate that rapid puffing tends to increase alertness. Alternatively, taking long drags and holding the smoke in the lungs achieves a sensation of relaxation.[19] Further, smokers unconsciously modify their smoking behaviors to achieve their desired dose of nicotine, regardless of the actual nicotine content of the cigarette they are smoking.

Moreover, cigarette smoking is a highly "overlearned" habit that is repetitively reinforced. Each day, a pack-a-day (20 cigarettes per pack) smoker who takes 10 puffs per cigarette, on average, delivers 200 "hits" of nicotine directly and immediately to the brain via the oral mucosa (no need to wait for nicotine to enter the bloodstream and circulate to the brain—which also happens—to get the sensation).

Susceptibility to developing smoking-related chronic diseases is variable and difficult to predict at the individual level. However, the relationship becomes quite clear when epidemiologic studies examine patterns in populations. One of the most robust findings is the appearance of a stair-step or dose–response relationship that predicts increasing risks for developing new disease in direct relation to an increasing cumulative dose of smoking over time. Many measures have been

(*continued*)

used to estimate dosage. Researchers use measures such as total years of smoking or packs per day. These time and quantity measures can be combined into hybrid indicators such as "lifetime pack-years" of smoking. The risk for future lung cancer, for example, is greater for the two-pack-a-day smokers compared to one-pack-a-day smokers, who, in turn, are at higher risk compared to half-pack-a-day smokers.

Equally relevant at the individual level are other metrics that assess dose in relation to the tar and nicotine content of the preferred cigarette brand or quantify dose as a combination of cigarettes per day, puffs per cigarette, and millimeters of cigarette smoked.

Also, at the individual level, certain smoking behaviors are causally implicated in specified health outcomes. For example, women who smoke during pregnancy are endangering their own health and the health of the fetus. Maternal smoking elevates risks for preterm birth, low birth weight, and pregnancy complications that, at the extreme, increase the likelihood for infant or even maternal death.

SOCIAL ECOLOGICAL PERSPECTIVE ON CIGARETTE SMOKING: BETWEEN FAMILIES AND SOCIAL NETWORKS

Cigarette smoking is a socially learned behavior often initiated with the first offer of a cigarette from a family member or peer. Having smoking role models in close social proximity increases the likelihood that children will experiment with cigarettes. Children observe and replicate the behavior of caregivers and older siblings; children living in households where family members smoke are more likely to start smoking themselves. Both smoking and drinking alcohol have been shown to aggregate in families owing to a combination of shared genetics and household environment.[20-24] When a parent smokes, and the child is provided with social temptations to smoke, the likelihood of adopting the smoking habit is greater than for children whose parents do not smoke.[24] Moreover, smoking in the household exposes all occupants, including the children, to the health hazard of secondhand smoke.

Adolescents experience a period when the peer network exerts considerable influence. Smoking by peers strongly incentivizes youth to engage in trial and experimentation with cigarettes, which may continue to regular use.[25] Studies of peer influences indicate that smoking by peers within an adolescent's friendship network predicts smoking onset, continuation, and possible later cessation.[22,26]

Social network influences induce smoking experimentation and may support progression to regular use while nicotine dependency acts to maintain the cigarette habit once started. Further, adoption of the smoking habit usually does not occur as an isolated behavior. Children and adolescents who smoke cigarettes frequently experiment with multiple substance use behaviors (drinking alcohol, trying illicit drugs). Worldwide, smoking and other substance use tend to occur together within the context of a range of problem behaviors.[27]

Smoking is reinforced not only through the direct role modeling by peers but also as a marker of group cohesiveness among those who are receiving less positive reinforcement for prosocial behaviors. Youth who smoke, as a group, tend to have poorer academic achievement while in school and diminished levels of overall educational attainment. This is due, in part, to the fact that low-performing

(*continued*)

youth who smoke have friendship ties with others who both smoke and perform poorly in school.[28] School burnout is another independent predictor of youth smoking.[29]

As part of the repertoire of problem behaviors, male youth who smoke tend to have more involvement in delinquency and antisocial activities.[30] Smoking may be socially valued as one identifying attribute among those who disavow traditional, achievement-oriented norms.

SOCIAL ECOLOGICAL PERSPECTIVE ON CIGARETTE SMOKING: NEIGHBORHOODS

At the neighborhood level, social connections expand upward and outward to include the local schools where youth spend most of their waking hours along with a range of community institutions that provide organized and supervised youth-focused programming. These include community centers, sports programs, group lessons for developing and refining artistic and athletic skills, clubs, and civic-sponsored or faith-based youth programs.

Engagement in some of these neighborhood-level institutions and activities decreases the likelihood of smoking. For example, schools are smoke-free facilities surrounded by smoke-free zones. Also, for youth who participate in athletics, tobacco use is proscribed.

Conversely, neighborhoods also provide plentiful opportunities and numerous venues where youth can socialize in unstructured and unsupervised settings ranging from street hangouts to friends' homes to shopping malls. Some of these settings facilitate the initiation and maintenance of smoking behaviors.

Smoking incidence and prevalence vary in relation to such neighborhood population characteristics as socioeconomic status, educational attainment, employment status, types of occupations, and proportion of recent immigrants and their degree of acceptance and acculturation. Smoking incidence prior to age 17 is twice as high for children growing up in disadvantaged neighborhoods.[31] Researchers attribute this finding both to the family socioeconomic position and—back to social networks—the "intergenerational transmission of smoking behavior from parents to children."

In this regard, smoking rates and cigarette brand preferences differ by residents' race and even country of origin. Tobacco companies are savvy to these microvariations in population makeup; tobacco advertising is targeted down to the level of the block, billboard, and bus stop. Cigarette product sales and direct person-to-person promotions ultimately take place at the neighborhood level[32] with menthol brands promoted to African American/Black populations and Camels featured in Latinx neighborhoods.[33] Moreover, tobacco advertising is paired with selected public events that are likely to attract subpopulations of youth who are more likely to experiment with tobacco products as well as adult members of their social networks.

SOCIAL ECOLOGICAL PERSPECTIVE ON CIGARETTE SMOKING: CITIES

It is at the level of the city or municipality where a degree of environmental control over smoking may be exerted. Many cities have enacted clean air ordinances that prohibit smoking in designated areas including school zones, shopping malls, construction sites (due to explosion risks), and government offices. Clean air laws

(continued)

and their enforcement differ regionally, particularly in relation to the presence or absence of tobacco cultivation or tobacco product manufacturing in the local area.

City health departments, local universities, and nongovernmental organizations actively engage in nonsmoking promotional activities. Citywide smoking restrictions are not limited to cities in the United States. The WHO has developed guidance and support for cities worldwide to go smoke-free as one element of the global tobacco-control strategy. The WHO has published case studies from diverse smoke-free cities such as Nakuru, Kenya; Almaty, Kazakhstan; Davao, Philippines; Recife, Brazil; and Mecca, Saudi Arabia.[34]

SOCIAL ECOLOGICAL PERSPECTIVE ON CIGARETTE SMOKING: STATES

Beginning in the 1980s, U.S. states began to raise excise taxes on cigarettes and tobacco products, arguing that the burden of smoking-related disease was impacting state funding for healthcare. These initiatives occurred at the state level. National legislation was impossible in the face of strong political and corporate opposition from tobacco-producing states. In contrast, legislation was possible initially in states like Minnesota and California that prioritized health and did not cultivate tobacco or manufacture cigarettes. Over the course of decades, taxation of cigarettes became a powerful disincentive for smoking onset and maintenance because, for youth with minimal disposable income, the cost of cigarettes became prohibitively expensive.[4] Minnesota simulated the effect of state-level policies (SimSmoke model), particularly taxation, to determine the effects on smoking rates.[35] The simulation accurately predicted smoking prevalence between 1993 and 2011 and demonstrated that tobacco-control policies, particularly taxes, substantially reduced smoking prevalence in the state. Moreover, these policies will avert 48,000 smoking-attributable deaths by 2041.

Many states have passed smoke-free laws that prohibit smoking in government offices and public venues. Some states have created antitobacco initiatives that promote nonsmoking. One example is Tobacco Free Florida, funded by the proceeds from the massive legal settlement between the State of Florida and the major tobacco companies.[36] Tobacco Free Florida is particularly well known for a series of provocative ads featuring former smokers who have developed severe, disfiguring, or grotesque medical conditions.

SOCIAL ECOLOGICAL PERSPECTIVE ON CIGARETTE SMOKING: COUNTRIES AND POLICIES

Globally, some low-income and middle-income countries are witnessing alarming increases in smoking rates.[37,38] The combination of aggressive tobacco marketing, providing financial incentives to political leadership (giving monies for valuable programs in exchange for open markets), blocking tobacco-control legislation, and advertising to youth has led to a tremendous growth market.[39,40] In these economically vulnerable countries, tobacco companies boost profits while accelerating population-level addiction by dumping inexpensive, high tar and nicotine content, tobacco products on the market.

Meanwhile, in high-income countries, the recent ascendency of e-cigarettes is a direct result of strategic marketing decisions to broaden the potential product set available to smokers in the face of growing disfavor of combustible cigarettes.

(continued)

The WHO continuously monitors tobacco-control strategies adopted by various nations worldwide. Approaches include smoke-free environments, taxation, mass media, warning labels, advertising bans, and smoking cessation programs.

On the plus side, national-level policies can be instrumental in restricting access to tobacco, enforcing clean air policies, and heavily taxing tobacco products based on the disproportionate expenses incurred by smokers who become ill and whose medical expenses are subsidized through government-supported healthcare delivery and payment mechanisms. Multiple nations are competing to be among the first to be officially designated as smoke-free countries. Finland is well on the way to complete eradication of smoking. The Philippines put a nationwide smoking ban in place in May 2017. In the Western Hemisphere, Costa Rica is taking steps to become a completely smoke-free nation, and 13 countries have 100% smoke-free laws in place: Argentina, Barbados, Brazil, Colombia, Ecuador, El Salvador, Guatemala, Panamá, Perú, Honduras, Trinidad and Tobago, Uruguay, and Venezuela.

SOCIAL ECOLOGICAL PERSPECTIVE ON CIGARETTE SMOKING: CLASSIFYING SMOKING PROMOTIVE FACTORS

As a wrap-up to this first case study on cigarette smoking, we summarize smoking promotive factors by social ecological level in **Table 5.1**. Examples of promotive factors are catalogued from the individual behavior level up to and including the global level.

TABLE 5.1 Social Ecological Perspective: Smoking Promotive Factors by Social Ecological Level	
SOCIAL ECOLOGICAL LEVELS	**SMOKING PROMOTIVE FACTORS**
Individual behavior	• Influence from role models for smoking within the household—smoking by parents, siblings • Influence from role models for smoking among the peer group and social networks • Engagement in other substance use and/or problem behaviors • Engagement in a range of risk-taking behaviors • Lower-income levels/poverty • Lower levels of educational attainment • Addiction to nicotine locks in the smoking habit and makes it difficult to successfully quit
Family	• Role models for smoking living in the household • Smoking seen as normative behavior • Smoking behavior associated with family activities, recreation

(continued)

TABLE 5.1 Social Ecological Perspective: Smoking Promotive Factors by Social Ecological Level (*continued*)

SOCIAL ECOLOGICAL LEVELS	SMOKING PROMOTIVE FACTORS
Social network	• Role models for smoking among peer network members • Smoking seen as normative behavior • Smoking behavior associated with peer group activities, socialization • Smoking in homes of peers, friends • Smoking with peers in clubs, malls, video arcades, or other hangouts • Engagement in other substance use and/or problem behaviors within the peer group (e.g., smoking and drinking) • Propensity for and promotion of risk-taking behaviors within the peer group • Attending activities with tobacco company sponsorship (e.g., NASCAR races) • Adults: working or socializing in settings where smoking is permitted
Neighborhood	• Prevalent smoking in the neighborhood • Targeted tobacco advertising on billboards, bus stops • Point-of-sale advertising in neighborhood stores • Lack of clean air laws or lax enforcement • Limited or lack of smoking bans in public places • Smoking as a normative behavior throughout the neighborhood
City	• Prevalent smoking in city public spaces, worksites • Widespread tobacco advertising on billboards, bus stops • Point-of-sale advertising in retail stores that sell tobacco products • Lack of clean air laws or lax enforcement • Limited or lack of smoking bans in public places • Smoking as a normative behavior throughout the city • Concerts, sporting events, and other mass gathering events where smoking is permitted
State	• Prevalent smoking throughout the state/province/territory • Governmental support for tobacco industry/farmers (e.g., price supports) in tobacco growing states • State income from tobacco crops and manufacturing • Employment and earnings for tobacco farmers and tobacco manufacturing workforces • Lobbying and donations from tobacco interests in exchange for protections/freedom to promote product • Widespread advertising

(*continued*)

TABLE 5.1 Social Ecological Perspective: Smoking Promotive Factors by Social Ecological Level (*continued*)

SOCIAL ECOLOGICAL LEVELS	SMOKING PROMOTIVE FACTORS
Country	• Prevalent smoking—smoking as a normative behavior nationally • National tobacco companies in several nations—full government support and major sources of income • Promotion of electronic vapor products (e-cigarettes) into youth markets • Promotion of electronic vapor products (e-cigarettes) into adult markets as "quit smoking" alternatives • Lobbying and donations from tobacco interests in exchange for protections/freedom to promote product • Widespread advertising • Powerful political involvement and support for candidates who favor the tobacco industry
Global	• Multinational tobacco companies with broad diversification into multiple industries • Financial support from the tobacco industry to governments to keep tobacco products available and open doors to trade • Global tobacco product promotion and advertising • Tobacco "dumping" of high tar/nicotine content cigarettes into new markets

LIFE COURSE PERSPECTIVE

We now introduce the second critical element for our population health framework. The life course perspective brings the time dimension to understanding how health is produced and how disease progresses. Four phases of the life course are highlighted: ages 0 to 14 years, covering the perinatal, infancy, and childhood periods; ages 15 to 24, the adolescent and young adult years; ages 25 to 64, adulthood; and ages 65 and beyond, older adulthood (**Figure 5.3**).

How does the time trajectory of life itself produce health or disease? We discuss three models through which exposures, both positive and negative, can influence the future likelihood for attaining optimal health or, alternatively, the onset and progression of disease. These models are critical and sensitive periods, chains of risk, and accumulation of risk.

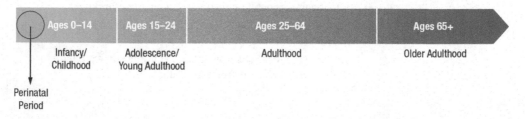

FIGURE 5.3 **The life course perspective with four life phases illustrated. Artistic credit: Parisa Varanloo.**

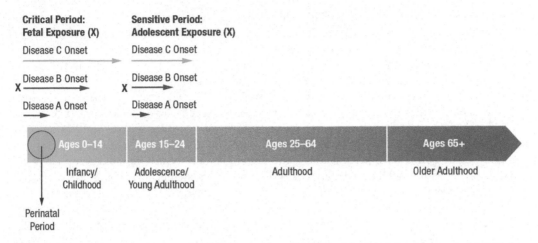

FIGURE 5.4 The life course and models of the production of health: critical and sensitive periods. Artistic credit: Parisa Varanloo.

CRITICAL AND SENSITIVE PERIODS

Figure 5.4 illustrates and differentiates critical and sensitive periods. The critical period model suggests that certain exposures, if they occur at a critical developmental moment, can strongly, perhaps singularly, influence future health outcomes. The period when the fetus is developing in utero is one particularly critical time. For example, mothers who regularly drink alcohol during pregnancy run the risk that their infants may be born with a fetal alcohol spectrum disorder (FASD). The features of FASD are often physically discernible due to the appearance and behavior of the infant and young child. This may include low body weight, short stature, small head size, lower intelligence, and problems with coordination. Fetal alcohol syndrome (FAS) is the most severe form of FASD. For youth born with FASD, problems may persist and multiply. These youth often struggle academically and are more prone to engage in higher risk behaviors and to develop substance use disorders.

In contrast to critical periods that are circumscribed to a single developmental period, sensitive periods (also described as susceptible or vulnerable periods) denote periods in the life span when exposures have greater impact than others. For example, thinking back to our youth, adolescence and early young adulthood is a period characterized by very active brain development. Exposures such as substance use during this sensitive period can short-circuit these vital neurological changes. This may lead to lifelong repercussions in terms of diminished educational achievement and career success that, in turn, carry implications for future health.

CHAINS OF RISK

Chains of risk involve exposures that occur in series (**Figure 5.5**). The term "chain" is appropriate for describing a domino-like sequence of risks. Multiple risks may add together in a relatively linear flow. Alternatively, one exposure may trigger multiple branching series of health consequences.

Some risk chains escalate, setting the individual on course toward a serious or fatal outcome. Consider youth who grow up in situations of social disadvantage. These individuals are more likely to experiment with tobacco smoking and develop regular smoking habits. Youth who smoke are

Chains of Risk:

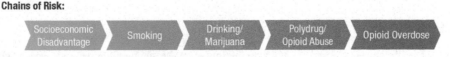

FIGURE 5.5 The life course and models of the production of health: chains of risk. Artistic credit: Parisa Varanloo.

more likely to drink alcohol. Smoking and drinking are regarded as common gateway behaviors for initiation of marijuana use. In turn, marijuana is frequently the first illicit drug tried and used regularly. However, youthful polysubstance users often do not stop with tobacco, alcohol, and marijuana. Instead, they may also experiment with a variety of harder drugs. In recent decades in the United States, based on drug availability, these adolescents and young adults have frequently tried opioid pain relievers that have been diverted to the illicit market. Mixing and matching opioids with street drugs elevates the risk for overdose. This has contributed to a recent surge in opioid overdose deaths.

The chains of risk model can also be usefully adapted to describe cascades of health-promoting behaviors. A talented subset of physically active youth who eat healthy diets and maintain normal body weight often become skilled in sports and athletic activities. Some develop sufficient prowess to be offered athletic scholarships in institutions of higher learning. Student athletes who perform well academically may graduate with prospects for well-paying careers and opportunities for advancement. These individuals tend to maintain their healthful lifestyles long term. Also, their professional trajectories create financial stability, which allows them to reside in safer neighborhoods that support healthy living.

ACCUMULATION OF RISK

The accumulation of risk model assumes that cumulative exposures or shocks throughout the life course increase the risk of diseases later in life, irrespective of timing (**Figure 5.6**). The model is well supported by numerous studies of lifestyle-related noncommunicable diseases (NCDs). Heart disease is one such example. Heart disease is strongly influenced by the social determinants of health including socioeconomic disadvantage.

Children who grew up in poor neighborhoods have fewer safe options for engaging in physical activity where they live. Considering our youth once again, children who engage in less physical activity are more prone to becoming overweight and developing obesity. Over a period of time, obesity increases risk for developing type 2 diabetes. High blood pressure is related to social disadvantage, physical inactivity, being overweight, and diabetes. The numbers of risk factors stack up. They accumulate. Risk factors cluster. They interact in a synergistic manner. This is the essence of the accumulation of risk model. Each and all of these risk factors elevate the likelihood for nonfatal heart disease episodes such as angina and heart attack. For many with this constellation of risk factors, the ultimate outcome is death from heart disease.

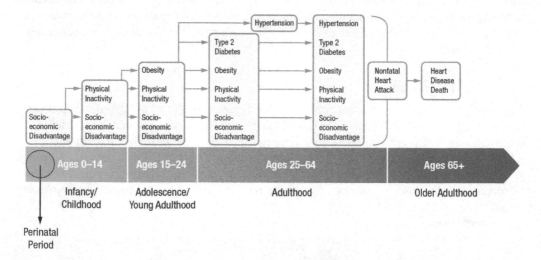

FIGURE 5.6 The life course and models of the production of health: accumulation of risk. Artistic credit: Parisa Varanloo.

CASE STUDY 5.2: CIGARETTE SMOKING: THE LIFE COURSE PERSPECTIVE

Now let us continue our exploration of cigarette smoking as a risk to population health, turning our focus toward the life course perspective. For this discussion, we describe the disease impact of cigarette smoking across the life span.

When discussing cigarette smoking, all three models just described—critical/sensitive periods, chains of risk, and accumulation of risk—are extremely salient. Cigarette smoking exerts its effects on health during critical periods (e.g., maternal smoking during pregnancy) and sensitive periods (e.g., peer modeling and encouragement for smoking experimentation in late childhood or early adolescence). As just noted, smoking cigarettes may be the first substance tried, acting as a "gatekeeper" for experimentation with alcohol and other drugs and setting off a cascade—or chain—of substance use and related problem behaviors. As we examine in detail, health risks associated with smoking accumulate over time to such an extreme that an estimated 50% of smokers will die from a smoking-related cause of death. We now visit each period of the life course in sequence, rappelling down into the health consequences of cigarette smoking.

LIFE COURSE PERSPECTIVE ON CIGARETTE SMOKING: PERINATAL PERIOD, INFANCY, AND CHILDHOOD (AGES 0–14)

Cigarette smoking by a pregnant mother affects the development of the fetus and influences pregnancy outcomes. Smoking by expectant mothers during pregnancy can be extremely detrimental to the health and survival of the developing fetus. In fact, maternal smoking has been described as the "first environmental risk factor of the unborn."[41]

Maternal smoking is causally related to short gestation and preterm birth and also to low birth weight regardless of the duration of the pregnancy. This places the fetus at a disadvantage for attaining viability. There is increased risk for fetal death, spontaneous abortion, and stillbirth.[42] These serious and deadly adverse outcomes relate to the dual actions of nicotine and carbon monoxide in cigarette smoke. While nicotine narrows blood vessels, including those in the umbilical cord, carbon monoxide binds to red blood cells, displacing oxygen. The combined effect is that of choking off the baby's oxygen supply.

Smoking doubles the rate of "short gestation/low birth weight" pregnancy outcomes. Babies who weigh less than 2,500 g (5.5 lb) at birth are considered to be low birth weight. Mothers who maintain a pack-a-day smoking habit during pregnancy truncate their babies' growth in the womb and, on average, their babies weigh one-half pound less at full term than babies of mothers who do not smoke.[43]

Maternal smoking increases the chances for maternal complications of pregnancy that can jeopardize the health of the fetus, the newborn, and the mother. Taken together, smoking poses significant risks to both mother and developing child. There is also a heightened likelihood of babies born with neurological deficits and congenital problems including heart defects. Nicotine crosses the placenta, so the newborn will also experience symptoms of nicotine withdrawal in the first days following birth. Pregnant smokers confer increased risks that their children will have lower IQs, learning disorders, and behavioral problems.

Breastfeeding infants whose lactating mothers smoke are exposed to nicotine in breast milk and experience changes in sleep patterns. On net, breastfeeding

(continued)

is protective for infants regardless of the smoking status of mothers, but smoking interferes with the lactational process, and smoking mothers are less likely to breastfeed and more likely to wean early.

Cigarette smoking by family members in the home produces secondhand (passive) smoking risks for all household members. Even if the mother does not smoke, her own health may be compromised during pregnancy by passive smoke exposure. A newborn is particularly susceptible to smoking by parents or household members. Passive smoking is a primary risk factor for sudden infant death syndrome (SIDS), a leading cause of infant death in the United States. Throughout childhood, youth who are exposed to environmental tobacco smoke are at greater risk for a range of respiratory conditions, including upper and lower respiratory infections, and also tuberculosis in areas of the world where the disease remains endemic. The onset and severity of asthma in childhood are related to, and exacerbated by, allergens in tobacco smoke.

Children exposed to passive smoking on the part of parents or household members are more likely to develop respiratory illnesses and miss more days of early childhood education, kindergarten, and primary grades than their peers who are not exposed to cigarette smoke at home.

Older childhood and early adolescence is a critical period for smoking initiation. Later childhood, ages 10 to 13, marks the period for "experimental" use of cigarettes, typically offered by same-age or older peers, at the developmental stage when children begin to migrate away from the parental sphere of influence. Tobacco companies astutely make high-nicotine, odorless "smokeless" alternatives to cigarettes that can addict adolescents to nicotine without detection by parents. Smokeless tobaccos have the social downside that users must chew and spit the product. So, within a few years, the transition is made to cigarettes; in fact, 95% of cigarette smokers initiate their tobacco habits prior to the age of 20 years. The introduction of e-cigarettes and vaping products has been rapidly supplanting the use of combustible cigarettes and, again, allows use by children and adolescents to go undetected.

LIFE COURSE PERSPECTIVE ON CIGARETTE SMOKING: ADOLESCENCE (AGES 15–24)

Early adolescence is the age when young people become addicted to cigarettes and when health risks transition from indirect, passive exposures to direct, self-inflicted, self-dosing exposures. Tobacco companies know that the great majority of regular smokers initiate smoking before age 20, and the product is heavily marketed, despite industry denials, to attract the adolescent market.[4] Enrolling youth into the ranks of active smokers is essential for tobacco companies to replenish their customer base, in part because older smokers die prematurely at higher rates than nonsmokers from smoking-related causes. Fortunately for the marketing of cigarettes, and unfortunately for the public's health, as youth continue to experiment with cigarettes, the habit rapidly becomes addictive. Once youth progress to regular smoking, quitting even a newly acquired habit is difficult and physiologically aversive. Specific to smoking-related diseases, respiratory illness is more common in adolescents and young adults who smoke or are regularly exposed to environmental tobacco smoke in home and other settings.

(continued)

LIFE COURSE PERSPECTIVE ON CIGARETTE SMOKING: ADULTS (AGES 25–64) AND OLDER ADULTS (AGES 65 AND OLDER)

Patterns of smoking-related illness and death extend throughout the entire life course. However, the greatest burden of illness, as well as premature death, due to smoking occurs during later adulthood and the older adult years. The adult years, ages 21 to 64, represent a period when many smokers maintain their addictive habits, dosing themselves daily with nicotine and progressively accumulating and concentrating cigarette smoke by-products in their oral and pharyngeal cavities, lungs, and other tissues. Frequently, decades of smoking are required to set off the specific carcinogenic changes that lead to a potentially fatal cancer. However, with most regular smokers beginning their habits in their teenage years, by the time smokers reach their later 40s and 50s, they have 30 or more "pack-years" of smoking exposure. Consider this: over a span of 30 years, a pack-a-day (20 cigarettes) smoker who averages 10 puffs per cigarette, will have self-administered 2,190,000 doses of nicotine and smoke by-products, certainly enough to damage tissues or trigger pathologic changes.

Mortality

Most nonsmokers sail through their adult years with minimal infirmity, and the large majority survive to become older adults. In the United States, while unintentional injury is the most common cause of death for all persons aged 20 to 44, cancer and heart disease take over as the leading causes of death during the 45 to 64 age period. Much of this very premature mortality, prior to the age of 65, is concentrated in the subpopulation of lifelong smokers.

One-in-two smokers will die from a tobacco-related cause of death. Beginning in the 40s, mortality rates for smokers exceed those for nonsmokers, and smoking-attributable mortality rates increase with age throughout the life span. Smokers die earlier in life than nonsmokers and have a shorter life expectancy. Their life course is truncated. Their longevity is time limited. Effectively, smokers come with an early expiration date.

Also notable, the insertion of cigarette smoking into the lifestyle has vaulted several diseases into prominence. Historically, some previously uncommon ailments contributed little to patterns of illness and death until the appearance of the cigarette. The two most notable examples are lung cancer and chronic obstructive pulmonary disease (COPD). Currently, for deaths from both lung cancer and COPD, the smoking-attributable fractions are close to 90%. This means that almost nine-in-10 deaths from these two causes are due to cigarette smoking. These are deaths that would not have occurred in a world without cigarettes, yet now, lung cancer and COPD rank among the leading causes of death worldwide.

Disease and Disability

Years-long patterns of exposure to the harmful effects of smoking produce life-changing and life-limiting disability. Nonfatal illnesses and not-yet-fatal episodes of chronic conditions related to smoking, such as heart disease, often precede

(*continued*)

death. Smokers are also more susceptible to infectious diseases and upper respiratory illnesses. They experience decreased pulmonary and cardiovascular function. This leads to more sick days, more work-loss days, decreased productivity, and decreased ability to participate in strenuous recreational activities and sports. Also, cigarette smoking is strongly associated with major depression. Debilitating depression is particularly problematic during the years of productive employment, leading to more work-loss and disability days, and decreased income and savings, at a critical point in the life cycle.

LIFE COURSE PERSPECTIVE ON CIGARETTE SMOKING: SUMMARIZING RISK BEHAVIORS AND DISEASE OUTCOMES BY LIFE COURSE PHASE

Bringing our journey through the life course to the close, we present a litany of smoking-related risk behaviors, diseases, and adverse health outcomes across the entire lifetime in **Table 5.2**.

TABLE 5.2 Life Course Perspective: Smoking Tobacco Cigarettes: Risk Behaviors and Disease Outcomes by Life Course Phase

LIFE COURSE PHASES	RISK BEHAVIORS	SMOKING-RELATED DISEASES AND ADVERSE OUTCOMES
Perinatal	• Expectant mother smoking cigarettes • Expectant mother: passive smoke exposure in home or worksite settings	• Ectopic pregnancy • Spontaneous abortion • Stillbirth and perinatal mortality • Maternal and fetal genetic polymorphisms • Low birth weight • Premature birth (short gestation) • Maternal complications of pregnancy • Birth defects (heart defects, clefting, clubfoot)
Infancy (first year of life)	• Infant: secondhand smoke exposure—mother, father, siblings, caregivers • Household members smoking cigarettes in home	• Nicotine in breast milk • Effects on neurocognitive development • SIDS • Increased frequency/severity of respiratory illness
Childhood (ages 1–14)	• Child: secondhand smoke exposure at home or in community settings	• SIDS • Increased frequency/severity of respiratory illness

(continued)

TABLE 5.2 Life Course Perspective: Smoking Tobacco Cigarettes: Risk Behaviors and Disease Outcomes by Life Course Phase (*continued*)

LIFE COURSE PHASES	RISK BEHAVIORS	SMOKING-RELATED DISEASES AND ADVERSE OUTCOMES
	• Older child: observing smoking by parents, siblings, older peers • First offer/trial of cigarettes • Early smoking habit	• Asthma • Elevated rates of ADHD, ODD, conduct disorder
Adolescence/young adulthood (ages 15–24)	• Peer role modeling of smoking • Transition to regular smoking • Addiction to nicotine • Increasing daily dose of cigarettes • Trial/possible adoption of drinking alcohol, and/or smoking marijuana, and/or other drug use • Polysubstance use • Possible engagement in problem behaviors • Early quit attempts	• Increased frequency/severity of respiratory illness • Asthma • Negative social stigma toward smokers
Middle adulthood (ages 25–44)	• Continued smoking • Repeated quit attempts • Periods of successful cessation • Relapse to smoking	• Increased frequency/severity of respiratory illness • Negative social stigma toward smokers • **Premature death**
Later adulthood (ages 45–64)	Varied smoking trajectories: • Continued smoking • Repeated quit attempts • Cycles of quitting and relapsing • Quitting after disease diagnosis • Successful long-term cessation	• **Cancers** of the lung, trachea, bronchus, lip, pharynx and oral cavity, esophagus, stomach, pancreas, larynx, cervix uteri (women), kidney and renal pelvis, liver, colon and rectum; acute myeloid leukemia • **Heart and vascular diseases:** coronary heart disease, stroke, rheumatic heart disease, pulmonary heart disease, atherosclerosis, aortic aneurysm, peripheral vascular disease, deep vein thrombosis

(continued)

TABLE 5.2	**Life Course Perspective: Smoking Tobacco Cigarettes: Risk Behaviors and Disease Outcomes by Life Course Phase (*continued*)**	
LIFE COURSE PHASES	**RISK BEHAVIORS**	**SMOKING-RELATED DISEASES AND ADVERSE OUTCOMES**
		• **Respiratory diseases:** COPD, respiratory infections, chronic bronchitis • **Other diseases:** diabetes mellitus, peptic ulcer, skin wrinkling and premature aging, infertility, erectile dysfunction • **Sense organs:** cataracts, macular degeneration, hearing loss, impaired sense of smell, impaired sense of taste • **Premature death**
Older ages (ages 65 and older)	Varied smoking trajectories: • Continued smoking • Repeated quit attempts • Cycles of quitting and relapsing • Quitting after disease diagnosis • Successful long-term cessation	• Same disease list as later adulthood, but higher rates and progressively more severe conditions with age • **Alzheimer's disease and other dementias** • **Premature death**

ADHD, attention deficit hyperactivity disorder; COPD, chronic obstructive pulmonary disease; ODD, oppositional defiant disorder; SIDS, sudden infant death syndrome.

CONSIDERING THE SOCIAL ECOLOGICAL AND LIFE COURSE DIMENSIONS TOGETHER

Now that we have discussed each framework, we can visually display both together. The multiple levels of the social ecological dimension can be considered to exert influences on population health throughout the entire life course. These dynamic interrelationships can be both health-promoting and health-compromising. Depending on the health issue, different levels within the social ecological sphere have greater or lesser influence during various phases in life.

We can create a matrix, showing the now-familiar phases of the life course timeline on the horizontal axis and multiple social ecological levels on the vertical axis. The number of life course phases and social ecological levels that appear in the matrix can be flexibly adapted depending on the application. As an illustration, in **Table 5.3**, we display five periods along the life course and we present four social ecological levels. This grid-like matrix structure allows us to visualize how health and disease are produced in populations at multiple levels in relation to phases of the life span.

We can also use this framework to plot the focus and the reach of interventions to promote health and mitigate disease risks. In quick succession, **Table 5.4** provides six examples that incorporate different social ecological levels and a variety of portions of the life course. We have intentionally selected a suite of intervention examples that do not overlap. Therefore, all six examples can be viewed simultaneously and compared in terms of their scope and range. We review all six examples in sequence.

TABLE 5.3   Matrix Displaying Social Ecological and Life Course Dimensions

SOCIAL ECOLOGICAL PERSPECTIVE	LIFE COURSE PERSPECTIVE				
	PERINATAL PERIOD	INFANCY AND CHILDHOOD	ADOLESCENCE AND YOUNG ADULTHOOD	ADULTHOOD	OLDER ADULTHOOD
Individual behavior					
Family/social networks					
Neighborhoods/cities					
Country/society					

TABLE 5.4   Six Examples of Public Health Interventions Presented on a Matrix Displaying Social Ecological and Life Course Dimensions

SOCIAL ECOLOGICAL PERSPECTIVE	LIFE COURSE PERSPECTIVE				
	PERINATAL PERIOD	INFANCY AND CHILDHOOD	ADOLESCENCE AND YOUNG ADULTHOOD	ADULTHOOD	OLDER ADULTHOOD
Individual behavior	Parental education and early childhood care guidance for new mothers			Supportive innovations for spouses and family members, caregivers of persons with Alzheimer's disease	
Family					
Social networks			Drug abuse prevention targeting adolescent peer groups		
Neighborhoods/ cities		Community-based childhood obesity prevention	Seat belt laws and legal penalties for drinking and driving, driving while texting		
Country/society	National and global initiatives and international alliances to combat the health effects of climate change				

First, consider *prenatal education and early childhood care guidance for new mothers.* Where would this fit in the matrix? In Table 5.4, this intervention is primarily targeted at the social ecological levels of individual behavior and family/social networks, intersecting with the perinatal, infancy, and very early childhood portions of the life course.

Second, consider *supportive interventions for spouses and family member caregivers of persons with Alzheimer's disease.* Table 5.4 displays this intervention at the individual behavior and family/social network levels, intersecting with the adult and older adult life course periods. Family caregivers to older adults with Alzheimer's disease tend to be similar-age spouses and next-younger-generation children of the affected parent.

Third, consider *drug abuse prevention targeting adolescent peer groups.* Table 5.4 portrays this intervention in a single cell of the matrix, representing the social network level for the adolescent/young adulthood age group.

Fourth, consider *community-based childhood obesity prevention.* Table 5.4 shows the social ecological level as neighborhoods and cities and childhood as the most relevant stage in the life course. Certainly, the public health professionals who design and deliver the intervention will be from an older generation, but the focus of the intervention itself is on children. If more details are provided indicating the explicit involvement of families or social networks, the scope could be expanded in the matrix.

Fifth, consider *seat belt laws and legal penalties for drinking and driving or drinking and texting.* Where would this fit in the matrix? These laws are enacted at state levels, including neighborhoods and cities, and administered by law enforcement personnel in municipalities. Licensed drivers include a wide age range, from adolescents to older adults.

Sixth, consider *national and global initiatives and international alliances to combat the health effects of climate change.* These initiatives, such as the annual Conference of the Parties (COP) summits, which include most nations worldwide as signatories, certainly fit well at the country and international levels and have health implications for citizens of all ages.

We conclude this section with two examples that display a broader range of social ecological levels and are based on existing operational programs. First, consider *an evidence-based, multilevel breastfeeding promotion program that has been developed to focus on low-income African American/Black women.*[44] The program incorporates both Healthy Start and the Baby-friendly Hospital Initiative. **Table 5.5** shows how this real-world program fits into the matrix. Notice that

TABLE 5.5 Two Examples of Public Health Interventions Extending Across a Range of Social Ecological Levels

SOCIAL ECOLOGICAL PERSPECTIVE	LIFE COURSE PERSPECTIVE				
	PERI-NATAL PERIOD	INFANCY AND CHILDHOOD	ADOLESCENCE AND YOUNG ADULTHOOD	ADULTHOOD	OLDER ADULTHOOD
Individual behavior	Evidence-based, multilevel breastfeeding promotion program		"This is not about drugs" program:		
Family			• Opioid prevention program for youth, grades 6–12 (ages 12–18)		
Social networks	Focus on low-income African American/Black women		• Focus on individuals, families, schools, communities in 18+ states		
Neighborhoods/cities	Involves Healthy Start, "Baby-friendly Hospital Initiative"		• 200+ delivery partners		
Country/society					

the perinatal period, infancy, and early childhood years are relevant to this intervention. This program spans a broad swath of the social ecological dimension, ranging from individual behavior up to the levels of neighborhoods and cities.

The second example is an ambitious *program aimed at prevention of opioid drug use by children and adolescents, ages 12 to 18 years (grades 6–12).*[45] The program goes by the name "This is not about drugs." This program explicitly claims to address individuals, families, schools, and communities. However, program administration goes as high as the city and state levels. In fact, this intervention is now adopted by about 20 states and is delivered by hundreds of community partners.

CASE STUDY 5.3: CIGARETTE SMOKING: CONSIDERING THE SOCIAL ECOLOGICAL AND LIFE COURSE DIMENSIONS TOGETHER

Our third rendition of a case study (Case Study 5.3), with a dedicated focus on cigarette smoking, is summarized in a detailed table. **Table 5.6** provides a detailed set of preventive actions and interventions, arrayed across our three life course phases. From the individual behavior level up to the city level of the social ecological dimension, separate examples are provided for each life course phase. At the state, country, and global levels, based on potential benefits derived by the whole of society, we provide examples of programs, policies, and interventions that cut across the entire life course.

This case study showcases how our two dimensions—social ecological and life course—fit together well in the matrix we have just introduced. The matrix itself (Table 5.6) effectively is the case study. You can access the podcast accompanying Case Study 5.3 by following the link to Springer Publishing Company Connect™ at http://connect.springerpub.com/content/book/978-0-8261-8043-8/part/part01/chapter/ch05).

TABLE 5.6 Combining the Social Ecological and Life Course Perspectives: Smoking Intervention Options by Social Ecological Level and Life Course Phase

SOCIAL ECOLOGICAL LEVELS	LIFE COURSE PHASES		
	PERINATAL PERIOD, INFANCY, CHILDHOOD, AND ADOLESCENCE	ADULTHOOD	OLDER AGE
Individual behavior	Childbirth counseling Quit programs for pregnant smokers Breastfeeding Well-baby visits Smoke-free home Prevention programs for school-age youth Health promotion education Tobacco age/sales restrictions Monitoring teen smoking trends Counteradvertising	Healthy lifestyle education targeted for adults Monitoring adult smoking trends	Health promotion education Engaging older adults to educate youth about tobacco risks

(*continued*)

TABLE 5.6 Combining the Social Ecological and Life Course Perspectives: Smoking Intervention Options by Social Ecological Level and Life Course Phase (*continued*)

SOCIAL ECOLOGICAL LEVELS	LIFE COURSE PHASES		
	PERINATAL PERIOD, INFANCY, CHILDHOOD, AND ADOLESCENCE	ADULTHOOD	OLDER AGE
Family	Smoke-free home Family support Support for nonsmoking	Partner/family support to quit/select healthful behaviors	Partner/children/family support to quit
Social network	Pregnant women: Socializing with nonsmokers Smoke-free worksites Nonsmokers in peer network Involvement in healthful peer activities	Peer support to live healthfully/quit smoking	Peer/community support to live healthfully/quit smoking
Neighborhood physicians/healthcare system	Prenatal visits Quit programs for pregnant smokers Pediatric visits Advice on preventing onset of smoking Adolescent health visits Guidance on nonsmoking, addiction, quitting	Guidance on addiction, quitting Rx for nicotine replacement Rx for quit programs	Guidance on addiction, quitting Rx for nicotine replacement Rx for quit programs
Neighborhood	Smoke-free norms, daycare, school zones, neighborhood public spaces	Smoke-free norms and neighborhood public spaces Community-based cessation options	Smoke-free senior centers Community-based cessation options
City	Smoke-free norms City clean air acts Smoke-free norms, schools, parks, malls, public spaces	City-supported cessation options Smoke-free norms, public spaces, malls City clean air acts	City-supported cessation options Smoke-free norms, public spaces, malls City clean air acts

(*continued*)

TABLE 5.6 Combining the Social Ecological and Life Course Perspectives: Smoking Intervention Options by Social Ecological Level and Life Course Phase (*continued*)

SOCIAL ECOLOGICAL LEVELS	LIFE COURSE PHASES		
	PERINATAL PERIOD, INFANCY, CHILDHOOD, AND ADOLESCENCE	ADULTHOOD	OLDER AGE
State	• Comprehensive state clean air laws • Smoke-free state government facilities • Tobacco litigation to fund state nonsmoking programs • Ongoing monitoring of smoking-attributable mortality, morbidity, economic costs • State taxation of tobacco products • Enforcement of tobacco sales, especially prohibiting sales to minors • Promotion of state-endorsed nonsmoking curricula for use in elementary through secondary schools • Tobacco counteradvertising • Monitoring of youth and adult smoking rates through the state health office		
Country	• Leadership to combat adoption of the tobacco habit from national health departments and ministries • Active participation by national organizations dedicated to specific disease prevention (e.g., cancer and heart associations) • National legislation for smoke-free environments/clean air regulations • Smoking prevention curricula • Physician-guided and community-based cessation programs • Mass media counteradvertising • National taxation of tobacco products • Tobacco advertising restrictions/bans		
	• Warning labels on tobacco products and electronic vapor products • Import bans on tobacco products • Sales restrictions including age restrictions and point-of-sale restrictions • Smoking-and-health research and dissemination of findings • Identification and promotion of evidence-based smoking prevention and intervention programs • Tobacco litigation to recoup the excess costs of smoking-related diseases • Smoke-free country designation (e.g., Costa Rica)		

(*continued*)

TABLE 5.6 **Combining the Social Ecological and Life Course Perspectives: Smoking Intervention Options by Social Ecological Level and Life Course Phase** (*continued*)

SOCIAL ECOLOGICAL LEVELS	LIFE COURSE PHASES		
	PERINATAL PERIOD, INFANCY, CHILDHOOD, AND ADOLESCENCE	ADULTHOOD	OLDER AGE
Global	• Leadership to combat adoption of the tobacco habit from World Health Organization and health-focused multinationals • Active participation by international organizations dedicated to specific disease prevention (e.g., cancer and heart associations) • Smoke-free environments/clean air regulations • Smoking prevention curricula • Physician-guided and community-based cessation programs • Mass media counteradvertising • Taxation of tobacco products • Import bans on tobacco products • Sales restrictions including age restrictions and point-of-sale restrictions • Smoking-and-health research and dissemination of findings • Identification and promotion of evidence-based smoking prevention and intervention programs • Promotion of smoke-free nations		

Rx, prescription.

SUMMARY

In public health, we routinely describe patterns of health and disease in terms of person, place, and time characteristics. Here we explain what causes the health of populations (the person dimension) by employing two frameworks. We examine the place dimension (both geographically and socially) using the multiple levels of the social ecological framework. For simplicity, we select three levels—individual behavior; family, social network, neighborhoods, and cities; and countries, policies, and health. In parallel, we examine the time dimension using the multiple phases of the life course. Again, for simplicity, we select three life periods: perinatal, infancy, childhood, and adolescence; adulthood; and older adult ages. In the realm of the life course perspective, we describe how health and disease are produced during critical or sensitive periods of life, and how risks may operate sequentially or accumulate over time to amplify the likelihood that disease will occur.

We use an expanded case study that applies our two frameworks to illustrate how cigarette smoking influences the production of health and disease at multiple social ecological levels across the entire life course. The social ecological and life course perspectives not only create a useful framework for understanding the production of health, but also interact in a dynamic manner. We use these social ecological and life course frameworks throughout this book to describe health behavior, the operation of risk factors, the diversity of disease patterns, and the development and targeting of interventions to improve and optimize health.

End-of-Chapter Resources

Access additional case study podcasts online at http://connect.springerpub.com/ content/book/978-0-8261-8043-8/

DISCUSSION QUESTIONS

1. What social ecological levels are most important in delivering interventions to prevent e-cigarette use among adolescents?
2. What social media channels would you use to encourage adolescents, adults, and older adults to get annual preventive medical checkups?
3. How do "chains of risk" and "accumulation of risk" apply to the risk of becoming addicted to opioids?

 A robust set of instructor resources designed to supplement this text is located at **http://connect.springerpub.com/content/book/978-0-8261-8043-8.** Qualifying instructors may request access by emailing **textbook@springerpub.com.**

REFERENCES

1. Keyes KM, Galea S. *Population Health Science.* Oxford University Press; 2016. https://global.oup.com/ academic/product/population-health-science-9780190459376?cc=us&lang=en&
2. World Health Organization. *Constitution of WHO: Principles*; 2016. https://www.who.int/about/governance/ constitution#:~:text=The%20Constitution%20was%20adopted%20by,are%20incorporated%20into%20this%20text
3. Krieger N. Epidemiology and the web of causation: has anyone seen the spider? *Soc Sci Med.* 1994;39:887-903.
4. Krieger N. Theories for social epidemiology in the 21st century: an ecosocial perspective. *Int J Epidemiol.* 2001;30(4):668-677. doi:10.1093/ije/30.4.668
5. Levins R, Lopez C. Toward an ecosocial view of health. *Int J Health Serv.* 1999;29(2):261-293.
6. Susser M, Susser E. Choosing a future for epidemiology: II. From black box to Chinese boxes and eco-epidemiology. *Am J Public Health.* 1996;86(5):674-677.
7. Kuh D, Ben-Shlomo Y, ed. *A Life Course Approach to Chronic Disease Epidemiology.* Oxford University Press; 1997.
8. Elder GH, Johnson MK, Crosnoe R. The emergence and development of life course theory. In: Mortimer JT, Shanahan MJ, eds. *Handbook of the Life Course.* Springer; 2003:3-19.
9. World Health Organization. *The History of Tobacco.* https://www.afro.who.int/sites/default/files/2017-09/ Chapter%2032.%20The%20history%20of%20tobacco.pdf
10. Samet JM, Thornton FL, eds. *The Health Consequences of Smoking—50 Years of Progress.* Centers for Disease Control and Prevention; 2014. https://www.ncbi.nlm.nih.gov/books/NBK179276
11. *WHO Global Report: Mortality Attributable to Tobacco.* World Health Organization; 2012. https://www.who .int/publications/i/item/9789241564434
12. *The rise and fall of tobacco advertising—in pictures. The Guardian.* Published January 22, 2015. https://www .theguardian.com/society/gallery/2015/jan/22/the-rise-and-fall-of-tobacco-advertising-in-pictures
13. Tobacco Prevention for K-12 Educators. *Tobacco industry and the connection to the military.* Published November 11, 2011. https://tobaccopreventionk12.wordpress.com/2011/11/11/tobacco-industry-and-the -connection-to-the-military
14. Gardner MN, Brandt AM. "The doctors' choice is America's choice": the physician in US cigarette advertisements, 1930–1953. *Am J Public Health.* 2006;96(2):222-232. doi:10.2105/AJPH.2005.066654
15. Surgeon General's Advisory Committee on Smoking and Health. *Smoking and Health: Report of the Advisory Committee to the Surgeon General of the Public Health Service.* Public Health Service Publication No. 1103. Office of the Surgeon General; 1964. https://profiles.nlm.nih.gov/ps/retrieve/ResourceMetadata/NNBBMQ
16. Reinhold R. *Surgeon General Report broadens list of cancers linked to smoking. New York Times.* February 23, 1982:1. https://www.nytimes.com/1982/02/23/science/surgeon-general-report-broadens -list-of-cancers-linked -to-smoking.html

17. National Institute on Drug Abuse. *Tobacco, nicotine, and e-cigarettes research report: is nicotine addictive?* Accessed January 2018. https://nida.nih.gov/publications/research-reports/tobacco-nicotine-e-cigarettes/nicotine-addictive

18. Hammond D, Fong GT, Cummings KM, Hyland A. Smoking topography, brand switching, and nicotine delivery: results from an in vivo study. *Cancer Epidemiol Biomarkers Prev.* 2005;*14*(6):1370-1375.

19. Center for Health Promotion and Education. *The health consequences of smoking: nicotine addiction: a report of the surgeon general.* Author; 1988. https://profiles.nlm.nih.gov/NN/B/B/Z/D

20. Bierut LJ, Dinwiddie SH, Begleiter H, et al. Familial transmission of substance dependence: alcohol, marijuana, cocaine, and habitual smoking: a report from the collaborative study on the genetics of alcoholism. *Arch Gen Psychiatry.* 1998;*55*(11):982-988. doi:10.1001/archpsyc.55.11.982

21. Boyle MH, Sanford M, Szatmari P, et al. Familial influences on substance use by adolescents and young adults. *Can J Public Health.* 2001;*92*(3):206-209. doi:10.1007/BF03404307

22. Smith KP, Christakis NA. Social networks and health. *Annu Rev Sociol.* 2008;*34*(1):405-429.

23. Avenevoli S, Merikangas KR. Familial influences on adolescent smoking. *Addiction.* 2003;*98*(suppl 1):1-20. doi:10.1046/j.1360-0443.98.s1.2.x

24. Wilkinson AV, Shete S, Prokhorov AV. The moderating role of parental smoking on their children's attitudes toward smoking among a predominantly minority sample: a cross-sectional analysis. *Subst Abuse Treat Prev Policy.* 2008;*3*(1):18. doi:10.1186/1747-597X-3-18

25. Chen PH, White HR, Pandina RJ. Predictors of smoking cessation from adolescence into young adulthood. *Addict Behav.* 2001;*26*(4):517-529. doi:10.1016/S0306-4603(00)00142-8

26. Kaplan CP, Nápoles-Springer A, Stewart SL, Pérez-Stable EJ. Smoking acquisition among adolescents and young Latinas: the role of socioenvironmental and personal factors. *Addict Behav.* 2001;*26*(4):531-550. doi:10.1016/S0306-4603(00)00143-X

27. Cai Y, Li R, Zhu J, et al. Personality, perceived environment, and behavior systems related to future smoking intentions among youths: an application of problem-behavior theory in Shanghai, China. *PLoS One.* 2015;*10*(3):e0122276. doi:10.1371/journal.pone.0122276

28. Robert P-O, Kuipers MAG, Rathmann K, et al. Academic performance and adolescent smoking in 6 European cities: the role of friendship ties. *Int J Adolesc Youth.* 2019;*24*(1):125-135.

29. Kinnunen JM, Lindfors P, Rimpelä A, et al. Academic well-being and smoking among 14- to 17-year-old schoolchildren in six European cities. *J Adolesc.* 2016;*50*:56-64. doi:10.1016/j.adolescence.2016.04.007

30. Sanchagrin K, Heimer K, Paik A. Adolescent delinquency, drinking, and smoking: does the gender of friends matter? *Youth Soc.* 2017;*49*(6):805-826. doi:10.1177/0044118X14563050

31. Morris T, Manley D, Van Ham M. Context or composition: how does neighbourhood deprivation impact upon adolescent smoking behaviour? *PLoS One.* 2018;*13*(2):e0192566. doi:10.1371/journal.pone.0192566

32. Seidenberg AB, Caughey RW, Rees VW, Connolly GN. Storefront cigarette advertising differs by community demographic profile. *Am J Health Promot.* 2010;*24*(6):e26-e31. doi:10.4278/ajhp.090618-QUAN-196

33. Dauphinee AL, Doxey JR, Schleicher NC, et al. Racial differences in cigarette brand recognition and impact on youth smoking. *BMC Public Health.* 2013;*13*(1):170. doi:10.1186/1471-2458-13-170

34. World Health Organization Centre for Health Development. *Making cities smoke-free.* 2011. https://www.who.int/publications/i/item/9789241502832

35. Levy DT, Boyle RG, Abrams DB. The role of public policies in reducing smoking: the Minnesota SimSmoke tobacco policy model. *Am J Prev Med.* 2012;*43*(5 suppl 3):S179-S186. doi:10.1016/j.amepre.2012.07.037

36. *Tobacco Free Florida.* 2023. http://tobaccofreeflorida.com

37. Wiblin R. *Smoking in the developing world.* 80,000 Hours. Published April 6, 2016. https://80000hours.org/problem-profiles/tobacco

38. World Health Organization. *WHO Report on the Global Tobacco Epidemic, 2008: the MPOWER package.* Published 2008. https://apps.who.int/iris/handle/10665/43818

39. Gilmore A. *Big tobacco targets the young in poor countries – with deadly consequences. The Guardian.* December 1, 2015. https://www.theguardian.com/global-development/2015/dec/01/big-tobacco-industry-targets-young-people-poor-countries-smoking

40. Sebrié E, Glantz SA. The tobacco industry in developing countries. *BMJ.* 2006;*332*(7537):313-314. doi:10.1136/bmj.332.7537.313

41. Mund M, Louwen F, Klingelhoefer D, Gerber A. Smoking and pregnancy—a review on the first major environmental risk factor of the unborn. *Int J Environ Res Public Health.* 2013;*10*(12):6485-6499.

42. Marufu TC, Ahankari A, Coleman T, Lewis S. Maternal smoking and the risk of still birth: systematic review and meta-analysis. *BMC Public Health.* 2015;*15*(1):239. doi:10.1186/s12889-015-1552-5

43. Miles K, Urang S (Medical Reviewer). *Smoking during pregnancy.* BabyCenter. https://www.babycenter.com/pregnancy/health-and-safety/how-smoking-during-pregnancy-affects-you-and-your-baby_1405720

44. Leruth C, Goodman J, Bragg B, Gray D. A multilevel approach to breastfeeding promotion: using healthy start to deliver individual support and drive collective impact. *Matern Child Health J.* 2017;*21*(suppl 1):4-10. doi:10.1007/s10995-017-2371-3

45. Overdose Lifeline. *This is not about drugs: an educational program designed to specifically address the opioid health crisis.* Published 2015. https://www.overdose-lifeline.org/opioid-heroin-prevention-education-program.html

A SOCIAL ECOLOGICAL APPROACH: WHAT CAUSES HEALTH AND WHAT WE CAN DO ABOUT IT

6

INDIVIDUAL BEHAVIOR

LEARNING OBJECTIVES

- Compare and contrast modifiable and nonmodifiable individual risk factors.
- Summarize reasons why individuals engage in unhealthy behaviors.
- Discuss how social, economic, and political factors interact with individual health behaviors.
- Discuss the underlying assumptions and purpose of the health belief model.
- Identify features of effective individual behavior change interventions.

OVERVIEW: HEALTH HAPPENS AND IS EXPERIENCED IN INDIVIDUALS

In population health science, we are concerned with the conditions that shape distributions of health across and within populations and how these conditions affect the health of individuals. As we discuss throughout this book, populations are composed of individuals with common characteristics or attributes (e.g., adults living in the United States, children born in Nigeria, and adolescents with attention deficit hyperactivity disorder). So, what makes an individual healthy? There are many ways to answer this question. We could say that to be healthy, we need to have a healthy diet, get regular exercise and annual physical examinations, have an active and supportive social network, set goals and boundaries, and have a positive outlook on life. The list could go on and on. And all of these are important elements indeed.

In this chapter, we (a) explain how individual behavior can create health and disease, (b) discuss how theories of behavior and behavior change inform our understanding of the interrelationship between behavior and health, (c) describe how public health interventions modify individual behavior and influence health, and (d) analyze why behavior change by itself is seldom successful without action on the other social ecological levels.

HEALTH BEHAVIORS AND THE CAUSES OF INDIVIDUAL HEALTH

UNDERSTANDING THE CAUSES OF INDIVIDUAL HEALTH

Individual causes of health can be broadly categorized as genetic and nonmodifiable biological factors versus factors that are modifiable and can, in theory, be changed by individuals. All of these factors, regardless of their classification, are called risk factors. When we talk of "risk factors," we do not imply only those factors that increase risk. Some risk factors are risk-elevating while others are risk-reducing and even protective. As such, having—or being exposed to—a risk factor does not signify that an individual will develop disease but rather that exposure to the risk factor modifies their future likelihood of developing disease.

Genetic and Other Nonmodifiable Risk Factors

Genetic risk refers to the impact that genes have on developing certain conditions and diseases. Individuals inherit genes from their parents, and dominant genes mask the effects of recessive genes. Consider for example an individual's eye color. It was once thought that an individual's eye color was determined by a single gene, with brown eye color being dominant and blue recessive. That would imply that two blue-eyed parents could never have a brown-eyed child. As it turns out, it is not quite as simple as that.[1] Eye color is based on inheritance of a combination of genes, and in fact, it is possible (albeit unlikely) for two blue-eyed parents to have a brown-eyed child.

Genetics represent an important determinant of individual health. Individuals who inherit specific genes may be at increased risk for developing certain diseases such as cardiovascular disease or breast cancer. Nevertheless, a specific genetic makeup influences, rather than mandates, that an individual will develop disease. The effects of genetics on both common and complex diseases are due to the interplay among many genes. Advances in technology such as whole genome sequencing have led to a dramatic increase in new discoveries of important genetic risk factors. Discoveries of effective interventions, however, have been slower to develop.

> **Genetics represent an important determinant of individual health. Individuals who inherit specific genes may be at increased risk for developing certain diseases such as cardiovascular disease or breast cancer.**

Beyond the potent influence of genetics, other prominent nonmodifiable risk factors include age, biological sex assigned at birth, and race/ethnicity. Moving along the life course stages, age tends to exert a risk-elevating influence, with risk for many unhealthy outcomes rising with increasing age. In fact, it may not be an individual's age that specifically causes disease but other changes that occur with aging.

Biological sex assigned at birth is a risk factor insofar as incidence and mortality rates for many diseases differ by sex. The impact of sex on disease risk may interact with other risk factors. For example, while males have a higher risk for incident cardiovascular disease compared with premenopausal females, this male–female risk differential disappears after women reach menopause. Gender, a social construct, brings with it other differential risks due to individual behavioral differences, and is not to be confused with biological sex.

Nonmodifiable risk factors often act as proxies or surrogates for other factors that cause or determine disease. For example, race/ethnicity is not modifiable, but there is much discussion about whether it is truly a risk factor for certain diseases or whether racism (structural, environmental, political) is the underlying risk factor.[2] Even when there are documented differences in a number of health outcomes by race/ethnicity (e.g., maternal mortality), we must be careful not to attribute differences in health outcomes to the color of one's skin or to certain cultural practices or experiences when it is actually something else.[3] Social context and exposures linked to race, including pervasive racism and discrimination that characterize our society, powerfully drive racial differences in health.

There are also documented differences in health outcomes by education and income. In theory, these are modifiable risk factors, but do some individuals actually have the opportunity or social power to modify them? This ultimately gets at the core role that context plays in shaping our health, as described by the social ecological model.

In population health science, we aim to uncover the true causes or determinants of health such as socioeconomic status and early influences in life (which we discuss in more detail when we delve into the life course) that are sometimes masked by characteristics such as sex and race/ethnicity.

Modifiable Risk Factors

Smoking, diet, and physical activity are examples of modifiable risk factors. Consuming a diet high in fat or smoking cigarettes are risk-elevating behaviors that increase the incidence and mortality rates for multiple diseases. Conversely, engaging in regular cardiovascular and resistance exercises as part of a physical activity regimen is a risk-reducing behavior that decreases disease incidence and mortality.

There is yet another category of metabolic risk factors that increase risk for many diseases. Elevations of blood pressure, low-density lipoprotein (LDL) cholesterol, and body mass index (BMI) increase risks for cardiovascular diseases. In other instances, abnormally low values of various factors may be associated with elevated rates of disease. Examples include low bone mineral density (a risk for osteoporosis), low high-density lipoprotein (HDL) cholesterol (a risk for heart disease), and low glomerular filtration rate (a risk for end-stage renal disease).

Some risk factors elevate incidence and mortality for multiple diseases. For example, cigarette smoking is a causal, risk-elevating factor for a broad range of cancers (cancers of the lung, trachea, bronchus, larynx, esophagus, oral cavity, stomach, pancreas, uterine cervix, bladder, liver, colon, and rectum; acute myeloid leukemia), coronary heart disease, diabetes mellitus, stroke, and chronic obstructive pulmonary disease, among other diseases.

There are complex relationships among different categories of risk factors. For example, environmental and social risk factors (e.g., education and income) interact with individual behavioral risk factors such as physical activity, diet, alcohol consumption, and other drug use, which in turn affect metabolic risk factors such as BMI, blood pressure, and cholesterol. All of these risk factors, taken together, affect the likelihood that an individual develops disease.

Risk Factor and Disease Cascades

Another dimension to consider is that some diseases, with their own sets of behavioral and social risk factors, are themselves risk factors for other diseases. How does this work? Consider obesity. About one-in-three Americans is clinically obese, with a BMI of 30 kg/m^2 or higher. Obesity is a diagnosable and treatable disease, with its own diagnosis codes and a set of definable risk factors including a diet high in calories from fats and carbohydrates coupled with physical inactivity.

However, obesity is also a primary risk factor for the later development of diabetes mellitus and hypertension. Now, along with obesity, both diabetes and hypertension are diseases, with their own diagnosis codes and sets of risk factors, but it does not stop there. Obesity, diabetes mellitus, and hypertension—all diseases in their own right—are also risk factors for coronary heart disease. So here we have a cascade of behavioral risk factors and diagnosable clinical diseases combining together to amplify the risks for severe downstream noncommunicable diseases (NCDs) like heart disease that have multifactorial causation.

Global Patterns of Risk Factors for Death in Relation to Country-Level Income Categories

On a global basis, the predominant risk factors associated with death vary by socioeconomic and income status of the country (**Table 6.1**). For example, in low-income countries, the leading risk factor for death is particulate matter pollution (air pollution) followed by low birth weight and short gestation, and high systolic blood pressure. In high-income countries, the leading risk

TABLE 6.1   Top 10 Risk Factors for Death Worldwide and for Low-, Middle-, and High-Income Countries, 2019

	GLOBAL
1	High systolic blood pressure
2	Smoking (tobacco use)
3	High fasting plasma glucose
4	Particulate matter pollution (air pollution)
5	High body mass index (obesity)
6	High LDL cholesterol
7	Kidney disfunction (impaired kidney function)
8	Alcohol use
9	Diet high in sodium
10	Diet high in whole grains
	LOW-INCOME COUNTRIES
1	Particulate matter pollution (air pollution)
2	Low birth weight and short gestation
3	High systolic blood pressure
4	Child growth failure
5	Unsafe water source
6	High fasting plasma glucose
7	Unsafe sanitation
8	Smoking (tobacco use)
9	No access to handwashing facility
10	High body mass index (obesity)
	MIDDLE-INCOME COUNTRIES
1	High systolic blood pressure
2	Smoking (tobacco use)
3	High fasting plasma glucose
4	Particulate matter pollution (air pollution)
5	High body mass index (obesity)
6	High LDL cholesterol

(*continued*)

TABLE 6.1   Top 10 Risk Factors for Death Worldwide and for Low-, Middle-, and High-Income Countries, 2019 (*continued*)

7	Kidney dysfunction (impaired kidney function)
8	Diet high in sodium
9	Alcohol use
10	Diet low in whole grains
HIGH-INCOME COUNTRIES	
1	High systolic blood pressure
2	Smoking (tobacco use)
3	High fasting plasma glucose
4	High body mass index (obesity)
5	High LDL cholesterol
6	Kidney dysfunction (impaired kidney function)
7	Alcohol use
8	Low temperature
9	Diet low in whole grains
10	Particulate matter pollution (air pollution)

Source: Data from GBD Compare—IHME Viz Hub. Institute for Health Metrics and Evaluation (IHME). https://vizhub .healthdata.org/gbd-compare/

factor for death is high systolic blood pressure, followed by smoking (tobacco use), and high fasting plasma glucose (see Table 6.1). This reality provides an insight into the interaction among multiple levels in our social ecological framework: individual risks, discussed in this chapter, are influenced by socioeconomic patterns at national and global levels.

Global Patterns of Risk Factors for Death in Relation to Age Category

Risk factors for death also vary by age (**Table 6.2**). Globally, for all ages combined, the top five risk factors for death are, in order, high blood pressure, smoking, air pollution (outdoor and indoor), high blood sugar, and obesity. However, when examined by age category, the leading risk factors are distinctly different for younger age groups. For example, the top five risk factors associated with infant and young childhood deaths under the age of 5 years are low birth weight, child wasting, household air pollution, unsafe water source, and poor sanitation.

Although the age categories include variable numbers of years, the burden of mortality increases with age, with most deaths concentrated in the 50 to 69 years and 70 and older age categories. For both of these age groups, five risk factors top the list–albeit in slightly different order: high blood pressure, smoking, high blood sugar, high cholesterol, and high BMI (obesity). Moreover, and not surprisingly, four of these five are precisely the four top risk factors found for all ages combined.

TABLE 6.2 Top Five Risk Factors of Death Worldwide, All Ages Combined and Selected Age Groups, 2019

	ALL AGES COMBINED
1	High blood pressure
2	Smoking
3	Air pollution (outdoor and indoor)
4	High blood sugar
5	Obesity
	AGES 0–4 YEARS
1	Low birth weight
2	Child wasting
3	Household air pollution
4	Unsafe water source
5	Poor sanitation
	AGES 5–14 YEARS
1	Unsafe water source
2	Poor sanitation
3	No access to handwashing facility
4	Indoor air pollution
5	Outdoor particulate matter pollution
	AGES 15–49 YEARS
1	High blood pressure
2	Alcohol use
3	Unsafe sex
4	High body mass index (obesity)
5	Smoking
	AGES 50–69 YEARS
1	High blood pressure
2	Smoking
3	High body mass index (obesity)
4	High blood sugar
5	High cholesterol

(*continued*)

TABLE 6.2 Top Five Risk Factors of Death Worldwide, All Ages Combined and Selected Age Groups, 2019 (*continued*)

AGES 70 YEARS AND OLDER	
1	High blood pressure
2	High blood sugar
3	Smoking
4	High cholesterol
5	High body mass index (obesity)

Source: Data from Ritchie H, Roser M. Causes of death. Our World in Data. Published February 2018. Updated December 2019. https://ourworldindata.org/causes-of-death

INDIVIDUAL HEALTH–RELATED BEHAVIORS

Injury, disease, and even death often result from the ways in which individuals live and behave. The most widely cited individual health-related behaviors include smoking, poor diet, physical inactivity, unsafe sexual practices, and consumption of alcohol and other drugs. Tobacco kills more than 8 million people each year. More than 7 million of those deaths are the result of direct tobacco use while around 1.2 million are the result of nonsmokers being exposed to secondhand smoke.[4]

Malnutrition

Malnutrition takes various forms including underweight (low weight for age), stunting (low height for age), wasting (low weight for height), and overweight and obesity. All forms of malnutrition place children under 5 years of age at increased risk for NCDs and death. Malnutrition confers long-lasting effects on individuals, communities, and societies.[5]

Over 460 million people worldwide are underweight with lower than expected weight for age. This includes 52 million children under 5 years of age who suffer from wasting. Another 155 million are stunted with lower height for age than expected. Approximately 45% of deaths in children under 5 years are linked to malnutrition, and these are concentrated in low- and middle-income countries.[5]

At the other end of the continuum, as diseases of overnutrition become increasingly prominent, in the very countries where subsets of the population currently suffer from underweight and nutritional deficiency diseases, the rates of adult and childhood overweight and obesity are rising.

Worldwide, obesity has nearly tripled since 1975.[6] Obesity is currently most prevalent in high-income countries. In 2016, more than 1.9 billion adults, 18 years and older, were overweight (BMI of 25 kg/m^2 and higher). Among these, 650 million were obese (BMI of 30 kg/m^2 and higher). Globally, 39% of all world citizens, ages 18 years and older, are overweight and 13% are obese. Obesity is directly linked to intake of calories and is, in theory, preventable.[7]

Worldwide, obesity has nearly tripled since 1975.[6] Obesity is currently most prevalent in high-income countries.

Insufficient Physical Activity

Insufficient physical activity is a leading risk factor for premature mortality and prominent NCDs including diabetes, cardiovascular disease, and cancer worldwide. Globally, one in four adults fail to meet the recommended physical activity guidelines. Importantly, from a life course perspective, more than 80% of adolescents do not meet physical activity guidelines, thereby increasing their risk for future health issues in their adult years.[8]

Sexually Transmitted Infections

Sexually transmitted infections (STIs) are transmitted through sexual contact and include chlamydia, gonorrhea, syphilis, herpes simplex virus (HSV), and human papillomavirus (HPV). There are approximately 376 million new (incident) cases of chlamydia, gonorrhea, syphilis, and trichomoniasis every year and a prevalence of 500 million HSV infections worldwide. HPV infection is the most transmitted STI, affecting more than 290 million women worldwide. HIV/AIDS has multiple modes of transmission and while not exclusively an STI, sexual transmission accounts for more cases of new infection and symptomatic HIV/AIDS illness than any other mode.

Pregnant women infected with an STI are at increased risk for a range of pregnancy complications, including preterm labor, and they also risk transmitting the infection to their newborn babies. Considering the life course perspective, some STIs produce serious reproductive health consequences beyond the immediate impact of the infection itself (e.g., infertility for the mother or mother-to-child transmission to the infant). Perhaps most concerning is that many STIs present no overtly detectable symptoms yet can still be transmitted to a sexual partner.[6]

Harmful Alcohol Use

Harmful, or excessive, alcohol use increases risk for NCDs including hypertension, cardiovascular disease, and cancer and also for infectious diseases such as tuberculosis and HIV/AIDS. Alcohol consumption, including binge drinking, increases risks for a range of unintentional injuries including motor vehicle crashes, drowning, intimate partner violence, and suicide. Harmful alcohol use accounts for 5.1% of all deaths worldwide and is particularly problematic for adults, ages 20 to 39 years, accounting for 13.5% of deaths in this age group. Harmful alcohol use is linked to poor performance at work and poor mental health. Some people drink alcohol to manage stress and anxiety yet find that alcohol use exacerbates these and other issues. Harmful alcohol use affects the individual very profoundly both directly and indirectly. Harmful alcohol use adversely affects family members, friends, coworkers, and neighbors in social, economic, and health-related terms.[9]

VARIABILITY IN THE INDIVIDUAL CAUSES OF HEALTH

Measuring Cigarette Smoking

The demographics of individuals who engage in these health-related behaviors vary widely. For example, there is considerable geographic variability throughout the United States in current combustible cigarette smoking rates by state (**Figure 6.1**).

Smoking rates vary by sex, race/ethnicity, poverty status, and education (**Figure 6.2**). The Centers for Disease Control and Prevention (CDC) provides fact sheets on numerous health behaviors, including smoking, which highlight the associations among risk factors and health behaviors.[10]

Health-related behaviors can be difficult to measure, leading to inaccuracies. Prevalence rates of engagement in risk-elevating or "problem" behaviors are typically underestimated.

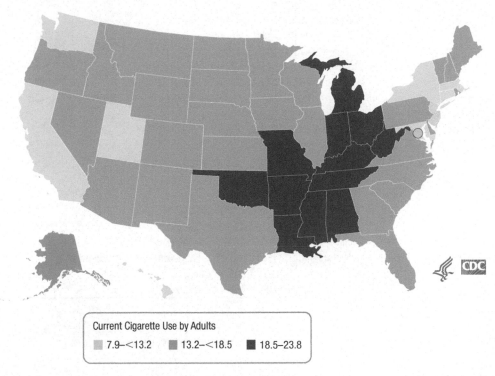

FIGURE 6.1 Current cigarette use among U.S. adults by state, 2019.
Source: From Centers for Disease Control and Prevention. State Tobacco Activities Tracking & Evaluation (STATE) system: map of current cigarette use among adults (Behavior Risk Factor Surveillance System) 2019. https://www.cdc.gov/statesystem/cigaretteuseadult.html

These behaviors are known to be unhealthy and are frequently underreported. For example, on the surface, smoking may seem like a very objective behavior to measure. Smoking is sometimes measured by the number of cigarettes smoked in the past day, week, or month. Alternatively, individuals are classified as never, former, or current smokers. There are individuals who occasionally smoke "socially" with friends or when they consume alcohol; they would never self-classify themselves as "smokers." Adding further complexity is the rapidly rising popularity of e-cigarettes and vaping products that are supplanting combustible cigarettes. Soaring rates of e-cigarette use have reversed the decades-long trend of decreasing prevalence rates of smoking and tobacco product use among youth.

Measuring Physical Activity and Diet

Physical activity is challenging to measure. Physical activity is sometimes measured as the number of minutes of vigorous activity per day—but the term "vigorous" is subject to interpretation. Also, there are individuals who engage in vigorous on-the-job manual labor, so how is this included in assessments of physical activity, if at all? Assessments of healthy or unhealthy diet are also quite difficult as they might ask individuals about consumption of specific food groups or nutrients or might focus on total caloric intake. Diets vary widely across geographic regions, so it is often difficult to compare populations in terms of diet and the impact of diet on health outcomes.

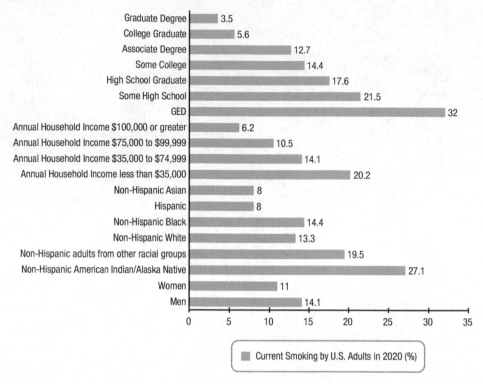

FIGURE 6.2 Current smoking by U.S. adults in 2020 by sex, race/ethnicity, poverty status, and education.
Source: From Centers for Disease Control and Prevention. Smoking and tobacco use: current cigarette smoking among adults in the United States. https://www.cdc.gov/tobacco/data_statistics/fact_sheets/adult_data/cig_smoking/index.htm

RISK-ELEVATING BEHAVIORS

Risk factors can be either risk-elevating or risk-reducing, depending on how individuals engage and behave. Risk-elevating behaviors are those that increase the risks for disease and death. Again, the most widely cited individual health-related behaviors are smoking, poor diet, physical inactivity, unsafe sexual practices, consumption of alcohol, and use of other drugs. There are a multitude of reasons why individuals engage in these behaviors, with many such precipitating factors occurring early in the life course. These include lack of parental supervision, difficulties in school, peer substance use, poverty, stress, mental health issues, neglect, and social isolation. If these issues persist into adolescence, they further increase the likelihood that individuals engage in and maintain their unhealthy behaviors.

Both the social ecological and life course perspectives, acting in tandem on health, are critical for understanding health behaviors. Adolescents, for example, take risks for several reasons. Perhaps the most important among these is the misperception that specific behaviors are not risky. Many adolescents experiment, yet there is a big difference between sneaking a drink of alcohol and shooting heroin—a difference with both health and legal implications. Adolescents' brains are still developing and are often not capable of the insight and self-control required to make healthy choices, particularly when influential others around them might be actively partaking in unhealthy behaviors. Adults also engage in unhealthy risk-elevating behaviors for a variety of reasons, including lack of knowledge about specific health risks and prioritizing short-term benefits over longer-term risks. And to further complicate this issue, individuals often engage in multiple risk-elevating behaviors concurrently, which is important as we aim to develop interventions to move individuals toward healthier behaviors.

RISK-REDUCING/PROTECTIVE BEHAVIORS

Protective or risk-reducing behaviors are those that decrease the risk of disease and death. Individuals with lower risk of disease and death are those who do not smoke, follow a healthy diet, get regular physical activity, practice safer sexual practices, and abstain from alcohol consumption and use of other drugs. There are a multitude of reasons why individuals engage in these risk-reducing behaviors including knowledge of risk behaviors and their consequences; skills in self-control and coping; choosing life experiences that are nurturing, supportive, and positive; and seeking health-promoting connections with peers through academics, school activities, athletics, social clubs, religious organizations, and the like.

CASE STUDY 6.1: MINDFULNESS PRACTICE: STRESS RELIEF FOR INDIVIDUALS

Stress is inherent at all stages in the life course and is experienced at multiple levels of the social ecological framework. Nevertheless, stress is one risk factor that can be dealt with effectively at the individual level. In recent decades, one approach for buffering stress that is supported by a growing evidence base is the practice of mindfulness.

Mindfulness has been described in several ways. According to researchers at the University of Calgary, mindfulness is "a mental state of focusing on the present moment and accepting the current state of the mind and body without judgment. Mindfulness meditation is a mental practice that helps achieve that state of mind."[11]

Brown University's Mindfulness Center starts with an elegantly simple definition, "paying attention on purpose, in the present moment, nonjudgmentally."[12] This definition combines two elements. The first element is *present moment awareness*, including awareness of our thoughts, emotions, and physical sensations—in the present. The second element is *quality of awareness*. Optimal awareness is nonjudgmental and possesses the attributes of curiosity, friendliness, and gentleness. This awareness is characterized by acceptance—accepting that this is just how things are in this moment.

Viewing the moment-by-moment world through the lens of mindfulness is not unlike the experience of an objective scientist who suspends judgment, observes what information is perceived through the senses, contemplates the information, and considers how to respond skillfully and creatively to what is observed.

According to the Yale Medicine clinicians, mindfulness may be a formal meditation—or not.[13] Dr. Auguste H. Fortin VI uses the analogy that meditation acts as a scaffold for developing mindfulness. "In meditation, your only job is to follow your breath and notice what your mind is doing while that's happening." His Yale colleague, Dr. Rajita Sinha provides the counterpoint that mindfulness practice does not need to occur in the context of meditation: "It is really about being in the moment, observing what's coming at you from the outside and what's coming up inside—taking it in and observing, and not reacting to it."

(continued)

MINDFULNESS TECHNIQUES

Mindfulness-Based Stress Reduction

Anne Dutton, director of the Yale Stress Center mindfulness education program teaches classes on Mindfulness-Based Stress Reduction (MBSR). She outlines three components that characterize mindfulness practice:

- Paying attention to what is happening in the present moment
- Paying attention purposely, deliberately, resolutely
- Staying with the mindfulness experience, pleasant or unpleasant

S.T.O.P.

Southern Utah University posted a series of helpful mindfulness techniques for college students, starting with the acronym S.T.O.P.:

- **S**top. Stop what you are doing and thinking. Dedicate a moment to mindfulness.
- **T**ake a deep breath.
- **O**bserve how you are feeling physically and emotionally.
- **P**roceed with the activity slowly and thoughtfully.[14]

Breathwork

Pause to focus on your breath. Observe the sensations of inhaling cooler air through your nose and exhaling warmer air through your mouth. Experiment with a variety of cycles of deep breathing to find one or several that work well for you.

- **Clear the mind**: Inhale for 4. Exhale for 4.
- **Calm down**: Inhale for 4. Exhale for 6.
- **Relieve stress** ("box breathing"): Inhale for 4. Hold for 4. Exhale for 4. Hold for 4.
- **Decrease heart rate and blood pressure**: Inhale for 4. Hold for 7. Exhale for 8.

Grounding, or 5-4-3-2-1 Practice

One way to alleviate stress and diminish worry thoughts about what happened in the past or what might happen in the future is to focus on the present, observing objects and sensations in real time. This can be done by focusing on your five senses in sequence.

- Name 5 things that **you can see**, that are not distressing.
- Name 4 things that **you can hear**, that are not distressing.
- Name 3 things that **you can touch**, that are not distressing.
- Name 2 things that **you can smell**, that are not distressing.
- Name 1 thing that **you can taste**, that is not distressing.

Body Scan

Lie down, close your eyes, and slowly scan your body mentally from head to toe — or start from the opposite direction — bringing your awareness to each part of the body without judging or trying to change anything.

(*continued*)

MINDFULNESS AND YOUNG ADULTS

Professionals from the Brown University Mindfulness Center have trained hundreds of students since the center's opening in 2015. Identified stressors for the college population include economic insecurity related to the burden of tuition payments, skyrocketing rent and housing prices, and rising prices for food and essentials. Social media has been a source of escalating stress involving many dimensions ranging from negative self-comparisons to popular influencers, to online bullying, to disclosure of sensitive personal information, to anxiety-inducing posts on such topics as body image and suicide.

Mindfulness Center staff outline three mechanisms through which mindfulness can effectively lower stress: self-awareness, attention control, and emotion regulation. Self-awareness, acquired and refined through mindfulness practice, allows individuals to engage in accurate self-observation of activities in real time and make choices to select and prioritize health-enhancing actions or to decline or stop participation in health-compromising behaviors. Attention control is valuable for making wise choices that are healthful both in terms of behaviors and interpersonal encounters. Regarding emotion regulation, mindfulness training alerts individuals to their emotional responses to stressful situations as they emerge in real time, providing a momentary pause to skillfully select how better to react.

Variations of mindfulness practice have been developed as smartphone applications (apps), and several of these were gaining popularity in the prepandemic era.[15] A small randomized controlled trial was conducted with college students who scored high on perceived stress.[16] The study was conducted using a randomized wait-listed control design. Intervention participants were asked to use a popular mindfulness smartphone app for 10 minutes daily over an 8-week period. At the conclusion of the study period, investigators reported significant decreases in self-reported stress, as measured on the Perceived Stress Scale, coupled with significant increases in mindfulness (using the Five Factor Mindfulness Questionnaire) and self-compassion (assessed with the Self-Compassion Survey—Short Form) for those who used a popular smartphone mindfulness app.

MINDFULNESS AND COVID-19

When COVID-19 arrived, mindfulness practice was adopted by many college students to deal with the burden of pandemic stress in the midst of university studies. In a study based at the University of Calgary, Alberta, Canada, Kam et al. examined whether 10 minutes of daily practice using a mindfulness meditation guided by a smartphone app "could cushion some of the negative effects of COVID-19 on emotional well-being."[17]

Participants were graduate university students from several North American universities who responded to an emailed invitation from the University of Calgary. This small scale, randomized, wait-listed control design was conducted very early in the pandemic, in May 2020. Two encouraging findings emerged following this brief, low-dose exposure to mindfulness practice. First, individuals in the intervention condition who used the app for 10 days reported a more positive affect (i.e., happier mood) than the wait-listed control participants. Second, students in the mindfulness app intervention were less negatively affected by exposure to

(continued)

COVID-19-related news that was proliferating at the time. Investigators suggested that mindfulness practice acted as a buffer against COVID-19 stress and emotional distress. The research team concluded that "guided mindfulness meditation holds promise as a simple-to-implement, cost-effective technique that can be practiced anywhere, anytime."[11]

Mindfulness practice gained followers across all age groups throughout the pandemic. Several extremely successful mindfulness smartphone apps came on the market. Meanwhile, mindfulness was increasingly documented to be beneficial for stress reduction in well-designed studies conducted with a wide variety of audiences.

For example, the nature of mindfulness overcomes the financial constraints often posed by costly mental health interventions, thereby prompting the increasing adoption of mindfulness techniques as an effective, affordable, "counter-stress" measure among students in low- to middle-income countries (LMICs).[18]

In the clinical realm, COVID-19 accelerated the wholesale switch to telehealth medical consultations. In that context, the pandemic prompted many clinicians to prescribe the use of mindfulness techniques and smartphone apps for their patients who were dealing with the compounding stressors of their disease diagnosis and the myriad challenges and life changes brought about by the COVID-19 pandemic.

Numerous applications of mindfulness practice are being evaluated for efficacy and effectiveness for individuals who encounter layers of stressors in their daily lives at home, work, and school.

UNDERSTANDING INDIVIDUAL BEHAVIOR

Given all of the data that link modifiable risk factors to poor health outcomes, why then do individuals engage in unhealthy behaviors?

Why do individuals smoke? There are over 1 billion smokers worldwide today, and for most, smoking initiation occurred in their early teen or even preteen years. Some individuals might have tried smoking as a rebellious act, thinking that they could experiment and quit at any time. Unfortunately, nicotine is powerfully addictive, and quitting is no easy task. Other individuals succumb to peer pressure or aggressive advertising or see an admired celebrity or influencer smoking, which seems appealing in some way.

Given all of the data that link modifiable risk factors to poor health outcomes, why then do individuals engage in unhealthy behaviors?

Why don't individuals eat a healthy diet? There is certainly ample, scientifically sound guidance available on healthy diet and nutritious food selections tailored to a variety of populations. The World Health Organization (WHO) offers specific nutritional guidelines for pregnant women, infants, and adolescents that include supplementation of vitamins and minerals and restrictions on sodium and sugars.[19] Also, the U.S. Department of Agriculture regularly updates and issues Dietary Guidelines for Americans (**Table 6.3**).

TABLE 6.3 Dietary Guidelines for Americans, 2020 to 2025, Ninth Edition

1	**Follow a healthy dietary pattern at every life stage.**
	All food and beverage choices matter.
	Choose a healthy eating pattern at an appropriate calorie level to help achieve and maintain a healthy body weight, support nutrient adequacy, and reduce the risk of chronic disease.
2	**Customize and enjoy food and beverage choices to reflect personal preferences, cultural traditions, and budgetary considerations.**
	Consider cultural and personal preferences to make these shifts easier to accomplish and maintain.
	Consider regional and seasonal food availability and incorporating a variety of fresh, frozen, dried, and canned options to fit a healthy dietary pattern within budgetary constraints.
3	**Focus on meeting food group needs with nutrient-dense foods and beverages, and stay within calorie limits.**
	To meet nutrient needs within calorie limits, choose a variety of nutrient-dense foods across and within all food groups in recommended amounts.
4	**Limit foods and beverages higher in added sugars, saturated fat, and sodium, and limit alcoholic beverages.**
	A healthy dietary pattern is designed to meet food group and nutrient recommendations while staying within calorie needs.
	Consume nutrient-dense food forms for around 85% of daily calories, with least amounts of added sugars, saturated fat, and sodium.

Source: Data from Brown Rodgers A, ed. *Dietary guidelines for Americans 2020–2025.* 9th ed. U.S. Department of Health and Human Services; 2020. https://www.dietaryguidelines.gov/resources/2020-2025-dietary-guidelines-online-materials

Given the wealth of information on healthy eating, why then do so many individuals struggle to follow the recommendations? Some individuals are unaware of the calories and fats in the foods they are eating. Many other individuals—and their families and communities—have limited access to healthy and affordable foods. Other individuals lack the time to prepare healthy meals and, seemingly by default, they rely on fast-food choices that are nutritionally deficient and fundamentally unhealthy.

Why don't individuals get regular physical activity? The U.S. Office of Disease Prevention and Health Promotion recommends that adolescents and adults get at least 60 minutes of physical activity per day, and this includes aerobic exercise along with muscle- and bone-strengthening activities.[20] The benefits of regular exercise are well documented, yet the vast majority of Americans do not meet these basic criteria. In fact, a substantial proportion of Americans are sedentary. Some lack motivation. Some have no access to safe spaces for exercise. Others juggle work, family, and other responsibilities, limiting their time to participate—and enjoy—endorphin-producing physical activity.

Why do individuals engage in unsafe sexual practices? Safer sexual practices involve taking steps to avoid contracting and spreading STIs. This requires an understanding of how STIs are spread person-to-person, and perhaps more importantly, open communication and negotiation with prospective and active sexual partners regarding experiences, expectations, and precautions for minimizing risks. However, opening conversations around safe-sexual practices can be difficult and uncomfortable. Many individuals fear rejection, which sometimes translates to skipping the conversation altogether.

Why do individuals use and abuse alcohol and other drugs? The National Institute on Alcohol Abuse and Alcoholism defines binge drinking as consuming five or more drinks for males and four or more drinks for females over approximately 2 hours. In the United States, approximately 17% of adults binge-drink every week. Binge drinking is especially popular among adults between the ages of 18 and 34 years. Most individuals under age 21 who drink alcohol—and do so illegally in the United States—meet the criteria for binge drinking.[21] Individuals drink alcohol because they like the taste, the sensation, and the decreased inhibitions; and alcohol is readily accessible for most adults—and most youth. Many individuals consume alcohol as a form of self-medication to handle stress while others fall prey to peer pressure.

For each of these individual risk factors, there is abundant evidence of their association with injury, disease, disability, and even death. There are real pressures and challenges to avoid smoking, eat a healthy diet, engage in regular physical activity, choose safer sexual practices, and minimize alcohol use and abstain from other drug use. Moderation is an option, and for many, a healthy choice. If we are to create conditions for all individuals to reach their health potential, we must understand individual behavior and evidence-based approaches for promoting healthful behavior change.

THEORIES OF BEHAVIOR AND BEHAVIOR CHANGE

The Health Belief Model (HBM) is a theoretical model that was developed by social psychologists in the U.S. Public Health Service in the 1950s to explain and predict individual health behavior and behavior change. The HBM is one of the most widely used models for understanding individual health behaviors. The model focuses on individual beliefs about health conditions (e.g., how susceptible am I to injury or disease, and how severe could it be?), which then influence specific health behaviors. The model is built on two underlying assumptions: (a) individuals wish to avoid injury and disease (or if already suffering from injury or disease, they wish to become well) and (b) specific health behaviors will prevent (or cure) disease. Individuals' selection of specific health behaviors depends on the perceived benefits of taking these actions (or engaging in these behaviors), perceived barriers to action, exposure to factors that prompt action, and confidence in their own abilities to be successful (self-efficacy). The HBM, like other health behavior models, is theoretical and does not offer specific strategies for changing individual health behaviors. To be successful, models or approaches to change individual health behaviors must account for the context and the social and environmental conditions that affect the ways in which individuals live and behave.

There are several other popular theories and models of individual behavior and behavior change such as social cognitive theory, the stages of change model (also called the transtheoretical model), and the theory of planned behavior/reasoned action. Each theory or model has a similar purpose: to move individuals away from unhealthy behaviors and toward adopting healthy behaviors. For example, the social cognitive theory addresses individual health behaviors as a function of individual experiences, interactions with others, and environmental forces. The social cognitive theory promotes health behavior change through setting expectations; developing skills; enhancing self-efficacy, self-control, and social support; learning from others; and rewarding behavior change.

The stages of change model examines individuals' readiness to modify their behavior and includes the following stages: precontemplation, contemplation, preparation, action, maintenance, and termination (defined here as the point at which individuals have no interest in returning to prior negative or unhealthy behaviors).

The theory of planned behavior is grounded on the assumption that individuals' behavior is based on their intention to engage in that behavior. Intention is predicted by individuals' attitudes toward behaviors and, more specifically, whether they feel that the health behaviors will positively affect health outcomes. As is the case with the HBM, individual attitudes are affected by the social and environmental context.

HOW PUBLIC HEALTH INTERVENTIONS CAN IMPROVE INDIVIDUAL BEHAVIOR AND IMPROVE HEALTH

Public health interventions designed to change individual behaviors focus on individual factors such as knowledge and beliefs, goal setting, linking goals to specific rewards, and applying techniques to monitor and reinforce healthy behaviors. Evidence shows that public health interventions based on social and behavioral theories of change, such as those outlined earlier, are more effective than interventions that lack a theoretical underpinning.[22] In practice, the HBM, social cognitive theory, and the stages of change model are among the most frequently applied theories in the field. Beyond these well-known, foundational theories, there is an upwelling of new adaptations that are specific to such wide-ranging health behaviors as disaster preparedness (the protective action decision model) and climate change adaptation (model of private proactive adaptation to climate change).[23,24]

Individual behavior change is a complex and multistage process. Interventions to change individual behaviors are most effective when they target individual knowledge, beliefs, and skills and when they move individual intentions to actions. That said, longer and more impactful changes are achieved when individual skill training and support is coupled with strategies and models to develop healthier policies, systems, and environments.

INDIVIDUAL BEHAVIOR AND BEHAVIOR CHANGE IN CONTEXT

There are documented associations between modifiable behavioral risk factors and adverse health outcomes (e.g., injury, disease, disability, and death). However, focusing on shifting individual behaviors and personal choices is important—but not sufficient—to improve population health. Individuals' choices are highly influenced by their social situations and the environments in which they work and live. Can all individuals truly choose healthy behaviors over unhealthy behaviors?

Individual health is shaped by population health and vice versa. Although individuals have preferences for health-related behaviors, their actual choices are often appreciably affected (and for some, severely limited) by their social and environmental surroundings. Arah tells a story of a young woman who breaks her leg in a motor vehicle accident.[25] This injury sharply and abruptly affects her individual health. Does it affect her population's health? As it turns out, this young woman was on her way to the hospital, as she was one of a few doctors serving her rural community. Furthermore, she was responding to an emergency call to assist her overtaxed colleagues. What happens now to her colleagues, to the patients they are caring for, and to the overall health of her population? Although this is a hypothetical case, it illustrates the many ways in which individual and population health interplay.

BEHAVIOR AND BEHAVIOR CHANGE REMAIN OF CORE IMPORTANCE FOR PUBLIC HEALTH

Public health is about preventing injury, disease, and disability in communities, and individual behaviors are key to this endeavor. Public health professionals focus on programs, policies, and services to educate and support individuals—and their encompassing communities—in engaging in healthy behaviors.

Consider now how individual behavior interacts with primary, secondary, and tertiary prevention. As described in Chapter 3, "At the Heart of Public Health: Prevention," primary prevention focuses on preventing the onset of risk behaviors and exposure to hazards in order to minimize disease incidence to the fullest extent possible. Secondary prevention involves screening for risk factors and early detection of subclinical conditions before target organ damage occurs. Secondary prevention interventions are targeted toward diminishing risk and restoring full health, thereby decreasing disease prevalence. Tertiary prevention focuses on containing or reducing the impact of diagnosed disease or injury once these have occurred, including actions to prevent reinfection, reinjury, or relapse. Tertiary prevention brings rehabilitation to the forefront, focusing on managing long-term consequences of disease and injury while optimizing quality of life and maximizing life expectancy.

Public health professionals often focus on primary prevention—preventing injury, disease, or disability before they happen. This is best accomplished with appropriately tailored and targeted individual communications, interventions, educational materials, programs, and services. To be effective, however, these tools and services must be coupled with structural changes in policies and systems at the community, city, national, and global levels—representing the encircling social ecological levels in which the individual is embedded.

INDIVIDUAL BEHAVIOR INTERSECTING WITH OTHER SOCIAL ECOLOGICAL DRIVERS OF HEALTH

Individual health–related behaviors are determined not only by the individual alone but across different social ecological levels. For example, a healthy diet is influenced by the individual's preferences and beliefs; social support (or lack thereof) from family, friends, and peers; availability of affordable foods at the community level; and food policies that govern national distribution and accessibility of staple foods.

Broadly speaking, public health focuses on communities while medicine is tailored toward individuals. Medical professionals have tended to focus on individual-level health behaviors driven by an individual's knowledge, beliefs, and skills, but these professionals are now considering a broader range of influencing factors across multiple social ecological levels. Recognition of the social, political, and environmental factors that affect an individual's choices and behaviors is essential to positively affect population health.

> **Broadly speaking, public health focuses on communities while medicine is tailored toward individuals.**

Population health is not merely the sum of the health of the individuals within the population. Population health is defined by the context in which people live, work, and play and the associated factors that affect health. Consider, for example, a population of children, ages 5 to 15 years, living in a particular geographic region. Suppose that each child in the population undergoes an extensive physical examination and no child is diagnosed with disease (this is unfortunately hypothetical!). On the surface, this seems like the perfectly healthy population. But what if these children are homeless, are hungry, have limited access to education, and lack social and parental support? Are they really healthy?

Individual behavior alone will never be sufficient for understanding or improving the health of populations. Health is produced in context. Consider the concentric layers of influence that were presented when the social ecological perspective was introduced in Chapter 5, "What Causes Health of Populations? A Social Ecological and Life Course Approach" (see Figure 5.1). Individual behavior is enveloped in families/social networks that occupy neighborhoods that are part of large cities or rural communities, which in turn are parts of larger nations and societies (**Figure 6.3**). Each of these social ecological levels exerts important influences on individual health.

We now turn to one of the most outwardly observable public health challenges—the United States obesity epidemic—to explore how policies that create health disparities come into play and ultimately influence individual behavior that may progressively lead to obesity (Case Study 6.2; you can access the podcast accompanying Case Study 6.2 by following this link to Springer Publishing Company Connect™: http://connect.springerpub.com/content/book/978-0-8261-8043-8/part/part02/chapter/ch06).

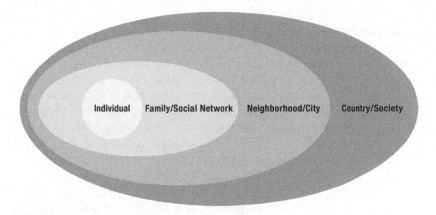

FIGURE 6.3 The multilevel social ecological perspective, highlighting the focus of this chapter: individual behavior. Artistic credit: Parisa Varanloo.

CASE STUDY 6.2: MEETING THE CHALLENGES OF OBESITY[26]

There is an obesity epidemic in the United States. In 2021, the prevalence of obesity among adults exceeded 30% in 40 states, 35% in 19 states, and 40% in two states—Kentucky and West Virginia (**Figure 6.4**).[27]

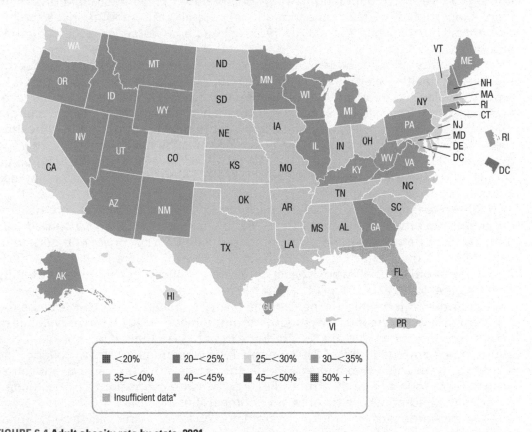

FIGURE 6.4 Adult obesity rate by state, 2021.
Source: Centers for Disease Control and Prevention. Adult Obesity Prevalence Maps. Updated September 27, 2022. https://www.cdc.gov/obesity/data/prevalence-maps.html

(*continued*)

Differences within the context of overall obesity have made this epidemic particularly devastating for a number of distinct socioeconomic and racial groups. These intergroup differences are a manifestation of social divides across the fundamental causes that shape individual well-being. These causes are shaped by access, or lack of access, to resources like wealth and social support.[28] Lack of access to these resources usually translates to poorer health, as in the case of obesity and associated conditions like heart disease, diabetes, and infant mortality.[29-31] Hence, when looking at obesity, we must also look at the unequal distribution of advantage in our society, and how that inequity drives the presence of health or the occurrence of disease in individuals who collectively comprise our populations.

A number of factors contributed to the dramatic rise in obesity. Over the past 20 years, food portion sizes in the American diet have greatly increased, doubling or in some cases tripling.[32] The increase is particularly noticeable in the sizes of sugary drinks.[33] In the 1950s, the average sugary drink was about seven ounces; it has since grown to an average of 42 ounces.

This upsizing has ramifications not only for how much we consume when we eat out, but for what we consider to be an appropriate amount of food to consume in a single sitting, even at home.[31] This problem is compounded by the fact that unhealthy foods are frequently much more affordable than healthier ones.[34] The affordability of cheap, energy-dense foods is a key driver of obesity among low-resource populations. Unfair disparities in healthy food affordability were exacerbated in 2022 with an inflationary spiral that sent food prices steeply upward at a time when the COVID-19 pandemic had worsened socioeconomic inequities.

The ubiquity of fast-food restaurants in poorer communities, compounded by the lack of healthy alternatives, also contributes to the rise of obesity.[34] Poorer families looking to improve their diets therefore face an uphill battle against economics, geography, and the social trends that have led over the decades to larger plates for all Americans. It has also become commonplace for high-fat, unhealthy foods to be marketed to children, inculcating unhealthy habits from an early age forward.[35] It is important to note that these obstacles have little to do with personal choice, or any of the "lifestyle" factors that are so central to American weight loss culture.

As these reasons amply suggest, obesity is closely tied to income and the conditions of poverty. In 2015, more than 35% of American adults who earned less than $45,000 per year were obese, compared with 25% of those who earned at least $65,000 per year.[36] From 2011 to 2014, 18.9% of children living at <130% FPL (federal policy level) were obese, compared to 10.9% of children with family incomes that were at >350% FPL (**Figure 6.5**).[37]

Lack of education, which is inextricably linked to poverty, also exacerbates the problem of obesity among low-resource communities.[35] In 2021, the prevalence of obesity among adults who did not graduate from high school or an equivalent was about 38%, compared with 26.3% among adults who graduated from college.[38] In a 2019 study, children who had an overweight parent with a high school education or less were found to be 80% more likely to become overweight or obese compared with children whose parents did not meet these criteria.[39]

As more Americans become overweight and obese, certain racial groups shoulder a disproportionate burden of this epidemic, driven largely by the higher rate

(*continued*)

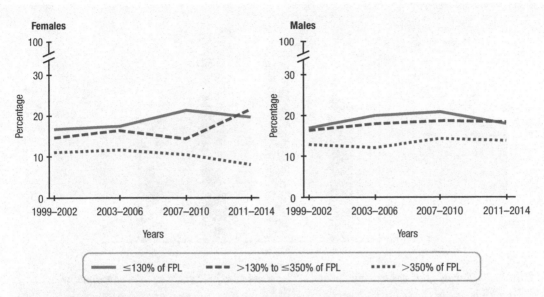

FIGURE 6.5 Trends in obesity prevalence among youths (persons aged 2–19 years), by household income—National Health and Nutrition Examination Survey, United States, 1999 to 2002 through 2011 to 2014. FPL, federal poverty level.
Source: Ogden CL, Carroll MD, Fakhouri TH, et al. Prevalence of obesity among youths by household income and education level of head of household—United States 2011–2014. *MMWR Morb Mortal Wkly Rep.* 2018;67:186–189. https://doi .org/10.15585/mmwr.mm6706a3

of poverty among these populations (**Figures 6.6 and 6.7**).[40] Particularly vulnerable are African American/Black and Latinx populations: as of 2020, the Black poverty rate was at 19.3% and the Latinx poverty rate was at 17%, compared to an 8.2% poverty rate for White Americans.[40] For 2017 to 2020, more than 4-in-10 U.S. adults

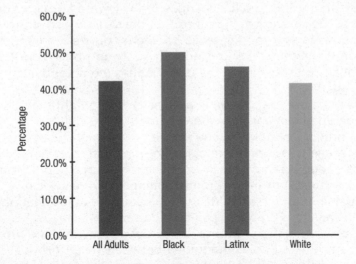

FIGURE 6.6 Obesity rates among adults by race and ethnicity (2017–2020).
Source: Centers for Disease Control and Prevention. National Health and Nutrition Examination Survey 2017–March 2020 prepandemic data files development of files and prevalence estimates for selected health outcomes. https://stacks.cdc .gov/view/cdc/106273

(continued)

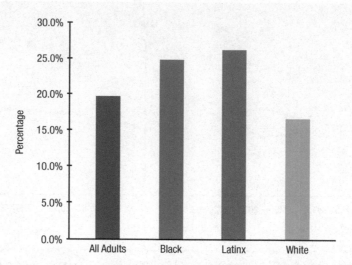

FIGURE 6.7 Obesity rates among children and adolescents aged 2–19 years by race and ethnicity (2017–2010).
Source: Centers for Disease Control and Prevention. National Health and Nutrition Examination Survey 2017–March 2020 prepandemic data files development of files and prevalence estimates for selected health outcomes. https://stacks.cdc .gov/view/cdc/106273

were obese (41.9% obese).[41] The highest burden of obesity was found for Latinx (45.6% obese) and African American/Black (49.9%) populations. White non-Latinx persons had an obesity prevalence of 41.4%. Yet the prevalence of obesity for Asians (16.1%) was only 38% of the overall rate for the nation, providing a contrasting case—within the U.S. population—that demonstrates that rising obesity is not inevitable.[41]

To meet the increasing challenges of obesity, public health professionals can focus on three areas. First, policy changes are warranted, for example, a tax on sugary drinks or the passage of laws that limit the serving size of these beverages. Taking tobacco taxes as a model, taxes on sugary drinks are intended to reduce consumption by increasing the unit price.[42] Applying portion controls to sugary drinks has proved controversial in the past, but has the potential to lessen obesity and improve health. [43,44]

Second, we must use the challenge of obesity to spotlight the role of economic inequality as an upstream source of health inequities. Given the link between obesity and the conditions of poverty, any attempt to tackle the root causes of obesity must address these conditions and come to grips with problems like food insecurity and lack of educational access among low-resource populations.[43] We must also push back against stigma by communicating how obesity is minimally a product of individual failings and principally a consequence of foundational drivers—a case that public health is uniquely positioned to make.[44]

Finally, we must situate our efforts against obesity within the broader context of our work to mitigate health inequities between racial groups. This strategy lies within the remit of public health as we move collectively toward achieving a population of less obese, healthier individuals inclusive of all races and ethnicities.

SUMMARY

Populations are composed of individuals, and individual health is determined by many factors, including individual health–related behaviors. Individual health behaviors can be classified as nonmodifiable (e.g., age) or modifiable (e.g., diet) and risk-reducing (e.g., regular physical activity) or risk-elevating (e.g., tobacco and other substance use). But individual health behaviors alone do not determine health. Social, environmental, and political systems and circumstances have a profound impact on individual health behaviors. In addition, individual risk behaviors change over time, and risk-elevating behaviors accumulate over the life course. This complexity makes changing individual health behaviors difficult. A multitude of forces, occurring at varying levels and intensities, influence individuals and how they behave. Public health interventions aim to prevent disease by changing unhealthy individual behaviors. Understanding what motivates individuals, along with the barriers and challenges they face in making healthy choices, is critical in designing effective public health interventions. Individuals' choices and behaviors are influenced by their social and environmental surroundings, the context in which they work, live, and play. The most effective interventions are based on sound theories and models, such as the HBM, that can address individual behavior within the context of multiple social ecological levels. To improve population health requires understanding and optimizing individual health while incorporating the wide array of social, economic, and political factors that produce population health.

End-of-Chapter Resources

Access additional case study podcasts online at http://connect.springerpub.com/ content/book/978-0-8261-8043-8/

DISCUSSION QUESTIONS

1. Think about individual behaviors related to anxiety in adolescents. Classify each individual behavior as risk-elevating or risk-reducing, and modifiable or nonmodifiable.
2. Explain the stages of change model in reference to an individual who is trying to quit the high-risk behavior of cigarette smoking.
3. Describe the stages of prevention—namely, primary, secondary, and tertiary—in the context of breast cancer.

 A robust set of instructor resources designed to supplement this text is located at **http://connect.springerpub.com/content/book/978-0-8261-8043-8**. Qualifying instructors may request access by emailing **textbook@springerpub.com.**

REFERENCES

1. MedlinePlus. *Is eye color determined by genetics?* https://medlineplus.gov/genetics/understanding/traits/eyecolor/
2. Sheets L, Johnson J, Todd T, et al. Unsupported labeling of race as a risk factor for certain diseases in a widely used medical textbook. *Acad Med.* 2011;86(10):1300-1303. doi:10.1097/ACM.0b013e31822bbdb5

3. Crear-Perry J. Race isn't a risk factor in maternal health. Racism is. *Rewire.News*. April 11, 2018. https://rewire
   .news/article/2018/04/11/maternal-health-replace-race-with-racism

4. World Health Organization. *Tobacco*. Published May 29, 2019. https://www.who.int/news-room/fact-sheets/
   detail/tobacco

5. World Health Organization. *Malnutrition*. Published February 16, 2018. https://www.who.int/news-room/
   fact-sheets/detail/malnutrition

6. World Health Organization. *Sexually transmitted infections (STIs)*. Published June 14, 2019. https://www.who
   .int/news-room/fact-sheets/detail/sexually-transmitted-infections-(stis)

7. World Health Organization. *Obesity and overweight*. Published February 16, 2018. https://www.who.int/news
   -room/fact-sheets/detail/obesity-and-overweight

8. World Health Organization. *Physical activity*. Published February 23, 2018. https://www.who.int/news-room/
   fact-sheets/detail/physical-activity

9. World Health Organization. *Alcohol*. Published September 21, 2018. https://www.who.int/news-room/fact
   -sheets/detail/alcohol

10. Centers for Disease Control and Prevention. *Smoking and tobacco use: fast facts and fact sheets*. https://www
    .cdc.gov/tobacco/data_statistics/fact_sheets/fast_facts/index.htm

11. University of Calgary. *Mindfulness meditation in brief daily doses can reduce negative mental health impact of
    COVID-19*. Published August 31, 2021. https://ucalgary.ca/news/mindfulness-meditation-brief-daily-doses
    -can-reduce-negative-mental-health-impact-covid-19-0

12. Brown University. *For young adults, mindfulness habits for life and the promise of better mental, physical health*.
    Brown University: News from Brown. Published April 12, 2022. https://www.brown.edu/news/2022-04-12/
    mindful-college-student

13. Katella K. *Mindfulness: how it can help amid the COVID-19 pandemic*. Yale Medicine. Published May 19, 2020.
    https://www.yalemedicine.org/news/mindfulness-covid

14. Bryers S. *Seven mindfulness techniques for college students*. Southern Utah University. Published October 20,
    2021. https://www.suu.edu/blog/2021/10/mindfulness-techniques-students.html

15. Hicks J. *College students are increasingly turning to mindfulness apps to ease stress*. Thrive Global. Published
    January 27, 2019. https://thriveglobal.com/stories/college-students-can-find-mindfulness-at-their-fingertips/

16. Huberty J, Green J, Glissmann C, Larkey L, Puzia M, Lee C. Efficacy of the mindfulness meditation mobile
    app "Calm" to reduce stress among college students: randomized controlled trial. *JMIR Mhealth Uhealth*.
    2019;7(6):e14273. doi:10.2196/14273

17. Kam JWY, Javed J, Hart CM, Andrews-Hanna JR, Tomfohr-Madsen LM, Mills C. Daily mindfulness training
    reduces negative impact of COVID-19 news exposure on affective well-being. *Psychol Res*. 2022;86(4):
    1203-1214. doi:10.1007/s00426-021-01550-1

18. An A, Hoang H, Trang L, et al. Investigating the effect of mindfulness-based stress reduction on stress level and
    brain activity of college students. *IBRO Neurosci Rep*. 2022;12:399-410. doi:10.1016/j.ibneur.2022.05.004

19. World Health Organization. Healthy diet. Published April 29, 2020. https://www.who.int/news-room/fact
    -sheets/detail/healthy-diet

20. Office of Disease Prevention and Health Promotion. *2008 physical activity guidelines for Americans*. 2008.
    https://health.gov/sites/default/files/2019-09/paguide.pdf

21. Centers for Disease Control and Prevention. *Fact sheets–binge drinking*. Published October 24, 2018. https://
    www.cdc.gov/alcohol/fact-sheets/binge-drinking.htm

22. Glanz K, Bishop DB. The role of behavioral science theory in development and implementation of public health
    interventions. *Annu Rev Public Health*. 2010;31(1):399-418. doi:10.1146/annurev.publhealth.012809.103604

23. Lindell MK, Perry RW. The protective action decision model: theoretical modifications and additional evidence.
    Risk Anal. 2012;32(4):616-632. doi:10.1111/j.1539-6924.2011.01647.x

24. Grothmann T, Patt A. Adaptive capacity and human cognition: the process of individual adaptation to climate
    change. *Glob Environ Change*. 2005;15(3):199-213.

25. Arah OA. On the relationship between individual and population health. *Med Health Care Philos*.
    2009;12(3):235-244. doi:10.1007/s11019-008-9173-8

26. Galea S. *Meeting the challenge of obesity*. Boston University School of Public Health. Published October 9,
    2016. https://www.bu.edu/sph/2016/10/09/meeting-the-challenge-of-obesity

27. The State of Obesity. *Adult*. Updated September 2018. https://stateofobesity.org/adult-obesity

28. Link B, Phelan J. Social conditions as fundamental causes of disease. *J Health Soc Behav*. 1995;Spec No:80-94.
    http://www.ncbi.nlm.nih.gov/pubmed/7560851

29. Klein S, Gastaldelli A, Yki-Järvinen H, Scherer PE. Why does obesity cause diabetes? *Cell Metab*.
    2022;34(1):11-20. doi: 10.1016/j.cmet.2021.12.012

30. World Heart Federation. *Diet, overweight and obesity*. 2011. https://world-heart-federation.org/wp-content/
    uploads/2017/05/Diet_overweight_and_obesity-2.pdf

31. Declercq E, MacDorman M, Cabral H, Stotland N. Prepregnancy body mass index and infant mortality in 38
    U.S. states, 2012–2013. *Obstet Gynecol*. 2016;127(2):279-287. doi:10.1097/AOG.0000000000001241

32. McCrory MA, Harbaugh AG, Appeadu S, Roberts SB. Fast-food offerings in the United States in 1986, 1991, and 2016 show large increases in food variety, portion size, dietary energy, and selected micronutrients. *J Acad Nutr Diet.* 2019;*119*(6):923-933. doi:10.1016/j.jand.2018.12.004

33. American Heart Association. *Extreme obesity, and what you can do.* https://www.heart.org/en/healthy-living/healthy-eating/losing-weight/extreme-obesity-and-what-you-can-do

34. Food Research & Action Center. *Low-income and food-insecure people are vulnerable to poor nutrition and obesity for a number of reasons.* https://frac.org/blog/whats-state-childhood-obesity/low-income-and-food-insecure-people-are-vulnerable-to-poor-nutrition-and-obesity-for-a-number-of-reasons

35. DoSomething.org. *11 facts about food deserts.* https://www.dosomething.org/us/facts/11-facts-about-food-deserts

36. Bentley RA, Ormerod P, Ruck DJ. Recent origin and evolution of obesity-income correlation across the United States. *Palgrave Commun.* 2018;4(146). doi:10.1057/s41599-018-0201-x

37. Ogden CL, Carroll MD, Fakhouri TH, et al. Prevalence of obesity among youths by household income and education level of head of household—United States 2011–2014. *MMWR Morb Mortal Wkly Rep.* 2018;67:186-189. doi:10.15585/mmwr.mm6706a3

38. Centers for Disease Control and Prevention. *Adult obesity prevalence maps.* 2022. https://www.cdc.gov/obesity/data/prevalence-maps.html

39. Healio. *Parental education levels, BMI influence childhood obesity risk.* 2019. https://www.healio.com/news/endocrinology/20190805/parental-education-levels-bmi-influence-childhood-obesity-risk#:~:text=Overall%2C%20children%20who%20had%20a,CI%2C%201.37%2D2.37)

40. Kandra J, Perez D. *By the numbers: Income and poverty, 2020.* Economic Policy Institute. Published September 14, 2021. https://www.epi.org/blog/by-the-numbers-income-and-poverty-2020/

41. Centers for Disease Control and Prevention. *Adult obesity facts.* National Center for Chronic Disease Prevention and Health Promotion, Division of Nutrition, Physical Activity, and Obesity. Updated May 17, 2022. https://www.cdc.gov/obesity/data/adult.html

42. Brownell KD, Farley T, Willett WC, et al. The public health and economic benefits of taxing sugar–sweetened beverages. *N Engl J Med.* 2009;*361*(16):1599-1605. doi:10.1056/NEJMhpr0905723

43. Levine JA. Poverty and obesity in the U.S. *Diabetes.* 2011;*60*(11):2667-2668. doi:10.2337/db11-1118

44. Puhl RM, Heuer CA. Obesity stigma: important considerations for public health. *Am J Public Health.* 2010;*100*(6):1019-1028. doi:10.2105/AJPH.2009.159491

7

FAMILIES, SOCIAL NETWORKS, NEIGHBORHOODS, AND CITIES

OVERVIEW: FAMILIES, SOCIAL NETWORKS, NEIGHBORHOODS, AND CITIES INFLUENCE HEALTH AND BEHAVIORS

We are not islands. As we move through the social ecological model, we come now to thinking about our networks and connections, about how we are connected to family and friends, and how those connections shape our health. We also recognize that as we move through the stages of the life course, the makeup of our important social networks changes. So, too, do our roles.

Further, the majority of the world now lives in cities, and more and more people will live in cities in the coming decades. City living is rapidly becoming the modal human experience and, as such, represents an important modifiable factor that could potentially improve the health of populations. Forces ranging from clean air to availability of healthy food, from public transportation to walkable environments, are all features of cities and can be changed to improve public health.

Our zip code can tell us more about our health than our genetic code. The place where we live shapes the air we breathe, the water we drink, and the food we eat. Places shape how we think, feel, and behave. Therefore, places represent a unique opportunity for the promotion of the health of populations. We mostly live in human-made environments creating even more of an opportunity for improving these environments toward improving the health of the public.

Our health is influenced by others around us, from the moment of conception forward.[1] When we consider the importance of individual behavior in producing health, we must also consider the context of those around us who are socially important and influential. These people are often geographically nearby, sometimes living under the same roof. This chapter moves beyond the individual, giving primary focus to our social networks and neighborhoods in which we live, work, and play.

In this chapter, we continue to expand the continuum of the social ecological dimension with a focus on families and social networks, neighborhoods, and cities (**Figure 7.1**). We (a) discuss what families and social networks are and how they influence individual behavior and health, (b) describe how families and social networks influence health in infectious and chronic disease, (c) highlight the role of vaccination as a public health tool, (d) explore how public health efforts influence network behaviors, (e) differentiate what is a neighborhood and a city in the United States and worldwide, (f) analyze how neighborhoods and cities influence health and disease, and how neighborhoods and cities can be modified to create the health of populations, and (g) examine public health efforts that have been used to improve health in neighborhoods/cities.

> **Our zip code can tell us more about our health than our genetic code. The place where we live shapes the air we breathe, the water we drink, and the food we eat. Places shape how we think, feel, and behave.**

> **Our health is influenced by others around us, from the moment of conception forward.[1]**

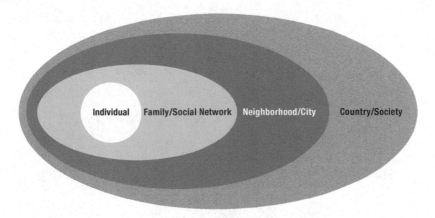

FIGURE 7.1 The multilevel social ecological perspective, highlighting the focus of this chapter: families, social networks, neighborhoods, and cities. Artistic Credit: Parisa Varanloo.

WHAT ARE FAMILIES/SOCIAL NETWORKS?

DYADS: THE BASIC BUILDING BLOCKS OF FAMILY/SOCIAL NETWORKS

The simplest form of a social network involves two people. We call this a social dyad. Two partners or spouses, a brother and sister, two classmates, two teammates, two colleagues—each of these pairs qualifies as a dyad. Social networks include at least two people, so the dyad represents the most basic element in its construction.

Social networks resemble elaborate molecular or matrix structures. Each individual is a node connected to at least one other person. When we draw a social network, there are no singletons, no lone individuals, floating around like disconnected atoms. By definition, every member of a social network has at least one connection. Consider the illustration in **Figure 7.2**. This web reveals readily how complicated social networks can get, very quickly. Some individuals are extraordinarily interconnected, while others are not. Later, we demonstrate how the actions and behaviors of those who are highly interconnected can influence others in their social networks.

DYADS AND BEYOND: DURING THE EARLIEST PHASES OF THE LIFE COURSE

The earliest phases of the life course, beginning with the perinatal period, depend on what happens between individuals. Often, this distills down to a sequence of essential pairings, or dyads.

Conceiving a child takes a dyad. This is followed by a 40-week pregnancy from conception to birth which also primarily involves a dyad. However, this dyadic relationship is very asymmetrical. The fetus is reliant on, and derives life from, the mother. The fetal period is one of complete fetal dependency on the mother. Studies have documented the importance of maternal–fetal attachment as a predictor of newborn and child health with potential lifelong ramifications.[2] Maternal–fetal attachment is outwardly manifested in the pregnant mother's caring behaviors that convey her commitment to the well-being of the fetus. These include the mother's own self-care behaviors such as maintaining a healthy diet, engaging in regular physical activity,

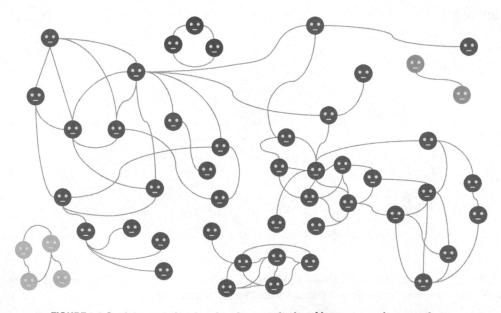

FIGURE 7.2 Social networks showing the complexity of interpersonal connections.

getting adequate rest, and abstaining from harmful substance use. Attachment is also observed in the form of comforting gestures (stroking the belly) and preparing for the baby's arrival (purchasing baby clothes, creating a nurturing space in the home).

In ideal contexts, the mother will receive care and support during pregnancy from her partner (dyad), her own parents, and perhaps a larger constellation of family members and friends, together fashioning an informal, expectant-mother–centered social network.

Then comes birth. Sustenance in the first few days and weeks of life takes two people—or more. The newborn depends on the parent for nutrition (breastfeeding in most cases) and comfort, a continuation of the ongoing dyadic relationship. Ideally there will be active participation from the partner and other family caregivers to meet the life-sustaining needs of the child—and provide relief and support for the parents. Although profoundly physically dependent, and cognitively undeveloped, under optimal conditions the newborn exists in a child-centric universe, safeguarded and nurtured by a social network of attentive caregivers.

DYADS AND BEYOND: DURING THE CHILDHOOD PHASE OF THE LIFE COURSE

Dyads are critical to social networks throughout the entire life course, starting from the earliest periods of life and continuing to the oldest ages. Positive, nurturing, caring home environments during infancy generate health during the first moments of a child's life that will ultimately propel positive benefits forward throughout the life course.

Unfortunately, some environments create the opposite dynamic. A robust and growing literature now describes the harmful effects of adverse childhood experiences (ACEs) on development and health lifelong. Exposure to ACEs often takes place within social networks. Among the most harmful of ACEs are physical, mental, verbal, and sexual abuse of young children by parents, older siblings, and relatives living in the home.

Households can face a myriad of other issues that impinge on the health of multiple family members. For example, parental health challenges may affect the physical or mental health of the children raised in the home even when loving care is provided and abuse is absent. Alternatively, having children in the home who themselves are living with a disability may have negative health effects on all members of the family unit.

DYADS AND BEYOND: DURING ADULT AND OLDER ADULT PHASES OF THE LIFE COURSE

Throughout the life course, the health of each partner in a dyad affects the other. Living in a positive and supportive spousal or partnered relationship increases health and life expectancy for both partners. As early as the 1850s, William Farr, one of the founding figures of public health, documented that married persons, especially married men, had a lower mortality rate than their unmarried counterparts,[3] a finding that has been related to evolutionary selection.[4]

Conversely, when one spouse becomes seriously ill, the burden associated with witnessing and supporting the suffering partner, providing hands-on care, and paying the medical bills may diminish the health and quality of life of the healthier partner, turned caregiver.[5,6] Most often, later in life, one partner dies first. We know that the loss of a spouse through death may diminish the health and hasten the death of the surviving partner.[5]

BEYOND DYADS: THE OVERARCHING POWER OF FAMILY/SOCIAL NETWORKS

We have described a series of social dyads, but it is important to know that the entire household is a social force to be reckoned with. As one example, use of tobacco and alcohol aggregates within families, and siblings track in similar trajectories into and through substance use behaviors.[7,8]

This suggests some combination of shared genetics and household social environment factors. Direct sibling influence clearly plays a role in substance use experimentation and adoption.[9,10]

Further, dietary and exercise behaviors surrounding weight loss or weight gain are socially transmissible via social networks. For example, the diagnosis of breast cancer in one woman can motivate another woman in this patient's family to seek breast cancer screening and counseling. The effects may be more widespread—neighborhood friends and office co-workers may likewise be prompted to undergo mammography or other cancer screening. Even impersonal social connections may be influential. High-social-influence celebrities who are diagnosed with breast cancer or who opt to undergo prophylactic surgeries may potentially influence the behavior of other women connected to them only through social media channels. The much publicized "Angelina Jolie effect" is a notable example. The actor's revelation that she underwent prophylactic mastectomy prompted a surge in women seeking screening for the *BRCA* breast cancer gene, although rates of preventive surgeries did not increase.[11]

PRESENTING FAMILY/SOCIAL NETWORKS VISUALLY

When seeking to spatially portray a social network, we envision ourselves, or the person of interest, as the center point, with members of the social network orbiting around the center. This conception resembles a tiny solar system. An alternative vision is a wheel-and-spoke configuration with the person of interest occupying the hub. Sounds egocentric? In fact, this is precisely the term used by sociologists, an egocentric network.[5] This method of visualizing social networks contrasts with the sociocentric network in which all network members and their interconnections are visualized at once, without giving priority to any one person. More on that conception is given later. Returning to the graphic we developed to display the social ecological perspective, we show how individuals are nested within multiple levels of influence; the family and social network level is highlighted in **Figure 7.3**.

Social networks are important influencers of health lifelong. Networks are not static. Even if the composition of a social network—such as a primary family unit—remains constant and unchanged in terms of its membership for years or even decades, each member is continuously interacting with the others, while all are simultaneously aging and moving along their life course paths. Understandably, the nature of the relationships within a network changes over time even if the cast of characters remains stable. It is, therefore, useful to consider social networks in the context and time sequence of the life course.

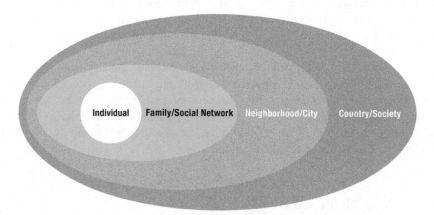

FIGURE 7.3 The multilevel social ecological perspective, highlighting the focus of this section: family/social networks. Artistic credit: Parisa Varanloo.

The influence that our most important networks have on each of us changes across the life course. The family often serves as the primary and most central social network, especially early in life. As an individual grows and moves through life, that individual's position within the family changes and so do the roles played. Not infrequently, the sequence goes something like this: parent cares for young child; child grows and becomes an independent, yet still connected, adult; parent and child live decades of adult life in a mutually supportive relationship; adult child partners and creates his or her own family, with parents assuming grandparenting roles; years later, adult child cares for elderly parents during their later life years. Thus, the reciprocal influences of family members on the health of other members are constantly reconfiguring over the life span.

Beyond the family and close household members, peer groups play a prominent role during adolescence. Later childhood and early adolescence are notable for the developmental transition from parents as primary influencers to peer groups holding increasing sway. This is sometimes a turbulent process, but ideally the resolution in young adulthood is the emergence of an autonomous individual who can balance roles effectively. Such an individual both derives benefits from, and contributes actively to, important networks of family, friends, coworkers, and colleagues. Family members and similar-age peers may be central to our lives over periods of decades. Other members of our social networks, such as memorable teachers or mentors, may take center stage for fleeting periods, yet leave lasting contributions. The makeup of our most important social networks shifts over time. This partially relates to our own developmental process. As we grow up, and as we invariably grow older, our roles within our primary networks necessarily change.

UNDERSTANDING THE ROLE OF FAMILY/SOCIAL NETWORKS

HOW FAMILY/SOCIAL NETWORKS INFLUENCE INDIVIDUAL BEHAVIOR AND HEALTH

Families and social networks produce effects on health in multiple ways (**Box 7.1**).[5,12]

First, *family/social networks serve as a source of perceived and practical social support.* An ever-expanding literature connects social networks to health-promoting and health-compromising behaviors, onset and progression of diseases and medical conditions, healthcare utilization, and compliance with prescribed medical regimens. One of the most solid findings is the tie-in between perceived social support and all-cause mortality. A meta-analysis of 148 studies demonstrated a 50% increased likelihood of survival for participants with stronger social relationships.[13] This increased life expectancy was found across a broad range of initial health status. What was particularly

---

BOX 7.1 FAMILY/SOCIAL NETWORKS PRODUCE EFFECTS ON HEALTH IN FIVE WAYS

Family/social networks produce effects on health in multiple ways

1. Family/social networks serve as a source of perceived and practical social support.
2. Family/social networks exert social influence, conveying norms and forms of social control.
3. Family/social networks provide a platform for social engagement.
4. Family/social network members include persons in close physical proximity.
5. Family/social networks provide access to resources, including shelter and financial support.

compelling was the finding that a lack of social connectedness increases the risk for premature death in a manner so potent that it is equivalent to a 15-cigarette per day smoking habit. Further, lack of social support was a stronger predictor of early death than obesity, physical inactivity, or alcohol abuse.

Across studies, perceived social support and, particularly, strong social relationships are remarkably consistent predictors of vibrant physical and mental health and increased life expectancy. In contrast, findings for received social support are much weaker and less conclusive. This tells us that, to favorably affect health, social support must be recognized, acknowledged, and consciously appreciated as valuable by the recipient. Conversely, for individuals lacking a strong perceived social support network, social isolation renders them less able to deflect life and health stressors. This absence of social support increases vulnerability to negative health outcomes—disease, disability, and death.

> **Across studies, perceived social support and, particularly, strong social relationships are remarkably consistent predictors of vibrant physical and mental health and increased life expectancy.**

Second, *family/social networks exert social influence, conveying norms and forms of social control.* This has been particularly well studied in men who have sex with men (MSM).[14] The health and well-being of MSM benefit from membership in social networks that feature pro-social norms and behaviors. These include disclosure of HIV status, negotiation for safer sex practices including every-time use of barrier protection, regular preventive medical exams, use of pre-exposure prophylactics (PrEP), and—for those who are seropositive—conscientious adherence to medication regimens that successfully lower chances of HIV transmission to noninfected partners.

Third, *family/social networks provide a platform for social engagement.* Friendship networks provide opportunities to participate in health-promoting activities while simultaneously enhancing the experience by adding the social dimension. For example, consider the experiential difference of solo exercise on a stationary cycle compared to instructor-motivated participation in a high-energy spinning class with regular class attendees you know. Actually, both options are healthy and there is a preferred time for each. However, not only can social engagement (e.g., attending a spinning class) spur friendly competition in physical activities, this attribute of social networks can also deepen and enrich social relations through shared pursuits.

It is now possible to harness the power of social media to prompt health-promoting behavior change.[15] In fact, during the COVID-19 pandemic, popular spinning classes were presented online, allowing a hybrid alternative—exercising "solo" and safely at home while participating in real time with an entire class of spinning enthusiasts from across the nation.

Fourth, *family/social network members are frequently the persons in closest physical proximity to the individual.* Network members may cohabit the same household or share the same classroom or workspace. This necessarily creates opportunities for person-to-person interaction. When it comes to sharing time and healthy activities with family and close friends, physical proximity is a bonus and a motivator. Contrastingly, physical closeness to members of one's social network increases the likelihood of exposure to communicable disease pathogens, secondhand cigarette smoke, or access to unlocked firearms.

Fifth, *family/social networks provide access to resources, including shelter and financial support.*[16] Pooling and sharing resources and skills confers health-related benefits on all network members. The ability to rely on each other often provides opportunities unattainable for isolated, unconnected individuals. This aspect of social networks is nothing less than lifesaving for populations living in impoverished or deprived conditions. The importance of this attribute of social networks becomes acutely apparent in humanitarian emergencies or the aftermath of a natural disaster when social networks pull together to help their members recover in situations of scarce resources and austere conditions.

UNDERSTANDING PUBLIC HEALTH APPROACHES TO INFLUENCE NETWORK BEHAVIORS

Health behavior change can successfully harness the power and the dynamics of social networks.[17] Researchers have developed social network interventions that have successfully modified dietary behaviors, cigarette smoking, physical inactivity, and high-risk HIV-transmission behaviors.[18] Such approaches have also favorably decreased bullying, supported mental health, and shaped family planning. Social network interventions are most effective when specific attributes of the social network are targeted to achieve a particular change in a health-related behavior. Successful social network interventions operate, and maintain their efficacy, by effectively channeling social influence mechanisms. These include applying health-promoting norms, modeling desired behaviors, modifying social identity, and dispensing social rewards. The use of peer influence leaders is well known and widely used for motivating change throughout a network.[19] Matching the best types of network interventions to the best-suited applications is an area of ongoing exploration. Among options that have shown promise are those that purposefully and cleverly "put the network in network interventions"; these interventions integrate the characteristics of social networks at their core.[19]

While health behavior change is possible, researchers continuously strive to increase intervention effectiveness and reach. Social environments are instrumental for the adoption and sustainability of health-enhancing behaviors and for discontinuing health-compromising behaviors. From a population health point of view, social network interventions—including modification of the social environment—can leverage more expansive and long-lasting behavior changes than individual-level interventions.

THE OPERATION OF SOCIAL NETWORKS IN INFECTIOUS DISEASE SPREAD

COMMUNICABLE DISEASE TRANSMISSION, PERSON TO PERSON

Sexually transmitted infections (STIs) provide a good example of the role of social networks and interpersonal connections in the transmission of disease. STIs are communicable diseases—such as chlamydia infection, gonorrhea, genital herpes, human papillomavirus (HPV) infection, syphilis, and HIV/AIDS infection—involving the transmission of an infectious agent from person to person through sexual contact. Sexually active persons are at risk for contracting STIs during vaginal, anal, or oral sex with a partner who is infected. Several STIs, particularly herpes and HPV infection, are also spread by skin-to-skin contact.[20] Using the United States as an example, STIs pose a present and growing danger to public health. Although youth risk behavior surveillance data showed a decrease from 1991 through 2019 in high school youth reporting that they are sexually active, rates of STIs have been rising. Specifically, according to the Centers for Disease Control and Prevention (CDC), from 2015 through 2019, rates of chlamydia, gonorrhea, and syphilis increased for males and females, aged 15 to 24.[21,22] This age group accounts for half of the 20 million new STI cases annually.[23] Forty percent of the U.S. adolescent and adult population, 110 million persons, are infected with an STI, so it is not surprising that one in two sexually active persons will contract an STI prior to age 25.[24] Nevertheless, according to a 2022 study, just one in five sexually active high schoolers reported being tested for STIs in the previous year.[25] Alarmingly, reports of drug-resistant strains of gonorrhea, chlamydia, and syphilis are increasing, and already, some cases of gonorrhea are untreatable with currently available medications. These concerning patterns of STI occurrence and spread reflect underlying trends in types and combinations of sexual behaviors.

One of the classic examples of person-to-person STI transmission involving social network influences was an anthropological study conducted in the 1980s. CDC researchers examined the spread of early cases of HIV/AIDS in San Francisco.[26] At that point in history, there were venues (bathhouses, the baths) in cities worldwide that provided sauna and pool facilities, open lounge areas, and private cubicles where men could congregate and engage in sexual contact with one or many other male partners. Frequently, the sexual couplings were anonymous. The bathhouse served as a "behavioral amplification system" that facilitated the overlap of HIV-infected and noninfected partners.[27,28]

Some men in the study were able to identify dozens of lifetime partners. The research team was able to partially map the network of sexual contacts and the overlaps among the partners. This study became notable for the identification of a highly sexually active male flight attendant who was named as a common sexual partner across multiple study subjects.[29] Moreover, this young man was linked to AIDS cases in the cities frequented in his travels, including Los Angeles, San Francisco, and New York City. His exploits led him to be erroneously described as "Patient Zero" in Randy Shilts's bestseller and film by the same name, *And the Band Played On.*[30]

This study reinforced the presumption that a core group of individuals who engage in high-frequency, multiple-partner sexual activity serves as the source of infection to lower activity groups and individuals. These cores become the primary reservoirs of STIs, and their existence sustains disease transmission in the larger population.

However, "core group theory" has not always been borne out. Indeed, other researchers found, for example, that adolescent affection and sexual networks in the U.S. Midwest tend to form a spanning tree with very limited overlap of partners.[31] In fact, sexual partnering seems to be guided by informal yet widely observed sexual mores such as a rule that holds, "Don't date your old partner's current partner's old partner."[31]

On the other side of the world, investigators studying HIV/AIDS in Malawi also found no evidence for active hubs of infected persons serving as a reservoir for sexual transmission of infection.[32] These conflicting findings suggest that it is critical to map broader networks. To make a finer point, what is needed is information on individuals' partners' partners. Lacking this information, it is impossible to discern whether a sexually active individual is at high risk based on having promiscuous partners with deep networks of sexual contacts or, conversely, at low risk because partners have few other contacts.[5]

UNDERSTANDING HOW SOCIAL NETWORKS INFLUENCE HEALTH IN INFECTIOUS DISEASE

One fascinating finding regarding transmission of STIs is the specificity and compartmentalization of disease transmission networks. Miami-Dade County has been an epicenter of the HIV/AIDS epidemic since its inception. One of the distinguishing features of Miami is that separate streams of HIV transmission take place in the same county, yet there is very little overlap. The first stream was the most predictable. Earliest cases were diagnosed in MSM. Social networks of gay men were frequenting the hub of gay clubs that proliferated on Miami Beach.

Back in the 1990s, as the HIV pandemic was spiraling upward, Miami's large population of homeless persons had the highest rate of HIV infection of any street-based population studied by the CDC. Almost one in four homeless people had HIV infection. Within the homeless encampments, a common mode of transmission was exchanging heterosexual sex for crack cocaine or money to buy crack. Miami was the locale where the U.S. crack epidemic originated. At one point, there were more than 700 active crack houses in operation in the city. Sexual exchange behaviors frequently took place on the premises of the crack houses or in nearby street venues.

Meanwhile, Miami had one of the largest networks of injection drug users with high rates of HIV infection. The most popular injection drugs were heroin, cocaine, and the combination of both together, called "speedballs." Drug injectors frequented settings called "shooting galleries" (the local Miami term was "get-off houses"), where they could rent paraphernalia (needles, syringes, cookers), inject, and if necessary, sleep off the effects in a wretched but supervised setting. Unfortunately, these sites facilitated the sharing of drug use paraphernalia that quickly became contaminated with the HIV-infected blood from other injectors. These sites were yet another example of a behavioral amplification system that accelerated the spread of HIV infection. These social networks were not necessarily composed of individuals known to each other, but they were linked instead by the commonality of sharing the venues and the rented injection equipment, a lethal combination.

County epidemiologists maintained ongoing surveillance on HIV/AIDS. For most years, Miami-Dade County ranked first in the nation on rates of new HIV infections and AIDS cases. What distinguished HIV/AIDS surveillance in Miami was that each of these streams—MSM, homeless crack smokers, and injection drug users—contributed to the countywide tally of cases. Yet the individuals participating in these networks were almost completely separate from one another. A proportion of MSM also injected drugs, but this was a small fraction of the county cases. Otherwise, these networks—each occupying a separate niche of Miami socially and geographically—were separate and nonoverlapping.

HOW HIGHLY NETWORKED INDIVIDUALS DRIVE INFECTIOUS DISEASE OUTBREAKS

One of the most remarkable findings is the dynamic nature of how social networks influence infectious disease outbreaks. Highly networked individuals, by virtue of their many connections, tend to become infected, ill, and infectious early in the outbreak. Also, based on their multitudinous connections, they become primary spreaders of disease.

This was demonstrated in real time and in a real-world scenario.[33] During the 2009 outbreak of H1N1 influenza, researchers tracked students on a college campus as the epidemic was unfolding. Investigators selected a large random sample of students and asked them to identify their friends. This seems deceptively simple. Researchers tracked both the original random sample and the subset of student-nominated friends throughout the course of the influenza epidemic.

The assumption was that the persons nominated as friends were more centrally located within the campus social networks and therefore had more social connections. This assumption proved to be correct. In the case of influenza, which is notable for the ease of widespread airborne respiratory transmission, socially connected individuals are extremely susceptible to infection. When put to the test, sure enough, the H1N1 epidemic swept through the socially connected friend group 14 days prior to reaching a peak within the larger randomly chosen sample (**Figure 7.4**).

These social network dynamics have implications for the early detection and intervention on infectious disease outbreaks. First, these findings indicate that the highly socially networked cores have connections that allow them, on the positive side, to be the early adopters of new "viral trends" and innovations. Afterall, these are the influencers that others watch and emulate. On the downside, when the viral trend is truly a virus, like H1N1 influenza, these trend-setting individuals are likely to be among the first to become ill.

Second, because these socially connected students were likely to become ill early in the outbreak, they effectively served as sentinels—or sensors—for the larger wave of epidemic illness to follow. Once infected, they were also extremely likely to infect each other right away.

Third, to the extent that highly connected individuals represent a socially talented and influential subset of the larger population, they will be at disproportionate risk of illness and death during a deadly outbreak. This suggests that in the realm of communicable disease outbreaks, individuals who are most socially gregarious are especially vulnerable.

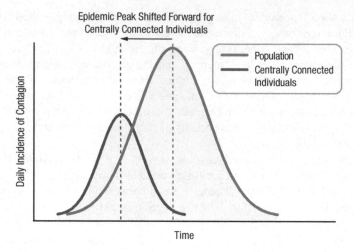

FIGURE 7.4 Epidemic curves for highly socially connected students and the general student population.
Source: From Christakis NA, Fowler JH. Social network sensors for early detection of contagious out breaks. *PLoS One.* 2010;5(9):e12948. doi:10.1371/journal.pone.0012948

CAPITALIZING ON SOCIAL NETWORK UNDERSTANDING TO IMPROVE THE HEALTH OF POPULATIONS

Highly Connected Network Members as Sentinels for Detecting Outbreaks

The methods used in the college campus study of H1N1 influenza through a student network can be repurposed to quickly detect an epidemic in the making and take preventive actions to shield the larger population.[33] There are several related strategies. Where social network mapping of a population has been conducted, it is possible to monitor and surveil those who are most central to the network to identify outbreaks rapidly. Remember that these individuals are the trendsetters, so they tend to receive attention and scrutiny for their social prominence. They also potentially serve as an early warning network for disease outbreaks. Finding early cases popping up among these network influencers may give public health officials weeks of advance lead time before the epidemic builds to a critical mass and case numbers surge upward. During this window of time, it may be possible to implement such public health strategies as social distancing, school and worksite closures, cancellation of mass gathering events, and population distribution of available vaccines or antiviral prophylactic medications.

High-Visibility Networks Uncovering Hidden Epidemics

Here is an historical disease outbreak example—predating social network research—of socially visible individuals putting us on the trail of a spreading epidemic. In a bygone era when commercial airlines served meals on flights, a ravenously hungry team of Minnesota Vikings professional football players boarded a charter flight heading home to Minneapolis following their preseason game against the Miami Dolphins.[34] Players downed quantities of sandwiches that had been prepared by the flight kitchen at the Minneapolis/St. Paul International Airport. Unfortunately, the sandwiches were heavily contaminated with *Shigella* bacteria. Within days, numerous members of the team were severely incapacitated with symptoms of fever, watery diarrhea, acute abdominal cramping, nausea, and in some cases, blood or pus in the stool. For a professional football team that was scheduled for rigorous practices and a big game the following week, these symptoms were crippling.

The Minnesota Department of Health immediately went into action, investigating the outbreak, tracing the source of *Shigella* to the flight kitchen, and identifying the specific foods contaminated with the bacteria. According to the investigators, confirmed or probable shigellosis was identified among 240 passengers on 219 flights to 24 states, the District of Columbia, and four countries. Extrapolating to all flights on which potentially contaminated food was served, thousands of passengers worldwide may have been exposed to the bacterial toxin. This epic foodborne outbreak of immense proportions might have gone undetected for weeks longer if one high-visibility social network—a team of professional football players—had not succumbed to illness and, in the process, alerted health officials to this potentially deadly epidemic.

Vaccinating Highly Connected Network Members to Achieve Herd Immunity

Vaccination is credited with saving hundreds of millions of lives and propelling life expectancy upward. In the realm of social networks, vaccination relates to breaking the chain of transmission. What do we know? When vaccination is used preventively, it is possible to achieve "herd" immunity even with less than perfect, 100% vaccine coverage. Social network scientists found that when preventive vaccination must be accomplished rapidly, or when vaccine stocks are insufficient to immunize the entire population, if it is possible to identify the core of highly connected persons in the social network and vaccinate them, vaccination of approximately 30% of the population—that includes the most connected persons—will safeguard the entire population as effectively as vaccinating more than 90% of the total population.[35] A truly astonishing finding.

THE OPERATION OF SOCIAL NETWORKS IN NONCOMMUNICABLE DISEASES

NONCOMMUNICABLE DISEASES ARE LINKED TO THE BEHAVIOR OF THOSE AROUND US

It is important to recognize that social networks do not impact population health only by influencing the transmission of communicable diseases. When it comes to noncommunicable diseases (NCDs), the influence of those around us operates in covert and subtle ways. As we will see, there can be many levels of influence that persist, or shift and change dynamically, along the life course. As we direct our attention to NCD transmission, the effects of social networks become much more nuanced and complex. Yet, understanding and invoking the power of social networks to address NCDs is a fairly new area of exploration.

It is important to recognize that social networks do not impact population health only by influencing the transmission of communicable diseases.

UNDERSTANDING HOW SOCIAL NETWORKS INFLUENCE HEALTH IN NONCOMMUNICABLE DISEASES

A global network design was used to demonstrate how obesity moves in epidemic fashion through a social network, resembling the spread of a communicable disease.[36] Researchers analyzed longitudinal data from 12,067 participants in the multigenerational, community-based

Framingham Heart Study. They fortuitously tracked body weight over a 32-year period during which the prevalence of obesity doubled in the United States.

All participants had body mass index (BMI) data available. Defining obesity as a BMI of 30 kg/m² or higher, researchers were able to examine associations between an individual's weight gain and the corresponding increases in weight among this person's friends, siblings, spouse, and neighbors. They could detect the moment when individuals crossed the BMI obesity threshold. All the while, they were examining the weight and BMI trajectory for each person in relation to what was happening during the same time periods to the persons composing their networks (**Figure 7.5**).

Results clearly demonstrated the person-to-person transmission of a biobehavioral trait.[5] Persons who became obese were embedded in social networks of persons who were likewise becoming obese. These were obesity clusters. BMIs continued to increase in many of these clusters as the entire network became progressively heavier over three decades of observation. Astonishingly, obesity clusters were apparent out to three degrees of separation. What this means is that an individual's BMI was predictable not only from the *BMIs of their closest friends*, but also from the *BMIs of the friends of their closest friends*—and even from the *BMIs of the friends of the friends of their closest friends*!

We conclude our discussion of social network dynamics with an examination of social media influences on health and mental health of youth and young adults who are active users of a variety of popular social media platforms. (Case Study 7.1; you can access the podcast accompanying Case Study 7.1 by following this link to Springer Publishing Company Connect™: http://connect.springerpub.com/content/book/978-0-8261-8043-8/part/part02/chapter/ch07).

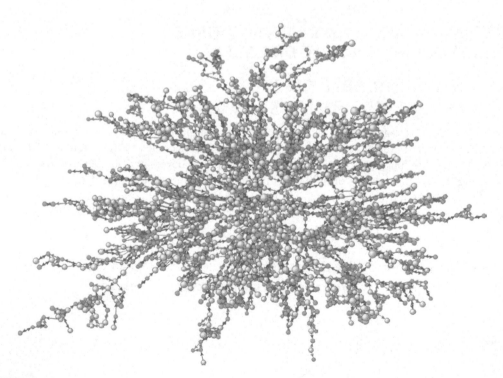

FIGURE 7.5 Obesity and normal weight clusters for individuals from the Framingham Heart Study and their social networks.
Source: Reproduced with permission from Smith KP, Christakis NA. Social networks and health. *Annu Rev Sociol.* 2008;34(1):405-429. doi:10.1146/annurev.soc.34.040507.134601

CASE STUDY 7.1: EVOLVING DIRECTIONS IN SOCIAL NETWORKS: HEALTH IMPLICATIONS FOR ACTIVE USERS OF SOCIAL MEDIA

Social networking is undergoing an extraordinary evolution. We are transforming the ways in which we relate and interact. In less than one-quarter century—basically a phenomenon of the millennium—the penetration of digital services has now reached the majority of world citizens. By early 2022, 62.5% of the world's population of 7.91 billion individuals were using the internet, and two-thirds (67.1%) were using mobile devices (**Table 7.1**).[37] Three in five subscribed to some form of social media. Facebook was the single most popular social media platform, with more than 2.9 million active users worldwide.[37] This is a generational phenomenon with about 60% of social media users in the 18- to 34-year age demographic (**Table 7.2**). Those who have grown up since their earliest years with this technology have been dubbed "digital natives." Almost 80% of subscribers use social media platforms daily or several times daily, and many use multiple social media platforms and applications each month. On average, users spend hours daily on social media and even more time using the internet.

TABLE 7.1   Global Penetration of Digital Technologies and Social Media, January 2022

TOTAL GLOBAL POPULATION	7,910,000,000	100.0%
TYPES OF DIGITAL USERS:		**PENETRATION (%):**
Internet users	4,950,000,000	62.5
Unique mobile users	5,310,000,000	67.1
Active social media users	4,620,000,000	58.4
SOCIAL NETWORKS:		
Facebook	2,910,000,000	36.8
YouTube	2,562,000,000	32.4
Instagram	1,478,000,000	18.7
TikTok	1,000,000,000	12.6
Twitter	436,000,000	5.5
LinkedIn	260,000,000	3.4
MESSENGER/CHAT APPLICATIONS:		
WhatsApp	2,000,000,000	25.3
WeChat	1,263,000,000	16.0
Facebook Messenger	988,000,000	12.5
Snapchat	557,000,000	7.0

Source: Data from Kemp S. Digital 2022: Another year of bumper growth. We Are Social. Published January 26, 2022. https://wearesocial.com/uk/blog/2022/01/digital-2022-another-year-of-bumper-growth-2/

(*continued*)

TABLE 7.2   Profiles of Facebook and Instagram Users, January 2018

AGE GROUP	FACEBOOK USERS (2.170 BILLION)			INSTAGRAM USERS (800 MILLION)		
	FEMALE (%)	MALE (%)	TOTAL (%)	FEMALE (%)	MALE (%)	TOTAL (%)
13–17 years	4	4	8	3	4	7
18–24 years	12	17	29	16	15	31
25–34 years	12	17	29	15	15	30
35–44 years	7	9	16	8	9	17
45–54 years	5	5	10	4	5	9
55–64 years	3	2	5	2	2	4
65+ years	2	2	4	1	1	2
Total	45	56	101	49	51	100

Source: Data from Kemp S. Digital in 2018: world's internet users pass the 4 billion mark. We Are Social. Published January 30, 2018. https://wearesocial.com/uk/blog/2018/01/global-digital-report-2018

The use of digital technologies has become normative, representing a behavior in which the majority of persons, across varied cultures, actively participate. Yet the time span since the introduction of these applications has been extremely brief. Moreover, the ongoing advancement of these products and services, made more complex by shifting preferences and patterns of use, has not allowed sufficient time for population health scientists to clearly evaluate the health implications. Only recently have studies begun to appear.[38] Not surprisingly, the results present a mixed picture. Active engagement with social media appears to produce both health benefits and risks, and both positive and negative health outcomes.[39]

The use of digital technologies has become normative, representing a behavior in which the majority of persons, across varied cultures, participate actively.

The Royal Society for Public Health explored the pros and cons of social media influences on the mental health of youth and young adults, aged 16 to 24 years.[39] Up front, the report explains, "social media has become a space in which we form and build relationships, shape self-identity, express ourselves, and learn about the world around us; it is intrinsically linked to mental health."

The report first examines the potential negative impacts of social media involvement on the mental health of youth. These include elevated rates of self-report of psychological distress—including symptoms of both anxiety and depression—among heavy users of social media.[40,41] In fact, the content of social media postings on Twitter and other platforms can even predict depression with moderate accuracy.

Another detrimental factor is that social media use, including use just before bedtime, is linked to decreased sleep time and diminished sleep quality.[42] In turn, shortened and disrupted sleep has direct links to both physical and mental

(*continued*)

health. The report also highlighted body image concerns that arise as youth scan the panoply of photos and images posted online, often making negative comparisons that can lead to lowered self-esteem or even prompt unhealthy dietary or exercise practices. Such effects have been documented as early as the pre-teen years.[43]

A direct offshoot of the digital age is the prevalent phenomenon of cyberbullying; a majority of teens have experienced some form of cyberbullying.[44] Victims may experience decreased academic performance, sleep disruption, and symptoms of anxiety and depression; some may engage in behaviors that are harmful to self or others.

Another emergent phenomenon, directly tagged to the use of social media, is "fear of missing out" (FoMO).[45] FoMO relates to the tension that is set in motion by hearing about the innumerable enjoyable activities that are taking place all at once. Yet each individual can participate in only a fraction of these events, owing to finite time and resources. Access to the internet and social media vastly amplifies the sense that an individual is missing out on so many opportunities, and this FoMO reality carries potential mental health consequences.

The report also highlights the flip side; social media can positively affect health in several ways. Among these is gaining access to the health-related experiences of peers; this goes beyond searching for expert health information and gives a personalized view. Some youth benefit from social support for specific personal health issues. Also available is community building and group support for members of subpopulations defined by race, ethnicity, gender, and sexual orientation who may be dealing with in-group issues with health overtones. Seven in 10 teens reported receiving support through social media channels when they were going through difficult personal challenges.

Social media also provides avenues for self-expression that may help youth navigate the tricky process of identity formation. Online expression is sometimes more comfortable than face-to-face peer encounters. Another benefit is the ease of communication that can help to solidify supportive friendships and relationships via frequent texting and other contact methods that were simply unavailable before the advent of these technologies.

After delineating 14 negative and positive features of active social media participation, researchers then mapped these factors for users of several popular platforms: YouTube, Facebook, Twitter, Instagram, and Snapchat. The study was conducted in 2018 and subject to change as platforms change in content, popularity, algorithms, and policies. With that caveat, for each factor, youth rated their social media experience in terms of making each of the 14 issues better or worse (ranging from −2, a lot worse, to +2, a lot better). For example, YouTube users indicated that their sleep was negatively impacted while awareness, self-expression, and community-building skills were improved, and overall there was a slight net positive rating for the use of YouTube. Instagram received the strongest net negative rating with sizable downside impacts noted for sleep, body image, FoMO, and bullying, along with worsening of anxiety and depression.

As a result of these findings, the Royal Society for Public Health, along with the Young Health Movement, is asking policy makers and social media companies to help promote the health-positive attributes of social media and to mitigate the health-negative consequences (www.rsph.org.uk/our-work/campaigns/status-of -mind.html). Several strategies have been endorsed including posting pop-up

(continued)

heavy usage warnings on the websites, signposting support to users with likely mental health problems, and alerting users to images that have been digitally manipulated.

Social media, as a relatively new and exponentially expanding domain of social networking, should be prioritized for concentrated research going forward in order to shape behaviors toward the most positive health outcomes. Evidence is just beginning to accrue regarding health outcomes associated with the already-rampant, and continuously expanding, use of social media.

WHAT IS A NEIGHBORHOOD? A CITY?

There is no perfect answer to the questions "What is a neighborhood?" or "What is a city?" Defining neighborhoods/cities is a challenge for many fields, including public health.[46] Administrative definitions (such as census tracts) and geographic information system (GIS)–based definitions are two of several approaches to define a neighborhood or a city; both have strengths and limitations. Most definitions of neighborhoods/cities in the scientific literature rely on geographic boundaries defined by administrative agencies.[38] In the public health literature, neighborhoods/cities usually refer to people's immediate residential environments that have both material and social characteristics related to health.[47]

UNDERSTANDINGS OF NEIGHBORHOODS/CITIES IN THE UNITED STATES

Census data and zip codes are two of the most widespread methods used to describe neighborhood boundaries in the United States. The Census Bureau publishes sample data on block groups; these are subdivisions of census tracts usually containing between 600 and 3,000 people, nested in the census tracts and representing small geographic units. Zip codes were created by the postal service in 1963 to facilitate more efficient delivery of mail.[46]

> Census data and zip codes are two of the most widespread methods used to describe neighborhood boundaries in the United States.

In 1880, the U.S. Census Bureau initially defined urban areas as communities with a minimum population of 4,000 individuals.[48] In 1910, the population threshold for an urban area was revised to 2,500 people. This is the currently used definition, and in 2015, 63% of the U.S. population lived in cities.[49]

UNDERSTANDING NEIGHBORHOODS/CITIES WORLDWIDE

Countries other than the United States also use diverse approaches to define neighborhoods/cities. For example, neighborhoods in China are assigned as part of the central administrative system of the country with anywhere from several hundred to more than 10,000 households in each neighborhood.[50,51] There is no official definition of neighborhoods in the United Kingdom; neighborhood boundaries are set through different methods including local services' catchment areas or through determining the homogeneity of communities occupying the area.[52] The county assembly of Nairobi, Kenya, defines neighborhoods based on groups representing common interests rather than people living in the same locality.[53]

There is general consensus that cities are places where large numbers of people live and work. Cities serve as hubs for government, transportation, and commerce. However, there are no global standards for determining the geographic boundaries of a city. Different countries employ different methods to define cities.

Generally, there are three approaches used to define a city. The "city proper" approach designates a city based on an administrative boundary. The "urban agglomeration" approach considers the extent of the contiguous urban area, or built-up area, to delineate a city's boundaries. The third approach is the "metropolitan area," which defines a city's boundaries according to the degree of economic and social interconnectedness of nearby areas.[54]

The 2014 World Urbanization Prospects report generally adhered to the concept of "urban agglomeration" in defining cities. However, the report also used the other two methods to provide a comprehensive list of cities around the world. Among the 1,692 cities with at least 300,000 inhabitants included in the report, 55% followed the "urban agglomeration" definition, 35% followed the "city proper" approach, and the remaining 10% were denoted as "metropolitan areas."[55]

About one-third of the world's urban population lives in slum conditions, primarily located in urban centers within low-income countries.[56] Slums are densely populated areas characterized by substandard housing conditions and low standards of living. Slums often lack a proper water supply, up-to-date sanitation, sufficient living area, durable construction, and security of tenure.[57] Between 2005 and 2010, the number of people living in slums in resource-limited countries increased by almost 50 million persons—reaching 828 million in just 5 years.[58]

CITY LIVING AS THE MOST PROMINENT DEMOGRAPHIC CHANGE OF OUR TIME

LIVING IN A CITY IS THE MODAL HUMAN EXPERIENCE

For the first time in history, the majority of people live in urban areas. The scale and pace of global urbanization over the past 50 years is unprecedented. At the beginning of the 20th century, only one in 10 people lived in an urban area, but by 2015, more than 50% of the population worldwide lived in urban areas.[59] The population size of urban centers is also increasing dramatically; in 2022, the 40 most populous cities in the world each had populations ranging in size from 9 to 37 million residents (Table 7.3).

TABLE 7.3   2022 Population of the World's 40 Most Populous Cities

RANK	CITY NAME	POPULATION	RANK	CITY NAME	POPULATION
1	Tokyo	37,274,000	21	Rio De Janeiro	13,634,274
2	Delhi	32,065,760	22	Lahore	13,541,764
3	Shanghai	28,516,904	23	Bangalore	13,193,035
4	Dhaka	22,478,116	24	Shenzhen	12,831,330
5	Sao Paulo	22,429,800	25	Moscow	12,640,818

(*continued*)

TABLE 7.3   2022 Population of the World's 40 Most Populous Cities (*continued*)

RANK	CITY NAME	POPULATION	RANK	CITY NAME	POPULATION
6	Mexico City	22,085,140	26	Chennai	11,503,293
7	Cairo	21,750,020	27	Bogota	11,344,312
8	Beijing	21,333,332	28	Paris	11,142,303
9	Mumbai	20,961,472	29	Jakarta	11,074,811
10	Osaka	19,059,856	30	Lima	11,044,607
11	Chongqing	16,874,740	31	Bangkok	10,899,698
12	Karachi	16,839,950	32	Hyderabad	10,534,418
13	Istanbul	15,636,243	33	Seoul	9,975,709
14	Kinshasa	15,628,085	34	Nagoya	9,571,596
15	Lagos	15,387,639	35	London	9,540,576
16	Buenos Aires	15,369,919	36	Chengdu	9,478,521
17	Kolkata	15,133,888	37	Nanjing	9,429,381
18	Manila	14,406,059	38	Tehran	9,381,546
19	Tianjin	14,011,828	39	Ho Chi Minh City	9,077,158
20	Guangzhou	13,964,637	40	Luanda	8,952,496

Source: Reproduced with permission from world city populations 2022. World Population Review. http://worldpopulation review.com

TREND TOWARD MORE PEOPLE LIVING IN CITIES WILL CONTINUE IN COMING DECADES

The pace of urbanization will accelerate over the coming decades. By 2030, six in 10 people will live in a city. By the mid-21st century, the global urban population will almost double, reaching 6.5 billion individuals.[55] Further, the United Nations projects that 90% of future global population growth will be in low- and middle-income countries.[59] Urban population growth will be principally concentrated in countries in Africa and Asia. Latin American countries will also see notable urban population expansion.[60] In terms of individual countries, urban population growth will be most pronounced in India, China, and Nigeria; these nations predict increases of 404 million, 292 million, and 212 million urban dwellers by 2050, respectively.[60] Meanwhile, high-income countries anticipate a more modest increase in urban residents, increasing from 900 million in 2005 to 1.1 billion by 2050.[61]

In 1990, there were only 10 megacities with populations exceeding 10 million inhabitants, and accounting for 7% of the world population.[60] By 2022, there were 32 megacities—many located in the Global South—with populations exceeding the 10 million threshold.[54] Currently, urban growth is rising most rapidly in cities with 500,000 inhabitants or less, accounting for about half of the world's urban population.[60]

HOW PLACES (NEIGHBORHOODS/CITIES) AFFECT OUR HEALTH

A large number of interconnected mechanisms operate together to produce the effects that neighborhoods and cities have on health outcomes.[62] Living in disadvantaged neighborhoods is associated with higher rates of cardiovascular disease and death.[63] Residents of neighborhoods with higher social cohesion are less likely to have hypertension.[64] Neighborhood conditions are also linked to obesity,[65] rates of smoking,[66] and mental health disorders.[67]

Cities are neither good nor bad for our health. Characteristics of cities simply influence health; some make our health better, others make it worse. For much of human history however, scholars and historians alike considered cities to be detrimental for health because cities were characterized by many features linked to poor health outcomes.[68] During the 19th century, unsafe water, improper waste management, poor handling of food, crowded unventilated housing, and a concentration of commerce all contributed to widespread infectious diseases in cities, especially in port cities.[69] As cities gained more importance in European society, they also witnessed an increase in population density, with attendant increases in the number of marginalized groups, pollution, and crime rates. In time, health indicators in cities became worse compared to rural areas.[68]

> Cities are neither good nor bad for our health. Characteristics of cities simply influence health; some make our health better, others make it worse.

The environment in many cities began improving dramatically in the mid-19th century to early 20th century. Sanitary reforms such as construction of sewers, pasteurization and disinfection of water, improvements in nutrition, and surveillance and quarantine or isolation of sick individuals all contributed to improving health within cities.[70,71] However, the mass departure of the middle class to suburban areas over the past half-century in the United States and other Western countries led to focalized poverty and racial segregation in cities. Later in the 20th century, cities had high rates of infant mortality, substance abuse, mental illness, HIV infections, asthma, and other health conditions.[72]

Currently, cities concentrate health hazards. Cities have finite health resources for large, heterogeneous, expanding populations. For example, crowded areas—such as slums—are conducive to the spread of communicable diseases. Moreover, the prevailing sedentary lifestyle in cities leads to increased rates of NCDs. Further, cities generally have high levels of crime.[56] These problems are usually compounded by poverty and occur systematically in low-income neighborhoods and populations. Disadvantaged populations generally have higher mortality and morbidity rates than the remainder of the population in high-, middle-, and low-income countries alike. These inequities in health tend to be more pronounced among those living in cities.[56] Despite the plethora of opportunities in cities, disparities in job opportunities and services, urban segregation, and heterogeneous socioeconomic characteristics all contribute to health inequities.[73] The key question for public health, and for public health action, is "How does living in a particular neighborhood or city affect our health?"

PLACES DEFINE OUR PHYSICAL ENVIRONMENT: THE AIR WE BREATHE, THE WATER WE DRINK, AND THE FOOD WE EAT

Neighborhood/city conditions shape the environmental atmosphere of a residential area. For example, geographic proximity to facilities that produce or store hazardous substances affects neighborhood air and water quality. In turn, poor air quality is linked to cardiovascular and respiratory diseases as well as higher mortality rates.[74] Moreover, substandard treatment of the water supply can expose residents to microbial, chemical, and radiological hazards for water-related diseases.[75]

There are profound racial, ethnic, and socioeconomic differences in neighborhood proximity to facilities that produce industrial pollutants in the United States.[76] Minority and lower socio-economic status neighborhoods are more likely to be located closer to sources of industrial pollutants than their counterparts.

Neighborhoods also determine the quality of the food we eat. There is a positive associa-tion between neighborhood availability of healthy foods and consumption of those foods by local residents. Low-income and minority neighborhoods often do not have adequate access to healthy foods.[77] Larger supermarkets, which are more likely to provide healthy food choices at a lower cost, are often not found in poor neighborhoods. Residents of low-income and minority-majority neighborhoods must resort to shopping at convenience stores that stock processed foods low in nutritional value.[78]

CASE STUDY 7.2: DYING FOR HEALTHY FOOD: FOOD DESERTS IN AMERICAN NEIGHBORHOODS

About 23.5 million people in the United States live in low-income areas where the nearest supermarket is more than a mile away. Such areas where sources of healthy foods are scarce are commonly referred to as food deserts.[79] In the 2008 Farm Bill, the U.S. Congress defined a food desert as an "area in the United States with limited access to affordable and nutritious food, particularly such an area composed of predominantly lower income neighborhoods and communities."[80] Food deserts generally lack access to healthy foods including, but not limited to, fresh fruit, vegetables, and dairy products. Moreover, food deserts are usually heavily dependent on local shops that sell processed foods loaded with sugar and fat.[81,82] Low-income zip codes have 30% more convenience stores, with fewer healthy food options compared to middle-income zip codes.[23]

The emergence and multiplication of food deserts was mostly driven by the growth of large chain supermarkets coupled with ever-changing demographics.[83] Large chain supermarkets, benefitting from an economy of scale, were able to provide better services, greater product variety, and longer hours of operation. This competitive environment forced the closure of many smaller grocery stores that once supplied local neighborhoods with healthy food choices.[84] As small gro-ceries closed, access to healthy foods became increasingly challenging for those who do not own a car or could not afford public transportation to reach the clos-est supermarket offering nutritious foods.[85] Moreover, between 1970 and 1988, more affluent households emigrated to suburban areas, and the shift created an economic segregation.[86] Eventually, with the median income decreasing in urban areas, about half of the supermarkets in the three largest cities in the United States closed while larger chains opened branches in suburban areas.[84]

Regardless of the precipitating factors, food deserts pose a challenge for the American population. Although food deserts are a nationwide issue, cities and urban areas suffer the most from lack of access to healthy food. A few examples are Detroit, New York City, Minneapolis, and Chicago. More than 550,000 of the residents of Detroit live in food deserts. In 2008, 3 million New York City residents lived in communities without easy access to supermarkets. More than half of

(continued)

Minneapolis is classified as a food desert, and in 2009, 36% of the corner stores in the city did not sell fresh produce. In Chicago, nearly 600,000 people live in food deserts.[87]

Regardless of the precipitating factors, food deserts pose a challenge for the American population. Although food deserts are a nationwide issue, cities and urban areas suffer the most from lack of access to healthy food.

Moreover, the extent of food deserts varies significantly between counties; in 2006, only 1.5% of households in wealthy suburban areas were located in food deserts compared to 5.9% of households in areas that have the lowest median income in the United States. These aggregate statistics understate the extent of the issue; in counties like Wilcox County, Alabama, and Holmes County, Ohio, the percentage of households living more than 1 mile from a supermarket and without access to a car are 18.6% and 27.9%, respectively.[88]

Minorities are more likely to live in a food dessert. African American/Black-majority neighborhoods have fewer options to obtain healthy food[89,90] compounded by a higher number of fast-food outlets.[91] In Detroit, in 2005, residents in majority poor African American/Black neighborhoods were 1.1 miles farther away from the nearest supermarket compared to residents in White-majority neighborhoods.[92] Nationally, in 2007, in majority African American/Black neighborhoods, availability of supermarket chains is only 52% of that in White-majority neighborhoods. Further, in majority Latinx neighborhoods, availability of supermarket chains is only 32% of that in majority non-Latinx neighborhoods.[93] Additional examples of food deserts with disparities in access to supermarkets and sources of healthy foods are presented in **Table 7.4**.[94]

Understandably, people generally choose foods that are available and accessible to them.[95] Hence, the lack of access to grocery stores, supermarkets, or other sources of healthy and nutritious food limits the ability of many Americans to eat a healthy diet.[96] This assertion is true regardless of the economic status of an individual. For example, among persons who participate in the food stamp program, easy access to supermarkets is associated with increased consumption of fruits and vegetables.[97] Lacking access to healthy food options creates a vast nutritional gap in food deserts where the void is filled with small convenience stores and fast-food restaurants. As the only walkable options available in local neighborhoods, these outlets charge high prices for their very limited selections of nutritionally deficient foods. As corroboration, in 2008, the Department of Agriculture reported that counties with more food deserts generally spend more per capita on fast food than their counterparts.[88]

The issue with food deserts is not just a matter of inconvenience; living in food deserts is also linked to a higher risk of NCDs including higher rates of obesity and type 2 diabetes.[98,99] The Department of Agriculture reported that counties with at least 10% of households living in food deserts had a 9% higher rate of adult obesity and a 5% higher rate of diabetes compared to counties with less than 1% of households living in food deserts.[88]

Public awareness of the impact of food deserts is growing and has led to a number of proactive policies.[100] The 2008 Farm Bill directed the Secretary of Agriculture

(*continued*)

TABLE 7.4   Examples of Neighborhoods/Communities with High Levels of Food Deserts in the United States

CITY/COMMUNITY	DATA ABOUT LIMITED ACCESS TO HEALTHY FOOD
	DISPARITIES IN ACCESS TO SUPERMARKETS
Los Angeles, California	• Low-poverty areas have 2.3 times as many supermarkets per household compared to high-poverty areas. • Predominantly White neighborhoods have 3.2 times as many supermarkets compared to predominantly African American/Black neighborhoods and 1.7 times as many supermarkets compared to predominantly Latinx neighborhoods.
West Louisville, Kentucky	In this low-income, predominantly African American/Black community, there is one supermarket for every 25,000 residents. This is compared to an average of one supermarket for every 12,500 residents in the county.
Washington, DC	One in five food stamp recipients lives in a neighborhood without a grocery store.
	DISPARITIES IN ACCESS TO HEALTHY FOODS AT NEIGHBORHOOD STORES
Albany, New York	Eight in 10 non-White residents live in a neighborhood that does not have any stores selling low-fat milk or high-fiber bread.
Baltimore, Maryland	In a survey of 226 stores, compared to 4% of predominantly White and 13% of higher income neighborhoods, 43% of predominantly African American/Black neighborhoods and 46% of lower income neighborhoods were in the bottom third of food availability.
Los Angeles, California	Three in 10 food stores in a predominantly African American/Black, high-poverty community lacked fruits and vegetables while nearly all of the stores in a low-poverty, predominantly White community sold fresh produce.

Source: Data from Treuhaft S, Karpyn A. *The Grocery Gap: Who Has Access to Healthy Food and Why It Matters.* PolicyLink; 2010. https://www.policylink.org/resources-tools/the-grocery-gap-who-has-access-to-healthy-food-and -why-it-matters

to address the issue of food deserts in the United States. The bill required more research on the causes and prevalence of food deserts and the impact of food deserts on populations. Moreover, the bill mandated the Department of Agriculture to provide recommendations to reduce and, ultimately, eliminate food deserts. The bill also encouraged community involvement and partnerships to address food deserts and provided incentives for opening food stores offering healthy and affordable selections in designated food deserts.[80]

Two years following the passage of the bill, the Obama Administration introduced a multiyear Healthy Food Financing Initiative to reduce numbers of neighborhoods with food deserts and encourage healthy food retailers to cater to underserved communities. Several states followed the federal government's

(continued)

example and launched measures to increase access to healthy food.[101] The ambitious goal of the national campaign, led by Michelle Obama, was to eradicate food deserts by 2017; alas, food deserts continue to exist in the United States still today.[102]

Food deserts continue to make people less healthy and contribute to widening the income gap in the country. Health problems associated with living in food deserts create the vicious cycle in which poorer communities are less capable of confronting their mounting health problems.[88]

PLACES PARTIALLY DEFINE OUR SOCIAL/BEHAVIORAL ENVIRONMENT, SHAPING HOW WE THINK, FEEL, AND BEHAVE

The social environment and the extent of cohesion within neighborhoods contribute to the overall health of residents. Characteristics of social cohesion include the strength of social relations as well as the degree of connectedness and mutual trust among residents. Close-knit neighborhoods generally maintain social control that discourages crime and other harmful behaviors that can directly or indirectly influence health. Children living in socially connected neighborhoods are less likely to engage in drinking, drug use, or gang activity.[103] Moreover, neighborhoods where residents express mutual trust and willingness to intervene for the public good have lower homicide rates.[104,105] Conversely, the lack of a socially cohesive neighborhood environment can exacerbate stress and increase rates of anxiety, depression, and related indicators of poor mental health.[106]

HOW PLACES SHAPE OUR ACCESS TO SALUTARY RESOURCES

Where we live influences our access to quality education, municipal services, public transportation, healthcare services, and employment opportunities. Such critical resources can affect health both directly and indirectly. For example, in the United States, poor and minority students who live in neighborhoods where schools are underfunded are more likely to receive lower quality education.[107] Quality of education is linked to health through several pathways, so expectedly, these students have poorer health across multiple indicators than their counterparts living in neighborhoods with better schools. Better education leads to healthier lifestyles.[108] Moreover, education affects health indirectly through providing access to better employment and, ultimately, improved economic conditions.[109]

IMPROVING NEIGHBORHOODS/CITIES TO ADVANCE THE HEALTH OF POPULATIONS

HUMAN-MADE ENVIRONMENTS PRESENT AN OPPORTUNITY FOR IMPROVING THE HEALTH OF THE PUBLIC

Human-made (or built) environments include buildings, structures, spaces, and products created or modified by humans. Improving the human-made environments is a feasible option for addressing the growing burden of chronic diseases. The built environment can be crafted to increase physical activity, reduce obesity rates, and decrease the risk of cardiovascular diseases and lung cancer.[89,110,111]

The purposeful design of modern parks provides a good example of how neighborhoods/cities can be modified to improve the health of populations. People living in neighborhoods that are safe and conducive for engaging in physical activity—particularly neighborhoods with parks and walking trails—are more likely to be active. In Los Angeles, building neighborhood parks contributed substantially to increased physical activity. Careful analyses were able to quantify substantial increases in moderate-to-vigorous physical activity by local citizens who used the park facilities.[112] Moreover, shifting neighborhood environments to be pedestrian-friendly can help improve the health of residents. For example, well-maintained footpaths, indoor walking areas, and street lights are positively associated with increased physical activity among older adults.[56] Providing walkable green spaces is also associated with higher functional status and lower risks for cardiovascular disease among neighborhood residents.[113,114]

> **The purposeful design of modern parks provides a good example of how neighborhoods/cities can be modified to improve the health of populations.**

EVIDENCE-BASED PUBLIC HEALTH EFFORTS THAT IMPROVE POPULATION HEALTH IN NEIGHBORHOODS/CITIES

There are many public health initiatives and policies to mitigate adverse neighborhood/city effects on health. For example, a few years ago, the U.S. Department of Housing and Urban Development (HUD) established a number of initiatives to offset adverse neighborhood effects. One is the Choice Neighborhood initiative, which aims to strengthen the underlying social structure of neighborhoods. The initiative provides grants for strategies to revitalize struggling neighborhoods. Projects funded by the initiative focus on improving housing conditions, education quality, commercial activity, and neighborhood safety.[115] Another example is the Moving to Opportunity program that gives families currently living in public housing in low-income neighborhoods the option to move to high-income neighborhoods. Adult participants who used the program showed a 20% reduction in depression symptoms compared to those who did not.[116]

Motivated by a Philadelphia study that found elevated rates of diet-related chronic diseases in areas with limited access to supermarkets that sell healthy foods, legislation was passed that supported the opening of 10 fresh food stores in underserved areas throughout the state of Pennsylvania.[117]

MUNICIPAL POLICY AND STRUCTURAL INTERVENTIONS

There is a long-standing connection between city planning and management and the health of urban populations. Municipal governments influence the health of city dwellers by providing services and regulating activities that affect health. Governments can modify both the physical and social environments of cities as well as oversee and deliver healthcare, social services, and public health interventions.[118]

> **There is a long-standing connection between city planning and management and the health of urban populations.**

Moreover, municipal governments can indirectly influence health through setting policies that promote health in areas such as transportation, recreation, public safety, criminal justice, welfare, housing, and employment.[118] For example, municipal transportation policies can affect health in a number of ways. Providing public transportation and regulating private transportation reduces air pollution. Public transportation also facilitates mobility in highly populated areas, which increases access to healthcare, employment, and fresh foods. Further, effective traffic management leads to decreased automobile-related injuries and deaths.[118] Regulating acceptable housing conditions is another example of how municipal governments affect health. Poor housing is linked to multiple health conditions including lead poisoning, asthma, respiratory infections, and injuries and can lead to adverse mental health outcomes.[119]

THE ROLE OF MUNICIPAL HEALTH DEPARTMENTS IN THE UNITED STATES

Municipal health departments play an important role in improving the health of city dwellers. Responsibilities of municipal health departments range from direct provision of healthcare services to prevention and health promotion initiatives. One example is the New York City Department of Health and Mental Hygiene, one of the largest public health agencies in the world. With an annual budget of $1.6 billion, the department coordinates the health agenda and policy decisions for New York City. The department provides a broad range of services including access to low-cost clinics, restaurant inspections, and investigations of disease clusters throughout the metropolitan area. The department works on initiatives to reduce the population health burden of obesity, diabetes, heart disease, HIV/AIDS, tobacco addiction, and substance abuse, and is always prepared, if necessary, to confront the threat of bioterrorism.[120]

The Chicago Department of Public Health provides another example of the important role health departments play in improving the health of city dwellers.[121] The department's mission is focused on engaging communities to enable residents to live healthy lives.[122] The department provides preventive and behavioral health services at no cost to those in need, and conducts food, housing, and environmental inspections. The department launched the Healthy Chicago 2.0 initiative with the goal of improving healthy equity throughout Chicago by 2020.[121]

CIVIL SOCIETY AND MOVEMENTS TOWARD HEALTHY CITIES

Civil society operates in all areas not controlled by the government or the market. Several forms of civil society can greatly influence health within a city. For example, community-based organizations—such as neighborhood associations and tenant organizations—have a long history of working to improve living conditions in cities.[118] Faith-based organizations also play a role in the movement toward healthy cities. They provide safe spaces, social support, and political leadership.[123,124] Organizations representing marginalized groups and residents of slums in both low- and high-income countries work to advocate on behalf of groups that might otherwise be left out of the broader conversation.[125] Further, over the second half of the 20th century, a number of social movements calling for equity emerged from urban settings. Examples include the civil rights, environmental, women's rights, and gay rights movements; all were associated with improved healthcare, reduced discrimination, stronger environmental protection, and higher levels of political participation.[118]

THE GLOBAL HEALTHY CITIES MOVEMENT

The World Health Organization (WHO) initiated the Healthy Cities movement to cope with the issues that are emerging with ever-expanding urbanization worldwide. According to the

WHO, a healthy city is "one that is continually creating and improving those physical and so-cial environments and expanding those community resources which enable people to mutually support each other in performing all the functions of life and developing to their maximum potential."[126]

The World Health Organization (WHO) initiated the Healthy Cities movement to cope with the issues that are emerging with ever-expanding urbanization worldwide.

A healthy city creates health-supportive environments, provides basic sanitation and hygiene, and ensures access for healthcare of its residents. Starting in 1986, Healthy Cities initiatives were launched in high-income European countries and in Canada, Australia, and the United States. In 1994, a number of resource-limited countries began their own Healthy City initiatives, adapting successful strategies from earlier implementations. Today, there are more than 1,000 cities from all WHO regions participating in the Healthy Cities network.[127]

In 2003, municipal governments, national governments, nongovernmental organizations (NGOs), the private sector, academic institutions, and international agencies founded the Healthy Cities Alliance. The alliance has been working to extend the concept of healthy cities beyond the scope of existing members.[128] Recently, the United Nations officially championed the Healthy Cities movement by including cities as one of the Sustainable Development Goals in 2015. Sustainable Development Goal 11 aims to "Make cities and human settlements inclu-sive, safe, resilient and sustainable" with a focus on reducing air pollution within cities. By the beginning of 2019, 150 countries had developed national-level urban policies to improve the conditions of their cities.[129]

ENVIRONMENTAL DETERMINANTS AND THEIR ROLE IN CREATING HEALTHY CITIES

Sources of urban environmental challenges differ among low-, middle-, and high-income coun-tries. For example, lack of access to water contributes to the environmental challenges in urban areas in resource-limited settings. In 2005, about half of the population in Africa, Asia, and Latin America suffered from infectious diseases due to lack of access to clean water and san-itation. More recently, Cape Town, one of the largest cities in South Africa, nearly ran out of water. In addition, many city dwellers in low-income countries use solid fuel, including biomass and coal, for their most basic energy needs. Burning solid fuel produces high levels of indoor air pollution.[130] Although cities in high-income countries are less susceptible to similar environ-mental stressors, they face their own challenges. Vehicle air pollution and use of lead-based and asbestos-contaminated building products are among the urban environmental hazards faced by cities in high-income countries.[131]

Sources of urban environmental challenges differ among low-, middle-, and high-income countries. For example, lack of access to water contributes to the environmental challenges in urban areas in resource-limited settings.

Cities are major contributors to greenhouse gas emissions and global climate change; ur-ban areas account for over 67% of energy-related greenhouse gas emissions worldwide and the percentage is expected to rise to 74% by 2030. Cities consume about 80% of the global energy production, and as the world becomes more urbanized, greenhouse gas emissions will primarily derive from energy production required for lighting, heating, and cooling urban areas.[132]

Moreover, the consequences of climate change on cities are overwhelmingly negative. Hundreds of millions of people in urban areas across the globe will be affected by episodes of extreme heat and cold, rising sea levels, inland floods, increased precipitation, and more frequent and stronger tropical cyclones and storms. In fact, many major cities, with 10 million residents or more, are already under threat. Further, climate change can also damage infrastructure and worsen access to basic services in cities.[133]

However, cities also represent the best opportunity to address climate change and environmental challenges. Cities can help reduce global greenhouse gas emissions through increasing urban density, which leads to lower per capita emission of greenhouse gases. Moreover, cities can improve urban design to reduce urban sprawl, invest in public transportation, change building practices, and identify and innovate new and renewable sources of energy.[132]

HOW CITIES INFLUENCE NEIGHBORHOODS AND MICROLEVEL PLACES

Neighborhood characteristics are one of the many mechanisms through which cities' living conditions influence health outcomes. Cities influence neighborhoods through multiple pathways ranging from municipal policies that distribute resources across neighborhoods, to city regulations that affect neighborhoods' living conditions.[134]

For example, one of the ways through which cities influence health is through housing regulations. Poor planning of housing conditions leads to significant physical and mental distress.[135] Cities can also influence neighborhoods through prioritization of public transportation systems over investing in infrastructure for private transportation. Policy makers in cities can invest in public transportation systems that reduce the growing reliance of city residents on private vehicles. Providing public transportation systems that are fairly distributed throughout urban neighborhoods is beneficial to those living in low-income neighborhoods. Available public transportation can lead to better access to healthy food and employment opportunities.[135]

CITIES INCLUDE THE KEY ELEMENTS AND RESOURCES THAT CONTRIBUTE TO URBAN RESILIENCE

Despite the concentration of hazards, overall, urban populations usually enjoy better health than their rural counterparts. Cities generally have better infrastructure than rural areas when it comes to provision of basic services such as clean water, sanitation services, and housing. Healthcare facilities, services, and personnel are more numerous and accessible in cities. Moreover, cities provide better quality education, employment, and public transportation than do non-urban areas.[56]

LIVING IN RURAL AREAS

The global population of rural areas is about 3.4 billion and, unlike the trend in cities, is expected to decrease to 3.1 billion by 2050.[60] It is worth noting that the clear systematic divide between rural and urban areas is more pronounced in high-income countries. This divide starts to get blurrier in low- and middle-income countries.

Geographic isolation, lower socioeconomic status, limited job opportunities, and higher rates of risky behaviors all contribute to poor health in rural areas.[136] For example, rural communities face challenges to accessing healthy food. In an analysis of 21 studies examining food access in rural communities in the United States, 20 had found significant food access challenges, mostly due to low population density and the longer distances between food retailers.[94]

Further, residents of rural areas face significant barriers to accessing healthcare that may affect health outcomes. These barriers include cultural attitudes toward illness and financial restraints, which are often compounded by lack of trained physicians, fragile infrastructure, limited availability of reliable high-speed internet, and fewer public transportation options.[137]

All of these factors contribute to the health disparities between rural and urban areas. Currently, rural populations experience significant health inequities compared to the general population. Such inequities produce such untoward outcomes as higher incidence of disease and disability, higher mortality rates, and lower life expectancy. (Case Study 7.3; you can access the podcast accompanying Case Study 7.3 by following this link to Springer Publishing Company Connect™: http://connect.springerpub.com/content/book/978-0-8261-8043-8/part/part02/chapter/ch07).

CASE STUDY 7.3: THE HEALTH OF BOSTON NEIGHBORHOODS

Massachusetts has about 315 doctors per 100,000 people—more than 10% higher than Maryland, the next closest state. Much of this is due to a remarkable density of physicians and trainees in Boston itself. The state also spends more on healthcare than any other state and has the lowest percentage of residents without health insurance (4.4%).[138] All of this might suggest that Boston would be a tremendously healthy city, a paragon of urban health. In many ways, it is. Prepandemic, life expectancy in Boston was 81 years, one of the highest of any U.S. city. But, like many U.S. cities, Boston also has some extraordinary inequities, both in health indicators and in the drivers of those indicators within its borders. To examine these inequalities, we "tour" the City of Boston courtesy of the venerable Massachusetts Bay Transportation Authority (MBTA) system, better known as "the T." We compare health and social indicators in the neighborhoods surrounding five T stops located throughout the Boston area: Arlington, Dudley Square, Fenway, Mattapan, and Maverick. We illustrate how different key health indicators are for Boston residents living near T stops that are geographically just a few miles apart (**Figure 7.6** and **Table 7.5**).

Starting with several core health indicators, the premature death rate per 100,000 is twofold higher for both the Roxbury (near the Dudley Square T stop) and Mattapan neighborhoods compared with the Back Bay area, which includes the Arlington T stop. Furthermore, compared to the areas around the Fenway or Maverick (in East Boston) T stops, the Mattapan neighborhood is notable for having more than twice the rate of low birth weight newborns, a key indicator that predicts a substantial burden of poor health and disability later in life. The rate of adult type 2 diabetes is more than three times higher in the vicinity of Roxbury (Dudley Square/Nubian T stop) compared to either the Back Bay (Arlington T stop) or Fenway neighborhoods. This disparity is even more pronounced for Mattapan, with rates of diabetes that are more than four times higher than Back Bay or Fenway.

These health indicators and outcomes are inexorably linked to a broad range of social indicators that are unevenly distributed across the city of Boston. Poverty is a frequently used summary indicator of socioeconomic position; it is well established as a marker of a broad range of other adversities. It is then not surprising that the proportion of residents below the poverty line is three times higher in Roxbury (Dudley Square/Nubian T stop) compared to Back Bay (Arlington T stop).

(*continued*)

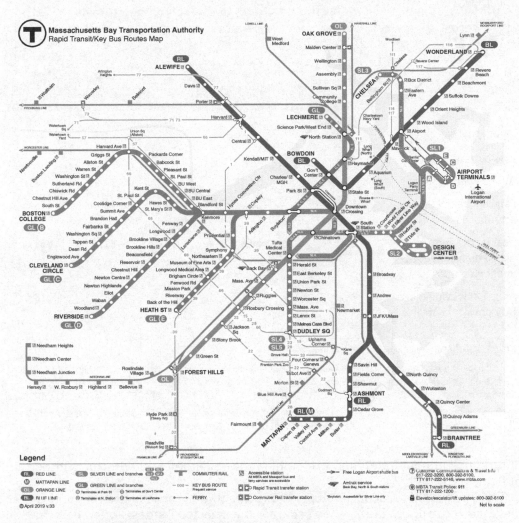

FIGURE 7.6 Selected Boston T stops for comparison of health indicators.
Source: Reproduced with permission from the Massachusetts Bay Transit Authority.

In contrast, the high proportion of residents who are below the poverty line in Fenway probably reflects the large population of students with minimal reported income who are living in proximity to the universities they are attending.

Other measures of socioeconomic position, such as education, track accordingly. While high school graduation rates are well above 90% in Back Bay (Arlington) and Fenway, they are 80% or less in Mattapan, Roxbury (Dudley Square/ Nubian), and East Boston (Maverick).

Further, these neighborhood differences are associated with commensurately poor health behaviors, such as physical inactivity. Achieving the CDC physical activity guidelines is substantially less likely for those living along the Red Line at Mattapan or the Blue Line at Maverick than for their counterparts on the Green Line near the Arlington T stop, for example. The question of how best to attribute

(continued)

TABLE 7.5 Comparison of Health Indicators for Selected Boston T Stops

HEALTH INDICATOR[a]	BOSTON T STOPS (NEIGHBORHOODS)				
	ARLINGTON (BACK BAY)	DUDLEY SQUARE/NUBIAN (ROXBURY)	FENWAY (FENWAY)	MATTAPAN (MATTAPAN)	MAVERICK (EAST BOSTON)
Premature deaths/100,000	149.0	296.4	197.7	302.7	180.8
Low birth weight	9%	10%	6%	13%	6%
Adults with diabetes	4%	14%	4%	17%	9%
Families below poverty line[b]	13%	37%	40%	20%	15%
Residents aged 25+ with a high school education or more	94%	79%	93%	80%	68%
Adults achieving the CDC physical activity guidelines	28%	20%	17%	18%	16%

CDC, Centers for Disease Control and Prevention.

[a]All health indicators listed are from the following source, unless otherwise indicated: Health of Boston 2016–2017. Boston Public Health Commission, Research and Evaluation Office. 2017. Accessed April 17, 2019: 112, 295, 334, 391, 557, 630. https://www.boston.gov/sites/default/files/file/2021/03/_HOB_16-17_FINAL_SINGLE%20PAGES-Revised%20Feb%202019.pdf

[b]Health of Boston 2014–2015. Boston Public Health Commission, Research and Evaluation Office. Accessed April 17, 2019: 94. https://www.boston.gov/sites/default/files/file/2021/03/FullReport_HOB_2014-2015-MSPDFforWeb.pdf

differences in health status to underlying socioeconomic differences is important but complex.[139,140]

The geographic space that hosts these health differences is remarkably small; distances of roughly 2 to 7 miles separate the selected T stops—often less than an hour's walk (**Table 7.6**). In many respects, it is remarkable that areas so close to one another should have such dramatically different health indicators.

Rounding this out brings us back to the fundamental condition of Boston discussed earlier—the incredible density of physicians, hospitals, and community health centers throughout the city. It is therefore not surprising that none of these T stops is particularly far from medical facilities. Clearly, medical centers differ in terms of populations served and variations in availability of specialty care, but there are negligible differences in the physical distances from each of these neighborhoods to quality medical care centers.

This tour of neighborhoods around several Boston T stops tells a story of a city richly characterized by top-of-the-line medical resources and overall health indicators that are enviably good, but that has, within it, substantial heterogeneity in those same health indicators. This heterogeneity is associated in large part with variations in the fundamental socioeconomic circumstances that produce health in populations. The challenge to public health is apparent and vivid—how do we

(continued)

TABLE 7.6   Distances between Boston T Stops as an Indicator of Geographic Proximity

BOSTON T STOP	AERIAL DISTANCE BETWEEN BOSTON T STOPS (MILES)				
	ARLINGTON	DUDLEY SQUARE/NUBIAN	FENWAY	MATTAPAN	MAVERICK
Arlington		1.8	1.9	6.0	2.0
Dudley Square	1.8		2.0	4.3	3.4
Fenway	1.9	2.0		5.5	3.7
Mattapan	6.0	4.3	5.5		6.8
Maverick	2.0	3.4	3.7	6.8	

contribute to the generation of knowledge that can bridge these health gaps and to the creation of conditions that produce health, not just for some but for all, across a city like Boston?

SUMMARY

Our health is influenced by others around us, from the moment of conception forward. As such, it is important to examine how family/social networks, neighborhoods, and cities shape health. Social networks include at least two people, or what we call a social dyad, starting from the prenatal period. One important dyadic relationship is the one between the fetus and the mother, which is a predictor of newborn and child health with potential lifelong ramifications. After birth, the focal relationship between mother and child includes bonding through breastfeeding, while care for the newborn extends to include the social network of family and household members. Networks of social relations expand rapidly as the child enters daycare and school environments. During adolescence, the social network of peers becomes salient and central for transitioning from parental influence, through the passage of identity formation, and on to independent functioning as an autonomous individual. Each of these critical social networks, and the complex relationships within them, changes constantly and dynamically over the life course.

Many health-related behaviors are socially transmissible via social networks. Social networks affect the health of an individual through (a) serving as a source of perceived and practical social support; (b) exerting social influence by conveying norms and forms of social control; (c) providing a platform for social engagement; (d) creating opportunities for person-to-person contact; and (e) providing access to resources, including shelter and financial support. Public health can intervene effectively in all these areas. Successful social network interventions—targeting both communicable and noncommunicable diseases—operate, and maintain their efficacy, by effectively channeling social influence mechanisms. From a population health point of view, social network interventions—including modification of the social environment—can leverage more expansive and long-lasting behavior changes than individual-level interventions.

Likewise, where we live determines the air we breathe, the water we drink, and the food we eat. It also affects how we think, feel, and behave. Moreover, where we live influences our access to quality education, municipal services, public transportation, healthcare services, and employment opportunities. Therefore, neighborhoods and cities largely shape our health, directly or indirectly. As such, public health interventions in neighborhoods—such as opening free food stores in low-income areas—represent a unique opportunity to promote the health of populations. The majority of people currently live in cities. Cities represent an important modifiable factor affecting the health of populations. Living in cities can influence health for better or worse. Cities have finite health resources for large, heterogeneous, expanding populations. They are also a major contributor to greenhouse emissions and climate change. Alternatively, cities generally have better infrastructure than rural areas when it comes to the provision of basic services such as clean water, quality healthcare facilities, education, employment, and public transportation. Cities also represent the best opportunity to address climate change and environmental challenges through interventions such as increasing urban density to lower per capita emission of greenhouse gases and improving urban design. Public health must act on social networks, neighborhoods, and cities to create healthier living environments that promote the health of populations.

End-of-Chapter Resources

Access additional case study podcasts online at http://connect.springerpub.com/ content/book/978-0-8261-8043-8/

DISCUSSION QUESTIONS

1. Once introduced, a new strain of influenza spreads at a high speed around the globe. During the deadliest global influenza outbreak on record in 1918 to 1919, more than one-third of the entire world population was infected. Based on your knowledge of the role of highly connected individuals in promoting infectious disease spread, what sort of social network intervention would you propose to limit the spread of influenza? Now think about the COVID-19 pandemic. What types of network interventions were applicable to mitigate the spread of that pandemic? How were they different than what might have worked in 1918?

2. Obesity provides a powerful illustration of the spread of a biobehavioral trait throughout a family/social network, with influences extending out to three degrees of separation. Provide one additional example of the spread of an NCD through a family or social network. Provide an example of the spread of some form of injury (unintentional or intentional) through a family or social network.

3. What is a major public health issue in your community—or in your country—that would benefit from a social network-based intervention? Explain why you selected this issue.

4. Identify any new policy implemented in your neighborhood or city and discuss how it has improved the health of the community.

5. There is an ongoing opioid epidemic in the United States. Discuss how living conditions in neighborhoods or cities can predispose a person to abuse opioids and other drugs and what could be done to combat this epidemic.

REFERENCES

1. Christakis N. *How do our social networks affect our health?* National Public Radio. Published March 4, 2016. https://www.npr.org/2016/03/04/468881321/how-do-our-social-networks-affect-our-health

2. Salisbury A, Law K, LaGasse L, Lester B. Maternal-fetal attachment. *JAMA*. 2003;*289*(13):1701-1701. doi:10.1001/jama.289.13.1701

3. Farr W. The influence of marriage on the mortality of the French people. In: Hastings GW, (Editor). *Transactions of the National Association for the Promotion of Social Science*. London, United Kingdom: John W Parker and Son; 1858.

4. Gellatly C, Störmer C. How does marriage affect length of life? Analysis of a French historical dataset from an evolutionary perspective. *Evol Hum Behav*. 2017;*38*(4):536-545. doi:10.1016/j.evolhumbehav.2017.02.002

5. Smith KP, Christakis NA. Social networks and health. *Annu Rev Sociol*. 2008;*34*(1):405-429. doi:10.1146/annurev.soc.34.040507.134601

6. Christakis NA, Iwashyna TJ. The health impact of health care on families: a matched cohort study of hospice use by decedents and mortality outcomes in surviving, widowed spouses. *Soc Sci Med*. 2003;*57*(3):465-475. doi:10.1016/s0277-9536(02)00370-2

7. Avenevoli S, Merikangas KR. Familial influences on adolescent smoking. *Addiction*. 2003;*98*(suppl 1):1-20. doi:10.1046/j.1360-0443.98.s1.2.x

8. Rajan KB, Leroux BG, Peterson AV Jr, et al. Nine-year prospective association between older siblings' smoking and children's daily smoking. *J Adolesc Health*. 2003;*33*(1):25-30. doi:10.1016/S1054 -139X(03)00044-2

9. Rende R, Slomkowski C, Lloyd-Richardson E, Niaura R. Sibling effects on substance use in adolescence: social contagion and genetic relatedness. *J Fam Psychol*. 2005;*19*(4):611-618. doi:10.1037/0893-3200.19.4.611

10. Low S, Shortt JW, Snyder J. Sibling influences on adolescent substance use: the role of modeling, collusion, and conflict. *Dev Psychopathol*. 2012;*24*(1):287-300. doi:10.1017/S0954579411000836

11. Troiano G, Nante N, Cozzolino M. The Angelina Jolie effect—impact on breast and ovarian cancer prevention: a systematic review of effects after the public announcement in May 2013. *Health Educ J*. 2017;*76*(6):707-715. doi:10.1177/0017896917712300

12. Berkman LF, Glass T, Brissette I, Seeman TE. From social integration to health: Durkheim in the new millennium. *Soc Sci Med*. 2000;*51*(6):843-857. doi:10.1016/s0277-9536(00)00065-4

13. Holt-Lunstad J, Smith TB, Layton JB. Social relationships and mortality risk: a meta-analytic review. *PLoS Med*. 2010;*7*(7):e1000316. doi:10.1371/journal.pmed.1000316

14. Amirkhanian YA. Social networks, sexual networks and HIV risk in men who have sex with men. *Curr HIV/AIDS Rep*. 2014;*11*(1):81-92. doi:10.1007/s11904-013-0194-4

15. Korda H, Itani Z. Harnessing social media for health promotion and behavior change. *Health Promot Pract*. 2013;*14*(1):15-23. doi:10.1177/1524839911405850

16. Berkman LF, Glass T. Social integration, social networks, social support, and health. In: Berkman L, Kawachi I, eds. *Social Epidemiology*. Oxford University Press; 2000:137-173.

17. Latkin CA, Knowlton AR. Social network assessments and interventions for health behavior change: a critical review. *Behav Med*. 2015;*41*(3):90-97. doi:10.1080/08964289.2015.1034645

18. Valente TW. Network interventions. *Science*. 2012;*337*(6090):49-53. doi:10.1126/science.1217330

19. Valente TW. Putting the network in network interventions. *Proc Natl Acad Sci USA*. 2017;*114*(36):9500-9501. doi:10.1073/pnas.1712473114

20. Centers for Disease Control and Prevention. *CDC fact sheet: information for teens and young adults: staying healthy and preventing STDs*. https://www.cdc.gov/std/life-stages-populations/stdfact-teens.htm

21. *Trends in the prevalence of sexual behaviors and HIV testing national YRBS: 1991–2019*. https://www.cdc.gov/healthyyouth/data/yrbs/factsheets/2019_sexual_trend_yrbs.htm

22. Centers for Disease Control and Prevention. *Sexually transmitted disease surveillance 2019*. U.S. Department of Health and Human Services; 2020. https://www.cdc.gov/std/statistics/2019/std-surveillance-2019.pdf

23. Centers for Disease Control and Prevention. *Sexual risk behaviors*. https://www.cdc.gov/healthyyouth/sexualbehaviors

24. Centers for Disease Control and Prevention. *CDC fact sheet: incidence, prevalence, and cost of sexually transmitted infections in the United States*. 2021. https://www.cdc.gov/nchhstp/newsroom/docs/factsheets/2018 -STI-incidence-prevalence-factsheet.pdf

25. Liddon N, Pampati S, Dunville R, Kilmer G, Steiner RJ. Annual STI testing among sexually active adolescents. *Pediatrics*. 2022;*149*(5):e2021051893.

26. Auerbach DM, Darrow WW, Jaffe HW, Curran JW. Cluster of cases of the acquired immune deficiency syndrome. Patients linked by sexual contact. *Am J Med*. 1984;*76*(3):487-492. doi:10.1016/0002-9343(84)90668-5

27. Latkin C, Weeks MR, Glasman L, et al. A dynamic social systems model for considering structural factors in HIV prevention and detection. *AIDS Behav*. 2010;*14*(suppl 2):222-238. doi:10.1007/s10461-010-9804-y

28. Elwood WN, Greene K, Carter KK. Gentlemen don't speak: communication norms and condom use in bathhouses. *J Appl Commun Res*. 2003;*31*(4):277-297. doi:10.1080/1369681032000132564

29. Doucleff M. *Researchers clear "patient zero" from AIDS origin story*. National Public Radio. Published October 26, 2016. https://www.npr.org/sections/health-shots/2016/10/26/498876985/mystery-solved-how-hiv-came-to-the-u-s

30. Spottiswoode R. *And the Band Played On*. Aaron Spelling, HBO; 1993.

31. Bearman PS, Moody J, Stovel K. Chains of affection: the structure of adolescent romantic and sexual networks. *Am J Sociol*. 2004;*110*(1):44-91. doi:10.1086/386272

32. Helleringer S, Kohler HP. Sexual network structure and the spread of HIV in Africa: evidence from Likoma Island, Malawi. *AIDS*. 2007;*21*(17):2323-2332. doi:10.1097/QAD.0b013e328285df98

33. Christakis NA, Fowler JH. Social network sensors for early detection of contagious outbreaks. *PLoS One*. 2010;5(9):e12948. doi:10.1371/journal.pone.0012948

34. Hedberg CW, Levine WC, White KE, et al. An international foodborne outbreak of shigellosis associated with a commercial airline. *JAMA*. 1992;*268*(22):3208-3212. doi:10.1001/jama.1992.03490220052027

35. Christakis N. *How social networks predict epidemics [video]*. TED. Published June 2010. https://www.ted.com/talks/nicholas_christakis_how_social_networks_predict_epidemics

36. Christakis NA, Fowler JH. The spread of obesity in a large social network over 32 years. *N Engl J Med*. 2007;*357*(4):370-379. doi:10.1056/NEJMsa066082

37. Kemp S. *Digital 2022: another year of bumper growth*. We Are Social. Published January 26, 2022. https://wearesocial.com/uk/blog/2022/01/digital-2022-another-year-of-bumper-growth-2/

38. Sampson RJ, Morenoff JD, Gannon-Rowley T. Assessing "neighborhood effects": social processes and new directions in research. *Annu Rev Sociol*. 2002;*28*(1):443-478. doi:10.1146/annurev.soc.28.110601.141114

39. Royal Society for Public Health. *#StatusofMind: Social Media and Young People's Mental Health and Wellbeing*. Author; 2017. https://www.rsph.org.uk/our-work/campaigns/status-of-mind.html

40. Sampasa-Kanyinga H, Lewis RF. Frequent use of social networking sites is associated with poor psychological functioning among children and adolescents. *Cyberpsychol Behav Soc Netw*. 2015;*18*(7):380-385. doi:10.1089/cyber.2015.0055

41. Lin LY, Sidani JE, Shensa A, et al. Association between social media use and depression among U.S. young adults. *Depress Anxiety*. 2016;*33*(4):323-331. doi:10.1002/da.22466

42. Woods HC, Scott H. #Sleepyteens: social media use in adolescence is associated with poor sleep quality, anxiety, depression and low self-esteem. *J Adolesc*. 2016;*51*:41-49. doi:10.1016/j.adolescence.2016.05.008

43. Tiggemann M, Slater A. NetTweens: the internet and body image concerns in preteenage girls. *J Early Adolesc*. 2014;*34*(5):606-620. doi:10.1177/0272431613501083

44. Anderson M. *A Majority of Teens Have Experienced Some Form of Cyberbullying*. Pew Research Center. Published September 27, 2018. https://www.pewresearch.org/internet/2018/09/27/a-majority-of-teens-have-experienced-some-form-of-cyberbullying/

45. Przybylski AK, Murayama K, DeHaan CR, Gladwell V. Motivational, emotional, and behavioral correlates of fear of missing out. *Comput Hum Behav*. 2013;*29*(4):1841-1848. doi:10.1016/J.CHB.2013.02.014

46. Duncan DT, Kawachi I, eds. *Neighborhoods and Health*. 2nd ed. Oxford University Press; 2018.

47. Diez Roux AV. Investigating neighborhood and area effects on health. *Am J Public Health*. 2001;*91*(11): 1783-1789. doi:10.2105/AJPH.91.11.1783

48. United States Census Bureau. *2010 Census urban area FAQs*. 2019. https://www.census.gov/programs-surveys/geography/about/faq/2010-urban-area-faq.html

49. United States Census Bureau. *U.S. cities are home to 62.7% of the U.S. population, but comprise just 3.5% of land area*. Published March 4, 2015. https://www.census.gov/newsroom/archives/2015-pr/cb15-33.html

50. Fu Q, He S, Zhu Y, et al. Toward a relational account of neighborhood governance. *Am Behav Sci*. 2015;*59*(8):992-1006. doi:10.1177/0002764215580610

51. China Legal Information Center. *What is the administrative division system of China?* Published June 16, 2017. http://www.chinadaily.com.cn/m/chinalic/2017-06/16/content_29770267.htm

52. Ministry of Housing Communities & Local Government. *Neighbourhood planning*. GOV.UK. Published March 6, 2014. Updated May 9, 2019. https://www.gov.uk/guidance/neighbourhood-planning-2

53. Republic of Kenya. The Nairobi City County Community and Neighbourhood Associations Engagement Bill, 2015. *Nairobi City Cty Gaz Suppl*. 2015;*17*(12):1-9. https://www.kpda.or.ke/documents/Policies/NCC%20Community%20and%20Neighbourhood%20Associations%20Engagement%20Bill,%202015.pdf

54. United Nations, Department of Economic and Social Affairs. *The World's Cities in 2016 Data Booklet*. United Nations; 2016. https://www.un.org/en/development/desa/population/publications/pdf/urbanization/the_worlds_cities_in_2016_data_booklet.pdf

55. United Nations. *Department of Economic and Social Affairs: Population Division. World Urbanization Prospects: The 2014 Revision*. 2014. https://population.un.org/wup/Publications/Files/WUP2014-Report.pdf

56. World Health Organization. *WHO Kobe*. https://extranet.who.int/kobe_centre/en

57. Friel S, Akerman M, Hancock T, et al. Addressing the social and environmental determinants of urban health equity: evidence for action and a research agenda. *J Urban Health*. 2011;*88*(5):860-874. doi:10.1007/s11524-011-9606-1

58. United Nations. *The Millennium Development Goals Report*. Author; 2008. https://www.un.org/en/development/desa/publications/millennium-development-goals-report-2008.html

59. Brockerhoff MP. Population Reference Bureau. Urbanizing World: Population Bulletin. Published September 1, 2000. https://www.prb.org/resources/urbanizing-world/

60. United Nations Department of Economic and Social Affairs. *World's population increasingly urban with more than half living in urban areas*. Published July 10, 2014. http://www.un.org/en/development/desa/news/population/world-urbanization-prospects-2014.html

61. Warah R, ed. *State of the World's Cities: Harmonious Cities 2008/2009*. UN-Habitat; 2008. https://unhabitat.org/books/state-of-the-worlds-cities-20082009-harmonious-cities-2

62. Diez Roux AV. Neighborhoods and health: what do we know? What should we do? *Am J Public Health*. 2016;*106*(3):430-431. doi:10.2105/AJPH.2016.303064

63. Diez Roux AV, Borrell LN, Haan M, et al. Neighbourhood environments and mortality in an elderly cohort: results from the cardiovascular health study. *J Epidemiol Community Health*. 2004;*58*(11):917-923. doi:10.1136/jech.2003.019596

64. Mujahid MS, Diez Roux AV, Morenoff JD, et al. Neighborhood characteristics and hypertension. *Epidemiology*. 2008;*19*(4):590-598. doi:10.1097/EDE.0b013e3181772cb2

65. Black JL, Macinko J. Neighborhoods and obesity. *Nutr Rev*. 2008;*66*(1):2-20. doi:10.1111/j.1753-4887.2007.00001.x

66. Chuang YC, Cubbin C, Ahn D, Winkleby MA. Effects of neighbourhood socioeconomic status and convenience store concentration on individual level smoking. *J Epidemiol Community Health*. 2005;*59*(7):568-573. doi:10.1136/jech.2004.029041

67. Truong KD, Ma S. A systematic review of relations between neighborhoods and mental health. *J Ment Health Policy Econ*. 2006;*9*(3):137-154. http://www.ncbi.nlm.nih.gov/pubmed/17031019

68. Vlahov D, Gibble E, Freudenberg N, Galea S. Cities and health: history, approaches, and key questions. *Acad Med*. 2004;*79*(12):1133-1138. http://www.ncbi.nlm.nih.gov/pubmed/15563646

69. Grob GN. *The Deadly Truth: A History of Disease in America*. Harvard University Press; 2005.

70. Hardy A. Edwin Chadwick Revisited—Christopher Hamlin, public health and social justice in the age of Chadwick: Britain, 1800–1854. *Med Hist*. 1999;*43*(2):255-259. doi:10.1017/s0025727300065145

71. Griscom JH. *The Sanitary Condition of the Laboring Population of New York: With Suggestions for Its Improvement*. Harper; 1845. https://archive.org/details/sanitaryconditi00grisgoog/page/n4

72. American College of Physicians. Inner-city health care. *Ann Intern Med*. 1997;*126*(6):485. doi:10.7326/0003-4819-126-6-199703150-00012

73. Vlahov D, Freudenberg N, Proietti F, et al. Urban as a determinant of health. *J Urban Health*. 2007;*84*(3 suppl):i16-i26. doi:10.1007/s11524-007-9169-3

74. Clougherty JE, Kheirbek I, Eisl HM, et al. Intra-urban spatial variability in wintertime street-level concentrations of multiple combustion-related air pollutants: the New York City Community Air Survey (NYCCAS). *J Expo Sci Environ Epidemiol*. 2013;*23*(3):232-240. doi:10.1038/jes.2012.125

75. World Health Organization. *Water Quality and Health Strategy 2013-2020*. Author; 2013. https://www.who.int/publications/m/item/water-quality-and-health-strategy-2013-2020

76. Crowder K, Downcy L. Inter-neighborhood migration, race, and environmental hazards: modeling microlevel processes of environmental inequality. *AJS*. 2010;*115*(4):1110-1149. doi:10.1086/649576

77. Larson NI, Story MT, Nelson MC. Neighborhood environments. *Am J Prev Med*. 2009;*36*(1):74-81. doi:10.1016/j.amepre.2008.09.025

78. Bower KM, Thorpe RJ, Rohde C, Gaskin DJ. The intersection of neighborhood racial segregation, poverty, and urbanicity and its impact on food store availability in the United States. *Prev Med*. 2014;*58*:33-39. doi:10.1016/j.ypmed.2013.10.010

79. Ver Ploeg M, Breneman V, Farrigan T, et al. *Access to Affordable and Nutritious Food: Measuring and Understanding Food Deserts and Their Consequences: Report to Congress*. United States Department of Agriculture; 2009.

80. Authenticated U.S. Government Information. *Pub L No. 110–246, 122 Stat 1651*. June 18, 2008. https://www.agriculture.senate.gov/imo/media/doc/pl110-246.pdf

81. Kim H. *Food Deserts: What Are They? Their Causes, Effects and Possible Solutions*. Sentient Media. Published July 8, 2022. https://sentientmedia.org/food-desert/#:~:text=While%20people%20living%20in%20so,stores%20and%20fast%2Dfood%20restaurants

82. Hendrickson D, Smith C, Eikenberry N. Fruit and vegetable access in four low-income food deserts communities in Minnesota. *Agric Human Values*. 2006;*23*(3):371-383. doi:10.1007/s10460-006-9002-8

83. Walker RE, Keane CR, Burke JG. Disparities and access to healthy food in the United States: a review of food deserts literature. *Health Place*. 2010;*16*(5):876-884. doi:10.1016/J.HEALTHPLACE.2010.04.013

84. Alwitt LF, Donley TD. Retail stores in poor urban neighborhoods. *J Consum Aff*. 1997;*31*(1):139-164. doi:10.1111/j.1745-6606.1997.tb00830.x

85. Guy C, Clarke G, Eyre H. Food retail change and the growth of food deserts: a case study of Cardiff. *Int J Retail Distrib Manag.* 2004;*32*(2):72-88. doi:10.1108/09590550410521752

86. Nyden P, Lukehart J, Maly MT, Peterman W. Chapter 1: neighborhood racial and ethnic diversity in U.S. cities. *Cityscape J Policy Dev Res.* 1998;*4*(2):1-17. https://www.huduser.gov/periodicals/cityscpe/vol4num2/ch1.pdf

87. *NewsOne Staff.* America's worst 9 urban food deserts. Published September 22, 2011. https://newsone .com/1540235/americas-worst-9-urban-food-deserts

88. Chinni D, Freedman P. *The socio-economic significance of food deserts. PBS News Hour.* Published June 29, 2011. https://www.pbs.org/newshour/arts/the-socio-economic-significance-of-food-deserts

89. Morland K, Wing S, Diez Roux A, Poole C. Neighborhood characteristics associated with the location of food stores and food service places. *Am J Prev Med.* 2002;*22*(1):23-29. doi:10.1016/S0749-3797(01)00403-2

90. Sloane DC, Diamant AL, Lewis LB, et al. Improving the nutritional resource environment for healthy living through community-based participatory research. *J Gen Intern Med.* 2003;*18*(7):568-575. doi:10.1046/j.1525-1497.2003.21022.x

91. Block JP, Scribner RA, DeSalvo KB. Fast food, race/ethnicity, and income: a geographic analysis. *Am J Prev Med.* 2004;*27*(3):211-217. doi:10.1016/j.amepre.2004.06.007

92. Zenk SN, Schulz AJ, Israel BA, et al. Neighborhood racial composition, neighborhood poverty, and the spatial accessibility of supermarkets in metropolitan Detroit. *Am J Public Health.* 2005;*95*(4):660-667. doi:10.2105/ AJPH.2004.042150

93. Powell LM, Slater S, Mirtcheva D, et al. Food store availability and neighborhood characteristics in the United States. *Prev Med.* 2007;*44*(3):189-195. doi:10.1016/j.ypmed.2006.08.008

94. Treuhaft S, Karpyn A. *The Grocery Gap: Who Has Access to Healthy Food and Why It Matters.* PolicyLink; 2010. https://www.policylink.org/resources-tools/the-grocery-gap-who-has-access-to-healthy-food-and-why-it-matters

95. Furey S, Strugnell C, McIlveen MH. An investigation of the potential existence of "food deserts" in rural and urban areas of Northern Ireland. *Agric Human Values.* 2001;*18*(4):447-457. doi:10.1023/A:1015218502547

96. United States Department of Agriculture Economic Research Service. *About the atlas.* https://www.ers.usda .gov/data-products/food-access-research-atlas/about-the-atlas

97. Rose D, Richards R. Food store access and household fruit and vegetable use among participants in the US Food stamp program. *Public Health Nutr.* 2004;*7*(08):1081-1088. doi:10.1079/PHN2004648

98. Allen LN, Feigl AB. What's in a name? A call to reframe non-communicable diseases. *Lancet Glob Health.* 2017;*5*(2):e129-e130. doi:10.1016/S2214-109X(17)30001-3

99. Mari Gallagher Research and Consulting Group. *The Chicago Food Desert Progress Report.* Author; 2011. https://www.marigallagher.com/2011/06/27/the-chicago-food-desert-progress-report-june-2011/

100. Food Empowerment Project. *Food deserts.* http://www.foodispower.org/food-deserts

101. Bell R, Lutz B, Webb D, Small R. *Discussion Paper: Addressing the Social Determinants of Noncommunicable Diseases.* United Nations Development Programme; 2013. https://www.undp.org/sites/g/files/zskgke326/files/ publications/Discussion_Paper_Addressing_the_Social_Determinants_of_NCDs_UNDP_2013.pdf

102. The White House President Barack Obama. *"You all took a stand."* Published February 20, 2010. https://obamawhitehouse.archives.gov/blog/2010/02/19/you-all-took-a-stand

103. Braveman P, Cubbin C, Egerter S, Pedregon V. *Neighborhoods and Health [Issue Brief #8].* Robert Wood Johnson Foundation; 2011. https://www.rwjf.org/content/dam/farm/reports/issue_briefs/2011/rwjf70450

104. Sampson RJ, Raudenbush SW, Earls FJ. Neighborhoods and violent crime: a multilevel study of collective efficacy. *Science.* 1997;*277*(5328):918-924. doi:10.1126/science.277.5328.918

105. Morenoff J, Sampson R, Raudenbush S. Neighborhood inequality, collective efficacy, and the spatial dynamics of urban violence. *Criminology.* 2001;*39*(3):517-558. doi:10.1111/j.1745-9125.2001.tb00932.x

106. National Research Council, Institute of Medicine. Physical and social environmental factors. In: Woolf S, Aron L, eds. *U.S. Health in International Perspective: Shorter Lives, Poorer Health.* National Academies Press; 2013:192-206. https://www.ncbi.nlm.nih.gov/books/NBK154491

107. Darling-Hammond L. Inequality in teaching and schooling: how opportunity is rationed to students of color in America. In: Smedley BD, Stith AY, Colburn L, Evans CH, eds. *The Right Thing to Do, the Smart Thing to Do: Enhancing Diversity in the Health Professions.* National Academies Press; 2001:208-233. https://www.ncbi.nlm .nih.gov/books/NBK223640

108. DeWalt DA, Berkman ND, Sheridan S, et al. Literacy and health outcomes. *J Gen Intern Med.* 2004;*19*(12):1228-1239. doi:10.1111/j.1525-1497.2004.40153.x

109. Ross CE, Wu C. The links between education and health. *Am Sociol Rev.* 1995;*60*(5):719-745. doi:10.2307/2096319

110. Handy SL, Boarnet MG, Ewing R, Killingsworth RE. How the built environment affects physical activity: views from urban planning. *Am J Prev Med.* 2002;*23*(2 suppl):64-73. doi:10.1016/S0749-3797(02)00475-0

111. Pope CA III, Burnett RT, Thun MJ, et al. Lung cancer, cardiopulmonary mortality, and long-term exposure to fine particulate air pollution. *JAMA.* 2002;*287*(9):1132-1141. doi:10.1001/jama.287.9.1132

112. Han B, Cohen DA, Derose KP, et al. How much neighborhood parks contribute to local residents' physical activity in the City of Los Angeles: a meta-analysis. *Prev Med.* 2014;*69*:S106-S110. doi:10.1016/J.YPMED .2014.08.033

113. Guralnik JM, Seeman TE, Tinetti ME, et al. Validation and use of performance measures of functioning in a non-disabled older population: MacArthur studies of successful aging. *Aging (Milano)*. 1994;6(6):410-419. http://www.ncbi.nlm.nih.gov/pubmed/7748914

114. Lee IM, Rexrode KM, Cook NR, et al. Physical activity and coronary heart disease in women: is "no pain, no gain" passé? *JAMA*. 2001;285(11):1447-1454. doi:10.1001/jama.285.11.1447

115. U.S. Department of Housing and Urban Development. *Choice neighborhoods.* https://www.hud.gov/program _offices/public_indian_housing/programs/ph/cn

116. Leventhal T, Brooks-Gunn J. Moving to opportunity: an experimental study of neighborhood effects on mental health. *Am J Public Health*. 2003;93(9):1576-1582. doi:10.2105/ajph.93.9.1576

117. Flournoy R, Treuhaft S, Bell J, et al. *Healthy Food, Healthy Communities: Improving Access and Opportunities Through Food Retailing.* PolicyLink; 2005. http://www.policylink.org/sites/default/files/HEALTHYFOOD.pdf

118. Galea S, Freudenberg N, Vlahov D. Cities and population health. *Soc Sci Med*. 2005;60(5):1017-1033. doi:10.1016/j.socscimed.2004.06.036

119. Krieger J, Higgins DL. Housing and health: time again for public health action. *Am J Public Health*. 2002;92(5):758-768. doi:10.2105/ajph.92.5.758

120. NYC Health. *About the NYC Department of Health and Mental Hygiene.* https://www1.nyc.gov/site/doh/about/about-doh.page

121. Chicago Department of Public Health. *Healthy Chicago 2.0.* https://www.chicago.gov/city/en/depts/cdph/provdrs/healthychicago.html

122. Chicago Department of Public Health. *Public health: mission.* https://www.chicago.gov/city/en/depts/cdph/auto_generated/cdph_mission.html

123. Thomas SB, Quinn SC, Billingsley A, Caldwell C. The characteristics of northern black churches with community health outreach programs. *Am J Public Health*. 1994;84(4):575-579. doi:10.2105/ajph.84.4.575

124. DeHaven MJ, Hunter IB, Wilder L, et al. Health programs in faith-based organizations: are they effective? *Am J Public Health*. 2004;94(6):1030-1036. doi:10.2105/ajph.94.6.1030

125. Burra S. Towards a pro-poor framework for slum upgrading in Mumbai, India. *Environ Urban*. 2005;17(1): 67-88. doi:10.1177/095624780501700106

126. Nutbeam D. *Health Promotion Glossary.* World Health Organization; 1998. https://academic.oup.com/heapro/article/13/4/349/563193

127. Ashton J, Tiliouine A, Kosinska M. The World Health Organization European Healthy Cities Network 30 years on. *Gac Sanit*. 2018;32(6):503-504. doi: 10.1016/j.gaceta.2018.03.005.

128. Alliance for Healthy Cities. *About the alliance.* https://www.alliance-healthycities.com/htmls/about/index_about.html#:~:text=The%20Alliance%20for%20Healthy%20Cities,approach%20called%20"Healthy%20Cities"

129. United Nation Sustainable Development Goals. *Goals: 11: make cities and human settlements inclusive, safe, resilient and sustainable.* https://sustainabledevelopment.un.org/sdg11

130. Garau P, Sclar ED, Carolini GY. *Improving the Lives of Slum Dwellers: A Home in the City.* Earthscan; 2005. https://www.mypsup.org/library_files/downloads/A%20Home%20in%20the%20City-%20Improving%20 the%20Lives%20of%20Slum%20Dwellers.pdf

131. Kjellstrom T, Friel S, Dixon J, et al. Urban environmental health hazards and health equity. *J Urban Health*. 2007;84(3 Suppl):86-97. doi:10.1007/s11524-007-9171-9

132. Hoornweg D, Sugar L, Freire M, et al. *Cities and Climate Change: An Urgent Agenda.* World Bank; 2010. https://openknowledge.worldbank.org/entities/publication/9dd0caa3-4a61-520e-8579-724d31f8a713

133. UN-Habitat. *Climate change.* https://unhabitat.org/urban-themes/climate-change

134. Freudenberg N, Galea S, Vlahov D. Beyond urban penalty and urban sprawl: back to living conditions as the focus of urban health. *J Community Health*. 2005;30(1):1-11. doi:10.1007/s10900-004-6091-4

135. Srinivasan S, O'Fallon LR, Dearry A. Creating healthy communities, healthy homes, healthy people: initiating a research agenda on the built environment and public health. *Am J Public Health*. 2003;93(9):1446-1450. doi:10.2105/ajph.93.9.1446

136. Rural Health Information Hub. *Rural health disparities.* 2019. https://www.ruralhealthinfo.org/topics/rural -health-disparities

137. Douthit N, Kiv S, Dwolatzky T, Biswas S. Exposing some important barriers to health care access in the rural USA. *Public Health*. 2015;129(6):611-620. doi:10.1016/J.PUHE.2015.04.001

138. Weigley S, Hess AEM, Sauter MB. *States with the fewest (and most) doctors.* 24/7 Wall St. Published October 19, 2012. https://247wallst.com/special-report/2012/10/19/states-with-the-fewest-and-most-doctors/5

139. Nandi A, Glymour MM, Subramanian SV. Association among socioeconomic status, health behaviors, and all-cause mortality in the United States. *Epidemiology*. 2014;25(2):170-177. doi:10.1097/EDE.0000000000000038

140. Lantz PM, House JS, Lepkowski JM, et al. Socioeconomic factors, health behaviors, and mortality: results from a nationally representative prospective study of US adults. *JAMA*. 1998;279(21):1703-1708. doi:10.1001/jama.279.21.1703

8

COUNTRIES, POLICIES, AND HEALTH

Salma M. Abdalla also contributed to this chapter

LEARNING OBJECTIVES

- Discuss why politics is inseparable from public health.
- Explain how political decisions shape causes of health at multiple levels down the social ecological causal chain.
- Provide examples of political decisions that resulted in healthier populations and the decisions that resulted in diminishing the health of populations.
- Discuss how organized public health efforts can engage political decision-making.
- Discuss the role corporations play in shaping the health of populations.

OVERVIEW: POLITICS AND POLICIES ARE INSEPARABLE FROM OUR HEALTH

When we think of health from a social ecological perspective, we inevitably arrive at thinking about the influence of countries on the health of populations (**Figure 8.1**). When we think about countries, we cannot but also think of politics. Politics, the practice of distributing resources to achieve collective goals, is inseparable from our health. Rudolf Virchow, one of the founding fathers of microbiology, famously said that "politics is nothing else but medicine on a large scale." In many ways, this is perhaps even more accurately said of public health. The health of populations depends on the social and economic structures around us. Politics and policies shape these social and economic structures. Political decisions determine resource allocations, and these resources in turn determine whether we are investing in a healthier world or not. In this chapter, we (a) discuss how political decisions can shape the determinants of health at other levels down the social ecological causal chain, (b) provide examples of political decisions that resulted in healthier populations, and the converse, (c) examine how organized public health efforts can engage political decision-making and encourage political action toward healthy populations.

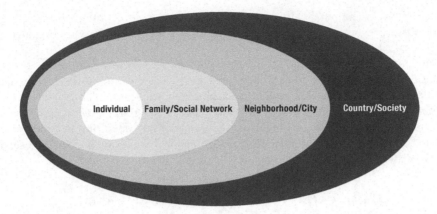

FIGURE 8.1 The multilevel social ecological perspective, highlighting the focus of this chapter: countries, politics, and policies. Artistic credit: Parisa Varanloo

THE INEXTRICABILITY OF HEALTH AND POLITICS: "POLITICS IS NOTHING ELSE BUT MEDICINE ON A LARGE SCALE"

In 1848, Virchow established the medical diagnosis of the typhus epidemic in Poland; he knew that this specific type of typhus was linked to hunger and war. In a report, he attributed the epidemic to social and, ultimately, political causes. He linked the epidemic to the multiyear famine in the country; which was precipitated by poverty, which was a direct result of the political oppression of peasants in the country. Virchow argued for the need to eliminate social inequities to prevent future epidemics of the disease.[1] Two centuries later, neither social inequities nor typhus has been eliminated.

There is abundant intuitive evidence that social, economic, and political factors influence health. In pre-COVID-19 pandemic times, a child born in Japan, Australia, or Switzerland could expect to live more than 80 years; in Fiji, 71 years; in Namibia, 64 years; and in many African countries, less than 60 years.[2] The differences are starker within countries worldwide. We can see the same dramatic variation, based on where an individual is born, in several other indicators of health and well-being. Around the world, illness and health follow a social gradient: Lower socioeconomic status generally translates to worse health outcomes. These systematic differences in health outcomes are expected given that social and economic structures and politics, from global to local, shape our health.[3]

> There is abundant intuitive evidence that social, economic, and political factors influence health.

WHY POLITICS IS INSEPARABLE FROM PUBLIC HEALTH

Politics defines who gets what, when, and how. Political decisions dictate policy priority areas: who is entitled to services, who delivers these services, who is subsidized, and how budgets are allocated.[4] Political decisions shape our social and economic living conditions which, ultimately, shape our health. As such, politics on all levels interact with the goals of public health to prevent disease, prolong life, and promote health through organized efforts in society.[5]

Governments can influence the health of populations directly through policies that regulate healthcare provision and public health measures such as safe drinking water, vaccination, or control of air pollution. Moreover, political decisions in which health might not be the main aim, such as housing, employment, and transportation, can strongly—in a positive or negative way— affect the health of populations and health equity.[3] Alternatively, decisions on a societal level can negatively affect the health of populations through major disruptions of social life such as the initiation of armed conflicts or the oppression of certain groups.[6]

HOW NATIONAL POLITICAL DECISIONS SHAPE THE DETERMINANTS OF HEALTH

POLITICAL DECISIONS SHAPING CAUSES OF HEALTH AT THE COUNTRY LEVEL

The nation state, clearly delineated by its geopolitical boundaries, is one of the most identifiable causes of health on a population level. The influence of a nation state on the health of its peoples starts with the form of the political system governing that country. For example, the political conditions in countries in Europe during the 20th century had a profound effect on the upward trajectories of life expectancy throughout the continent. The convergence and divergence of life expectancy in different countries were linked to their formation and dissolution. Moreover, overall, life expectancy was higher among democratically governed states compared to authoritarian states.[6]

Access to healthcare is an important factor in the health of populations. Based on whether access to healthcare is considered a human right in a nation state, there are a variety of healthcare delivery models that a country can adopt. Governments can implement public systems in which healthcare is available to all, such as in Canada, or systems in which individuals are ultimately responsible for their own healthcare, such as in the United States. Regardless of the specific system, the health of populations is dependent on more than just healthcare. Legislation and budget allocations can create, regulate, and maintain public goods that impact health such as access to quality education or investments in public transportation versus roads and highways designed for private transportation. Political decisions can impose regulations on natural resources to limit exposure to pollutants. Laws, and law enforcement agencies, can affect health positively through mandating and implementing requirements to protect individuals, such as seat-belt laws.[7] However, law enforcement entities at different levels along the social ecological chain, including states, cities, and counties, can also affect the health of populations negatively if they are discriminating against, and disproportionally targeting, segments of the population. For example, police killings of unarmed African American/Black citizens have an adverse effect on the mental health of the African American/Black population in general, regardless of whether a specific person knows a victim of the police-involved shooting or not.[8]

Access to healthcare is an important factor in the health of populations. Based on whether access to healthcare is considered a human right in a nation state, there are a variety of healthcare delivery models that a country can adopt.

POLITICAL DECISIONS SHAPING CAUSES OF HEALTH AT OTHER LEVELS DOWN THE SOCIAL ECOLOGICAL CAUSAL CHAIN

Political decisions shape causes of health on many levels along the social ecological causal chain, which can improve or worsen health outcomes and may exacerbate health inequity. For example, national and state urban planning policies driven by favoritism toward one group over others based on sociodemographic characteristics can produce neighborhoods that are substantially different in their access to local amenities such as safe and affordable housing and public transportation. In turn, such discriminatory practices can affect access to healthcare, availability of healthy food, employment opportunities, and ultimately, health outcomes.

National policies can have an impact on the behaviors of individuals. For example, national taxation policies that elevate the price of tobacco products by 50% have been shown to consistently reduce smoking and tobacco consumption by 20% in low-, middle-, and high-income countries alike.[9]

POLITICAL DECISIONS SHAPING DETERMINANTS OF HEALTH AT MULTINATIONAL AND GLOBAL LEVELS

While nations are responsible for protecting and improving the health of their populations, globalization has introduced social determinants of health that operate beyond the control of a single government. In response to multinational and truly global health concerns, there are now several international entities that regulate policies to improve health worldwide. The World Health Organization (WHO) was founded as a neutral body in 1948 to provide global leadership on matters critical for health as well as set and promote standards for health.[10]

Unfortunately, global health decisions are also affected by political power disparities, particularly when contrasting high-income countries with low- and middle-income countries. This asymmetry sometimes leads to global-priority setting in health that is largely determined by countries with the greatest economic and political clout. For example, in 1994, the World Trade Organization (WTO) adopted an agreement to protect subsidized agriculture in high-income countries. While this policy was not intended to affect health, the consequence of its implementation was that small-scale farmers in resource-limited countries could not compete effectively, leading to a cascade of negative health outcomes including food insecurity and malnutrition in poorer countries.[11]

When it comes to aid, power asymmetries between donor and recipient countries can also shape health policies. For example, the United States' political positions regarding sexual and reproductive health have affected funding for overseas aid organizations providing women's health services without recipient countries having much say in the policy changes. Specifically, the global gag rule is a law that prohibits the U.S. government from providing funding to organizations that offer abortion services or even provide information about the procedure. Over decades, this gag rule, prohibiting funding to providers of reproductive services that include abortion, has been put in place during Republican Party–controlled administrations and repealed when the Democratic Party holds power. Following U.S. national elections that result in changes in political parties, abrupt shifts in allowable funding for reproductive services immediately impact the recipient countries. For example, the transition from the Obama (Democrat) to the Trump (Republican) presidencies in early 2017 resulted in the sudden closure of many women's health clinics serving some of the world's most vulnerable populations.[12]

EXAMPLES OF POLITICAL DECISIONS THAT MODIFIED POPULATION HEALTH

POLITICAL DECISIONS THAT RESULTED IN HEALTHIER POPULATIONS

Title X Family Planning Program

The United Nations Population Fund (UNFPA) defines sexual and reproductive health as:

> a state of complete physical, mental, and social well-being in all matters relating to the reproductive system. This implies that people are able to have a satisfying and safe sex life, the capability to reproduce, and the freedom to decide if, when, and how often to do so. [13]

There is a clear connection between reproductive health and the well-being of individuals, their families, and populations across generations. [14] Reproductive rights worldwide are inextricable from gender equality and human rights, particularly the human rights of women. [15]

There has been substantial and dramatic progress on reproductive health worldwide over the past few decades. For example, globally, the number of women who died in pregnancy or childbirth decreased by almost half over the past 25 years. [16] In the United States, the teenage pregnancy rate in 2013 reached a record low, recording a 10% drop over the previous year, attributed in no small part to birth control used by sexually active teens throughout the country. [17] As a testament to U.S. success in promoting overall reproductive health, abortion rates decreased from 2002 to 2011 for women in all age groups 15 years and older, although rates increased for adolescent females younger than 15. [18]

There has been substantial and dramatic progress on reproductive health worldwide over the past few decades.

Enacted in 1970 as part of the Public Health Service Act, Title X is a grant program aiming to provide comprehensive family planning and reproductive health services that prioritize low-income individuals and those not eligible for Medicaid. [19] Title X services are overseen by the Office of Population Affairs, U.S. Department of Health and Human Services (HHS). Title X does not fund abortions. However, Title X supports a range of counseling services, contraceptive methods, cancer screening, pregnancy testing, HIV testing, and screening and treatment for sexually transmitted infections (STIs).

Title X–funded services reach about 4.5 million clients a year. Providers of Title X services include state, county, and local health departments; community health centers; Planned Parenthood centers; and hospital-based, school-based, faith-based, and other private nonprofit organizations. [19] Public expenditures for family planning services in the United States overall totaled $2.37 billion in 2010, with Medicaid supporting 75% of total expenditures, state appropriations supporting 12%, and Title X supporting 10%. [20]

Two straightforward pieces of evidence readily showcase the contribution to population health made by Title X. First, clients who access Title X reproductive services are primarily poor, young women from minority communities. These women need access to safe, effective reproductive health services that would be unavailable to them without Title X funding support. Among the 20 million women in need of publicly funded contraceptive care, 77% are considered low-income. Between 2000 and 2010, the proportion of Latinx women seeking these services increased by 47%; the proportion of African American/Black women increased by 17%; and the proportion of White women increased by 4%. [20]

Second, it is estimated that every public dollar spent on contraceptive services in 2008 resulted in a cost savings of $3.74 that would have been spent on Medicaid costs related to prenatal care, delivery, and newborn healthcare throughout infancy.[19]

In the United States, the strength of reproductive rights and the quality of reproductive health vacillate based on changeable political and legal currents. Shifts in political power can significantly impact the funding appropriations provided for core programs that promote population health such as Title X.

As the political landscape of the United States changes over time, one would rather not contemplate the implications of a regressive government for the health of the U.S. population. However, this very real prospect clarifies the need for resolute public health voices advocating for action by all three branches of the government to consistently promote women's reproductive health.

Roe v. Wade and Access to Sexual and Reproductive Health in the United States[21]

About half of all pregnancies in the United States each year are unplanned. Over their lifetimes, almost one-third of U.S. women will have an abortion, usually during their adolescent and young adult years of life. In 2011, adolescents, aged 15 to 19 years, accounted for 14% of U.S. abortions. The largest proportion of abortions were performed for women in their 20s (58%). Among abortion recipients, 69% were economically disadvantaged.[18]

The provision of safe abortions is a core reproductive right that remains elusive for women in many countries in the world, not the least of which is the United States. Access to safe abortions dramatically reduces the number of unsafe, medically incompetent abortions, which are linked with higher risks of death, injury, and infertility in women who have the procedure. In fact, on January 22, 1973, *Roe v. Wade* transformed reproductive health in the United States, ruling unconstitutional a state law that banned abortions for any reason other than saving the life of the mother.[22] The decision declared that states were only allowed to regulate abortions after the first trimester of pregnancy, and only in cases explicitly related to maternal health or when laws protecting the lives of fetuses during the third semester were in force in the jurisdiction. The *Roe v. Wade* lawsuit was brought by a pregnant woman in Dallas, "Jane Roe," whose lawyers argued that the Texas ban on abortions was violating her constitutional rights.[23] The majority opinion for the Supreme Court's 7 to 2 decision was written by Justice Harry Blackmun.

Blackmun argued that contraception and childbirth are covered in constitutional "zones of privacy" and are therefore protected by the First, Fourth, Ninth, and Fourteenth Amendments. The decision in a companion case, *Doe v. Bolton*, was released on the same day, overturning the Georgia abortion law that required a licensed physician to perform an abortion only under their "best clinical judgment," among many other statutes surrounding the practice.[24]

Although *Roe v. Wade* was transformative, providing abortion care remained challenging, and frequently challenged, in the United States. The Hyde Amendment, which was originally passed in 1976 and has been updated since, bans the use of federal funds for abortion services in all but extreme circumstances such as rape, incest, or life endangerment.[25] Many states defied the decision of *Roe v. Wade* outright by passing new laws that prohibited abortions, while others put logistical hurdles in place for women seeking abortions.

In 1982, Pennsylvania passed the Abortion Control Act, which required women to give informed consent, and minors to get informed consent from their parents (except in cases of "hardship") and placed a 24-hour waiting period on abortions while women were given information about the procedure.[23] The act also stipulated that a wife must inform her husband of her plans to abort, except in medical emergencies. Further, all Pennsylvania abortion clinics are required to report themselves to the state. In 1992, *Planned Parenthood v. Casey* affirmed the *Roe v. Wade* basic ruling. This case prohibited states from placing unnecessary burdens or obstacles on women seeking abortions. However, it also said that states may outlaw abortions of "viable" fetuses and ruled that most of Pennsylvania's laws were in fact constitutional. In 2015, in the Supreme Court case, *Whole Woman's Health v. Cole*, the Court ruled 5 to 3 that the State of Texas cannot place unreasonable restrictions on access to, and delivery of, abortion services.

Roe v. Wade came at a time when most states had strict abortion policies and bans that made obtaining an abortion difficult for all, and impossible for many. Given this highly restrictive underpinning, the freedoms accorded under the *Roe v. Wade* decision represent critical elements that protect the population reproductive health of women.

Roe v. Wade became the center of attention again when the U.S. Supreme Court heard oral arguments for the landmark *Dobbs v. Jackson Women's Health Organization* case in December, 2021. The case questioned the constitutionality of a 2018 Mississippi state law that banned most abortion operations after the first 15 weeks of pregnancy. A draft opinion, written by Justice Samuel Alito, was leaked in May 2022 prompting nationwide discussion on the issue. On June 24, 2022, the. Supreme Court issued its decision on the *Dobbs* case and overturned *Roe v. Wade* and *Planned Parenthood v. Casey,* in a 6 to 3 majority opinion. The Court's decision terminated access to constitutionally protected abortions in the United States. Determining both the legality of abortion and access to abortion services had been turned over to the discretion of each state. While this decision does allow individual states to protect access to abortions, much of the focus was directed toward legislation that was already crafted in many states that would impose total or near-total abortion bans, which might also extend to include severe restrictions on pregnancy-terminating "medication abortions."

The 14th Amendment and the Effect of Discrimination on the Health of Populations

In 2010, White families in the United States were six times wealthier than minority families. The African American/Black–White gap in access to resources is amplified by differences in employment rates; the African American/Black unemployment rate has remained twice that of the White unemployment rate for more than three decades.[26] Moreover, substantial disparities in access to health-promoting resources such as healthy foods, medical care, and safe neighborhoods also add to this gap.[27] This leaves little mystery, then, as to why people concentrated in lower income neighborhoods (mostly minorities) have consistently higher mortality rates than those who live in wealthier ones.[28] The real question becomes instead: Where does this disparity originate? Why do we have poor and wealthy neighborhoods to begin with, rather than integrated communities that represent the spectrum of wealth within a region?

The 14th Amendment to the U.S. Constitution is part of the answer to that question. "All persons born or naturalized in the United States" begins Section I, going on to grant citizenship and guarantee equal protection under the law to all such individuals, including, for the first time in the nation's history, recently freed slaves. The amendment was ratified in 1868[29]–although it would be followed by nearly a century of institutionalized inequality before crucial Supreme Court cases and laws, such as *Brown v. Board of Education* and the Civil Rights Act of 1964, ended legally sanctioned segregation and discrimination. While the Civil Rights Act prohibited openly discriminatory actions, it did not prohibit policies that indirectly perpetuated discrimination. Thus, it fell to the courts to determine what could be legally labeled discrimination and what was merely disparate impact.

An early case confronting this question was brought by two African American/Black applicants for police officer positions in 1976, who sued District of Columbia officials for what they considered to be racially discriminatory recruitment and hiring practices. Their case, *Washington v. Davis*, focused specifically on an examination that was administered to all police applicants that was structured in a manner that resulted in failure rates that were four times higher for

African American/Black applicants. They argued that as a result of this examination, the District of Columbia police force did not resemble or reflect the city's demographic makeup.

The Court ruled against the plaintiffs, citing that while the 14th Amendment's equal protection clause prohibits discrimination, there were no previous cases—no legal precedents—that had found statutes unconstitutional solely on the basis of a disproportionate impact on a particular group.[30] The Court determined that in order for an action to violate the equal protection clause, it would need to be shown to have "discriminatory purpose." In other words, the impact of an action was not sufficient proof of discrimination. In order to overturn a policy resulting in disproportionate effects on a particular group, plaintiffs needed to prove something far more challenging: intent.

The *Washington v. Davis* decision, while necessitating proof of intent in cases of discrimination, did not provide a means for determining the said intent. It was a year later, in *Village of Arlington Heights v. Metropolitan Housing Development Corporation*, that the Court defined a series of methods that lower courts and plaintiffs could use to determine whether a discriminatory purpose existed. However, notably, these methods did not include foreseeability of disparate impact. The blunt outcome was to render invalid the traditional "presumption, common to the criminal and civil law, that a person intends the natural and foreseeable consequences of his voluntary actions."[31]

By 1979, when Helen Feeney brought her case against the Personnel Administration of Massachusetts to the Supreme Court, intent to discriminate needed to be clear and uncontestable—impact mattered less.[32] Feeney's argument was that a Massachusetts state law that provided preference to veterans for civil service positions was inherently discriminatory, as its benefits tremendously favored males. Yet expanding upon previous definitions, the Court felt such a fact was insufficient in proving discrimination. The Court ruled against Feeney, and further tightened its interpretation of discrimination. The Court recognized that the adverse effects toward women were undoubtedly known and accepted by legislators of the Massachusetts law. However, it also deemed that for an act to have "discriminatory purposes," it must be that the policy makers chose to adopt such an act "because of" its discriminatory impact, rather than "in spite of" the said impact.[31]

It is easy to see the conflict that justices must have faced in Feeney's case. It is a largely universal opinion that veterans deserve help in reentering domestic life, and it seems likely that the intention of the law was just that. Moreover, it seems likely that the subsequent impact on women was a side effect—unavoidable in terms of the legislation. However, it is cases like Feeney's that create interpretations that prevent laws from being wholly utilized by the populations they were written for. The worry in such cases would appear to be that we are harming one marginalized group (veterans) in an effort to protect another (women). Nonetheless, such cases need not be reduced to a binary choice between help and harm. For example, rather than restrict a law that is crucial to maintaining the rights of marginalized individuals, a program to prepare veterans for the domestic workforce could be instituted. Veterans are still receiving vital help, but no longer to the detriment of others. Solutions like this could be found for many of the fringe cases that make defining discrimination such a challenging topic, rather than allowing such cases to circumscribe the interpretation of laws meant to protect vulnerable individuals.

In 2015, the Supreme Court made a decision that has the potential to turn the tide on these past decades of restricted interpretations. In *Texas Department of Housing and Community Affairs (TDHCA) v. Inclusive Communities Project, Inc. (ICP)*, the Court ruled against the TDHCA, supporting ICP's claim of discrimination in housing practices under the 14th Amendment and the Fair Housing Act.[33] The ICP argued that the TDHCA had been effectively buttressing segregation policies in Dallas by placing subsidized housing projects in predominantly low-income and minority neighborhoods. This practice prevented individuals in need of subsidized housing from moving into more middle-class, majority-White neighborhoods. While there was no evidence of an active intent on the part of TDHCA, the Court ruled that the impact was sufficient to be considered in violation of the law.[34] This case has the potential to reverse the precedents outlined earlier and return some power to marginalized groups in defending themselves against discrimination under the U.S. Constitution.

The Texas practices renounced by the Court helped clarify segregation's ability to persist in American society despite all efforts to extinguish it. Schools today are more segregated than they were 40 years ago, a reflection not only on the education sector but on our society as a whole.[35] We have created a system in which subtle discrimination, intentional or not, marginalizes minorities from the outset, funneling those populations into lower paying jobs and, in turn, lower income housing in neighborhoods with other struggling people. Thus, this legally sanctioned discrimination allows segregation to continue, perpetuating inequities in health through inequalities in access to everything from jobs to healthcare. It is entirely reasonable that individuals who are daily faced with adverse circumstances and who have fewer avenues for coping would be more likely to partake in risky behaviors, like smoking and heavy drinking, and less likely to partake in health-promoting behaviors. It is hard to ask someone to go for a walk around the neighborhood when gunshots are ringing out across the street.

POLITICAL DECISIONS THAT RESULTED IN DIMINISHED POPULATION HEALTH

Mental Health and Incarceration in the United States

Today, the U.S. prison population is roughly seven times what it was in 1980. This increase, and the subsequent toll on the health of not only those who are imprisoned, but their families and communities, is largely due to policy changes on both the state and federal levels. These decisions were often made in moments of public outcry, such as that over the conditions of mental health institutions, enacted without thorough research or foresight, and the system that developed from them is one riddled with injustice and ineffectiveness.

The increase of mentally ill inmates can be traced back to 1955, with the discovery and subsequent widespread use of chlorpromazine as an antipsychotic in mental institutions.[36] The drug inspired hope for the possibility of successful mental health treatment at home, and between 1955 and 1965, the number of patients in institutional psychiatric wards dropped by 15%.[37] With the intent of building on this national shift away from institutionalized treatment toward more rounded, community-based care, President John F. Kennedy signed the Community Mental Health Act of 1963. This came about in a period of growing public awareness and subsequent unrest regarding the conditions in, and ineffectiveness of, state-run psychiatric institutions. The act was meant to encourage a transition away from institutionalized care via federal funding for the construction and maintenance of community-based facilities and services, but much of this funding was stripped away before the bill was passed. Despite this, focus remained on decreasing the institutionalized population, and in keeping with that agenda, when Medicaid was passed in 1965, it included a mandate that denied funding to "institutions for mental diseases," thereby rapidly accelerating the process of deinstitutionalization.[38] Thus, while psychiatric wards continued to be shut down, more and more patients were ousted with nowhere to go.[39]

Deinstitutionalization was occurring at a remarkable rate and, within a decade, shifts began to surface in other populations. In 1975, the number of patients living in psychiatric wards had decreased by 60%[37] while the prison population had increased by 14%. By 1980, with only a quarter of the population of U.S. psychiatric wards remaining institutionalized, the U.S. prison population increased by 50%.[40]

The reverse correlation between the numbers of incarcerated prisoners in the correctional system and institutionalized psychiatric patients is not new: In 1939, Lionel Penrose observed this phenomenon in European countries, calling it the "balloon theory." His theory was later corroborated by George Palermo, who analyzed statistics on the U.S. mental health and prison systems between the years 1904 and 1987.[36] Today, the three largest public mental health providers are correctional systems: Rikers Island, Cook County, and Los Angeles County.[39] In Cook County alone, one in every three inmates has a mental disorder.[41] It is understandable, then, that so much funding should be required by a correctional system that it is charged not only with punishing and rehabilitating individuals, but with caring for the mentally ill as well. What should be examined, rather, is how these mentally ill arrived in the wrong system to begin with.

From 2009 to 2012, U.S. state legislators slashed a total of $4.5 billion from mental health services at the same period when Americans were still reeling from the Great Recession, and many had lost jobs and homes. These cuts often manifested in the closing of mental health clinics and hospitals, leaving patients without access to care. As more centers were shuttered, more of the mentally ill began to be sent to prisons rather than clinics, continuing the national trend. As the system operates today, incarcerated individuals are the only American citizens possessing a constitutional right to healthcare, and, under such laws, prisons are the most accessible avenues to mental healthcare for many populations.[41] Policies and programs like these, and the budgetary decisions that finance them, lead to a remarkably high prevalence of mental illness among the incarcerated population. Among male inmates, the prevalence of mental illness is more than quadruple that of their nonincarcerated community counterparts. For female inmates the difference is sixfold.[42] In examining these institutional relationships, the funding stripped from mental health appears to have been reallocated to the prison system, rather than saved.

One challenge presented by policies such as these is their intermingled nature. In the current system, mental health facilities have been deprived of funding and, as a consequence, many have closed their doors, leaving their patients without quality, timely access to much-needed care and medication. These closures likely disproportionately affect lower income populations, who do not have the ability to finance other means of treatment or seek out other clinics that may be distant from their community. This disaffected population is left on its own, meaning that those with fewer resources turn to other options. Whether through attempting to self-medicate or to get by without treatment, many of the choices left to these individuals land them in jail, contributing to the growing population within prisons. Many lose homes or jobs while being held, and upon release are provided no means to reenter their communities. Without treatment on the outside or a means of obtaining it, most continue in a cycle of incarceration and release. Beyond this, the fundamental cause of their incarceration, their mental health issues, has not been addressed. (Case Study 8.1; you can access the podcast accompanying Case Study 8.1 by following this link to Springer Publishing Company Connect™: http://connect.springerpub.com/content/book/978-0-8261-8043-8/part/part02/chapter/ch08).

CASE STUDY 8.1: MASS INCARCERATION AS A SOCIAL JUSTICE ISSUE AND A PUBLIC HEALTH CRISIS

"The United States is the epicenter of mass incarceration," according to The Vera Institute of Justice.[43] The Vera Institute tracks trends in incarceration and proactively advocates for evidence-based reforms.

The demographics and dynamics of imprisoned populations vary over time. Even with a drop in incarcerations during the first year of the COVID-19 pandemic, as of spring 2021, 1.9 million people were incarcerated in the United States. However, this is just a snapshot at a single point in time. Actually, people are sent to U.S. jails and prisons more than 11 million times each year. Some individuals cycle in and out of jail multiple times during a single year.

The United States incarcerates more people than China, a nation with four times the U.S. population. In fact, while the country has 4% of the world's 8 billion people, the United States accounts for 16% of all people incarcerated worldwide.[44] Sixteen percent is equivalent to one in every six incarcerated people.

(continued)

The United States incarcerates more people per capita than any other high-income country. In late 2022, according to the World Prison Brief, the only nations that ranked slightly above the United States per capita incarceration rate were Cuba, El Salvador, Rwanda, and Turkmenistan (plus the U.S. territory of American Samoa).[44]

Mass incarceration was not always a prominent feature of the American landscape. A sharp upward inflection in the number of U.S. inmates began around the 1970s, accelerating steeply for four decades to a peak in 2009. Numbers of incarcerated people tapered for a decade and dipped momentarily during the COVID-19 years, only to rise again as the pandemic receded.[45]

Jail incarceration declined in large U.S. metropolitan areas during the early 2000s, but was offset by dramatic rises in smaller cities and rural areas, now accounting for roughly half of incarcerated people. Furthermore, the Vera Institute indicates that there are vast inconsistencies given the variability in local policies for the more than 3,000 local jails and justice systems operating nationwide.[46]

Particularly troubling is the tenfold increase in the number of women incarcerated in local jails and prisons, especially in rural counties, during recent decades. The Vera Institute illuminates the disproportionate vulnerabilities of women inmates. High proportions of incarcerated women have been victims of multiple adverse childhood experiences, trauma, and abuse. Among women inmates there is a high prevalence of mental illness and substance use disorders. Moreover, many imprisoned women are single mothers whose incarceration has ripple effects for the health and well-being of their children.[47]

The dramatic upsurge in incarceration since the 1970s reflects an extension of patterns that are deeply rooted in American history.[48] The Vera Institute describes this powerfully, "from America's founding to the present, there are stories of crime waves or criminal behavior and then patterns of disproportionate imprisonment of those at the margins of society." Incarcerated women and men share distinguishing demographic characteristics. Simply stated, inmates predominantly come from low-income communities of color.

Among those currently overrepresented among the incarcerated population are those who are African American/Black, American Indian/Alaska Native, immigrants, and refugees. Over the 80-year period extending from the Civil War through the 1940s, almost half of the incarcerated population in the United States was comprised of racial and ethnic minorities and persons who were foreign-born, including non-English-speaking European immigrants. This situation has worsened thereafter; African American/Black residents currently make up 13.4% of the population but account for 37.6% of those who are incarcerated. Latinx residents represent 18.3% of the population but account for 31.8% of those who are in jails and prisons. Thus, African American/Black and Latinx residents, who together account for one-third of the general population, make up more than two-thirds of those who are incarcerated. In response, the Marguerite Casey Foundation is funding projects that are advancing a policy of "decarceration."

The much-heralded "crime waves" that are showcased in political rhetoric to justify locking people up change with the times. Yet, the Vera Institute rebukes the U.S. criminal justice system where "more than 80% of all arrests are for low-level, nonviolent offenses and conduct related to poverty."[49] The system operates to essentially criminalize poverty by jailing people who do not have the financial means to pay minor fees or fines.

(continued)

One of the principal dynamics propelling the incarceration surge that started in the 1970s was the War on Drugs.[50] Many people have been imprisoned not for drug dealing but, in many cases, for the mere possession of small quantities of "illicit" substances. Alleged drug crimes have created such an enormous back-log in the criminal justice system that it is estimated that more than 80% of the jailed population has never been convicted of the crime they were purported to have committed. Many low-income, minority persons who are jailed on unproven charges are convinced by their attorneys to plea bargain for a light sentence and relatively short jail terms—despite not having committed a crime. Lawyers sug-gest this strategy to clients to avoid prolonged waits in jail for a jury trial to be scheduled and to avoid taking a chance that the outcome of the trial—based on the nature of the case, the quality of their legal representation, and the makeup of the jury—will result in conviction and long-term imprisonment.

Against this backdrop, mass incarceration poses a variety of serious threats to public health. The incarcerated population has a high prevalence of substance use disorders, estimated at two-thirds of jail inmates (68%) and half of persons in state prisons (50%), in stark contrast to an overall population prevalence of 9%.[51] One in seven men in jails and almost one in three women in jails have a diagnosable serious mental illness—compared to 3.2% of men and 4.9% of women in the non-incarcerated general population.[52] Noncommunicable diseases (NCDs) are also more common among prisoners and are especially prevalent in persons ages 55 and older. Imprisoned persons over the age of 55 increased by 550% in the 20-year span, 1992 to 2012![53]

Injuries are a prominent feature of life in correctional facilities. One in six (15%) state prisoners reported violence-related intentional injuries while more than one in five (22%) reported nonintentional "accidental" injuries. Moreover, suicide is the cause of one-third of deaths in jails.[54]

The nature of confinement is highly conducive for communicable disease spread. Jails and prisons are notorious for the concentrated spread of HIV, hep-atitis C, and a variety of STIs related to coerced or situational sexual contact. HIV rates in the incarcerated population are two to seven times greater than in the gen-eral population. Also, consider the reverse: One in six U.S. residents living with HIV will pass through a correctional facility each year.[55] The prevalence of hepatitis C among incarcerated people is an alarming eight to 21 times higher than for non-incarcerated persons. More imprisoned people die from hepatitis C than from HIV.

Women who are imprisoned frequently have a history of sexual trauma or abuse and many have engaged in sex work. Not surprisingly, therefore, incarcer-ated women have high prevalence rates of chlamydia, gonorrhea, and syphilis compared with women not behind bars.

In 2020, during the first year of the COVID-19 pandemic when no vaccines were available, prisons became primary sources of rampant outbreaks, including super-spreader events and case clusters. It was not possible to achieve social dis-tancing and observe hygienic conditions in correctional facilities. As of June 2022, just over 2 years since the arrival of COVID-19 in the United States, nearly 600,000 people who have been incarcerated in U.S. prisons had a documented case of COVID-19 and more than 2,900 had died.[56]

Advocates for social justice and prison reform are seeking proactive solutions for confronting the social injustices of the system, including the elevated risks to life and health for incarcerated persons. Among a broad variety of programs that

(continued)

are being implemented or proposed are expanding higher education programs, including implementing degree-earning programs in prisons; introducing diversion programs to decrease encounters with the legal system and keep people in communities; decreasing the detention of immigrants; advocating to reduce "overpolicing" of minority neighborhoods and racial stereotyping; and decriminalizing some types of substance use. These activities will be challenged by an entrenched, for-profit prison industry and historical legislative traditions that are heavy on punishment in a manner that is heavily skewed toward locking up individuals from communities targeted for marginalization. Nevertheless, there are ample opportunities for motivated champions of social justice to make a difference—and public health professionals need to be in the vanguard.

Exempting Firearms From Oversight and Regulation

Guns kill more and more Americans by the year.[57] Lack of gun regulation and oversight are major contributors to the problem. Many of the firearm-related deaths can be linked to accidental discharges and faulty equipment or, in other words, a simple lack of consumer-oriented safety standards. Between 2005 and 2010, about 3,800 people died from unintentional shootings. Moreover, a federal study showed that about 8% of these fatalities resulted from shots fired by children under the age of 6.[58]

There is no question that firearms are consumer products. Per capita firearm ownership more than doubled between 1968 and 2012 to 310 million firearms or one gun per person in the United States.[59] Moreover, one-in-three households has a firearm.[60] And, like other consumer products, firearms are advertised in both mainstream media outlets and specialty publications.[61] However, firearms, unlike most other products, are specifically designed to kill or at least injure individuals. They might, by far, be the most hazardous products in the American marketplace. As such, requiring at least the same regulatory standards set for other products is a logical conclusion, yet, unlike with other consumer products, firearm manufacturing and distribution are not regulated.

Following the creation of the Consumer Product Safety Commission in 1972, lawmakers worked tirelessly to ensure the exclusion of firearms from the mandate of the commission, mostly citing fear of a slippery slope of hindering the Second Amendment (the right to bear arms).[62] In 1976, the Consumer Product Safety Act was amended. In part, the amendment read, "The Consumer Product Safety Commission shall make no ruling or order that restricts the manufacture or sale of firearms, firearms ammunition, or components of firearms ammunition including black powder or gunpowder for firearms."[63] Because this amendment was passed, no federal agency has a mandate to oversee how firearms are built. Further, while some special consumer products are regulated by product-specific agencies such as the Food and Drug Administration (FDA) for food products, medications, and medical devices, there is no comparable oversight agency for firearm production. The Bureau of Alcohol, Tobacco, Firearms and Explosives (ATF) focuses on regulating the illegal use of firearms; it does not, however, regulate safety requirements for firearm production.[64] Some state legislators even try to work around the minimal oversight role of the ATF. For example, the state of Texas legislature proposed a law that firearms made and sold in Texas do not have to comply with federal regulations such as the 1994 ban on assault weapons (that expired in 2004 and has not been renewed).[65] At the same time, Congress continues to pass legislation that limits the ATF's ability to carry out its existing mission of preventing violence.[66] In addition to the lack of oversight on firearm safety, Congress passed the Protection of Lawful Commerce in Arms Act in 2005, which exempted gun manufacturers from the majority of tort lawsuits.[67] As of today, the federal government is incapable of recalling defective firearms. The federal government can, however, recall polluting cars and unsafe toys. Moreover, there is no system to track deaths due to malfunctioning firearms.[62]

With lack of oversight and laws regulating the safety of firearms, manufacturers have been reluctant to incorporate technologies that improve firearm design and increase safety. Technologies to manufacture child-resistant handguns have existed since the late 1800s. Moreover, there are multiple technologies that allow only authorized users to operate firearms.[68] For example, adding a childproof gun safety device and a chamber load indicator to alert the user when bullets are in the firearm would prevent about 31% of unintentional firearm deaths.[69] Yet, the industry is not obligated, nor motivated, to adopt protective measures that reduce gun-related accidents. Governmental incentives for manufacturers to design and build safe firearms are almost nonexistent. Moreover, as interested parties and insurers have no reason to worry about financial liability, there is no pressure on gun manufacturers to improve safety standards.

All of these dynamics created an industry that is self-policing.

Unintentional firearm discharges represent a relatively small but preventable subset of firearm deaths in the United States each year. Mass shootings in school settings represent a high-visibility contributor to the firearm death toll. Although they represent a relatively small proportion of total firearm deaths, these events galvanize the national conversation around firearm oversight and regulation.

More than 20 years have elapsed since the shooting massacre at Columbine High School in Littleton, Colorado, on April 20, 1999. During these two decades, an additional 240 multiple-victim shootings have occurred in U.S. schools, most resulting in fatalities. In fact, 32 episodes of mass shootings in schools occurred in the 14 months between the massacre at Marjorie Stoneman Douglas High School in Parkland, Florida, on Valentine's Day 2018, and the observance of the 20th anniversary of Columbine in April 2019. **Table 8.1** lists and ranks the eight deadliest mass shootings in schools during the first 23 years of the post-Columbine era.

TABLE 8.1 Rank Ordering of the Eight Deadliest U.S. School Shootings Following the Columbine School Massacre, April 20, 1999

SCHOOL NAME, CITY, STATE	DATE	DEATHS	INJURIES
Virginia Tech University Blacksburg, VA	April 16, 2007	32	17
Sandy Hook Elementary School Newtown, CT	December 14, 2012	27	2
Robb Elementary School Uvalde, TX	May 24, 2022	21	18
Marjory Stoneman Douglas High School Parkland, FL	February 14, 2018	17	17
Columbine High School Littleton, CO	April 20, 1999	13	24
Santa Fe High School Santa Fe, TX	March 18, 2018	10	13
Umpqua Community College Roseburg, OR	October 1, 2015	9	8
Red Lake Indian Reservation/School Red Lake, MN	March 21, 2005	9	5

HOW ORGANIZED PUBLIC HEALTH EFFORTS CAN ENCOURAGE POLITICAL ACTION TOWARD HEALTHY POPULATIONS

As a discipline, public health aims to improve and protect the health of populations, which, on many occasions, depends on engaging politicians to take actions. By way of example, one of the major successes for public health was the organized campaign advocating for tobacco control. During the first half of the 20th century, smoking was a fashionable and increasingly popular social norm in the United States; the annual per capita cigarette consumption increased from 54 cigarettes in 1900 to 4,345 cigarettes in 1963[70] (**Figure 8.2**). Public health efforts such as publishing epidemiologic evidence on the links between smoking and lung cancer, coupled with media campaigns to educate the public, led to pressure on politicians to pass legislation to reduce cigarette consumption on a population level. Political actions ranged from the release of the landmark 1964 Surgeon General report on the harms of cigarettes, to legislation to increase taxes on cigarettes, to banning smoking in public places (the Clean Air Act legislation). These political actions—allied with other public health interventions—ultimately led to a reversal in the trend; annual per capita consumption of cigarettes dropped to 2,261 in 1998[70] and 1,078 in 2015.[71]

> As a discipline, public health aims to improve and protect the health of populations, which, on many occasions, depends on engaging politicians to take actions.

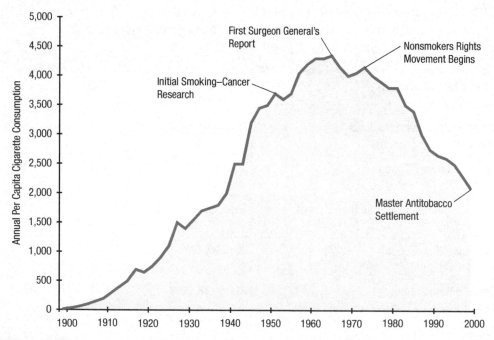

FIGURE 8.2 Annual adult per capita cigarette consumption and major smoking and health events: United States, 1900–1998.
Source: Centers for Disease Control and Prevention. Achievements in public health, 1900–1999: tobacco use—United States, 1900–1999. *Morb Mortal Wkly Rep.* 1999;48(43):986-993.

THE ROLE OF CORPORATIONS IN SHAPING POLICIES THAT AFFECT POPULATION HEALTH

Corporations affect almost all aspects of human experiences—ranging from eating habits, to personal identity, to lifestyle—in multiple ways, often through advertising and marketing their products. Moreover, corporations determine the working conditions for a significant percentage of the population. They also play a central role in shaping policies regulating tax systems, welfare, healthcare, trade, and the environment. Through these multiple pathways, corporations' impact on health is on the rise.[72] More directly, corporations affect the health of populations through their products. For example, consumer products such as tobacco, low-nutrient foods, and firearms are major contributors to the burden of disease and injury. However, such adverse health impacts are not always a deterrent; production decisions by corporations are often largely, if not solely, based on the best methods to maximize profit. Case Studies 8.2 and 8.3 provide examples of the impact corporations have on setting health-related policies.

> **Corporations affect almost all aspects of human experiences—ranging from eating habits, to personal identity, to lifestyle—in multiple ways, often through advertising and marketing their products.**

CASE STUDY 8.2: CONTINUING USE OF LEAD BY CORPORATIONS DESPITE SAFETY CONCERNS

One example of how corporations ignore evidence of the harmful health effects of certain substances is the history of using lead in consumer products. Lead, an elemental heavy metal and known human toxin, has been an integral part of human history and development over millennia.[73] The compound's versatility, ductile nature, and corrosion resistance explain its widespread use in everything, from art to infrastructure, in early human societies.[74] And while acute lead poisoning— resulting from large, concentrated exposures through food or manufacturing— was noted early on, it was not until the 19th century that the possibility of other forms of hazardous lead contact began to be explored.[75]

The evidence-based revelation of lead's toxicity, even with low-dose exposures, did not halt its use. Following the discovery of lead's detrimental effects on children through contact with lead-based house paints, many countries, such as France and Austria, opted to ban its use in interior paints—but the United States forged ahead with lead production and use.[76] Before the 1950s, an American can of paint could contain as much as 70% lead.[77] By 1990, more than a decade after the United States had finally banned the use of lead in interior paints—more than half a century after many other high-income nations had imposed similar bans[78]—some 64 million housing units nationwide were still contaminated with the substance.[77]

By the 1970s, when the newly minted Environmental Protection Agency (EPA) initiated efforts to eradicate environmental lead, it was apparent just how ubiquitous the substance had become in the modern American landscape. This was not always the case, and the litigation against lead was, in some cases, responding to public anxieties that dated back more than a century. As early as 1859, there

(continued)

was documented public concern regarding the use of lead piping in city plumbing. Lacking robust scientific data to support this concern, lead pipes were indeed installed.

As lead-poisoning fatalities climbed, however, research tracing the connections between lead plumbing and the rising death toll proliferated. As early as the 1920s, state officials began to edit plumbing codes to prevent further use of lead piping—and lead manufacturers took notice. In 1928, the Lead Industries Association (LIA) was established and set out on what would be more than half a century of campaigning for the continued use of lead in products ranging from piping to paint.[79]

Even as a debate was waged over lead plumbing, lead was already creeping into other manufacturing sectors. In 1921, Thomas Midgley, Jr., an engineer for General Motors (GM), realized that tetraethyl lead could be used to diminish engine "knocking" (the tendency of the air–fuel mixture to ignite off-cycle instead of in response to the spark plug firing; this leads to "pinging" and inefficient combustion that could ultimately damage the engine).

Although tetraethyl lead had been discovered more than 60 years earlier, it had not been marketed owing to health concerns regarding lead poisoning. However, the research division of GM where Midgley worked was in a bind. GM was undergoing a major ownership and management shake-up and every department was under scrutiny to prove itself to be profitable. Midgley's boss, Charles Kettering, saw an opportunity to save the research division with this discovery, and quickly passed it up the chain to company officials. Lead was appealing for use in the automobile industry, in part, because the process of isolating the tetraethyl compound was patentable, unlike the process used in creating its closest competitor chemical, ethanol. Shifting to tetraethyl compound promised huge profits for GM. Moreover, discontinuing the research experiments with ethanol appealed to the nation's big oil producers, who had already been fighting the possible emergence of ethanol as an alternative fuel to gasoline. And so, by 1923, lead had found its way into the air by way of automobiles.[80]

What makes lead of particular interest in the history of health regulation is the industry's success in stifling the voice of public health from the outset. By 1922, lead was a known toxin, and one that deeply troubled public officials. It was known that poisoning was not merely due to a single exposure to purified lead but more often resulted from the accumulation of repeated milder exposures. Knowledge of lead's toxicity prompted a U.S. Public Health Service (USPHS) professional, William Mansfield Clark, to write to the Assistant Surgeon General, A.M. Stinson, requesting that the use of tetraethyl lead in gasoline be investigated before its widespread distribution began. The surgeon general's request for an investigation yielded no results, however, because collecting the necessary data was deemed beyond the remit of the USPHS. Instead, the responsibility for investigating health effects was delegated to the automobile industry, effectively asking these for-profit manufacturers to self-regulate.[80]

As the number of industries capitalizing on this versatile substance continued to grow, stories of lead poisoning reached the national news and frightening symptoms began to surface. Credit for expanding the use of lead in a growing roster of products can be largely ascribed to the success of the LIA. The LIA deftly maneuvered the compound into all manner of products. Capitalizing on the shifting tides of consumer interest, from increased homeownership to hygiene, the LIA ensured that lead found its way into each new fixture of American life.[77] By the late

(continued)

1920s, this included nearly every part of an individual's environment, from children's toys, to the washing machines that cleaned the clothes, to the light bulbs on the ceilings, to the paint on the walls, and down to the very air people breathed.[77] The LIA even managed to counteract the apprehension that had swelled around lead plumbing in the early 1920s, successfully sowing doubt as to the purported (actually, very real) relationship between lead piping and tainted water supplies.[79] The LIA was a master at lobbying and produced publications touting the material's myriad advantages and useful applications. LIA officials manipulated both public and private images of lead and its effects; quieting public anxieties around the fatalities of factory workers manufacturing tetraethyl lead[80]; blaming the mounting rates of lead poisoning in children on their lower class, "ineducable" parents; and relegating the issue to a back burner by associating it with minorities in inner-city slums.[77]

Capitalizing on bigotry and ignorance, the industry staved off legal intervention for decades. Use of leaded gas, releasing nearly 200,000 tons of toxic metal particles per year in the United States alone, continued into the 1970s before a government-mandated phase-out began.[81] The atmospheric lead released by gas combustion was infiltrating not just our air, but the soil, groundwater, and croplands worldwide.[81] In 2000, it was estimated that 5% of U.S. children had subclinical lead poisoning.[76] Today, the most sustained risks of lead exposure are concentrated in poor minority populations, living in aging homes built before bans on lead were implemented.[82]

In January 2016, President Obama declared a state of emergency in Flint, Michigan, due to the lead leeching into the city's water supply from an outdated lead plumbing system and a change in water sourcing.[83] Cases like that of Flint are illustrative of a history of disparities in health protections provided to different communities, as well as the lasting ramifications of industrial and governmental decisions made without considerations for population health.

CASE STUDY 8.3: CORPORATIONS, HYDROFRACKING, AND POPULATION HEALTH

In 1947, in a gas field in Kansas, Floyd Farris of the Stanolind Oil and Gas Corporation carried out the first hydraulic fracturing of a limestone deposit 2,400 feet below the earth's surface. Having explored the relationship between pressure and the functionality of wells, Farris designed the practice hoping to increase well production. While his initial experiment was not successful, the method was published and refined, resulting in a patent by Halliburton Oil Well Cementing Company in 1949. Halliburton's improved methodology commercialized hydrofracking, and within a decade the company had increased well treatments 10-fold.[84] By 2015, 51% of crude oil[85] and more than 67% of natural gas produced in the United States came from hydraulically fractured wells (**Table 8.2**).[86] This unfettered expansion has raised questions, however, as to the potential effects on population health, and the relative dearth of data on such effects.

These doubts, few of which have been adequately assuaged in the view of public health officials, fuel much of the public debate that continues to surround

(continued)

TABLE 8.2 Oil and Natural Gas Production in the United States and Proportion From Hydralically Fractured Wells ("Fracking"), 2000–2015

| | OIL PRODUCTION | | | NATURAL GAS PRODUCTION | | |
| | TOTAL OUTPUT | OUTPUT FROM HYDRAULICALLY FRACTURED WELLS | | TOTAL OUTPUT | OUTPUT FROM HYDRAULICALLY FRACTURED WELLS | |
YEAR	MILLION BARRELS/ DAY	MILLION BARRELS/DAY	PERCENTAGE OF TOTAL (%)	BILLION CUBIC FEET/DAY	BILLION CUBIC FEET/ DAY	PERCENTAGE OF TOTAL (%)
2000	5.8	0.1	2	55	4	7
2001	5.7	0.2	3	56	6	11
2002	5.6	0.2	4	54	8	15
2003	5.5	0.3	5	54	8	19
2004	5.3	0.3	6	53	11	21
2005	5.0	0.3	6	52	14	27
2006	4.9	0.4	8	53	16	30
2007	4.9	0.5	10	55	20	36
2008	4.8	0.6	12	58	25	43
2009	5.2	0.7	14	59	27	46
2010	5.3	0.9	17	61	31	51
2011	5.5	1.2	22	66	37	56
2012	6.3	2.1	33	69	41	59
2013	7.3	3.0	41	70	44	62
2014	8.7	4.2	48	75	49	65
2015	9.1	4.6	51	78	52	67

Source: Data from The U.S. Energy Information Administration (EIA). Hydraulically fractured wells provide two-thirds of U.S. natural gas production. 2016. https://energycentral.com/c/ec/hydraulically-fractured-wells-provide-two-thirds-us-natural-gas-production

fracking. Such reservations are particularly pronounced regarding the methods of extraction. In order to release an oil or gas reserve, generally 6,000 to 10,000 feet beneath earth's surface, companies must drill to that depth and implant vertical columns of pipe through which fuel can rise to the surface. Once the drilling operation has reached the subterranean reserve, explosives are detonated to fracture the shale formation that holds the oil or gas. These

(*continued*)

fractures are expanded and held open by fracking fluid, which is injected at high pressure, allowing the fuel reserves to be released and carried up through the pipework.[87]

Fracking has raised concerns about its potential cancer-causing effects. A review of the chemicals released into the water and air by the fracking process found that 55 may cause cancer.[88] In recent years, the use of carcinogens has only been exacerbated with an EPA report identifying 1,600 chemicals employed in drilling and fracking or fracking wastewater, of which 200 were regarded as carcinogens or toxic to human health.[89] The use of such chemicals is another source of conflict. Beyond tensions regarding the industry's power of choice in disclosing chemical use, hydrofracking is exempt from EPA regulations mandated by the SDWA. Many have voiced concerns over this practice, as fracking fluid is disposed of in wastewater wells, which have been known to leak.[90]

It is not just the wanton disregard for known public health risks that angers many of those who oppose fracking, but the industry's dismissal of health concerns. An independent and objective evaluation of the health consequences seems critical, given both the lack of knowledge regarding the long-term effects of fracking and the obvious geographic proximity of fracking fluids and products to a vital public good, drinking water. Adding to the frustrations is the history of policy decisions that have allowed fracking to sidestep regulatory measures traditionally applicable in such scenarios.

The exemption of fracking from the SDWA has been contentiously challenged for decades. Since its origin in 1974, the SDWA has explicitly not regulated hydraulic fracturing, which would otherwise fall under the underground injection control regulations mandated by the SDWA. While the reason behind the original distinction is unclear, when it was challenged in 1997, in *Legal Environmental Assistance Foundation, Inc. v. U.S. Environmental Protection Agency* (*LEAF v. EPA*), the EPA claimed that the underground injection control programs were meant to regulate only the fluids pumped underground by wells for which this was the "principal function." The 11th Circuit Court ruled in favor of LEAF, stating that hydrofracking clearly fell within the SDWA's definition of underground injection as "the subsurface emplacement of fluids by well injection," regardless of other purposes served by the wells. This interpretation, along with the subsequent ruling by the court that the use of hydrofracking in Alabama for coal bed methane fell into the definition of a Class II well and was therefore required to meet the regulations therein, had the potential to open a larger dialogue regarding national regulation of hydraulic fracturing.

Before this could occur, however, an amendment was made to the SDWA in 2005. This amendment, called the Energy Policy Act of 2005, clarified in plain language that hydrofracking, except that which involved diesel fuel, was exempt from all underground injection regulation.[91] Thus, the fracking industry was effectively released from any federal oversight regarding ground water supplies. The amendment drew public suspicion, however, because of the relationship between President George W. Bush's administration and fracking corporations. Bush's Vice President, Dick Cheney, had been CEO of Halliburton—the first company to patent hydraulic fracturing—prior to joining the Bush Administration.[92]

(continued)

Lack of industry transparency and absence of government oversight make it difficult to investigate the public health ramifications of hydrofracking. While longitudinal data are absent, however, there is evidence to merit further investigation regarding the health risks of the process. Residential populations living close to the fracking sites are at elevated risk for respiratory complications due to pollutants released by the process, as well as drinking water contamination from poor well construction, and soil contamination from spills.[93] While oil and gas reserves reside well below the deepest regions of our water table,[94] the vertical fracking pipes pass through the ground water supplies on their way into the deeper earth. This becomes problematic when coupled with methane migration—a process in which methane drifts up to the surface from deep within the earth. Methane migration occurs naturally, but the process of hydrofracking accelerates the process over time by creating fractures and rifts through which the methane can escape. This drifting can contaminate wells and groundwater supplies, making sources of drinking water unusable.[95] Methane poses additional environmental risks; methane is a greenhouse gas, estimated to be as much as 105 times more potent than carbon dioxide (CO_2) when released into the atmosphere.[96]

Public health concerns are heightened by the societal impacts of fracking at the community level. Communities close to fracking sites suffer from increased stress and increased traffic flow, as well as strain on resources. Some studies have found a correlation between certain birth complications and proximity to fracking sites, and many show increases in a plethora of symptoms, such as nosebleeds and dizziness, among residents near worksites.[93]

Jobs in the fracking industry are well paid. This may lead to an influx of less educated skilled and semiskilled laborers coming to the area for work, and most are male. For example, the population of western North Dakota has been significantly transformed by the introduction of the hydrofracking industry. To handle the acute rise in population, the early phase of a new fracking site is likely to see the formation of "man camps" where workers bivouac during their off hours in dormitory-like quarters.[97] This has led to a proliferation of prostitution, increased rates of STIs, overuse of alcohol, and periodic episodes of violence.[98]

As of 2018, nine of every 10 new oil and gas wells use fracking.[99] Because of lack of federal oversight, though, regulatory decisions fall to the states. In New York, the debate was particularly contentious, considering that some of the state's most economically depressed regions sit atop one of the largest natural gas deposits in the world.[100] The revenue that could have been generated by fracking in those regions, as well as the energy that would have been produced, further complicated the decision. The eventual choice to ban fracking in New York was not made on the basis of the information uncovered by a state-run health investigation into the practice, as the information found was incomplete. The health risk to residents could not be accurately evaluated, and without adequate proof in either direction, the risk was deemed too great.[101] Such a decision has the potential to set a precedent. It did not dismiss hydrofracking unequivocally but rather put the ball in the industry's court. Rather than placing an evidentiary burden on the public to correlate ill-health and fracking, the burden now rests with the industry to acknowledge and address public concern and establish a verifiable lack of such correlation.

SUMMARY

The health of populations depends on the social and economic structures around us. Around the world, illness and health follow a social gradient: Lower socioeconomic status generally translates to worse health outcomes. Politics and policies, on both the national and international levels, shape these socioeconomic structures. Accordingly, politics on all levels interact with the goals of public health to prevent disease, prolong life, and promote health through organized efforts in society.

Governments' influence on the health of their populations extends beyond policies that regulate healthcare provision and public health measures to social determinants of health such as housing, public transportation, employment policies, or even decisions to initiate an armed conflict or oppress a subset of the population.

Political decisions shape causes of health at other levels across the social ecological causal chain from the structure of the healthcare system down to individual behaviors. On a global level, globalization has introduced social determinants of health that operate beyond the control of a single government. The WHO is the global body that provides leadership on matters critical for health and sets and promotes standards for health worldwide. Corporations are another important actor in shaping the social determinants of health in populations. Corporations affect almost all aspects of human experiences in multiple ways, ranging from marketing and lobbying efforts to continuing to produce harmful products such as tobacco to influencing individual behavior.

End-of-Chapter Resources

Access additional case study podcasts online at http://connect.springerpub.com/ content/book/978-0-8261-8043-8/

DISCUSSION QUESTIONS

1. Discuss differences in life expectancies globally. In your discussion, consider the political system, access to medical services and prevention programs, as well as environmental conditions, housing, and food quality.
2. Identify a national political decision/policy that did not directly address the healthcare system but had an impact on the overall health of the population in your country.
3. Consider two different approaches to distributing health resources that vary by country. Describe the different approaches and how they affect health inequities in each country.
4. Consider two different policies designed to address health inequities that vary by country. Describe the different policies and how they affect health inequities in each country.

REFERENCES

1. Mackenbach JP. Politics is nothing but medicine at a larger scale: reflections on public health's biggest idea. *J Epidemiol Community Health*. 2009;63(3):181-184. doi:10.1136/jech.2008.077032

2. Central Intelligence Agency. *The world factbook*. 2019. https://www.cia.gov/the-world-factbook/

3. Commission on Social Determinants of Health. *Closing the Gap in a Generation Health Equity Through Action on the Social Determinants of Health*. World Health Organization; 2008. https://apps.who.int/iris/bitstream/handle/10665/43943/9789241563703_eng.pdf

4. Glassman A, Buse K. Politics, and public health policy reform. In: Heggenhougen K, Quah S, eds. *International Encyclopedia of Public Health. Vol 5*. Academic Press; 2008:163-170. https://www.brookings.edu/wp-content/uploads/2016/06/09_public_health_glassman.pdf

5. World Health Organization Regional Office for Europe. *About WHO/Europe*. https://www.who.int/europe/about-us/about-who-europe

6. Mackenbach JP. Political conditions and life expectancy in Europe, 1900-2008. *Soc Sci Med*. 2013;82:134-146. doi:10.1016/j.socscimed.2012.12.022

7. Galea S. *Injuries and the Health of the Public*. Published August 25, 2017. https://www.bu.edu/sph/news/articles/2017/injuries-and-the-health-of-the-public/

8. Bor J, Venkataramani AS, Williams DR, Tsai AC. Police killings and their spillover effects on the mental health of black Americans: a population-based, quasi-experimental study. *Lancet*. 2018;392(10144):302-310. doi:10.1016/S0140-6736(18)31130-9

9. Jha P, Peto R. Global effects of smoking, of quitting, and of taxing tobacco. *N Engl J Med*. 2014;370(1):60-68. doi:10.1056/NEJMra1308383

10. World Health Organization. *What we do*. https://www.who.int/about/what-we-do

11. Ottersen OP, Dasgupta J, Blouin C, et al. The political origins of health inequity: prospects for change. *Lancet*. 2014;383(9917):630-667. doi:10.1016/S0140-6736(13)62407-1

12. Quackenbush C. *The impact of President Trump's "global gag rule" on women's health is becoming clear. Time*. February 2, 2018. http://time.com/5115887/donald-trump-global-gag-rule-women

13. United Nations Population Fund. *Sexual & reproductive health*. https://www.unfpa.org/sexual-reproductive-health

14. Karolyne Q, Ejlak J. *Women's sexual and reproductive health: a literature review*. 2008. https://apo.org.au/node/8609

15. United Nations Population Fund. *Gender equality*. https://www.unfpa.org/gender-equality

16. World Health Organization. *Millennium Development Goals (MDGs)*. Published February 19, 2018. https://www.who.int/news-room/fact-sheets/detail/millennium-development-goals-(mdgs)

17. Centers for Disease Control and Prevention. *Reproductive health: teen pregnancy*. https://www.cdc.gov/teenpregnancy

18. Pazol K, Creanga AA, Burley KD, Jamieson DJ. Abortion surveillance—United States, 2011. *MMWR Surveill Summ*. 2014;63:1-41. https://www.cdc.gov/mmwr/preview/mmwrhtml/ss6311a1.htm

19. HHS.gov. *Title X service grants*. https://www.hhs.gov/opa/title-x-family-planning/index.html

20. Guttmacher Institute. *Publicly supported family planning services in the United States*. Published September 2016. https://www.guttmacher.org/fact-sheet/publicly-funded-family-planning-services-united-states

21. Galea S. *Reproductive health on the anniversary of Roe v. Wade*. Boston University School of Public Health. Published January 24, 2016. https://www.bu.edu/sph/2016/01/24/reproductive-health-on-the-anniversary-of-roe-v-wade

22. *Roe v. Wade 410 U.S. 113* 1973.

23. McBride A. *Expanding civil rights: landmark cases: Roe v. Wade (1973)*. Thirteen/WNET. https://www.thirteen.org/wnet/supremecourt/rights/landmark_roe.html

24. Cornell Law School Legal Information Institute. *Mary DOE et al., Appellants, v. Arthur K. BOLTON, as Attorney General of the State of Georgia, et al*. 1973. https://www.law.cornell.edu/supremecourt/text/410/179

25. Congress.gov. *S.142 - Hyde Amendment Codification Act*. 2013. https://www.congress.gov/bill/113th-congress/senate-bill/142

26. Irwin N, Miller CC, Sanger-Katz M. *America's racial divide, charted*. New York Times. August 19, 2014. https://www.nytimes.com/2014/08/20/upshot/americas-racial-divide-charted.html?_r=0

27. Williams DR, Mohammed SA. Discrimination and racial disparities in health: evidence and needed research. *J Behav Med*. 2009;32:20-47. doi:10.1007/s10865-008-9185-0

28. Farley T, Cohen DA. *Prescription for a Healthy Nation: A New Approach to Improving Our Lives by Fixing Our Everyday World*. Beacon Press; 2005.

29. National Constitution Center. *14th amendment: citizenship rights, equal protection, apportionment, civil war debt*. https://constitutioncenter.org/the-constitution/amendments/amendment-xiv#:~:text=No%20State%20shall%20make%20or,equal%20protection%20of%20the%20laws

30. FindLaw. *Washington v. Davis 426 U.S. (1976)*. https://caselaw.findlaw.com/us-supreme-court/426/229.html

31. Kobick J. Discriminatory intent reconsidered: folk concepts of intentionality and equal protection jurisprudence. *Harv Civ Rights-Civil Lib Law Rev*. 2010;45(2):517. https://www.researchgate.net/publication/265046266_Discriminatory_Intent_Reconsidered_Folk_Concepts_of_Intentionality_and_Equal_Protection_Jurisprudence

32. Cornell Law School Legal Information Institute. *Personnel administrator of massachusetts et al, appellants v. Helen B. Feeney. 442 U.S. 256 (1979)*. 1979. https://www.law.cornell.edu/supremecourt/text/442/256

33. Harvard Law Review. *Texas department of housing & community affairs v. inclusive communities project, Inc.* 2015. https://harvardlawreview.org/2015/11/texas-department-of-housing-community-affairs-v-inclusive -communities-project

34. Crampton L. *Supreme court sides with opponents of Texas housing program. The Texas Tribune.* June 25, 2015. https://www.texastribune.org/2015/06/25/supreme-court-rules-dallas-fair-housing-case

35. Orfield G, Lee C. *Historic reversals, accelerating resegregation, and the need for new integration strategies.* University of California. Published August 29, 2007. https://civilrightsproject.ucla.edu/research/k-12-education/ integration-and-diversity/historic-reversals-accelerating-resegregation-and-the-need-for-new-integration -strategies-1

36. Public Broadcasting System. *Deinstitutionalization: a psychiatric "Titanic."* January 13, 2017. https://www.pbs .org/wgbh/pages/frontline/shows/asylums/special/excerpt.html

37. Harcourt BE. *Reducing mass incarceration: lessons from the deinstitutionalization of mental hospitals in the 1960s.* University of Chicago Law & Economics, Olin Working Paper No. 542; University of Chicago, Public Law Working Paper No. 335. January 26, 2011. doi:10.2139/ssrn.1748796

38. Jaffe D. *Medicaid, mentally ill, and state hospitals.* Mental Illness Policy Org. http://mentalillnesspolicy.org/imd/ imd-medicaid-mentally-ill.html

39. Young Minds Advocacy. *The community mental health act of 1963.* https://www.youngmindsadvocacy.org/the -community-mental-health-act-of-1963

40. Bureau of Justice Statistics. *Prisoners 1925–81.* U.S. Department of Justice; 1982. https://www.bjs.gov/ content/pub/pdf/p2581.pdf

41. Ford M. *America's largest mental hospital is a jail. The Atlantic.* June 8, 2015. https://www.theatlantic.com/ politics/archive/2015/06/americas-largest-mental-hospital-is-a-jail/395012/

42. Cloud D. *On Life Support: Public Health in the Age of Mass Incarceration.* Vera Institute of Justice; 2014. https://www.vera.org/publications/on-life-support-public-health-in-the-age-of-mass-incarceration

43. Vera Institute. *Ending mass incarceration.* https://www.vera.org/ending-mass-incarceration?ms=awar_comm _all_grant_BS22_ctr_AP2&utm_source=grant&utm_medium=awar&utm_campaign=all_AP2&gclid= EAIaIQobChMIr9zZobbj-gIV_4laBR0Q0gitEAAYASAAEgIf-PD_BwE

44. World Prison Brief. *Highest to lowest–prison population rate.* https://www.prisonstudies.org/highest-to-lowest/ prison_population_rate?field_region_taxonomy_tid=All

45. Bureau of Justice Statistics. *National prisoner statistics, United States, 1978-2020. Inter-University consortium for political and social research.* Published December 16, 2021. https://doi.org/10.3886/ICPSR38249.v1

46. Washington M. *Jails in the United States.* Vera Institute. Published November 2021. https://www.vera.org/ beyond-jails-community-based-strategies-for-public-safety/jails-in-the-united-states

47. Vera Institute. *Overlooked: women and jails in an era of reform.* Published August 2016. https://www.vera.org/ publications/overlooked-women-and jails report

48. Delaney R, Subramanian R, Shames A, Turner N. *American history, race, and prison.* Vera Institute: Reimagining Prison Web Report. https://www.vera.org/reimagining-prison-web-report/american-history-race -and-prison

49. Vera Institute. *Criminalization & racial disparities.* Published November 2021. https://www.vera.org/ criminalization-racial-disparities

50. History. *War on drugs.* Updated December 17, 2019. https://www.history.com/topics/crime/the-war-on-drugs

51. Vera Institute. *The burden of mental illness behind bars. Vera Institute of justice.* Published June 21, 2016. http://humantollofjail.vera.org/the-burden-of-mental-illness-behind-bars/

52. Treatment Advocacy Center. *Serious mental illness prevalence in jails and prisons.* Published September 2016. https://www.treatmentadvocacycenter.org/evidence-and-research/learn-more-about/3695

53. Zaitzow BH, Willis AK. Behind the wall of indifference: prisoner voices about the realities of prison health care. *Laws.* 2021;*10*(1):11. doi:10.3390/laws10010011

54. Wang L. *Rise in jail deaths is especially troubling as jail populations become more rural and more female.* Prison Policy Initiative. Published June 23, 2021. https://www.prisonpolicy.org/blog/2021/06/23/jail_mortality/

55. Maruschak LM. *HIV in prisons, 2020–statistical tables.* Bureau of Justice Statistics. Published May 2022. https://bjs.ojp.gov/library/publications/hiv-prisons-2020-statistical-tables

56. Kwan A, Garcia-Grossman I, Sears D, Bertozzi SM, Williams BA. The impact of COVID-19 on the health of incarcerated older adults in California state prisons. *Health Aff.* 2022;*41*(8):1191-1201. doi:10.1377/hlthaff .2022.00132

57. LaFraniere S, Palmer E. *Guns in America. New York Times.* October 21, 2016. https://www.nytimes.com/ spotlight/gun-violence

58. Giffords Law Center. *Statistics.* https://lawcenter.giffords.org/gun-deaths-and-injuries-statistics

59. Krouse WJ. *Gun Control Legislation.* CreateSpace Independent Publishing Platform; 2012.

60. Horsley S. *Guns in America, by the numbers. National Public Radio.* June 5, 2016. https://www.npr.org/2016/ 01/05/462017461/guns-in-america-by-the-numbers

61. Saylor EA, Vittes KA, Sorenson SB. Firearm advertising: product depiction in consumer gun magazines. *Eval Rev*. 2004;*28*(5):420-433. doi:10.1177/0193841X04267389

62. Li O. *Cars, toys, and aspirin have to meet mandatory safety standards. Guns don't. Here's why. The Trace*. Published January 19, 2016. https://www.thetrace.org/2016/01/gun-safety-standards

63. National Shooting Sports Foundation. *Writer's guide to firearms and ammunition*. 2015. https://www.nssf.org/media/writers-guide-and-glossary

64. CNBC. *Why guns can only be recalled by manufacturer*. October 19, 2010. https://www.cnbc.com/id/39743850

65. Guy C. *Proposed state law would exempt Texas-made guns from federal regulation*. Beaumont Enterprise. May 9, 2009. https://www.beaumontenterprise.com/news/article/Proposed-state-law-would-exempt-Texas-made-guns-745828.php

66. Beyer DS Jr. *Let's end gun safety hypocrisy and pass the ATF Enforcement Act. Washington Post*. April 13, 2016. https://www.washingtonpost.com/opinions/lets-end-gun-safety-hypocrisy-with-the-atf-enforcement-act/2016/04/11/2769c910-fffe-11e5-b823-707c79ce3504_story.html?utm_term=.80de481c6262

67. Chu VS. *The Protection of Lawful Commerce in Arms Act: An Overview of Limiting Tort Liability of Gun Manufacturers*. Congressional Research Service; 2012:1-8. https://fas.org/sgp/crs/misc/R42871.pdf

68. Defrancesco S, Lester KJ, Teret SP, Vernick JS. *A Model Handgun Safety Standard Act*. 2nd ed. The Johns Hopkins Center for Gun Policy and Research; 2000. https://www.jhsph.edu/research/centers-and-institutes/johns-hopkins-center-for-gun-violence-prevention-and-policy/_archive-2019/_pdfs/Model_Law_2ed.pdf

69. U.S. Government Accountability Office. *Accidental Shootings: Many Deaths and Injuries Caused by Firearms Could Be Prevented*. Author; 1991. https://www.gao.gov/assets/160/150353.pdf

70. Centers for Disease Control and Prevention. Achievements in public health, 1900–1999: tobacco use—United States, 1900–1999. *MMWR Morb Mortal Wkly Rep*. 1999;*48*(43);986-993. https://www.cdc.gov/mmwr/preview/mmwrhtml/mm4843a2.htm

71. Statista. *Per capita cigarette consumption in the United States from 1900 to 2015*. 2016. https://www.statista.com/statistics/261576/cigarette-consumption-per-adult-in-the-us

72. Florey LS, Galea S, Wilson ML. Macrosocial determinants of population health in the context of globalization. In: Galea S. ed. *Macrosocial Determinants of Population Health*. Springer; 2007. doi:10.1007/978-0-387-70812-6_2

73. Needleman HL. *Human Lead Exposure*. CRC Press; 1992.

74. International Lead Association. *Why lead matters*. https://www.ila-lead.org/lead-facts/history-of-lead

75. Hernberg S. Lead poisoning in a historical perspective. *Am J Ind Med*. 2000;*38*(3):244-254. http://www.ncbi.nlm.nih.gov/pubmed/10940962

76. Markowitz G, Rosner D. "Cater to the children": the role of the lead industry in a public health tragedy, 1900-1955. *Am J Public Health*. 2000;*90*(1):36-46. doi:10.2105/ajph.90.1.36

77. Rosner D, Markowitz G. Building the world that kills us: the politics of lead, science, and polluted homes, 1970 to 2000. *J Urban Hist*. 2016;*42*(2):323-345. doi:10.1177/0096144215623954

78. United States Environmental Protection Agency. *Protect your family from sources of lead*. https://www.epa.gov/lead/protect-your-family-exposures-lead#water

79. Rabin R. The lead industry and lead water pipes: a modest campaign. *Am J Public Health*. 2008;*98*(9):1584-1592. doi:10.2105/AJPH.2007.113555

80. Kitman JL. *The secret history of lead. The Nation*. March 20, 2000. https://www.thenation.com/article/archive/secret-history-lead/

81. Landrigan PJ. The worldwide problem of lead in petrol. *Bull World Health Organ*. 2002;*80*(10):768. http://www.ncbi.nlm.nih.gov/pubmed/12471395

82. Kathuria P, Rowden AK. Lead toxicity. In: Ramachandran TS, ed. *Medscape*. Updated April 23, 2018. https://emedicine.medscape.com/article/1174752-overview#a5

83. Kennedy M. *Lead-laced water in Flint: a step-by-step look at the makings of a crisis*. National Public Radio. Published April 20, 2016. https://www.npr.org/sections/thetwo-way/2016/04/20/465545378/lead-laced-water-in-flint-a-step-by-step-look-at-the-makings-of-a-crisis

84. Montgomery CT, Smith MB, NSI Technologies. *Hydraulic Fracturing—History of an Enduring Technology*. Society of Professional Engineers; 2010. https://www.ourenergypolicy.org/wp-content/uploads/2013/07/Hydraulic.pdf

85. The U.S. Energy Information Administration. *Hydraulic fracturing accounts for about half of current U.S. crude oil production*. Published March 15, 2016. https://www.eia.gov/todayinenergy/detail.php?id=25372

86. Energy Central. *Hydraulically Fractured Wells Provide Two-Thirds of U.S. Natural Gas Production*. Published May 6, 2016. https://energycentral.com/c/ec/hydraulically-fractured-wells-provide-two-thirds-us-natural-gas-production

87. FracFocus Chemical Disclosure Registry. *Hydraulic Fracturing*. https://fracfocus.org/learn/hydraulic-fracturing

88. Vogel L. Fracking tied to cancer-causing chemicals. *CMAJ*. 2017; 189(2): E94–E95. doi: 10.1503/cmaj.109-5358

89. U.S. Environmental Protection Agency. *U.S. EPA. Hydraulic Fracturing for Oil and Gas: Impacts from the Hydraulic Fracturing Water Cycle on Drinking Water Resources in the United States (Final Report).* EPA/600/R-16/236F, 2016.

90. Lustgarten A. *Are fracking wastewater wells poisoning the ground beneath our feet? Scientific American.* June 21, 2012. https://www.scientificamerican.com/article/are-fracking-wastewater-wells-poisoning-ground-beneath-our-feeth

91. Vann A, Murrill BJ. *Hydraulic Fracturing: Selected Legal Issues.* Congressional Research Service; 2014. https://fas.org/sgp/crs/misc/R43152.pdf

92. Rosenbaum DE. *A closer look at Cheney and Halliburton. New York Times.* September 28, 2004. https://www.nytimes.com/2004/09/28/us/a-closer-look-at-cheney-and-halliburton.html

93. Zucker HA, Dreslin S. *A Public Health Review of High Volume Hydraulic Fracturing for Shale Gas Development.* Department of Health; 2014. https://www.health.ny.gov/press/reports/docs/high_volume_hydraulic_fracturing.pdf

94. U.S. Geological Survey. *General facts and concepts about ground water.* https://pubs.usgs.gov/circ/circ1186/html/gen_facts.html

95. StateImpact Pennsylvania. *Tap water torches: how faulty gas drilling can lead to methane migration.* https://stateimpact.npr.org/pennsylvania/tag/methane-migration

96. McKibben B. *Global warming's terrifying new chemistry. The Nation.* March 23, 2018. https://www.thenation.com/article/archive/global-warming-terrifying-new-chemistry/

97. Adams-Heard R. *Welcome to the 'man camps' of West Texas. Bloomberg Businessweek.* August 7, 2018. https://www.bloomberg.com/news/articles/2018-08-07/welcome-to-the-man-camps-of-west-texas

98. Loyola University Chicago Undergraduate Admission. *Oil, fracking and man camps: human health along the pipelines [Video].* YouTube. Published April 16, 2018. https://www.youtube.com/watch?v=DGzZRlgnD0I

99. American Petroleum Institute. *Hydraulic fracturing.* https://www.api.org/oil-and-natural-gas/wells-to-consumer/exploration-and-production/hydraulic-fracturing#sort=date%20descending

100. Institute for Energy Research. *Marcellus Shale Fact Sheet.* Author; 2012. https://instituteforenergyresearch.org/wp-content/uploads/2012/08/Marcellus-Fact-Sheet.pdf

101. Kaplan T. *Citing health risks, Cuomo bans fracking in New York State. New York Times.* December 17, 2014. https://www.nytimes.com/2014/12/18/nyregion/cuomo-to-ban-fracking-in-new-york-state-citing-health-risks.html

ACROSS THE LIFE COURSE: WHAT CAUSES HEALTH AND WHAT WE CAN DO ABOUT IT

9

THE PERINATAL PERIOD, INFANCY, CHILDHOOD, AND ADOLESCENCE

LEARNING OBJECTIVES

- Explain the importance of the life course framework when discussing the health of populations.

- Describe the importance of early life exposures and experiences for setting up the trajectory of lifelong health.

- List the five domains of nurturing care and explain how each of these supports healthy child development.

- Outline the most prominent and impactful adverse childhood experiences (ACEs) and discuss ACEs as threats to child health and development.

- Analyze current patterns of health-related behaviors for adolescents/young adults in the United States in the realms of diet, exercise, and obesity; tobacco, alcohol, and other substance use; injury, violence, and suicide; and sexual risk behaviors.

- Explore successful public health interventions for (a) promoting health-enhancing behaviors and (b) intervening on health-compromising behaviors—among adolescents and young adults.

- By integrating the multiple levels of the social ecological framework, describe both favorable and unfavorable influences of family/social networks, neighborhoods, and cities from birth through 24 years of age.

OVERVIEW: THE LIFE COURSE PERSPECTIVE

Our focus, in Chapters 9 to 11, is on tracking health across the life course. This traces the second of the two conceptual lenses we take in this book: the life course perspective, complementing the social ecological perspective that we discussed in Chapters 6 to 8. In this chapter, we begin with the earliest years (the perinatal period, infancy, childhood, adolescence, and the transition to adulthood (ages 0–24); we then move, in Chapter 10, "Adulthood," to health throughout four decades of adult life (ages 25–64), and we conclude this section in Chapter 11, "Older Age" with health in the older adult years (ages 65 and beyond). We begin our life course explorations in this chapter starting before birth and extending through the formative years of childhood and into adolescence and young adulthood.

Life course thinking, as an approach to describing population health, continues to gain momentum. The Pan-American Health Organization (PAHO) notes:

> *In the life course approach, the health of individuals and populations is conceived as the result of dynamic interaction between exposures and events throughout life, conditioned by mechanisms that embody the positive or negative influences that shape individual trajectories and the development of society as a whole. According to this conceptual framework, health is a fundamental dimension of human development and not merely an end in itself.[1]*

The life course approach focuses on the flow of health from the earliest years into later years and represents one aspect of upstream–downstream thinking. Health influences that are encountered upstream, earlier in life, exert immediate effects and also set in motion currents of downstream influences that play out throughout subsequent years. In some cases, early influences make an imprint that continues to be experienced lifelong.

The life course approach focuses on the flow of health from the earliest years into later years and represents one aspect of upstream–downstream thinking.

Here is a powerful motivating force for examining the first years of life through a life course lens.[2] An estimated 250 million children worldwide—43% of those younger than 5 years of age living in low- and middle-income countries—are currently at risk of not reaching their developmental potential. These children may experience suboptimal health early in life along with cognitive and intellectual deficits that may limit their abilities to become fully functional and productive adults.

All children require nurturing care.[2] The five essential domains of nurturing care form the underpinning for children to acquire the essential competencies and skills for healthy development. These elements are responsive caregiving, nutrition, early learning, safety and security, and health (**Figure 9.1** and **Table 9.1**).

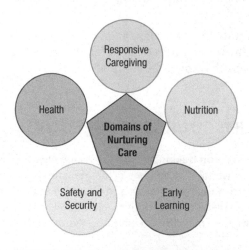

FIGURE 9.1 The five domains of nurturing care.

Nurturing care can help overcome disadvantages for children growing up in poverty and hardship. For children with more resources, nurturing care can springboard them toward optimal development and ongoing achievement.

In this chapter, we (a) describe how health is generated perinatally, throughout infancy, childhood, and adolescence in a way that can affect populations throughout the life course, (b) delineate the threats in each period that can harm health, (c) explain how public health can mitigate these threats in each period, and (d) provide successful examples of public health efforts to improve health through action early in the perinatal period, infancy, childhood, and adolescence.

TABLE 9.1 Five Components of Nurturing Care

COMPONENTS	ACTIONS TO OPTIMIZE NURTURING CARE BENEFITS FOR THE CHILD
Good health	• Monitoring children's physical and emotional condition • Giving affectionate and appropriate responses to children's daily needs • Protecting young children from household and environmental dangers • Having hygiene practices that minimize infections • Using promotive and preventive health services • Seeking care and appropriate treatment for children's illnesses *Note: These actions depend on caregivers' physical and mental well-being.*
Adequate nutrition	• Mother's nutrition during pregnancy affects her own health and well-being • Mother's nutrition during pregnancy affects the developing child's nutrition/growth • Young children flourish on exclusive breastfeeding from birth to 6 months • Infant/mother skin-to-skin body contact during breastfeeding is nurturing • After 6 months: breastfeeding and diverse, complementary foods that are rich in micronutrients are needed for the rapid growth of body and brain *Note: Food safety and family food security are essential for adequate nutrition.*

Responsive caregiving	• Observing/responding to children's movements, sounds, gestures, verbal requests
	• Responsive feeding
	• Caregiver/child engagement: cuddling, eye contact, smiles, vocalizations, gestures:
	  o Create an emotional bond
	  o Stimulate connections in the brain
	• Forms the basis for:
	  o Protecting children against injury and the negative effects of adversity
	  o Recognizing and responding to illness
	  o Enriched learning
	• Building trust and social relationships

(continued)

TABLE 9.1 Five Components of Nurturing Care (*continued*)

COMPONENTS	ACTIONS TO OPTIMIZE NURTURING CARE BENEFITS FOR THE CHILD

Opportunities for early learning	• Learning is a built-in mechanism for human beings
	• Begins at conception as a biological mechanism called epigenesis
	• Earliest years: skills acquired interpersonally, relating to others:
	  o Smiling and eye contact
	  o Talking and singing
	  o Modeling and imitation
	  o Simple games
	• Caregiver roles that stimulate child learning:
	  o Talk/interact with a child during feeding, bathing, household tasks
	  o Provide affectionate secure caregiving from adults in a family environment
	• Guide children in daily activities and relationships with others

Security and safety	• Young children cannot protect themselves
	• Children are vulnerable to unanticipated danger, physical pain, emotional stress
	• Extreme poverty and low income diminish safety and security
	• Pregnant women and young children: most vulnerable to environmental risks
	• Unclean or unsafe environment is full of potential threats
	• Children can experience extreme fear when people abandon them
	• Severe punishment of children has multiple consequences:
	  o Emotional, mental, and social maladjustment
	  o Mistrust of adults
	  o Fear, which may be acted out as aggression toward other children
	Note: Nurturing care includes making sure that defenseless young children feel safe and secure.

Source: WHO 2018 nurturing care for early childhood development: a framework for helping children survive and thrive to transform human potential. https://apps.who.int/iris/bitstream/handle/10665/272603/9789241514064-eng.pdf

HOW HEALTH IS GENERATED DURING THE EARLIEST PHASES OF THE LIFE COURSE

GENERATING HEALTH PERINATALLY

Throughout pregnancy, the womb environment provides the developing fetus with physical protection and all means of sustenance. However, the fetus is also confined to the womb and is therefore susceptible to, and unable to escape from, a range of potentially harmful exposures. The pregnant mother's moment-by-moment experience is, in a real sense, instantaneously transmitted to her fetus.

Specific environmental exposures—some even preceding conception—affect the viability, health, and development of the fetus in the womb. The intertwined physiologies of the pregnant mother and fetus react in tandem to how a mother rests; how she moves; and what she breathes, eats, drinks, or smokes. Every physical action, every environmental exposure, every human interaction, and every emotional response of the mother is experienced by the fetus as a reactive alteration of the womb environment. This intricate, intimate connection of mother and fetus presents opportunities for the pregnant mother to promote fetal health during pregnancy, supported by a network of persons, resources, and services available within the family and community.

Specific environmental exposures—some even preceding conception—affect the viability, health, and development of the fetus in the womb.

The pregnant mother safeguards her fetus. Under optimal circumstances, when supplies of food are ample, a mother who eats a healthy diet and observes a regular exercise regimen will consume sufficient calories to maintain her own health and transfer a balanced blend of nutrients that allow the fetus to thrive. The placenta, the only organ shared by more than one human, serves as the passageway for oxygen and vital nutrients needed by the fetus. The womb itself provides a cushioning, protective cocoon to shield the infant from physical buffeting and potentially injurious agents, for example, by prohibiting the entry of various disease and immune factors. These protections are afforded to all fetuses, courtesy of the mother's highly evolved human physiology.

In contrast, protecting the fetus from other harmful exposures relies on maternal behavior and decision-making. With good maternal behavioral choices, the fetus will not be exposed to radiation, toxins, tobacco smoke, alcohol, illicit drugs, and certain forms of prescription medication. Also, ideally for the health of the fetus, but outside the pregnant mother's direct control, the mother will not be exposed to physical abuse, gender-based violence, armed conflict, natural disaster, or other potentially injurious or traumatic shocks during the pregnancy (Case Study 9.1).

For pregnant mothers, it is important that nutritional needs are met for both mother and child. To optimize the expectant mother's health during pregnancy, she should eat a diet that balances energy and protein intake.[3] The American College of Obstetrics and Gynecologists recommends a healthy diet, regular exercise, and plenty of rest. Avoidance of alcohol, tobacco, and drugs is particularly important because of the adverse effects on the health of the fetus.

Ensuring nutrient uptake is particularly important, which is why prenatal vitamin supplementation is recommended. In particular, women with nutritional deficiencies should take micronutrients to decrease the risk for fetal growth restriction.[4] Folic acid (vitamin B9) is particularly important[5] and a daily dose of 600 mcg is strongly recommended during pregnancy to reduce the risk of brain and spinal birth defects.[6] Increased maternal intake of iron is critical[7]; as pregnancy progresses, the mother's blood volume will almost double and iron supplementation is needed to prevent anemia. Vitamin D supplementation is also recommended.[8]

And finally, we know that when pregnant mothers have common mental disorders such as depression, there may be negative outcomes for the newborn and young child.[9] These include preterm birth, low birth weight, diminished cognitive development, behavioral and emotional problems during early childhood, and difficulty forming secure attachment to the mother and caregivers.

CASE STUDY 9.1: TWO WOMEN'S STORIES

During the gestational period, representing the earliest stages of human development, the health of the fetus is primarily determined by the womb environment. In turn, the health of the mother and her environment translate directly to the conditions experienced by the fetus. Consider two pregnant women in the vicinity of San Diego, California, close to the border with Tijuana, Mexico, in the spring of 2018.

The first is a 27-year-old married expectant mother living in suburban San Diego who has two children (ages 2 and 6). She is a middle-class, U.S.-born White Latinx citizen who is college-educated and bilingual (English/Spanish native fluency). She is a working professional who has health insurance, a primary care provider, and an OB/GYN physician who provides prenatal care. Her childbirth experience is elected and preplanned at the local hospital birth center where her young children were born previously. She goes to her neighborhood health club four times weekly, does not smoke, abstains from alcohol, observes a healthy diet, and maintains normal weight. In addition to her husband, she has supportive family members living nearby.

The second is Gabriela Hernandez, a 27-year-old, pregnant Honduran mother of two boys (ages 2 and 6) who has just caravanned more than a thousand miles through Central America and across all of Mexico to reach the U.S. border at Tijuana. She and her young boys are sleeping on the ground alongside the United States–Mexico border barriers, peering into San Diego. The border itself is heavily guarded.

Gabriela is hoping to be given the opportunity to plead for entry into the United States and to seek asylum from the violence in her home country that has threatened her children's lives. She knows she will face hostility and that receiving permission to live in the United States is uncertain. Nevertheless, the extremity of the interpersonal and gang violence in Honduras has propelled her to leave everything behind and to make this dangerous journey, even while pregnant.

For these two women who do not know each other but whose paths have placed them in geographic proximity, the pregnancy experiences, and the resultant womb environments for their unborn children, are likely to be very different. The upcoming childbirth experience and the subsequent infancy of their two offspring will be very different as well.

This illustration is based on the true story of a single migrant woman whose saga was followed on national television, juxtaposed alongside her fictitious—but realistically described—U.S. citizen counterpart.[10] However, this is not an isolated story at any time in history. Contemporaneously with ongoing violence throughout portions of Central America prompting migration to the United States at a time of immigration controversy, the population health equivalent plays out with large migrating groups elsewhere around the globe. This includes massive numbers of Syrian conflict refugees seeking safe haven and attempting to make a new life throughout Europe and the Middle East and hundreds of thousands of U.S.-citizen Puerto Ricans relocating to the United States following the island-wide devastation wrought by Hurricane Maria in September 2017. More recently, in 2022 and beyond, this includes the exodus of millions of Ukrainian women and their children escaping the unprovoked Russian invasion and crippling destruction of residential areas, while the men remain inside Ukraine to defend their nation. On an ongoing

(continued)

basis, this also includes rising numbers of climate migrants whose habitats of origin are no longer livable owing to sea level rise, extreme heat, desertification, drought, and famine. Under each of these scenarios, pregnant women are among the most vulnerable migrants.

The health of young children is strongly influenced by the degree to which parents are able to remain healthy and functional and provide nurturing care. The case of Gabriela illustrates a very strong mother who is determined to seek a better life for her family. Nevertheless, she faces myriad obstacles related to her status as a single mother who has been exposed to atrocities in her home country, has endured the rigors of migration, and now faces the uncertainty of admission to the United States based on the processing of her asylum plea. She has left her social support network and all worldly possessions behind. She arrives without resources or employment prospects. These harsh exposures to trauma, loss, and life change certainly challenge Gabriela's personal health and abilities to provide care and sustenance for her children.

GENERATING HEALTH IN INFANCY

Generating health in infancy acts as a slingshot for propelling health forward throughout the life course. This is no more emphatically illustrated than by graphically comparing the share of persons surviving to successive ages over the span of 180 years (**Figure 9.2**).

In the 1850s, 30% of the population died before the age of 10 with most of these deaths occurring in the first year of life (infancy) or shortly thereafter. The graphic depicts this for England

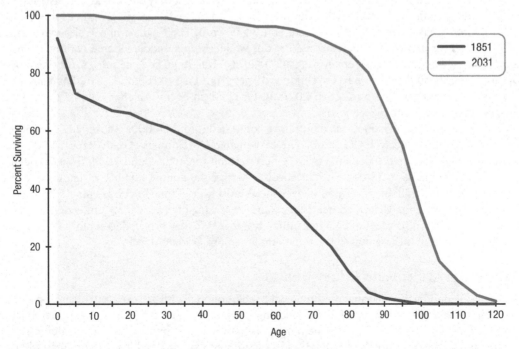

FIGURE 9.2 Share of persons living to successive ages for persons born in 1851 and 2031, England and Wales.
Source: Data from Ortiz-Ospina E. "Life expectancy"-what does this actually mean? Our World in Data. Published August 28, 2017. https://ourworldindata.org/life-expectancy-how-is-it-calculated-and-how-should-it-be-interpreted

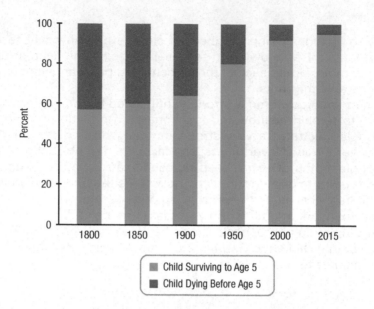

FIGURE 9.3 Global under-5 child survival and mortality, 1800 to 2015.
Source: Data from Roser M. Child & infant mortality. Our World in Data. Published 2019. https://ourworldindata.org/child-mortality

and Wales by showing the survival curve for persons born in 1851 plunging downward from 100% at birth (age 0) to 70% by age 10. In contrast, for the cohorts born in the 2000s, mortality is minimal in the first years of life and throughout the age range 0 to 14 years, the focus of this chapter. In fact, more than 90% of the entire group survives not only childhood, but also adolescence, young adulthood, and middle adulthood, living to the age of 60 years and beyond. Moreover, the maximal age of human survival is shifting upward. The England and Wales experience is replicated throughout the high-income nations while low-and-middle-income nations are also experiencing favorable improvements in childhood survival. In just two centuries, the likelihood of surviving throughout the earliest childhood ages from birth through 4 years has increased from a probability of less than six in 10, even for children born in higher income nations, to greater than 97 in 100 (**Figure 9.3**).

Sharp declines in childhood mortality have continued into the 2000s. In the 2021 report of the United Nations Secretary General, The Sustainable Development Goals Report 2021, the under-5 mortality rate had declined by 50% between the years 2000 and 2019, from 76 deaths per 1,000 live births to 38 deaths.[11] In absolute terms, the annual number of under-5 deaths dropped from 9.9 million to 5.6 million over this relatively brief time interval. This startling combination of decreasing childhood death rates and increasing life expectancy underscores how a healthier childhood provides a lifelong health advantage. We now proceed to explore factors that promote health, and those that threaten health, at a more granular level.

Factors That Promote Infant Health

Meeting the child's foundational physiological needs, coupled with attentive nurturing, optimize infant growth and maturation while diminishing risks for childhood diseases. As critical dimensions of infant health, the brain and the nervous, endocrine, and immune systems undergo expeditious development during early childhood as the infant explores and learns from the richness of its environment. Therefore, effective childcare during infancy, followed by early childhood educational opportunities during the front end of the life span, pay dividends toward lifelong health promotion and disease prevention.

Breastfeeding is prevalent across cultures and confers health benefits to both the child and mother alike. Extending into early childhood, breastfed children benefit from decreased rates of such common conditions as eczema and obesity and more serious diseases, including type 2 diabetes and childhood-onset leukemia. Less robust findings link breastfeeding to lower incidence rates of both type 1 diabetes and asthma.

On the other side of the mother–infant dyad, mothers who breastfeed for a lifetime total of 12 months or more have improved cardiovascular disease risk profiles, including lower rates of elevated cholesterol and hypertension. Followed prospectively through the life course, these women experience lower rates of onset of type 2 diabetes and cardiovascular diseases than do their counterparts who did not breastfeed.

Consistent with this cluster of favorable findings, the U.S. Preventive Services Task Force (USPSTF) explicitly recommends that primary care clinicians support and encourage their pregnant patients to breastfeed their infants. The USPSTF concludes that support from clinicians is influential in women's decisions to initiate and continue breastfeeding for their newborns and infant children.

Breastfeeding creates extended benefits that are measurable over the life course. One example is demonstrated by a 2015 cohort study with 3,493 subjects who were enrolled as infants and followed for 30 years.[12] Detailed information was recorded regarding breastfeeding from the subjects. Breastfeeding, predominant breastfeeding (breastfeeding as the main form of nutrition), and a longer duration of breastfeeding were all associated with higher IQ scores, higher levels of educational attainment, and increased income in young adults.

The flip side to these positive benefits that can accrue to a child who is well-fed and nourished is that the primary causes of stunting during the first years of life are a combination of poor nutrition and exposure to infectious diseases.[13] In turn, poverty and low socioeconomic status[14] are among the social determinants of health most strongly linked to both poor nutrition and poor sanitation that contribute to growth retardation and stunting. The negative effects of poverty travel along multiple pathways of influence.[15] For example, poverty is associated with lower educational attainment for mothers, compounded by higher levels of maternal stress,[16] leading to less nurturing care provided to the young child. Poverty may be associated with fewer opportunities to enroll children in high-quality early childhood and primary education. This composite of risks can severely thwart child development and decrease the acquisition of language and cognitive skills.[13]

GENERATING HEALTH IN CHILDHOOD AND PREADOLESCENCE

Social support and social interaction contribute to the well-being of young children. Healthy child development depends on social interactions especially with the mother, but also with the father (or other parents or caregivers), siblings, nurturing relatives, and peers and their parents during child-focused activities (e.g., "play dates"). Engagement with in-home and community-based caregivers adds another dimension to the child's social network. The reverse is that social isolation of young children is extremely detrimental to health.[17] Taking a life course view, social isolation of children is related to lower levels of educational performance and attainment, lower socioeconomic status, and higher rates of psychological distress in adult life.[18]

Young children depend on the adults in their lives to provide for their survival needs and for social interaction. Not surprisingly, the evolution of the child's own behavior is shaped by how well the family is functioning. As an illustration, following the devastation of a disaster, resulting in community-wide destruction and school closures, one of the strongest predictors of children's social and mental health is how well their parents cope, function, and meet the needs of their families despite adversity.[19]

Lifelong health, learning, well-being, productivity, and attainment are set in motion and shaped by early childhood experiences. In a structural sense, stability is foundational for child-hood development.[20] In contrast, instability during early formative years can be extremely dis-ruptive. Positive development relies on such pillars of stability as a nurturing home environment and skilled and loving parenting provided by mentally healthy parents. Contributors to a stable base on which children can thrive include (a) family income that is comfortably above the pov-erty line, (b) esteem-building and well-paying employment for parents, (c) supportive relation-ships with emotionally available and child-attentive parents and caregivers, (d) safe and secure housing, and (e) quality educational opportunities in home, childcare, early childhood educa-tion, and school settings. Added to this—to ensure optimal physical health—children also need regular meals that feature healthy and nutritious foods, and access to medical care, including immunizations and regular preventive checkups.

Parents play a guiding role in the formation and solidification of children's health-related behav-ioral patterns.[21] They do so in several complementary ways. Parents serve as primary role models for healthful behavior.[22] They influence attitudes and actions by discussing desirable health behav-ior choices with their children. They encourage and support the formation of health-promoting habits during early phases of trial and adoption of these new behaviors. Parents provide pathways for children to increasingly gain independence, self-control, and decision-making abilities as chil-dren adopt, practice, and progressively gain mastery of newly acquired health behaviors.

Childhood development exerts life-shaping leverage on the future health of each individual and collectively, on similar-age cohorts around the globe. Childhood development is "a matura-tional and interactive process, resulting in an ordered progression of perceptual, motor, cogni-tive, language, socio-emotional, and self-regulation skills."[23] Across cultures, children worldwide follow similar sequences of skill acquisition, but context matters and influences the speed and completeness with which children achieve developmental benchmarks.[24]

Childhood sets the pace for physical, cognitive, emotional, and social dimensions of being. What is necessary to propel young children toward successful attainment of this repertoire of capabilities? In some ways this can be summarized as "nurturing care."[25] Much of this nurtur-ing can be provided within a child-sensitive and supportive home environment that promotes health, provides wholesome nutrition and responsive feeding,[26] and protects children from harm. Within such a home, caregivers are attentive, emotionally available, and attuned to the child.[27] Another optimal quality is providing the young child with opportunities for exploratory and imaginative play activities that also stimulate language development.[28] In addition to the immediate home environment, nurturing care is supported by a range of contexts that span much of the social ecological continuum. This includes parental occupational settings, childcare venues, early childhood education opportunities, formal schooling, community-sponsored youth activities, and child-focused policy initiatives.[29]

For children who are raised with nurturing care, the young person's capabilities will have broadened expansively on all fronts by the age of 3 years. During this short interval, the child will have transformed from the total dependency of a newborn into a multitalented, increasingly independent, and quite sophisticated young human. The healthy 3-year-old is a high-stamina, im-mensely mobile, verbal, problem-solving creature. The 3-year-old actively engages in, and man-ages, relationships with parents, siblings, teachers, peers, and other significant persons. This represents an extraordinary developmental achievement, and one that is within the grasp of chil-dren worldwide who are provided with caring and capable nurturing and a healthy environment.

GENERATING HEALTH IN ADOLESCENCE

Throughout most of human history, the human life span was characterized by a combination of high birth rates and high death rates and a relatively brief average span of life in between. What is remarkable to contemplate is that, prior to the industrial and postindustrial eras, adolescence was not even a defined phase of life. Simply put, physical maturation was followed within a few short years by parenthood. Now, especially in high- and middle-income countries, parenthood is typically delayed by a gap of 10 to 15 years. People live longer and live through a clear phase of adolescence and early adulthood that was not previously part of the life course. In the scheme of human history, adolescence is a new and novel insertion into the human life experience.[1]

Adolescence: A Pivotal Point for Lifelong Health

Adolescence constitutes the healthiest period of life, with the lowest death rates. It is a pivotal time in development that establishes life's future trajectory and potential. During this period, physical maturation coupled with prolific brain development plots the future course for an individual's cognitive, social, and interpersonal capabilities for the remainder of the life span.

Conversely, adolescence is also the period of life when an individual may engage in behaviors that may inflect the life course in an unhealthy manner. Adolescence is also the phase of life when "health capital" either expands or contracts. Health capital is "the set of resources that determine trajectories of health across the life course."[30] Future health, well-being, life satisfaction, and longevity are determined by how life is lived in adolescence and young adulthood.

Adolescent health therefore is relevant (a) in the present, focusing on the health of today's adolescents; (b) throughout future phases of the life course, as a legacy of adolescent life and health choices projected forward; and (c) into the next generation, as today's adolescents assume future parenting roles.[31]

Adolescence is the foremost transition phase of life, moving youth out of the parental sphere of influence, passing through the phase where peer influences are central, and eventually emerging as relatively autonomous individuals. During adolescence, many individuals focus most hours of the day on formal, and often advanced, education. They navigate through early occupational experiences, interning or apprenticing to gain skills, and come away with marketable vocational or professional capabilities and roles. In tandem with acquiring cognitive and emotional skills, adolescents engage in a spectrum of social relationships with the possibility of forming lasting friendships and long-term partnerships.

Secondary and higher education is concentrated in this life phase. Notably, adolescent years are those when peers exert their most pronounced influence on development. The shift from family of origin to "family of one's own" during adolescence is clearly illustrated. The initial on-ramp into employment frequently occurs during this period of the life course. The roles of prolific media consumption and intensive social media engagement are prominent, evolving, and expanding throughout this life phase.

The adolescent health advantage is characterized by a combination of rapid physical maturation and sophisticated neurological development occurring during the healthiest, most disease-free era of life. Adolescents have already survived earlier, more precarious life phases, including fetal development, childbirth, infancy, and childhood. If early childhood is about learning survival skills, then the youth and young adult years are about learning life and social skills. The second burst of physical growth that occurs during adolescence is accompanied by neurological changes that bring off an extraordinary expansion of brain function. Cognitive abilities continue their ascent throughout adolescence and beyond, peaking in the third decade of life.

> The adolescent health advantage is characterized by a combination of rapid physical maturation and sophisticated neurological development occurring during the healthiest, most disease-free era of life.

Adolescence is all about behavioral experimentation and creating capabilities. Health and well-being during adolescence, and beyond, are substantially shaped by the opportunities that are made available (e.g., education, social support, civic interaction) and by the behavioral choices that are made. This active experimentation is taking place while simultaneously, the individual's physical, cognitive, and emotional capabilities are undergoing rapid transformation.[32]

Not only is adolescence the second most active period for development of neural systems (infancy is first), but brain changes are different structurally and they occur in different regions of the brain than during the first years of life. If childhood can be seen as stimulating a proliferation of brain matter, then adolescent brain development may be envisioned as an act of trimming and shaping the brain to acquire and refine social, emotional, and interpersonal skills. Adolescence, therefore, is an exquisitely sensitive period for brain development. Brain modifications during adolescence are also instrumental for the sociocultural processing that is needed to form healthy relationships with peers and to successfully master the interpersonal aspects of a youth's educational and early occupational roles.[1,33-35]

The developmental processes of adolescence are determined by an entire spectrum of factors, including family, peer group, social network, school, community, media, social media, cultural, and societal influences. One of the distinguishing features of adolescence is the process of branching out socially beyond the immediate family orbit. Adolescents learn to interact interpersonally with peers and, ultimately, with broader social networks. This is a period of behavioral experimentation during which a spectrum of social encounters present opportunities for youth to try on and test out new roles, values, and lifestyles. Bonds formed within the peer group provide the chance to gradually let go of the family, as the primary unit of social influence, while having something else—peers—to hold onto. This creates a sort of rung-over-rung progression toward achieving independence and autonomy.[36]

> **The developmental processes of adolescence are determined by an entire spectrum of factors, including family, peer group, social network, school, community, media, social media, cultural, and societal influences.**

At this time in history, the ecology of adolescent existence has expanded at an accelerating pace. Youth today are more engaged educationally than ever before while encountering global megatrends that are changing continuously. This is evident in the generational self-labeling of successive waves of adolescents. The current generation of "millennials" has supplanted the previous Generation X cohort. Millennials themselves are being supplanted by their successors, Generation Z. Today, adolescence is embedded in a mix of countercurrents that include widespread and instantaneous information access, constantly evolving and highly interactive new media, increasing varieties of educational channels, opportunities for international travel and cultural exchange, career invention, and rapid technological advances. Meanwhile, these youth lifestyle transformations are further modified by ongoing trends of urbanization, globalization, climate crises, conflict, and political upheaval. The COVID-19 pandemic precipitously upended the developmental course of youth and young adults, creating roadblocks and detours whose consequential effects are not yet fully realized.

As one example, these phenomena came to the forefront following the rampage mass shooting at Marjory Stoneman Douglas High School, in Parkland, Florida, on Valentine's Day, 2018. The surviving high school students converted their personal tragedy into a nationwide movement (The March for Our Lives) that focused political advocacy on the need for stricter gun laws. The students used a variety of social media tools to organize their own leadership activities and to coordinate nationwide sister marches and events.

Adolescents depend on a stable social environment to facilitate optimal brain development that will ensure their own well-being—physical, social, and emotional—during their adult years.

Many adolescents are initially protected by the safety net of their family structure. The protection afforded by the home environment persists even as adolescents are increasingly socializing with friends and becoming sensitized to school, community, and work settings. The recent explosive growth of varied media communications is creating influences on youth that are, at best, incompletely defined and continuously in flux. Social media influences on adolescents' health-related knowledge, attitudes, beliefs, values, and most importantly, behaviors, are pervasive but only vaguely understood.

Youth now have easy access to the latest and most evidence-based scientific health information. Yet, the production of misinformation is proliferating, pumped out by an explosion of influencers and special interests, obscuring what is true and confronting what is scientifically grounded. With equal ease, adolescents can access, view, and be influenced to participate in high-risk behaviors while using the same media channels that promote safe, health-promoting behaviors. Risk-elevating activities that are discussed or portrayed through social media range from extreme sports, to various forms of substance use, to unsafe sex, to eating disorders, to self-harm, or even to suicidal behaviors.[1,37-39] Risk-taking leading to harm and injury is an important influence on the health and well-being of youth. Harm may take the form of unintentional injuries, interpersonal violence, self-harm including suicidal actions, substance abuse, and risky sexual behaviors. In turn, these risk-related behaviors shape patterns and trends of adolescent morbidity and mortality at national levels and worldwide. Physical risks are closely tied to behavioral choices.

UNDERSTANDING THREATS TO HEALTH

DEFINING THREATS TO PERINATAL AND INFANT HEALTH THAT MAY EXTEND THROUGHOUT THE LIFE COURSE

Mortality in Early Childhood

When we consider health threats, we must consider the leading causes of death during the fetal period, infancy, and childhood. Considering the overarching life course theme that flows through this sequence of three chapters (Chapters 9–11), deaths in the earliest days or years of life short-circuit the life course entirely.

> When we consider health threats, we must consider the leading causes of death during the fetal period, infancy, and childhood.

Appropriately, much of the emphasis within the past 150 years of modern public health has been devoted to decreasing life-threatening—and life-taking—childhood conditions. The successful conquest of infectious diseases, the development of vaccines and childhood immunizations, and improvements in child—and maternal—health are credited with effecting the most precipitous drop in early life mortality rates in human history (**Figure 9.4**). Steeply plummeting child mortality rates have been observed worldwide. While decreases in early life mortality have occurred across the entire socioeconomic spectrum in recent decades, they have been most pronounced in lower-income countries. Although high-income nations still have the lowest absolute child mortality rates, the gap is narrowing.

The United States spends a higher proportion of its national gross domestic product (GDP) on healthcare than any other nation, so a logical question to ask is whether these hefty expenditures translate into best-of-class health indicators. In the case of infant the mortality rate (IMR), the answer is emphatically "no." Infancy is defined as the first year of life. The IMR is a leading

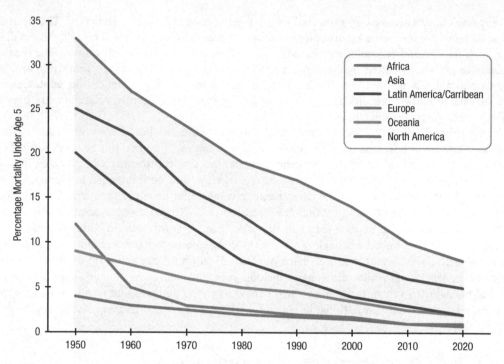

FIGURE 9.4 Child mortality: share of children dying before they reach the age of 5, by continent and decade, 1950 to 2020.
Source: Data from Roser M. Child & infant mortality. Our World in Data. Published 2019. https://ourworldindata.org/childmortality

health indicator, measured for all nation states, and computed as deaths before the first birthday per 1,000 live births. The U.S. Central Intelligence Agency (CIA) World Factbook provides a rank ordering of 225 nations on the IMR measure. The U.S. rank is 170, with a lower IMR than 169 other nations. However, 45 additional nations have a lower IMR than the United States.[40] In fact, the majority of high-income nations worldwide have lower IMRs than the United States. At 5.80 infant deaths per 1,000 live births, the U.S. IMR is about three times higher than that of Monaco (with the lowest IMR in the world, 1.80) or Japan (with an IMR of 2.00).

One contributor to the overall poor showing of the United States on IMR in comparison with other high-income countries is the continuation of sharp race/ethnic inequities.[41] Although the IMR has been declining for all race/ethnicity categories for years, the IMR for non-Latinx African American/Black infants remains much higher than that for other subgroups. IMRs are also elevated for U.S. citizens of American Indian or Alaskan Native origin. IMRs are almost identical for Latinx and non-Latinx Whites. IMR varies by country of origin for Latinx. The lowest of all is the IMR for the Asian or Pacific Islander subcategory of the U.S. population; this represents a desirable benchmark for achievable decreases in U.S. infant mortality.

Causes of Mortality in Early Childhood

Understanding early childhood mortality is important for defining the preventable fraction of these deaths and taking steps to continue the downward trajectory in child mortality worldwide.[42] On a global scale, there is mixed news. Infectious diseases and complications of childbirth still feature prominently as causes of early life mortality. Globally, the top five causes of death for children under 5 years are lower respiratory infections, neonatal preterm complications, diarrheal diseases, neonatal asphyxia and trauma, and congenital birth defects. These are preventable causes of early childhood death and, indeed, the death rates for these causes are moving downward during the early decades of the 2000s.

Higher income nations have eliminated or significantly controlled communicable diseases. This signals that, ultimately, these diseases should be either preventable or effectively controlled worldwide. Indeed, over the 25-year span from 1990 to 2015, child deaths from the world's deadliest infectious diseases declined.

Also, bringing focus to a period of exquisite vulnerability for the newborn, the first month of life, it is apparent that neonatal mortality (mortality during the first 28 days postpartum) is related to potentially preventable preterm and intrapartum birth complications and sepsis. We can expect further reductions in neonatal mortality in the short-term future, over and above the quantum decreases already achieved during the 1900s.

In the United States, in 2021, congenital malformations and low birth weight were the two major causes of infant death. Sudden infant death syndrome, unintentional injuries, and maternal complications of pregnancy rounded out the top five causes of infant death. Even extending to include the entire top 10 medical conditions that contributed to the U.S. IMR, the only infectious disease cause of death was bacterial sepsis, seventh on the list. This is in sharp contrast to global mortality patterns in which infectious diseases contribute substantial numbers of deaths both during infancy and throughout the first 5 years of life.

Certainly, the abrupt insertion of the COVID-19 pandemic into the conversation has affected mortality patterns for all ages worldwide, but fortunately, death rates from this disease are lowest for the youngest of the young. COVID-19 was not in the top 10 causes of infant mortality in the United States during either 2020 or 2021, the first 2 years of the pandemic.

THREE SENTINEL THREATS TO CHILDHOOD THAT CAN HARM HEALTH

Although there are many threats to childhood that can harm health, we talk about three of them here, seeing them as key threats to the health of children globally.

Poverty

The effects of poverty on child health are pervasive.[43] Socioeconomic status is a key determinant for mortality, as just observed, and for a range of health and disease indicators for children who survive. Poverty influences child development, including access to education and school performance. Access to educational opportunities represents one potential escape route from the suppressive effects of poverty on attainment of lifelong health and well-being. Optimally, early childhood education should be available from the first years of life forward to provide young children with a jump start toward school readiness. Ideally, making quality early childhood education and school offerings available is a key component of a comprehensive poverty alleviation strategy, coupled with establishing community opportunity structures and promoting family empowerment.

Adverse Childhood Experiences

An ever-expanding research literature has identified the role of children's early life exposures to ACEs in relation to harmful effects on future health throughout the life course (**Figure 9.5**). Commonly studied ACEs include childhood physical abuse; household substance abuse; childhood sexual abuse; household mental illness; exposure to domestic violence; emotional, psychological, or verbal abuse; parental separation or divorce; household criminality; and neglect (**Table 9.2**). Across a large body of studies, ACEs are associated with future problematic drug use, interpersonal and self-directed violence, problematic alcohol use, sexual risk taking, diagnosed mental illness, smoking, heavy alcohol use, poor self-rated health, cancer, heart disease, and respiratory disease. When considering health throughout the life course, the research on ACEs provides solid evidence linking early life experiences to negative future health outcomes.

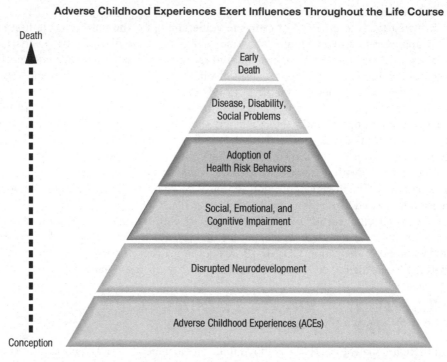

Adverse Childhood Experiences Exert Influences Throughout the Life Course

FIGURE 9.5 **How ACEs can influence health throughout life. ACEs, adverse childhood experiences.**
Source: Adapted from Felitti et al. 1998. https://www.ajpmonline.org/article/S0749-3797(98)00017-8/fulltext

TABLE 9.2 Characteristics and Correlates of Adverse Childhood Experiences	
ACEs	Direct personal harm and neglect ACEs:
	• Physical abuse
	• Sexual abuse
	• Emotional abuse
	• Physical neglect
	• Emotional neglect
	Household member ACEs:
	• Intimate partner violence
	• Mother treated violently
	• Substance misuse within household
	• Household mental illness
	• Parental separation or divorce
	• Incarcerated household member

(continued)

TABLE 9.2 Characteristics and Correlates of Adverse Childhood Experiences (*continued*)

Defining characteristics of ACEs	ACEs are common: • More than one in four report childhood physical abuse • More than one in five report childhood sexual abuse ACEs are clustered: • 40% report two or more ACEs • 12% report four or more ACEs ACEs have a dose–response relationship with health problems: • Cumulative ACEs score: strong, graded relationship to numerous health, social, and behavioral problems over the life course • Problems related to ACEs tend to be comorbid (co-occurring)
ACEs and substance use	ACEs are related to: • Early initiation of **alcohol use** (earlier age of drinking onset) • Higher risk of **mental/substance use disorders at ages 50+ years** • Continued **tobacco use** during adulthood • **Prescription drug use** (62% increase in drug prescriptions for each additional ACE) • Lifetime **illicit drug use**, drug dependency, and self-reported addiction (each ACE increases the likelihood of early initiation into illicit drug use by two- to fourfold)
ACEs and behavioral problems	ACEs are related to: • **Suicide attempts:** ACEs in any category increased the risk of attempted suicide by two- to fivefold across the life span • **Lifetime depressive episodes:** ACEs may increase the risk of depression diagnosis during young adult and adult years • **Sleep disturbances** in adults • **High-risk sexual behaviors** • **Fetal mortality** attributed to adolescent pregnancy related to ACEs • **Adverse pregnancy outcomes:** low birth weight, prematurity • **Lifelong negative physical health outcomes**

ACEs, adverse childhood experiences.
Source: https://www.cdc.gov/violenceprevention/aces/index.html

Poor Education

Education provides a direct conduit to quality jobs, higher income, and access to resources for optimizing personal and family health. These resources include healthy foods, exercise facilities, green outdoor spaces for safe physical activity and recreation, access to preventive healthcare including prenatal care for expectant mothers, and transportation. Educated youth acquire health knowledge and skills, and they live in healthier neighborhoods. Educated youth experience reduced psychological stress, increased opportunities to learn and refine life skills, and enriched social networks of persons who both provide social interaction and create opportunities. The consequences of poor education, often in tandem with living in poverty, are associated with the reverse constellation of attributes.

HEALTH BEHAVIORS THAT THREATEN ADOLESCENT HEALTH

In the United States, a year-over-year national snapshot of youth health risks and behaviors is performed continuously by the Centers for Disease Control and Prevention (CDC) through the mechanism of the Youth Risk Behavior Surveillance System (YRBSS). The YRBSS monitors priority health risk behaviors that include physical inactivity, unhealthy dietary behaviors, substance use (tobacco, alcohol, and other drug use), behaviors that elevate risks for unintentional injury, behaviors that contribute to violent injury, and sexual behaviors that increase transmission risks for sexually transmitted infections (STIs) or elevate rates of unplanned pregnancies.[44]

YRBSS data chronicle patterns of diet and physical exercise annually and over multiple years for school-based youth in the United States. Lifestyle eating and activity patterns adopted during childhood and adolescence strongly predict the onset and severity of cardiovascular diseases and some cancers (e.g., colorectal cancer) later in adult life. However, one outcome of the combination of overnutrition and physical inactivity during the first decades of life is the trend toward increasing obesity among U.S. adolescents.

SUBSTANCE USE BEHAVIORS

One of the hallmarks of adolescence is experimentation with new behaviors. This is the period in the life course when youth are likely to begin to use a variety of addictive substances, with the potential for progressing to regular use. Substance use includes the use or misuse of products containing tobacco, alcohol, illicit or diverted prescription drugs, or combinations. These products operate on the reward circuitry in the brain, frequently leading to addiction. These substances, at a minimum, modify human physiology, and they often influence motor skills, mood, cognition, and social interactions.

In the United States, common adolescent substance use includes tobacco and nicotine products, alcohol, and other drugs. E-cigarettes and vaping products have become extremely popular, with an estimated 2.5 million youth in the United States using these products, equivalent to 14% of high school students and more than 3% of middle school students. E-cigarette and vaping product sales increased steadily throughout the early years of the COVID-19 pandemic.

The earliest experimentation with substance use often takes place in the later years of childhood. The first offer of a cigarette frequently occurs during the elementary school years. First experiences of drinking alcohol or smoking marijuana may happen several years later, and not infrequently, initiation occurs before the age of 13. It should be noted that underage use of both tobacco and alcohol is technically illegal in the United States, but, with the exception of retailers selling these products to minors, it is almost never prosecuted.

The period of adolescence frequently marks the age when early trial behaviors that began in childhood shift toward regular use, powered by addiction. From a population health perspective, this is the life era during which patterns of use develop, driven by many factors, including family and peer influences, community availability of substances, and tolerance for experimentation. Adolescence is the time when a drug-using "career" solidifies and takes hold.

Youth who smoke tend to drink. Youth who smoke and drink tend to try other substances. There is no lockstep sequence for trying various types of addictive substances. However, research suggests a possible "gatekeeper" pathway whereby adolescents start with cigarettes, alcohol, or both before trying stronger drugs. Where e-cigarettes and vaping products fall in this sequence is currently being explored. Marijuana is commonly the first illicit drug tried. There is a well-known and clearly documented clustering effect of so-called "problem behaviors." Youth who engage in one substance use behavior have a much greater-than-chance likelihood that they will use multiple substances. Polysubstance use is normative among adolescents who use at least one substance.

The public health consequences of substance use are multidimensional. The pharmacological properties of substance use, and the actions of these substances on the dopaminergic reward pathways in the brain, create an extremely high likelihood that the adolescent will become addicted. Indeed, addictive substance use behaviors have only recently been properly recognized and explained as brain diseases.

Cigarette smoking is recognized as the chief preventable cause of death in the United States. A lifetime of regular smoking that begins during the teen years greatly amplifies the risks for premature, severe, and deadly chronic diseases throughout the duration of the life span. Adolescents who drink alcohol and drive motor vehicles are at elevated risk for road traffic accidents that may result in death, life-changing injury, or criminal conviction. And, perhaps most alarmingly, the United States is, by far, the major consumer nation for illicit drugs. Taking drugs, possessing quantities of drugs, and especially dealing drugs, are criminal behaviors that may be prosecuted. The national drug crisis, in turn, has led to draconian penalties and mandatory sentencing guidelines that have spawned a flourishing, for-profit criminal justice enterprise. Consequently, the United States has the highest proportion of incarcerated citizens per capita of any nation on earth, with prisons overflowing with persons who have been sentenced based on drug charges, often in the absence of conviction (see Case Study 8.1, "Mass Incarceration as a Social Justice Issue and a Public Health Crisis"). So, the spin-offs of substance use have led to compounding societal problems of public health significance that extend far beyond the debilitating effects of the drugs themselves on human physiology.

Tobacco Use Trends

Tobacco use among U.S. adolescents has changed much in recent decades. The picture for tobacco use is complicated because of the ongoing introduction of a variety of nicotine delivery devices that are available to youth. While the **prevalence** of cigarette smoking has declined sharply, the advent of electronic vapor products (including e-cigarettes, e-cigars, e-pipes, vape pipes, vaping pens, e-hookahs, and hookah pens) has ushered in new means to foster nicotine addiction.

According to 2019 YRBSS data, almost one in two (48.2%) students in grades 9 through 12 used cigarettes, smokeless tobacco, cigars, or electronic vapor products on at least 1 day during the 30 days prior to completing the survey, including 52.1% of male and 43.8% of female students. The percentage of current users of any of these nicotine products climbed in an upward stair-step fashion by grade, from 34.6% of 9th graders to 63.4% of 12th graders.

There has been a proliferation of youth experimenting with some form of electronic vapor products; 50.1% reported ever trying electronic vapor products, with almost equal percentages of males (49.6%) and females (50.7%). With increasing grade, increasing percentages of youth reported trying these products, rising to 60.1% of 12th graders. The rate of current use, defined as using any electronic vapor product on at least 1 day during the 30 days before the survey, was 32.7%—almost one in three. These vapor products are, therefore, contributing more than any other type of tobacco use to the overall percentage of youth who reported current use of a nicotine or tobacco product.

Specific to tobacco cigarettes, around one-fifth (24.1%) of youth, grades 9 through 12, had ever tried a cigarette, 6% smoked on at least 1 day (the criterion for a current smoker), 1.3% smoked on 20 or more days, and 1.1% smoked daily during the 30 days prior to the survey.

About half (47.6%) of current smokers had tried to quit. The CDC trend data document a very significant decline in the percentage of youth experimenting with cigarettes and adopting a regular cigarette smoking habit dating at least from 1991.

Smokeless tobacco products (e.g., chewing tobacco, snuff, or dip) had been used by 3.8% of respondents, and 5.7% had smoked cigars, cigarillos, or little cigars on at least 1 day during the 30 days before the survey.[45,46]

CASE STUDY 9.2: E-CIGARETTES AS GATEKEEPERS FOR COMBUSTIBLE CIGARETTE SMOKING

In frigid January 2022, a New York Times online edition banner read, *That Cloud of Smoke Is Not a Mirage*, attracting readers to a story by lifestyle reporter John Ortved. The same tale came out one day later in the print edition with an equally intriguing alternative title, *The Urge for a Smoke Swirls Back*.[47] Ortved described how young adults were stepping out to catch a smoke in social settings, even if that meant outdoors in winter due to clean indoor air restrictions. Nicotine vaping was surging, but Ortved was describing a different phenomenon, the return of the traditional tobacco cigarette asking, "Have cigarettes, those filthy, cancer-causing things—and still the No. 1 cause of preventable death in the United States, according to the Centers for Disease Control and Prevention—lost their taboo?"[48]

For context, cigarette smoking rates had been trending downhill since the release of the first Surgeon General's report on smoking and health back in 1964 (**Figure 9.6**).[49] So too have cigarette pack and total sales figures (**Figure 9.7**). Coupling together the effects of powerful scientific research substantiating the health harms of tobacco, stringent clean air legislation, spiking prices on top of hefty taxation, and tobacco litigation lawsuits that extracted crippling financial penalties from the industry—along with the pervasive negative perceptions of the stench of tobacco smoke—the traditional tobacco cigarette seemed immensely unpopular and unlikely to resurrect.

Cigarette consumption and sales may have declined, but nicotine addiction is steadily on the rise.

Dented but undaunted, the tobacco industry, the purveyors of the most profitable legal addictive drug on the planet, experimented with numerous variations of nicotine delivery devices that could attract young users and circumvent bans, restrictions, and public disfavor. They struck it rich with the introduction of e-cigarette and vaping products, sometimes called "electronic nicotine delivery systems," and cloaked their new devices in the mystique of harmlessness, even healthfulness.

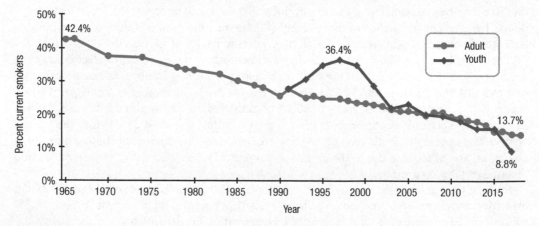

American Lung Association analysis of CDC data: NHIS 1965–2018. YRBSS 1995–2017.

FIGURE 9.6 Cigarette smoking rates have fallen significantly for both youths and adults. NHIS, National Health Interview Survey; YRBSS, Youth Risk Behavior Surveillance System.
Source: American Lung Association. Overall Tobacco Trends. https://www.lung.org/research/trends-in-lung-disease/tobacco-trends-brief/overall-tobacco-trends#

(continued)

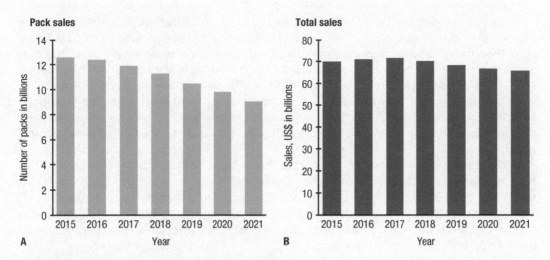

FIGURE 9.7 U.S. cigarette pack and total sales, 2015 to 2021.
Source: Data from Ali FRM, Seaman EL, Schillo B, Vallone D. Trends in annual sales and pack price of cigarettes in the US, 2015–2021. *JAMA Netw Open.* 2022;5(6):e2215407. doi:10.1001/jamanetworkopen.2022.15407

Introduced in 2003, e-cigarette and vaping products continue their multigenerational evolution[50]:

- Generation 1: disposable e-cigarettes
- Generation 2: e-cigarettes with prefilled or refillable cartridges
- Generation 3: tanks or mods
- Generation 4: pod mods

Promoting e-cigarettes and vaping products employed highly effective marketing.[51] Youth, ages 13 to 17, who had never used e-cigarettes, but were exposed to e-cigarette advertising, perceived nicotine vaping to be less addictive, safer than combustible cigarettes, cooler, more fun, and more enjoyable than youth who had not viewed the ads.[52,53] Youth who had seen the ads came away with impressions that e-cigarettes could be used where cigarette smoking is prohibited; that, unlike traditional cigarettes, using e-cigarettes would pose no harm to persons nearby who breathed the vapors they had exhaled; and that using e-cigarettes was a means for expressing personal independence.[52,53]

Vaping has made progressive inroads over a decade with rising sales coinciding with consistently rising prevalence among youth. While trends in vaping have been surfing a rolling wave of misinformation about the relative safety, the appeal of a rainbow assortment of flavors, and the generational acceptance of a new trend that conveys coolness, sales of combustible smokes have been tapering.

Studies of the health effects of e-cigarettes and vaping products are ongoing. Clearly, users are exposed to the highly addictive properties of nicotine and a variety of potentially harmful chemicals in the vapor. CDC continues to elucidate the nature, severity, and frequency of E-cigarette or Vaping use-Associated Lung Injury (EVALI) for users of e-cigarettes.[54]

However, there is one finding that suggests that the upward trend in e-cigarette consumption could wrap around to boost the use of traditional cigarettes.[55]

(continued)

A study conducted by researchers at the Boston University School of Public Health found that about one in five youth, aged 12 to 15 years, whose first foray into nicotine products was an e-cigarette, later went on to smoke traditional cigarettes and sometimes very soon after first trying e-cigarettes.[56,57] When the research team extrapolated their findings to the estimated national numbers of youthful e-cigarette users, they found that tens of thousands may springboard to smoking traditional cigarettes after initially experiencing the rapidly addictive properties of nicotine while experimenting with one or more varieties of vaping products.

To add nuance to the findings, researchers determined that there was a three-fold higher likelihood for youth who started with nicotine vaping to progress to smoking cigarettes than for youth to start smoking cigarettes straightaway.[56,57] Particularly concerning was the finding that this vaping-to-combustible cigarette smoking transition was more pronounced for youth actually deemed to be at lower risk for smoking initiation.

These findings are reminiscent of the "Gateway Hypothesis," first popularized decades ago by Denise and Eric Kandel, suggesting that early life experimentation and adoption of the cigarette smoking habit—along with attendant nicotine addiction—was often the pathway to using alcohol, marijuana, other "illicit" drugs, and engaging in problem behaviors.[58] Consistent with the gateway notion, Grant and colleagues found that e-cigarette use preceded subsequent alcohol use and opiate use, and was associated with mental health histories of attention deficit hyperactivity disorder (ADHD), posttraumatic stress disorder (PTSD), anxiety, and impulsivity and low self-esteem.[59] The Boston University study adds another potential step to the sequence: e-cigarette/nicotine vaping as a gatekeeper to cigarette smoking.[56,57]

Use of e-cigarettes and nicotine vaping skyrocketed during the decade preceding the COVID-19 pandemic. Particularly steep rises in daily, 30-day, and lifetime e-cigarette prevalence rates were noted for the period 2017 through 2019 when patterns were assessed in a nationally representative sample of 10th grade and 12th grade students enrolled in the Monitoring the Future study.[60] Rising prevalence rates were not observed in 2020, perhaps related to publicity about some of the concerning health effects of vaping, but also very likely related to marked changes in lifestyle, socialization, and mobility during the first year of the COVID-19 pandemic.[61] In 2020, vaping prevalence was 22% for past 30-day use. Youth reported decreased accessibility for some vaping products compared to previous years, and higher levels of perceived health risk associated with vaping.

Nevertheless, e-cigarette and vaping product unit sales have continued to escalate throughout the peak years of the pandemic (**Figure 9.8**).[62] What has changed, however, is the mix of e-cigarette and vaping products. The market appears extraordinarily resilient. When the Food and Drug Administration instituted a federal e-cigarette flavor ban on the sale of flavored prefilled cartridges but exempted disposable devices and menthol and tobacco prefilled cartridges, in February 2020, sales diminished only momentarily. Disposable devices surged almost instantaneously and took over the market. Meanwhile, the flavor favorites morphed as mint and menthol flavors supplanted the fruit flavors.

Even as the market dynamics ebb and flow with new products coming online, the trend in e-cigarette and vaping product use is up. These products are becoming so popular that they threaten to actually turn around the decline in traditional

(continued)

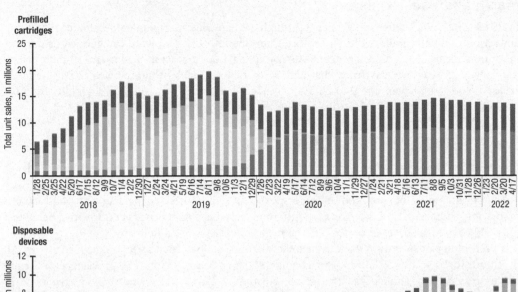

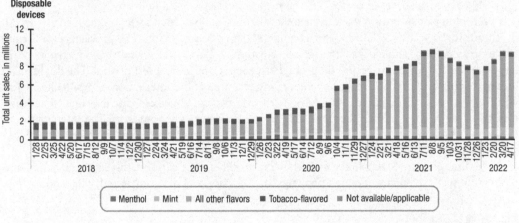

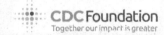

FIGURE 9.8 Cigarette smoking rates have fallen significantly for both youths and adults.
Source: Data from CDC Foundation. Monitoring U.S. e-cigarette sales: national trends data brief. Published April 17, 2022.
https://www.cdcfoundation.org/National-E-CigaretteSales-DataBrief-2022-April17?inline

cigarette use as more e-cigarette users adopt—or re-adopt—the combustible smoking habit, perhaps buoyed by edgy trends to socialize with a vengeance as pandemic restrictions wane.

Alcohol Use Trends

In 2019, almost two-thirds (63%) of students in grades 9 through 12 had tried alcohol at least once while almost one-third (29.2%) had consumed at least one drink of alcohol on at least 1 day during the 30 days before the survey (current user). This included 26.4% of males and 31.9% of females. Prevalence of current (past-month) drinking increased with increasing grade and age, from 19% in grade 9 to 39.9% in grade 12. The prevalence of current drinking for African American/Black adolescents (16.8%) was lower than for either White (34.2%) or Latinx adolescents (28.4%). Around one in seven (13.7%) reported having five or more drinks in a row on one occasion, and rates of this "binge drinking" behavior increased with each increasing grade from 7.3% in grade 9 to 22.4% in grade 12.

Marijuana Use Trends

In 2019, 36.8% of students in grades 9 through 12 had tried marijuana at least once, including almost half of 12th graders (48.7%). More than one-fifth (21.7%) were categorized as current marijuana users based on self-reported use on at least one occasion during the 30 days before the survey. Prevalence was somewhat higher for males (22.5%) than females (20.8%) and increased from 14.6% in grade 9 to 28.3% in grade 12. Prevalence was relatively similar for African American/Black (21.7%), Latinx (22.4%), and White non-Latinx students (22.1%).

UNINTENTIONAL INJURIES[63]

Unintentional injuries are common and usually nonfatal but are also the leading cause of death for adolescents. Many of these injuries are related to popular activities and newly acquired risky behaviors including contact and extreme sports, driving without using seat belts, and experimentation with substance use. Cycling without a helmet is a dangerous yet normative behavior; fully 81% of youth surveyed on the YRBSS never or rarely wore a helmet.

Often injury ensues from various behavioral combinations such as texting while driving. Almost four in 10 youth (39%) report engaging in texting while driving. The prevalence of texting while driving rises with increasing grade level from 17.2% in grade 9 to 59.5% in grade 12, in large part owing to the correspondingly higher proportions of licensed drivers. The dual behaviors of driving and texting present an interesting example of the interaction of new technologies with injury risks. First, adolescents have been driving motor vehicles for less than a century, a small sliver of human time. Second, texting is a far newer phenomenon. The intersection of these two behaviors has sharply elevated the risk that youth who attempt to do both behaviors simultaneously will be involved in an injurious or fatal motor vehicle crash.

As further examples, substance use behaviors modify injury patterns through such behavioral combinations as driving while high on drugs, or the trifecta of drinking and driving and texting.

INTERPERSONAL VIOLENCE

Interpersonal violence, including assaults and abuse, also factors into the patterning of physical risks. Gang violence, community violence, gender-based violence, and even radicalization or forced recruitment of youth to serve in situations of armed conflict are observed worldwide.

These behaviors produce unique constellations of injury, and when fatal, translate into homicide statistics. YRBSS respondents were asked a battery of questions relating to exposure to violence. For example, 21.9% reported having been in a physical fight, with more males (28.3%) than females (15.3%) responding affirmatively. Physical fighting is one risk behavior for which prevalence decreases steadily with increasing grade, from 25.8% in grade 9 to 17.6% in grade 12. Almost one in five (19.5%) reported having been bullied on the school premises, but for this question, the prevalence was much higher for female students (23.6%) than for males (15.4%).

The YRBSS continuously updates questionnaire items to keep up with the salient issues of the times. Electronic bullying is a newly recognized violence issue; one-sixth (15.7%) of students report cyberbullying, including 20.4% of females. The YRBSS began to ask about sexual dating violence, which is reported by three times more female respondents (12.6%) than males (3.8%), even before the #MeToo movement gained momentum.

SEXUAL RISK BEHAVIORS

Adolescence is the primary life period for sexual initiation and experimentation. It is also the time when partnering relationships tend to be brief in duration and often nonexclusive. This is a life era when sexual experimentation steeply increases risks for STIs based on partner choice, partner numbers, brevity of relationships, engagement in riskier and unprotected forms of sexual contact, and a high frequency of contacts between persons who are and who are not infected with a transmissible disease.

In the YRBSS sample, the proportions of youth who reported having ever had sexual intercourse (38.4%) and who were currently sexually active (27.4%) rose steeply and steadily with increasing grade in school. Among 12th graders, 56.7% reported having sex, including 42.3% who were currently sexually active.

Sexual activity carries concomitant risks for STIs and unplanned pregnancy. YRBSS assessed the prevalence of several behaviors that are known to increase sexual risks. One in five (21.2%) surveyed youth reported using alcohol or drugs prior to engaging in sex and 8.6% reported having sex with four or more partners.

Since the 1990s, U.S. adolescents have been using condoms and contraceptives more often but still inconsistently. Only about half of sexually active youth (54.3%) reported using a condom the last time they had sexual intercourse. Although 11.9% of sexually active YRBSS respondents reported using no method to prevent pregnancy, 30.9% reported using some specific method other than condoms (birth control pills, birth control ring, implant or intrauterine device, shot, or patch) to prevent pregnancy the last time they had sexual intercourse.[44] The gender differential was notable; 35.2% of females versus 25.9% of males reported using some method to prevent pregnancy. Furthermore, the percentage of White non-Latinx (39.5%) adolescents was twice that for African American/Black (19.7%) and Latinx adolescents (18.2%).

Globally, the implications of sexual activity have important ramifications for women's health. Complications of pregnancy and childbirth represent the leading cause of death for adolescent females, ages 15 to 19 years, who account for 11% of all births worldwide, primarily in low- and middle-income countries. Globally, the adolescent birth rate (44 births per 1,000 adolescent females, ages 15–19) has been declining markedly since 1990.[64]

MENTAL HEALTH

Many adolescents exemplify vibrant mental health and resilience. Nevertheless, one in five adolescents has some form of mental disorder. Half of the mental health problems have their onset, and are recognized, prior to age 15. Fortunately, prevention of the onset of mental health problems is possible for some youth, while the combination of early detection, intervention, and effective treatment can minimize negative impacts of mental health problems on the lives of adolescents.[65,66]

The most common mental disorder affecting youth in the United States, as well as globally, is depression. The numbers of U.S. adolescents who are experiencing major depressive episodes has increased substantially in the decade from 2005 to 2014. In 2020, more than one in six (17%) young adults aged 18 to 25 years reported a major depressive episode in the past year.[67]

CASE STUDY 9.3: COVID-19 STRESSORS AND THE MENTAL HEALTH OF U.S. ADOLESCENTS

The COVID-19 pandemic has created a multiplicity of stressors for adolescents globally. In the United States, the CDC recognized that youth were experiencing pandemic-induced exposures to trauma, loss, and life change that were invariably linked to mental health and well-being. Moreover, these experiences are likely to influence health for this cohort that will extend into adult life.[68]

To explore the ramifications of the COVID-19 pandemic, the CDC launched the Adolescent Behaviors and Experiences Survey.[69] This online survey was conducted

(continued)

with a nationally representative, probability-based, sample of 7,707 U.S. public- and private-school students in grades 9 to 12. The CDC fielded the survey from January through June 2021.

CDC investigators described the range of stressors these youth faced in the first years of the pandemic with the potential to influence mental health.[68] School closures were a prominent feature that related to pervasive experiences of social isolation. Many youth received their instruction online with variable internet connectivity while living in an environment that was not conducive to being able to focus on the material being presented. Furthermore, adolescents were cooped up in stressful home environments while some family members lost jobs, others attempted to work from home, and entire households faced economic hardships.

A high proportion of youth personally became ill with COVID-19 and often reported that family members were severely ill. Indeed, some family members required hospitalization, intensive care stays, and mechanical ventilation. Some family members and close friends died. Access to healthcare was limited.

Other studies have expanded the list of stressors to include child abuse and violence in the home, along with a broad spectrum of ACEs.[70] Mental health during the pandemic appears to be worse for children and adolescents in low-income households, and this is coupled with decreased access to mental health services.[70]

On the CDC survey, a set of five items looked at mental health and suicidality[68]:

- *During the COVID-19 pandemic, how often was your mental health not good?*
- *During the past 30 days, how often was your mental health not good?*
- *During the past 12 months, did you ever feel so sad or hopeless almost every day for two weeks or more in a row that you stopped doing some usual activities?*
- *During the past 12 months, did you ever seriously consider attempting suicide?*
- *During the past 12 months, how many times did you actually attempt suicide?*

The findings were eye-opening.

Almost three in eight students reported experiencing poor mental health during the COVID-19 pandemic.[68] This was not restricted to an initial spike in poor mental health during the early lockdown months but instead persisted. One year into the pandemic, fully 31.1% of adolescent respondents reported poor mental health during the 30 days prior to taking the survey.

More than four in 10 (44.2%) described consistent feelings of sadness or hopelessness for a duration of 2 weeks or more during the 12 months prior to the survey as COVID-19 was actively circulating. During the prepandemic years 2018 and 2019, U.S. adolescents aged 12 to 17 years already self-reported substantial prevalence rates of anxiety symptoms (13%) and depression symptoms (7%). The 44.2% figure from the CDC survey conducted in early 2021, one year into the pandemic, portrays a stratospheric rise in depression symptoms compared to the prepandemic baseline rates.

Particularly alarming were two related findings. One in five youth (19.9%) indicated that they had seriously considered attempting suicide in the preceding 12 months.[68] Even more sobering, one in 11 (9.0%) had actually attempted suicide—one or more times during the pandemic.

(continued)

These findings for youth were not limited to adolescence but were recorded in the context of a global pandemic that had produced a startling upsurge in symptoms of depression, anxiety, trauma- and stress-related disorders, increased substance use, and suicidality in the adult population, with steepest rises on all measures among emerging adults, ages 18 to 29.[71] These findings from the Adolescent Behaviors and Experiences Survey indicate that the burden of mental disorders in youth is also shared by young and middle-aged adults.[72-74] In consequence, youth who are struggling and might understandably turn for help to older family members, friends, and role models may be seeking support from others who are likewise experiencing poor mental health.

Throughout the pandemic, both COVID-19 illness and common mental disorders were co-occurring within families and social networks.

CDC investigators also explored the possible buffering effects of closeness and connectedness with school-age peers and with a broader array of family, friends, and other supports by asking two questions[68]:

- *Do you agree or disagree that you feel close to people at your school?*
- *During the COVID-19 pandemic, how often were you able to spend time with family, friends, or other groups, such as clubs or religious groups, by using a computer, phone, or other device?*

Results were encouraging and suggest that closeness and connectedness is helpful for maintaining—or possibly regaining—mental health and resilience. Closeness and connectedness, assessed on these two items, were found to consistently predict better scores for each of the five items used to assess mental health and suicidality.[68]

First, when compared to youth who did not feel close to persons at school, those students who did experience closeness had a lower prevalence of self-reported poor mental health throughout the first year of the pandemic (28.4% versus 45.2%) and also, during the previous 30 days (23.5% versus 37.8%).[68]

While an alarming 35.4% of students—more than one in three—who did indicate they felt close to persons at school nevertheless reported persistent feelings of sadness or hopelessness, this troubling finding contrasts with an even higher percentage of youth who did not feel close to persons at school reporting they were feeling sad and hopeless—52.4%—more than one in two!

Regarding suicidality, the differentials for students who felt close to school peers, versus those who did not feel close, were large. More than one-quarter of youth who lacked a feeling of closeness to people at school (25.6%) reported that they seriously considered attempting suicide, compared to 14.0% who did experience closeness. The proportion who lacked closeness and reported attempting suicide (11.9%) was more than double the proportion who experienced closeness yet nevertheless reported attempting suicide (5.8%).

Second, although the differences were of smaller magnitude, students who were virtually connected to others fared better on all five mental health/suicidality measures than their counterparts who did not report having online, phone, or cellular connections to family, friends, or other groups, such as clubs or religious groups.[68]

When contrasting the virtually connected to not virtually connected subsets, the comparison figures for the three mental health items were as follows: poor mental health during the pandemic (35.5% versus 42.0%), poor mental health

(continued)

during the past 30 days (28.7% versus 36.8%), and persistent sadness or hope-lessness (41.9% versus 51.7%).

Regarding suicidality, virtual connectedness appears to exert a possible protective effect. When contrasting the virtually connected to not virtually connected subsets, the comparison figures for the two suicidality items were as follows: seriously considered attempting suicide (18.4% versus 24.9%) and reporting one or more actual suicide attempts (8.0% versus 12.2%).

The survey was conducted during the first half of 2021, at the time when COVID-19 variants were emerging and circulating. The B.1.1.7 (Alpha) variant became predominant during the time of the survey but did not cause a major surge in the United States. Nevertheless, 2021 proved to be a year of multiple pandemic surge events involving the Alpha, Delta, and Omicron variants.

Later in 2022, populations in the United States and worldwide experienced periods of considerable freedom to socialize and congregate, attend school and work with minimal precautions or restrictions, and resume many in-person activities. This change toward living resiliently with COVID-19 may persist.

Meanwhile, regardless of the future COVID-19 pandemic patterns, the CDC authors of the Adolescent Behaviors and Experiences Survey advocate for developing strategies and approaches to enhance feelings of closeness and connectedness—in-person or virtually—among youth in school settings, and within their families and social networks. Such strategies hold promise for buffering against COVID-19 stressors and hardships and for safeguarding mental health and well-being.[68]

HOW PUBLIC HEALTH CAN MITIGATE THREATS TO HEALTH DURING THE EARLIEST PHASES OF THE LIFE COURSE

Understanding how health is produced early in childhood, how can public health act to promote childhood health toward creating health throughout the life course? This depends on a range of actions at multiple levels of the social ecological framework. Such approaches must address health and development across the life course and understand the impact of forces over various settings (what we describe as the social ecological perspective) and a range of social determinants. Examples of these approaches follow.

BEFORE PREGNANCY

At the front end of this timeline, the health of the mother-to-be is primary. Preventive interventions provided during adolescence focus on family planning, healthy sexual choices, and healthy lifestyles to optimize maternal health during pregnancy. Healthy nutrition for expectant mothers, including dietary supplementation, is strongly advocated.

DURING PREGNANCY

As the expectant mother navigates her pregnancy, interventions vary by trimester. Maternal nutrition and scheduled prenatal care are fundamental to ensure a healthy pregnancy. Prevention, detection, diagnosis, and treatment of maternal infections are critically important. This is of life-and-death importance for the health of the fetus in cases of maternal infections with HIV or sexually transmitted diseases. As the pregnancy progresses, the focus shifts increasingly toward assessment and management of fetal health and growth. Management of pregnancy complications is important close to the time of childbirth especially for high-risk expectant mothers.

LABOR AND DELIVERY

Infant viability and survival are safeguarded by having competent obstetrical and perinatal care during labor, childbirth, and the first days following birth. When necessary, this is the crucial phase for managing birth complications for mother and infant.

FIRST 24 MONTHS OF LIFE

During the first 2 years of life, child development can be optimized in multiple ways. In the earliest months of life, options include neonatal disease prevention and treatment, nurturing care for the infant from parents and family, nutritional support for the mother, and breastfeeding for the infant. Later in the first year and throughout the second year, the young child should be provided with healthy dietary offerings, quality early childhood care in home and community settings, and ideally, early childhood education programs if the child is cared for outside the home.

MONTHS 25 TO 60 (UP TO AGE 5)

During the following 3 years of the young child's life span, priorities to maintain health include prevention, detection, and timely management of infectious diseases and childhood illnesses. At this stage, many children will receive a combination of in-home and out-of-home care. The availability of quality early childhood education programs may be a differentiating factor in terms of the child's advancement along multiple domains of development.

EXAMPLES OF PUBLIC HEALTH ACTIONS TO IMPROVE HEALTH EARLY IN THE LIFE COURSE

Evidence-based interventions that can optimize early child health and have positive effects throughout the life course exist. These interventions can be sequentially delivered beginning prior to pregnancy and moving forward throughout the birth and newborn phases, through the period of infancy, and into the early childhood years. Timed, tailored packages of interventions enhance the child's progression through the staged developmental tasks across multiple domains. Interventions also optimize nutrition and growth, and decrease rates of child death, disease, injury, and disability.

> **Evidence-based interventions that can optimize early child health and have positive effects throughout the life course exist.**

We can think about these sequentially, both across the life course and across the social ecological framework. First, the most essential public health needs must be met, including access to sanitation, clean water, and nutritious foods, along with practicing hygienic behaviors when caring for the young child. Second, physical and social protection must be ensured. Third, parenting programs teach skills for positive parenting; psychosocial stimulation of, and responsivity to, the young child; and prevention of exposures of children to maltreatment and adverse experiences. Monitoring maternal mental health, coupled with detecting, and intervening on, maternal depression or other mental health disorders is critical for mother and child alike.

Given the extensive litany of available interventions, efficiencies are critical for grouping, disseminating, and delivering these programs to large numbers of children who can benefit from them (Case Study 9.3). Experts have already weighed in on how to group the interventions, suggesting three specific packages of approaches, described in the following three sections, that can be adopted broadly to improve health.[25]

FAMILY SUPPORT AND STRENGTHENING

Mothers and other family caregivers benefit from guided training and practice on the set of skills that comprise nurturing care. Family support also includes facilitated access to prenatal care during pregnancy, obstetrical or midwife support during childbirth, directed education about breastfeeding and maternal and child nutrition, and pediatric care during the child's early years that includes the full complement of childhood immunizations. Another component is family support policies, safety networks, and various forms of social protection, aligned with the local culture.

CARING FOR THE CAREGIVER

These programs and services span two generations. Protecting parents'—and caregivers'—well-being, including both physical and mental health, is one component, in tandem with programs that expand parents' capabilities to consistently provide nurturing care to their young children.

EARLY LEARNING AND PROTECTION

These programs encompass a larger realm of social ecological influences, going beyond the immediate family and primary caregivers. Included here are broader interventions to optimize the provision of a nurturing care "environment" in daycare and early childhood education centers by supporting a range of caregivers—parents, extended family members, teachers, and their assistants. These programs focus both on empowerment of caregivers and teachers and child protection.

CASE STUDY 9.4: THE FINNISH BABY BOX

Some public health actions to improve health in early life literally involve the "packaging" of an intervention; one example is the Finnish baby box. This is a proven intervention with history and longevity, conceived long before the formalization of programs targeted to enhance child development. This intervention has become the national standard in Finland, and the benefits for newborns and their caregivers are unequivocal. The nation of Finland introduced a public health measure to enhance newborn care more than 80 years ago.[75] As described, "it's a tradition that dates back to the 1930s and it's designed to give all children in Finland, no matter what background they're from, an equal start in life." The Finnish baby box is not only egalitarian; it is practical and it works. Expectant mothers receive a large cardboard box from the government lined with a formfitting mattress. The box also comes with bodysuits, a sleeping bag, outdoor gear, bathing products for the baby, nappies, and bedding. Most babies across Finland, regardless of social class, sleep in the baby box for the early months of life. To add to the public health value of the national program based at the Social Insurance Institution of Finland, eligibility to receive the box is very simple but pragmatic; mothers must have visited a physician or a prenatal clinic in their municipality prior to the fourth month of pregnancy. So, seeking timely prenatal care is incentivized. Moreover, this has now evolved to become a valued national tradition.

The Finnish baby box represents a deceptively simple intervention, yet it is normative and broadly endorsed by the population. Through the use of this approach, almost all mothers do seek prenatal care that carries lifesaving potential for both mother and baby.

SCALING UP INTERVENTIONS FOR GLOBAL DISSEMINATION

One of the most glaring gaps—and barriers—to bringing evidence-based programs to one-quarter billion at-risk children is the failure to amplify and scale programs for mass distribution and adoption. Knowledge is at hand; effective evidence-based early childhood development programs exist. However, they have not been bundled and delivered at scale. Only a trickle of children who could benefit have these programs available. So, the major issue is how to ramp up and expand programs to reach children in need.

Fortunately, we can identify a number of programs that are true exemplars of how to scale operations in a manner that successfully delivers services to large numbers of recipients. Several characteristics distinguish successful programs. First, they have reached the level of political priority. Second, they are supported by legislation, statute, policy, or government strategy. Third, they scale up by tapping into existing systems and funding sources, most often governmental or sometimes civil society organizations. Fourth, child development is positioned as a solution to compelling issues of pervasive poverty or inequality, or social exclusion. Fifth, they effectively integrate and showcase the multigenerational benefits to the children, their parents (or caregivers), and their extended families and social networks.

At the community and societal levels, environments that generate healthy populations have many attributes. These include supporting the health of expectant mothers by providing them with diets rich in plant-source nutrients from fruits, vegetables, and grains; opportunities for cardiorespiratory exercise; prioritization of restful sleep; availability of prenatal care; access to obstetrical services to ensure a safe delivery; teaching about and support for breastfeeding after childbirth; and paid parental leave—ideally for both parents.

> **At the community and societal levels, environments that generate healthy populations have many attributes.**

During infancy and early childhood, children should receive regular medical checkups, a full course of childhood vaccinations and immunizations, and rapid detection and effective intervention for acute childhood illnesses. Children should ideally be able to live in environments that minimize exposure to dust and pollutants. Their diets should be rich in plant-source foods with very limited intake of unrefined sugars and foods containing high proportions of fats and sodium. Children need ample opportunities for physical activity and active play in safe and supervised settings. Particularly influential is early childhood education that prioritizes healthy socialization with same-age youth and provides guided instruction across a range of verbal and motor skills to stimulate brain development. The more enriched the child's environment during the earliest years of life, the greater will be the range of capacities developed. Getting such a healthy start launches children toward the healthiest attainable future life course.

Thus, the public health approach, using the mainstream social networks surrounding the child, has also been described in the social ecological section of this book. Healthy children come from healthy families, supplemented by healthy early childhood educational opportunities and a variety of social-skill-focused community activities that promote stimulation of mind and body.

Unfortunately, there are also instances where government policies are scaled up in a manner that actually perpetuates ACEs (Case Study 9.5; you can access the podcast accompanying Case Study 9.5 by following this link to Springer Publishing Company Connect™: http://connect .springerpub.com/content/book/978-0-8261-8043-8/part/part03/chapter/ch09).

CASE STUDY 9.5: SEPARATING CHILDREN AND PARENTS AT THE BORDER: WHEN SCALING UP A GOVERNMENT PROGRAM IS ANTITHETICAL TO POPULATION HEALTH

Health is more than what happens to us in the here and now. Our early exposures shape our health throughout our life and the lives of our children. This case study describes how a governmental policy had the effect of creating extremely adverse and harmful childhood experiences for families seeking entry and asylum in the United States after escaping atrocities in their countries of origin in Central America.

In 2017 and 2018, during a time when U.S. border security and immigration policy was a salient and strongly contested political issue, a carryover from a major theme during the 2016 presidential election, the Trump Administration implemented a harsh "zero-tolerance" policy to deter immigration to the United States from Central America by taking children from their families at the U.S. border.

Viewed through a population health and life course lens, this policy is likely to have undermined the health of children and parents alike for multiple generations. During 2018, much was rightly written about the forced separation of families and children at the U.S. border. As details of the separations emerged, it became clear that we were witnessing acts of wanton cruelty. Many of the detained children were being held in warehouse facilities; some were, appallingly, placed in cages.

The currents of social justice and public health are fully intermingled; the stated perspectives on the fundamental wrongness of the "zero-tolerance" policy carry overtones of population health. These separations jeopardized the health of young children and their family members. The unfolding public health and mental health crisis triggered a proliferation of statements from professional medical associations that were unified and vocal in condemning this health-compromising policy.

The American Public Health Association (APHA) and Trust for America's Health directly invoked the life course point of view when they published a news release, "Separating parents and children at U.S. border is inhumane and sets the stage for a public health crisis."[76] The statement opened with, "The Trump administration's policy of separating parents and children at the U.S.-Mexico border will have a dire impact on their health, both now and into the future."

The American Medical Association (AMA) asked the administration to withdraw this policy of separating children from caregivers.[77] One of its board members noted "Children leaving the chaos of their home countries should not be further traumatized by the U.S. government policy of separating children from their caregiver. It's inhumane and risks scarring children for the rest of their lives."

The president of the American Academy of Pediatrics minced no words when she stated, "These children have been traumatized on their trip up to the border, and the first thing that happens is we take away the one constant in their life that helps them buffer all these horrible experiences. . . . That's child abuse."[78] The American Psychiatric Association's statement opposing the policy highlights the mental health consequences; "Any forced separation is highly stressful for children and can cause lifelong trauma, as well as an increased risk of other mental illnesses, such as depression, anxiety, and posttraumatic stress disorder (PTSD)."[79]

This is echoed by the position statement from the American Academy of Child and Adolescent Psychiatry (AACAP), a psychiatric subspecialty dealing with the mental health of children and youth. AACAP states, "we know that children who experience sudden separation from one or both parents, especially under

(continued)

frightening, unpredictable, and chaotic circumstances, are at higher risk for developing illnesses such as anxiety, depression, posttraumatic stress disorders (PTSD), and other trauma-induced reactions."[80]

In parallel, the president of the American Psychological Association wrote:

The administration's policy of separating children from their families as they attempt to cross into the United States without documentation is not only needless and cruel, it threatens the mental and physical health of both the children and their caregivers. Psychological research shows that immigrants experience unique stressors related to the conditions that led them to flee their home countries in the first place.[81]

Taken together, the public health and mental health perspectives present a compelling case. The persons who are presenting themselves at U.S. borders, supplicating the Department of Homeland Security personnel for entry and protection, have already experienced multiple phases of potentially traumatizing exposures and profound losses. First, many have experienced structural violence in their countries of origin where physical and sexual violence, gang violence, intimate partner and gender-based violence, assassinations, and threats to family members are rampant. In making the choice to abandon their home communities, they know that they are losing all material possessions and leaving the lives and livelihoods they have known. Second, many have encountered a grueling journey while traversing Central America and Mexico, often punctuated by trauma, hardship, exploitation, and abuse while in transit. Third, they arrive at the U.S. border to encounter extreme uncertainty; calculated delay and deterrent tactics; and brutal environmental conditions without respite from the elements and hunger. They face the likely prospect that during processing they will be separated from family members, including minor children, detained, and prejudicially prosecuted at the border. These tactics of institutionalized hostility strip human dignity and feed discriminatory, anti-immigrant sentiments.

Immigration policies have strong proponents and staunch opponents. Border security issues are controversial and stir strong feelings on both sides. What is stated here is that, apart from political implications, these policies are antithetical to the public's health and the precepts of social justice. This case study is placed here because of the pervasive and prolonged negative effects these policies have on child health and child development. Health consequences will ripple throughout the entire life course for those children—and their parents—who experienced a terrifying family separation in what was, at that moment, a strange and foreign land. These policies have been unanimously decried by the public health, medical, psychiatric, and psychological professions and by human rights organizations.

These people are fleeing to the United States, long a bastion of liberty and a refuge for oppressed peoples. How ironic then that the United States was promulgating policy in 2018 that drew the condemnation of Amnesty International and other advocates for human rights because the United States was in violation of its own laws and also international human rights laws.[82,83] The government agenda has continued to mislead. In 2022, Florida governor Ron DeSantis approved a budget allocating $12 million to transport unauthorized migrants out of Florida to places such as Martha's Vineyard in Massachusetts.[84] Government employees misled migrants promising aid, employment, safe shelter, and meals, while deceiving them and shuttling them toward the northeast.

EXAMPLES OF PUBLIC HEALTH ACTIONS TO IMPROVE ADOLESCENT HEALTH

Public health can be instrumental in mitigating threats to the health of adolescents. Once again, comprehensive responses can be considered at multiple levels. In fact, these complementary strategies are absolutely necessary to effect meaningful change in health threats. Here we summarize and provide examples of wide-ranging approaches to health promotion and threat prevention for adolescents.

STRUCTURAL INTERVENTIONS

As we have seen, major themes in adolescent health include diet and nutrition, substance use, motor vehicle safety, sexual and reproductive health, interpersonal violence, and self-harm. To address the salient adolescent health issues requires interventions from across the social ecological spectrum. These interventions, including programs and policies for families, communities, schools, and health services, must be specifically targeted and appropriate for adolescents. Structural interventions include sound governance, extending to legislation, taxation, youth education, and policies that enable health promotion while restricting access to harmful products and engagement in harmful behaviors.

MEDIA AND SOCIAL MARKETING

One of the most powerful influences on youth at this time is the expansive growth of social media, which increasingly opens new communication channels that influence norms, attitudes, and behaviors. Increasingly, adolescents want to control and shape the nature of their social media engagement. So, it will be necessary going forward to fully include youth as architects and creators of social media that favorably influence healthy behaviors while effectively mitigating against threats to health. In addition to social media, today's youth are computer savvy and electronically literate. Adolescents are facile at searching immediately and reflexively for information. This makes online interventions particularly amenable, reachable, and highly appropriate for the youth audience. Effective online interventions ideally should involve youth in the development and vetting of the materials.

> **One of the most powerful influences on youth at this time is the expansive growth of social media, which increasingly opens new communication channels that influence norms, attitudes, and behaviors.**

COMMUNITY INTERVENTIONS

Behavioral choices are influenced by norms and attitudes, but it is primarily the behaviors themselves that determine the patterns of health and risk for adolescents and young adults worldwide. Community interventions therefore must be tailored to the most compelling health issues within the local culture, religions, and value systems. Universally, qualities that define effective community programs are those that demonstrably shift behaviors and health outcomes in a favorable direction while promoting life skills, self-esteem, youth engagement, and effective problem-solving. Hallmarks of efficacious programs include drawing upon community assets, incorporating science-based education and information that moves youth toward higher levels of health and well-being, and using a multifaceted set of program elements. The Communities That Care initiative is a prime example of such a program that has been used effectively across international settings.[85,86]

SCHOOL-BASED INTERVENTIONS

Schools represent the primary venue outside of the family where youth spend much of their time and develop important relationships with friends and teachers. Schools represent a point of access to a large proportion of the youth population, and as sites of education, schools are a primary conduit for teaching about behaviors that ensure or threaten optimal health. The ability to follow cohorts of students over time enhances the value of school-based interventions that can be tested for efficacy, refined, and made better. Until recently, schools were generally considered safe venues for students. We must now factor in the shifting student perceptions of school safety in an era of gang violence, rampage shootings, and school lockdowns.[87]

HEALTH SERVICES

Access to, and availability of, quality healthcare presents an additional opportunity for prevention education and early detection of critical health issues for adolescent patients. Ideally, healthcare providers maintain a nonjudgmental and proactive attitude, and become trusted confidants and advocates for their adolescent patients.

RAMPING UP TO THE NATIONAL LEVEL

Programs and interventions that are found to be beneficial and protective of adolescent health can only be made broadly available if they can be adopted and scaled up to serve the larger youth population. This requires a mechanism for funding, supporting, and promulgating best practices in order to magnify the beneficial effects.

EXAMPLES OF SUCCESSFUL PUBLIC HEALTH PROGRAMS

Here are examples of successful programming at the national and international levels. The National Adolescent and Young Adult Health Information Center (NAHIC) at the University of California San Francisco actively catalogues exemplary evidence-based programs for youth. What is immediately apparent is that different groups have specialized in identifying best practice programs in specific areas. The NAHIC serves as a major trunk line to other programs that specialize in a particular area of adolescent health and risk.

For example, Advocates for Youth focuses its work on identifying science-based programs with a track record of success in the area of "helping young people prevent pregnancy, HIV, and STDs." Advocates for Youth has evaluated programs both in the United States and in low- and middle-income countries.

In parallel, the NAHIC directs interested persons to Blueprints for Healthy Youth Development, a research project based at the Center for the Study and Prevention of Violence at the University of Colorado Boulder. The purpose of Blueprints is "to identify evidence-based prevention and intervention programs that are effective in reducing antisocial behavior and promoting a healthy course of youth development."

Similarly, the NAHIC funnels adolescent health program experts to a series of U.S. government branches for information on school health programs (CDC's Division of Adolescent and School Health), tobacco control (CDC's Office on Smoking and Health), and unintentional injuries (CDC's National Center for Injury Prevention and Control).

These are just a few of the many linkages referenced by the NAHIC. What is evident is that the range of programs is vast, the science is solid, and the best approach is to specify the topic area of interest and then seek out evaluated resources of documented high quality.

Despite successes on many fronts, important challenges to adolescent health remain. Here we describe current patterns of adolescent and young adult suicide that call out for urgent attention (Case Study 9.6; you can access the podcast accompanying Case Study 9.6 by following this link to Springer Publishing Company Connect™: http://connect.springerpub.com/content/book/978-0-8261-8043-8/part/part03/chapter/ch09).

CASE STUDY 9.6: ADOLESCENT SUICIDE: RISING RATES AND PROLIFERATING RISKS

Our earlier discussion of mortality patterns in adolescents highlighted the prominence of unintentional and intentional injury deaths. Of particular concern are the rising rates and risks for "intentional self-harm"—suicide.

According to the CDC, in 2020, suicide accounted for more than 45,000 deaths, ranking ninth among leading causes of death.[88] The annual suicide rate increased by 24% over 15 years and is almost four times higher for males.[88] Firearms represent the major lethal means for committing suicide (24,292 deaths in 2020), followed by suffocation (12,495 deaths).[89]

Adolescent suicide is the third leading cause of death among youth 10 to 19 years of age. In 2020, there were 2,797 suicides in this age group. This included 1,293 firearm suicides, 1,095 suffocations, and 214 suicide poisonings.[88] The risk landscape for suicidal thoughts and behaviors is more nuanced for adolescents and young adults than for older persons.[90] Moreover, there are emerging behavioral patterns and new technologies that are enlarging the spectrum of suicide risks for this age group.

Data from the Minnesota Student Survey identified multiple risk-elevating factors for adolescent suicidality: history of self-injurious behavior (a measure that strongly differentiates adolescents who actually attempt suicide), running away from home, history of childhood abuse or victimization, bullying and fighting behavior, dating violence, same-sex sexual attraction, anxiety, depression, impulsiveness, weight dissatisfaction, personal substance use, and parental substance abuse.[91] Regarding bullying, an extensive review documented a strong relationship between bullying victimization (and also perpetration in males) in relation to elevated rates of suicidal ideation and behavior.[92]

Also identified was an opposing cluster of risk-reducing, protective factors that safeguard youth from suicidal ideation and actions. These include successful academic achievement, school engagement and enjoyment, sports involvement, supportive friendships, and connectedness to parents and trusted adults. These factor clusters are robust and predictive; the combination of lowest risk factors/highest protective factors characterized youth with "no history of suicidality," while the reverse pattern (high-risk factors/low protective factors) was evident in youth who had actually attempted suicide (with intermediate levels for students reporting suicidal ideation).

Risks for adolescent suicide are ever-expanding. Recent research has examined nonsuicidal self-injury (NSSI) as a risk factor for both suicidal ideation and suicide attempts.[93,94] NSSI refers to the intentional destruction of body tissue without suicidal intent through episodes of cutting, burning, scratching, banging, or hitting. Most adolescents who engage in NSSI use multiple methods.[95] Suicidal and nonsuicidal self-injurious thoughts and behaviors (SITBs) are interconnected and pose risks to adolescent health. In a 2017 study, adolescents in outpatient and inpatient treatment settings reported both NSSI and suicidal thoughts.[96] There was a relatively consistent temporal sequence for the appearance of these thoughts and behaviors. Thoughts of NSSI and suicidal ideation tend to occur first. Then, in relatively predictable sequence, these thoughts are followed by NSSI behaviors, suicide plans, and finally suicide attempts that sometimes result in completed suicides.

(continued)

Another recent finding is that a subset of adolescent males (who are already four times more likely than females to die from suicide) experience transient periods of high-severity suicidal ideation. These brief bursts of intensive ideation are difficult to detect on screening but may serve as triggers that precipitate suicide attempts.[93]

Further, under investigation worldwide are internet use and playing video games for five or more hours daily. These online activities frequently lead to suicide-related searches, sometimes including views of prosuicide websites. Together, these web-based activities are predictive of elevated risks for suicidal behaviors and possible suicide completion.[97-99]

In response to the rising rates of adolescent suicide, the CDC has released a package of policies, programs, and practices on teen suicide prevention.[100] The comprehensive public health approach includes screening to identify youth at risk, lessening harms, intervening on risk factors using evidence-based programs, and promoting the constellation of protective behaviors, with special emphasis on connectedness. School-based programs are at the forefront.

SUMMARY

The life course approach focuses on the flow of health from the earliest years into later years. This chapter leads off with a discussion of what produces health and what threatens health during the period of fetal development, the moment of childbirth, the first year of life (infancy), and throughout the years of childhood, adolescence, and young adulthood through the age of 24 years.

Ideally, the perinatal period will be optimized by having the pregnant mother engaging in healthful behaviors, observing a nutritious diet, exercising regularly, getting restful sleep, avoiding use of harmful substances, and minimizing stressful exposures. Immediately following birth, breastfeeding confers health benefits to infant and mother alike. To acquire the skills for healthy development, children rely on an early life environment that provides the five domains of nurturing care: responsive caregiving, nutrition, early learning, safety and security, and health. If these elements are consistently provided, the child is likely to thrive, achieve and exceed developmental benchmarks, and grow in health.

Unfortunately, many children are deprived of nurturing care and instead face one or more of three salient threats to health: poverty, poor education, and ACEs. Fortunately, evidence-based interventions have been shown to promote child health and offset the detrimental effects of limited income and education and even exposure to ACEs. These interventions focus on family support and strengthening, caring for the caregiver, and prioritizing early learning and protection. These interventions can be customized and adapted for a variety of settings and cultures and can be scaled up for widespread dissemination.

The period of adolescence marks the emergence of the individual—identity formation—and the course can be smooth or not. The chances of experiencing a healthful adolescence that serves as a launchpad for a healthy adult life are greater for youth growing up in higher income nations than for those who live in multiburden or injury-excess nations. Effective interventions to optimize the health of adolescents differ by nation and culture, but draw upon available structural resources, media and social marketing, community settings, school venues, and health services.

End-of-Chapter Resources

 Access additional case study podcasts online at http://connect.springerpub.com/content/book/978-0-8261-8043-8/

DISCUSSION QUESTIONS

1. Education can be a great equalizer—in terms of health and opportunity for advancement—even for children who are born into disadvantage. In your home community, what strategies could be implemented to provide quality and equitable educational opportunities for children across the family income spectrum?

2. ACEs create a cascade of negative health consequences lifelong. Discuss your ideas for innovative interventions that could be implemented to prevent or diminish the impact of ACEs.

3. "The mission of the U.S. Department of Health and Human Services (HHS) is to enhance the health and well-being of all Americans."[101] However, HHS ran the shelters for immigrant children who were forcibly separated from their parents at the U.S. southern border and were therefore seen as "complicit" in these acts of child endangerment. How can HHS be true to its mission in situations in which political decisions endanger the public's health?

4. Although earliest experimentation may start in childhood, regular use of addictive substances (tobacco, alcohol, illicit and diverted prescription drugs) tends to solidify in adolescence. Recently, the use of electronic vapor products (e-cigarettes, vaping) has become increasingly popular. Given common beliefs about the relative safety of these products, despite the high level of nicotine content and addiction potential, how would you design an effective intervention to discourage experimentation and use of these products?

5. At any given time, some populations of adolescents and young adults are living in areas of active armed conflict or extreme poverty. Discuss how you would design programs to optimize the health of these populations of youth and young adults who are exposed to violence and disruption. Is this even possible?

 A robust set of instructor resources designed to supplement this text is located at **http://connect.springerpub.com/content/book/978-0-8261-8043-8**. Qualifying instructors may request access by emailing **textbook@springerpub.com**.

REFERENCES

1. Pan American Health Organization. *Building health throughout the life course.* 2019. https://www.paho.org/salud-en-las-americas-2017/pv-course.html#:~:text=In%20the%20life%20course%20approach,of%20society%20as%20a%20whole

2. *Advancing early childhood development: from science to scale.* An executive summary for the Lancet's series. Lancet. 2016. https://www.thelancet.com/pb-assets/Lancet/stories/series/ecd/Lancet_ECD_Executive_Summary.pdf

3. Imdad A, Bhutta ZA. Maternal nutrition and birth outcomes: effect of balanced protein-energy supplementation. *Paediatr Perinat Epidemiol.* 2012;26:178-190. doi:10.1111/j.1365-3016.2012.01308.x

4. Haider BA, Bhutta ZA. Multiple-micronutrient supplementation for women during pregnancy. *Cochrane Database Syst Rev.* 2015;*2015*(11):CD004905. doi:10.1002/14651858.CD004905.pub4

5. Imdad A, Yakoob MY, Bhutta ZA. The effect of folic acid, protein energy and multiple micronutrient supplements in pregnancy on stillbirths. *BMC Public Health.* 2011;*11*(suppl 3):S4. doi:10.1186/1471-2458-11-S3-S4

6. American Pregnancy Association. *Pregnancy vitamins and nutrients.* http://americanpregnancy.org/pregnancy-health/nutrients-vitamins-pregnancy

7. Peña-Rosas JP, De-Regil LM, Garcia-Casal MN, Dowswell T. Daily oral iron supplementation during pregnancy. *Cochrane Database Syst Rev.* 2015;*2015*(7):CD004736. doi:10.1002/14651858.CD004736.pub5

8. Hollis BW, Johnson D, Hulsey TC, et al. Vitamin D supplementation during pregnancy: double-blind, randomized clinical trial of safety and effectiveness. *J Bone Miner Res.* 2011;*26*(10):2341-2357. doi:10.1002/jbmr.463

9. Stein A, Pearson RM, Goodman SH, et al. Effects of perinatal mental disorders on the fetus and child. *Lancet.* 2014;*384*(9956):1800-1819. doi:10.1016/S0140-6736(14)61277-0

10. Shah K, Krupa M. *Migrants picked this pregnant mother of 2 to go to the front of the asylum line.* CNN. Published May 1, 2018. https://www.cnn.com/2018/05/01/americas/mom-migrant-caravan-asylum/index.html

11. Jensen L, ed. *The Sustainable Development Goals Report 2021.* United Nations; 2021. https://unstats.un.org/sdgs/report/2021/The-Sustainable-Development-Goals-Report-2021.pdf

12. Victora CG, Lessa Horta B, Loret De Mola C, et al. Association between breastfeeding and intelligence, educational attainment, and income at 30 years of age: a prospective birth cohort study from Brazil. *Lancet Glob Health.* 2015;*3*(4):c199-c205. doi:10.1016/S2214-109X(15)70002-1

13. Grantham-McGregor S, Cheung YB, Cueto S, et al. Child development in developing countries 1: developmental potential in the first 5 years for children in developing countries. *Lancet.* 2007;*369*:60-70. https://www.thelancet.com/pdfs/journals/lancet/PIIS0140-6736(07)60032-4.pdf

14. Bradley RH, Corwyn RF. Socioeconomic status and child development. *Annu Rev Psychol.* 2002;*53*(1): 371-399. doi:10.1146/annurev.psych.53.100901.135233

15. Paxson C, Schady N. *Cognitive Development Among Young Children in Ecuador: The Roles of Wealth, Health and Parenting.* World Bank; 2005. doi:10.1596/1813-9450-3605

16. Baker-Henningham H, Powell C, Walker S, Grantham-McGregor S. Mothers of undernourished Jamaican children have poorer psychosocial functioning and this is associated with stimulation provided in the home. *Eur J Clin Nutr.* 2003;*57*(6):786-792. doi:10.1038/sj.ejcn.1601611

17. No Isolation. *How does social isolation affect a child's mental health and development?* Published June 21, 2017. https://www.noisolation.com/global/research/how-does-social-isolation-affect-a-childs-mental-health-and-development

18. Lacey RE, Kumari M, Bartley M. Social isolation in childhood and adult inflammation: evidence from the national child development study. *Psychoneuroendocrinology.* 2014;*50*:85-94. doi:10.1016/j.psyneuen.2014.08.007

19. Shaw JA, Espinel Z, Shultz JM. *Care of Children Exposed to the Traumatic Effects of Disaster.* American Psychiatric Association Publishing; 2012.

20. Sandstrom H, Huerta S. *The Negative Effects of Instability on Child Development: A Research Synthesis.* Urban Institute; 2013. https://www.urban.org/sites/default/files/publication/32706/412899-The-Negative-Effects-of-Instability-on-Child-Development-A-Research-Synthesis.PDF

21. Stafford F, Chiteji N. Shaping health behavior across generations: evidence from time use data in the panel study of income dynamics and its supplements. *Ann Econ Stat.* 2012;*105*:185-208. http://www.ncbi.nlm.nih.gov/pubmed/24443703

22. Webley P, Nyhus EK. Parents' influence on children's future orientation and saving. *J Econ Psychol.* 2006;*27*(1):140-164.

23. Black MM, Walker SP, Fernald LCH, et al. Early childhood development coming of age: science through the life course. *Lancet.* 2017;*389*(10064):77-90. doi:10.1016/S0140-6736(16)31389-7

24. Sameroff AJ, ed. *The Transactional Model of Development: How Children and Contexts Shape Each Other.* American Psychological Association; 2009.

25. Britto PR, Lye SJ, Proulx K, et al. Nurturing care: promoting early childhood development. *Lancet.* 2017;*389*(10064):91-102. doi:10.1016/S0140-6736(16)31390-3

26. Black MM, Aboud FE. Responsive feeding is embedded in a theoretical framework of responsive parenting. *J Nutr.* 2011;*141*(3):490-494. doi:10.3945/JN.110.129973

27. Singla DR, Kumbakumba E, Aboud FE. Effects of a parenting intervention to address maternal psychological wellbeing and child development and growth in rural Uganda: a community-based, cluster-randomised trial. *Lancet Glob Health.* 2015;*3*(8):e458-e469. doi:10.1016/S2214-109X(15)00099-6

28. Bradley RH, Putnick DL. Housing quality and access to material and learning resources within the home environment in developing countries. *Child Dev.* 2012;*83*(1):76-91. doi:10.1111/j.1467-8624.2011.01674.x

29. Shonkoff JP, Phillips DA. *From Neurons to Neighborhoods: The Science of Early Childhood Development.* National Academies Press; 2000. doi:10.17226/9824

30. Grossman M. On the concept of health capital and the demand for health. *J Polit Econ.* 1972;*80*(2):223-255. https://pdfs.semanticscholar.org/e656/466bba4f898ad560498998639eb147f62396.pdf

31. Patton GC, Sawyer SM, Santelli JS, et al. Our future: a Lancet commission on adolescent health and wellbeing. *Lancet.* 2016;*387*(10036):2423-2478. doi:10.1016/S0140-6736(16)00579-1

32. Nussbaum MC. *Creating Capabilities the Human Development Approach.* Belknap Press; 2011.

33. Blakemore SJ, Mills KL. Is adolescence a sensitive period for sociocultural processing? *Annu Rev Psychol.* 2014;*65*(1):187-207. doi:10.1146/annurev-psych-010213-115202

34. Andersen SL, Teicher MH. Stress, sensitive periods and maturational events in adolescent depression. *Trends Neurosci.* 2008;*31*(4):183-191. doi:10.1016/j.tins.2008.01.004

35. Viner RM, Ozer EM, Denny S, et al. Adolescence and the social determinants of health. *Lancet.* 2012;*379*(9826):1641-1652. doi:10.1016/S0140-6736(12)60149-4

36. Crone EA, Dahl RE. Understanding adolescence as a period of social–affective engagement and goal flexibility. *Nat Rev Neurosci.* 2012;*13*(9):636-650. doi:10.1038/nrn3313

37. Patton GC, Coffey C, Cappa C, et al. Health of the world's adolescents: a synthesis of internationally comparable data. *Lancet.* 2012;*379*(9826):1665-1675. doi:10.1016/S0140-6736(12)60203-7

38. DiIorio C, Kelley M, Hockenberry-Eaton M. Communication about sexual issues: mothers, fathers, and friends. *J Adolesc Health.* 1999;*24*(3):181-189. doi:10.1016/S1054-139X(98)00115-3

39. Fall CHD, Osmond C, Haazen DS, et al. Disadvantages of having an adolescent mother. *Lancet Glob Health.* 2016;*4*(11):e787-e788. doi:10.1016/S2214-109X(16)30263-7

40. Central Intelligence Agency. *The World Factbook 2016-17.* 2016. https://www.cia.gov/the-world-factbook/

41. Mathews TJ, Driscoll AK. Data Brief 279: trends in infant mortality in the United States, 2005–2014. *NCHS Data Brief.* 2017;*279*:1-8. https://www.cdc.gov/nchs/data/databriefs/db279_table.pdf#1

42. Roser M. *Child and infant mortality.* Our world in data. 2019. https://ourworldindata.org/child-mortality

43. Engle PL, Black MM. The effect of poverty on child development and educational outcomes. *Ann N Y Acad Sci.* 2008;*1136*(1):243-256. doi:10.1196/annals.1425.023

44. Centers for Disease Control and Prevention. *Youth Risk Behavior Surveillance System (YRBSS).* www.cdc.gov/yrbs

45. Centers for Disease Control and Prevention. *Tobacco use and United States students.* 2016. https://www.cdc.gov/healthyyouth/data/yrbs/pdf/2015/2015_US_Tobacco.pdf

46. Centers for Disease Control and Prevention. *Trends in the prevalence of tobacco use: national YRBS: 1991–2015.* 2016. https://www.cdc.gov/healthyyouth/data/yrbs/pdf/trends/2015_us_tobacco_trend_yrbs.pdf

47. Ortved J. *That cloud of smoke is not a mirage: cigarettes, once shunned, have made a comeback with a younger crowd who knows better.* New York Times. Published January 12, 2022. https://www.nytimes.com/2022/01/12/style/smoking-cigarettes-comeback.html

48. Centers for Disease Control and Prevention. *Current cigarette smoking among adults in the United States.* https://www.cdc.gov/tobacco/data_statistics/fact_sheets/adult_data/cig_smoking/index.htm#references

49. American Lung Association. *Overall tobacco trends.* https://www.lung.org/research/trends-in-lung-disease/tobacco-trends-brief/overall-tobacco-trends#

50. Centers for Disease Control and Prevention. *E-cigarette, or vaping, products visual dictionary.* https://www.cdc.gov/tobacco/basic_information/e-cigarettes/pdfs/ecigarette-or-vaping-products-visual-dictionary-508.pdf

51. Collins L, Glasser AM, Abudayyeh H, Pearson JL, Villanti AC. E-Cigarette marketing and communication: how e-cigarette companies market e-cigarettes and the public engages with e-cigarette information. *Nicotine Tob Res.* 2019;*21*(1):14-24. doi:10.1093/ntr/ntx284

52. Duke JC, Allen JA, Eggers ME, Nonnemaker J, Farrelly MC. Exploring differences in youth perceptions of the effectiveness of electronic cigarette television advertisements. *Nicotine Tob Res.* 2016;*18*(5):1382-1386. doi:10.1093/ntr/ntv264

53. Farrelly MC, Duke JC, Crankshaw EC, et al. A randomized trial of the effect of e-cigarette TV advertisements on intentions to use e-cigarettes. *Am J Prev Med.* 2015;*49*(5):686-693. doi:10.1016/j.amepre.2015.05.010

54. Centers for Disease Control and Prevention. *Outbreak of lung injury associated with the use of e-cigarette, or vaping, products.* https://www.cdc.gov/tobacco/basic_information/e-cigarettes/severe-lung-disease.html#overview

55. Baenziger ON, Ford L, Yazidjoglou A, Joshy G, Banks E. E-cigarette use and combustible tobacco cigarette smoking uptake among non-smokers, including relapse in former smokers: umbrella review, systematic review and meta-analysis. *BMJ Open.* 2021;*11*(3):e045603. doi:10.1136/bmjopen-2020-045603

56. Samuels M. *Teens who vape are more likely to start smoking.* Boston University. Published February 1, 2019. https://www.bu.edu/sph/news/articles/2019/teens-who-vape-are-more-likely-to-start-smoking/

57. Berry KM, Fetterman JL, Benjamin EJ, et al. Association of electronic cigarette use with subsequent initiation of tobacco cigarettes in US youths. *JAMA Netw Open.* 2019;*2*(2):e187794. doi:10.1001/jamanetworkopen.2018.7794

58. Kandel D, Kandel E. The gateway hypothesis of substance abuse: developmental, biological and societal perspectives. *Acta Paediatr.* 2015;*104*(2):130-137. doi:10.1111/apa.12851

59. Grant JE, Lust K, Fridberg DJ, King AC, Chamberlain SR. E-cigarette use (vaping) is associated with illicit drug use, mental health problems, and impulsivity in university students. *Ann Clin Psychiatry.* 2019;*31*(1):27-35.

60. Miech R, Johnston L, O'Malley PM, Bachman JG, Patrick ME. Trends in adolescent vaping, 2017-2019. *N Engl J Med.* 2019;*381*(15):1490-1491. doi:10.1056/NEJMc1910739

61. Miech R, Leventhal A, Johnston L, O'Malley PM, Patrick ME, Barrington-Trimis J. Trends in use and perceptions of nicotine vaping among US youth from 2017 to 2020 [published correction appears in JAMA Pediatr. 2021 Mar 1;175(3):328]. *JAMA Pediatr.* 2021;*175*(2):185-190.

62. CDC Foundation. *Monitoring U.S. e-cigarette sales: national trends data brief.* Published April 17, 2022. https://www.cdcfoundation.org/National-E-CigaretteSales-DataBrief-2022-April17?inline

63. Centers for Disease Control and Prevention. *Trends in the Prevalence of Behaviors that Contribute to Violence on School Property National YRBS: 1991–2019.* https://www.cdc.gov/healthyyouth/data/yrbs/factsheets/2019_violence_school_property_trend_yrbs.htm

64. World Health Organization. *Adolescent and young adult health.* Published December 13, 2018. https://www.who.int/en/news-room/fact-sheets/detail/adolescents-health-risks-and-solutions

65. National Institute of Mental Health. *Mental illness.* Updated February 2019. https://www.nimh.nih.gov/health/statistics/mental-illness.shtml

66. Ahrnsbrak R, Bose J, Hedden SL, et al. *Key Substance Use and Mental Health Indicators in the United States: Results from the 2016 National Survey on Drug Use and Health.* Center for Behavioral Health Statistics and Quality, Substance Abuse and Mental Health Services Administration; 2017.

67. National Institute of Mental Health. *Major depression.* Updated February 2019. https://www.nimh.nih.gov/health/statistics/major-depression.shtml

68. Jones SE, Ethier KA, Hertz M, et al. Mental health, suicidality, and connectedness among high school students during the COVID-19 pandemic–adolescent behaviors and experiences survey, United States, January-June 2021. *MMWR Suppl.* 2022;*71*(3):16-21. doi:10.15585/mmwr.su7103a3

69. Rico A, Brener ND, Thornton J, et al. Overview and methodology of the adolescent behaviors and experiences survey–United States, January-June 2021. *MMWR Suppl.* 2022;*71*(3):1-7. doi:10.15585/mmwr.su7103a1

70. Panchal N, Kamal R, Cox C, Garfield R, Chidambaram P. *Issue Brief: Mental Health and Substance Use Considerations Among Children During the COVID-19 Pandemic.* KFF; 2021. https://www.kff.org/coronavirus-covid-19/issue-brief/mental-health-and-substance-use-considerations-among-children-during-the-covid-19-pandemic/

71. Czeisler MÉ, Lane RI, Petrosky E, et al. Mental health, substance use, and suicidal ideation during the COVID-19 pandemic–United States, June 24-30, 2020. *MMWR Morb Mortal Wkly Rep.* 2020;*69*(32):1049-1057. doi:10.15585/mmwr.mm6932a1

72. Ettman CK, Abdalla SM, Cohen GH, Sampson L, Vivier PM, Galea S. Prevalence of depression symptoms in US adults before and during the COVID-19 pandemic. *JAMA Netw Open.* 2020;*3*(9):e2019686. doi:10.1001/jamanetworkopen.2020.19686

73. Abdalla SM, Ettman CK, Cohen GH, Galea S. Mental health consequences of COVID-19: a nationally representative cross-sectional study of pandemic-related stressors and anxiety disorders in the USA. *BMJ Open.* 2021;*11*(8):e044125. doi:10.1136/bmjopen-2020-044125

74. Ettman CK, Cohen GH, Abdalla SM, et al. Assets, stressors, and symptoms of persistent depression over the first year of the COVID-19 pandemic. *Sci Adv.* 2022;*8*(9):eabm9737. doi:10.1126/sciadv.abm9737

75. Lee H. *Why Finnish babies sleep in cardboard boxes. BBC News.* June 4, 2013. https://www.bbc.com/news/magazine-22751415

76. American Public Health Association. *Separating parents and children at US border is inhumane and sets the stage for a public health crisis.* Published June 15, 2018. https://docs.house.gov/meetings/IF/IF14/20180627/108510/HMKP-115-IF14-20180627-SD016.pdf

77. O'Reilly KB. *Doctors oppose policy that splits kids from caregivers at border.* American Medical Association. Published June 13, 2018. https://www.ama-assn.org/delivering-care/population-care/doctors-oppose-policy-splits-kids-caregivers-border

78. O'Connor L. *President of American academy of pediatrics calls Trump border policy "child abuse." Huffington Post.* June 18, 2018. https://www.huffpost.com/entry/pediatrics-academy-border-separation-child-abuse_n_5b27f437e4b0783ae12bfe6d

79. The American Psychiatric Association. *APA statement opposing separation of children from parents at the border.* Published May 30, 2018. https://docs.house.gov/meetings/IF/IF14/20180719/108572/HHRG-115-IF14-20180719-SD005.pdf

80. Wagner KD. *President's statement: separating children from families.* American Academy of Child and Adolescent Psychiatry. Published May 2018. https://www.aacap.org/AACAP/Latest_News/2014/President_Statement_Separating_Children.aspx

81. American Psychological Association. *Statement of APA president regarding the traumatic effects of separating immigrant families.* Published May 29, 2018. https://www.apa.org/news/press/releases/2018/05/separating-immigrant-families.aspx

82. Amnesty International. *Amnesty USA reaction to government report on family separations.* Published January 17, 2019. https://www.amnestyusa.org/press-releases/amnesty-usa-reaction-to-government-report-on-family-separations

83. Amnesty International. *USA: "you don't have any rights here."* https://www.amnesty.org/en/latest/research/2018/10/usa-treatment-of-asylum-seekers-southern-border

84. Sandoval E, Jordan M, Mazzei P, Goodman JD. *The story behind DeSantis's migrant flights to Martha's Vineyard. The New York Times.* Published October 2, 2022. https://www.nytimes.com/2022/10/02/us/migrants-marthas-vineyard-desantis-texas.html

85. Catalano RF, Fagan AA, Gavin LE, et al. Worldwide application of prevention science in adolescent health. *Lancet.* 2012;379(9826):1653-1664. doi:10.1016/S0140-6736(12)60238-4

86. Fagan AA, Catalano RF. What works in youth violence prevention: a review of the literature. *Res Soc Work Pract.* 2013;23(2):141-156. doi:10.1177/1049731512465899

87. PBS NewsHour. *Last school year, 4 million students were on lockdown. [Video].* Published January 27, 2019. https://www.youtube.com/watch?v=tdQJMZLcbbo

88. Centers for Disease Control and Prevention. *Leading causes of death reports, 1981-2020.* https://wisqars.cdc.gov/fatal-leading

89. *Centers for Disease Control and Prevention.* Suicide and Self-Harm Injury. https://www.cdc.gov/nchs/fastats/suicide.htm

90. Hedegaard H, Curtin SC, Warner M. Suicide rates in the United States continue to increase. *NCHS Data Brief.* 2018; 309:1-8. https://www.cdc.gov/nchs/data/databriefs/db309_table.pdf#2

91. Taliaferro LA, Muehlenkamp JJ. Risk and protective factors that distinguish adolescents who attempt suicide from those who only consider suicide in the past year. *Suicide Life Threat Behav.* 2014;44(1):6-22. doi:10.1111/sltb.12046

92. Klomek AB, Sourander A, Gould M. The association of suicide and bullying in childhood to young adulthood: a review of cross-sectional and longitudinal research findings. *Can J Psychiatry.* 2010;55(5):282-288. doi:10.1177/070674371005500503

93. Bloch MH. Editorial: reducing adolescent suicide. *J Child Psychol Psychiatry.* 2016;57(7):773-774. doi:10.1111/jcpp.12585

94. Glenn CR, Kleiman EM, Cha CB, et al. Implicit cognition about self-injury predicts actual self-injurious behavior: results from a longitudinal study of adolescents. *J Child Psychol Psychiatry.* 2016;57(7): 805-813. doi:10.1111/jcpp.12500

95. Klonsky ED, Victor SE, Saffer BY. Nonsuicidal self-injury: what we know, and what we need to know. *Can J Psychiatry.* 2014;59(11):565-568. doi:10.1177/070674371405901101

96. Glenn CR, Lanzillo EC, Esposito EC, et al. Examining the course of suicidal and nonsuicidal self-injurious thoughts and behaviors in outpatient and inpatient adolescents. *J Abnorm Child Psychol.* 2017;45(5):971-983. doi:10.1007/s10802-016-0214-0

97. Shain B. Committee on adolescence. Suicide and suicide attempts in adolescents. *Pediatrics.* 2016;138(1):e20161420. doi:10.1542/peds.2016-1420

98. Durkee T, Hadlaczky G, Westerlund M, Carli V. Internet pathways in suicidality: a review of the evidence. *Int J Environ Res Public Health.* 2011;8(10):3938-3952. doi:10.3390/ijerph8103938

99. Messias E, Castro J, Saini A, et al. Sadness, suicide, and their association with video game and internet overuse among teens: results from the youth risk behavior survey 2007 and 2009. *Suicide Life Threat Behav.* 2011;41(3):307-315. doi:10.1111/j.1943-278X.2011.00030.x

100. Stone D, Holland K, Bartholow B, et al. *Preventing Suicide: A Technical Package of Policy, Programs, and Practices.* National Center for Injury Prevention and Control, Centers for Disease Control and Prevention; 2019. https://www.cdc.gov/violenceprevention/pdf/suicideTechnicalPackage.pdf

101. *U.S. Department of Health and Human Services.* https://www.hhs.gov/about/strategic-plan/2022-2026/introduction/index.html

10

ADULTHOOD

LEARNING OBJECTIVES

- Outline the three roles and responsibilities of adulthood that shape current and future health patterns and trends.

- Describe the relationship of income and education to the production of health and disease.

- Summarize the complex interrelationships among risk factors that together predict the likelihood of future disability and mortality from noncommunicable diseases (NCDs) during adulthood and beyond.

- Appraise the burden of nonfatal disease that is primarily concentrated in the adult years in relation to the social ecological levels using the example of depression.

- Explain the multigenerational set of responsibilities taken on by the adult "sandwich" generation.

OVERVIEW: HEALTH DURING THE ADULT YEARS

We now focus on adulthood. The period of adulthood extends across four decades, equivalent to half of the human life span. We principally examine adults ages 25 to 64 years, although the discussion sometimes focuses on ages that reach back into younger adult years ("emerging adulthood") or extend forward into later decades of life. The adult years represent critical transitions in terms of roles and responsibilities in three interrelated areas, all of which carry implications for health. These areas are (a) developing skills and contributing productively to one's community, (b) partnering and parenting, and (c) living a lifestyle that optimizes health and well-being throughout the adult years.

In this chapter, we (a) examine the health challenges of adulthood, from emerging adulthood to the mid-60s, including the cumulative effects of unhealthy behavior and exposures, (b) explore how public health can mitigate these threats, and (c) provide successful examples of public health efforts to improve health through action in emerging adulthood and adult life.

TRANSITIONS AND IMPLICATIONS FOR HEALTH

GENERATING INCOME AND CONTRIBUTING TO THE PRODUCTIVITY OF SOCIETY

The first thing adulthood represents is a period of peak productivity. This is the period for generating income so that adults can support themselves and their family's economic needs. In turn, individual output contributes to population prosperity. Adult years also represent a period for creative and inventive contributions. Individuals create their legacies in their productive adult years more than in any other period of life.

Populations are largely dependent on the economic output of the adult workforce. Adults straddle and provide economic and instrumental support for three generations. It is not uncommon for adults in their 40s and 50s to simultaneously provide financially for their aging parents, their growing children, and themselves, a situation that has led these adults to be described as the "sandwich" generation.

Throughout this chapter, we examine the bidirectional health–wealth relationship, showing how health increases productivity and how the output of productive work, notably income and wealth accumulation, influences health.

PARTNERING AND PARENTING

The second thing adulthood represents is a period for forming long-term partnerships, creating families, and child-rearing. In terms of raising a family, the health of adult mothers is especially critical to the health of their newborns and young children. Adult parents are centrally the providers of nurturing care that is essential for healthy child development. Parents largely determine the health of their children's environment, and simultaneously, they role model and impart health behaviors to their children.

LIFESTYLE BEHAVIORS AND THE EMERGENCE OF CHRONIC DISEASES

Third, in the chronology of the life course, adulthood is the longest life period. Throughout life, individuals make health-promoting or health-compromising behavioral choices, sometimes on a moment-by-moment basis (e.g., buckling the seat belt) and sometimes on a habitual basis (e.g., eating a healthful diet). Health-influencing choices, at individual and community levels, shape health and disease states, going forward throughout the adult, as well as older adult, life phases.

From a life course perspective, adults in their mid-20s and 30s generally enjoy relatively disease-free good health and low mortality. This age cohort has successfully navigated through the higher mortality first years of life and the higher risk adolescent years.

However, how adults in their 20s and 30s live, and the behavioral choices they make, sets currents in motion that will mold future health throughout the remainder of their adult years. Lifestyle behaviors include such fundamentals as daily dietary and physical activity choices. Over years and decades of adulthood, lifestyle behaviors modify human physiology and affect organ systems. At the population level, social determinants of health, interacting with habitual lifestyle behaviors, as practiced by adults in the community, influence the health and disease states that come increasingly to the forefront with increasing age.

If health-promoting behaviors are adopted and embraced by adults in the community and supported by systems, structures, and policies at the community, state, and national levels, these adults can look forward to ongoing vibrant health throughout their adult years, continuing into older adulthood. In the most literal sense, time will tell. Indeed, during the later decades of the adult years, especially for persons in their 50s and early 60s, the cumulative and residual effects of their lifelong behavioral choices, individually and collectively, coupled with environmental exposures, become outwardly manifest in terms of continued health or emerging disease.

In populations in which many individuals adopt health-compromising choices, these behaviors transform into diagnosable clinical disorders and disease conditions within a few short decades. Two examples illustrate this point. First, consider how the mass marketing and adoption of the wildly popular new product of the early 1900s, the tobacco cigarette, not only propelled lung cancer from obscurity to prominence (as the leading cancer killer of Americans) but actually created a new disease, chronic obstructive pulmonary disease (COPD), now more commonly referred to as chronic lower respiratory disease (CLRD). The point is that COPD/CLRD was unidentified, unnamed, and virtually nonexistent before the cigarette came on the market; now COPD/CLRD ranks high among leading causes of death in the United States and globally.

> **In populations in which many individuals adopt health-compromising choices, these behaviors transform into diagnosable clinical disorders and disease conditions within a few short decades.**

Second, consider the situation in Russia where more than 30% of all-cause mortality is attributable to alcohol consumption, prompting one journalist to write, "Russia is quite literally drinking itself to death."[1] No other country comes close to this level of alcohol-induced disease burden. Not only does alcohol-related premature mortality occur at exceedingly high rates, but the signature feature of drinking behavior in Russia is excessive consumption of vodka.[2]

ADULT LIFE ROLES AND HEALTH

Adulthood comes laden with life roles and responsibilities. These include the three transitional areas just described, each of which can be described in terms of responsibilities. Adulthood is a time of (a) becoming financially responsible and productive, (b) being responsible for others as a partner and parent (taking care of spouse, partner, children, or parents), and (c) being responsible for self and personal health–related actions that will define the contours of personal and community health and well-being.[3]

In the following sections, we delve more deeply into some of the forces that ultimately produce health in adulthood, building upon a lifetime of experience.

HEALTH IN RELATION TO THE RESPONSIBILITIES OF ADULTHOOD

ADULTHOOD AS A PERIOD FOR MAXIMUM PRODUCTIVITY AND WAGE GENERATION: HEALTH IMPLICATIONS

Adulthood is the period of life characterized by entry into the workforce or a profession, occupational advancement, wage generation, and productive contribution to society. At the front end of this process is what some researchers have described as an interceding life phase, "emerging adulthood," extending across the curious age range of 18 to 29 years.[4] Based on the life course periods presented here, emerging adulthood overlaps with the latter portion of young adulthood and the first years of what we describe as adulthood.[5] Emerging adulthood represents a newly defined life phase characterized by accepting responsibilities, taking on new roles, making in-dependent decisions, and achieving a degree of self-sufficiency.[6] Emerging adulthood varies by culture and is most clearly observable in high-income countries.

Not unlike adolescence, emerging adulthood is also a time of transition, but the tasks here are different. Many emerging adults complete their educational and practical preparations that form a foundation for the rest of their lives. This may entail vocational studies or graduate-level education, specialized training, and professional internships. Emerging adulthood represents a precarious time of considerable stress and instability as individuals enter the workforce, trying on first jobs and new occupational roles with variable degrees of success.

> **Not unlike adolescence, emerging adulthood is also a time of transition, but the tasks here are different.**

Income Production and Health Correlates

Income and socioeconomic status (SES) are among the most thoroughly researched social de-terminants of health (SDOH—see Chapter 4, "At the Heart of Public Health: Social Determi-nants of Health and Health Equity").[7] This research reveals that there is an unequal world out there for adults who are shouldering their occupational and parenting roles, and this results in the transmission of advantage, or disadvantage, over generations. Social disadvantage creates a "health gap" for those adults who occupy lower SES strata.[8] The Millennium Cohort Study demonstrated that social conditions that either support or impede parenting affect both the adults who are actively engaged in raising their children and their children's own developmen-tal potential.[9] Even parents who engage in positive parenting practices cannot fully overcome the detrimental effects of social disadvantage on child development.[10] This means, in practical terms, that the social gradient that caps the parents' upward mobility most often gets passed down to their children.

In terms of earning a living, health is critical for maximizing adult output and productivity. The relationship between health and income generation is bidirectional.[11] First, persons who en-joy good health generally are able to earn more income. Second, increased income is associated with lower rates of disease, disability, and premature death.[12] Third, persons with higher income levels have better health across a range of indicators than those who have lower incomes.[13] Fourth, health status is influenced by both income (annual earnings and other money acquired) and wealth (net worth and assets).[14] Fifth, lower income is a social determinant of poor health and a risk factor for early death.[15]

For example, in the United States, there is a clear relationship between income and self-reported health.[16] Simply summarized, persons with lower incomes are much more likely to report poor health than those with higher incomes, who report less psychological distress, sadness, hopelessness, and worthlessness.

As another example, the prevalence of a wide range of noncommunicable diseases (NCDs) that are common in adults and older adults is demonstrably higher in lower income households (**Table 10.1**). This is plainly illustrated in the U.S. National Health Interview Survey findings.[11,16] The prevalence of multiple leading causes of disease and death in the United States is 50% to 100% higher for families with an annual income below $35,000 compared to those with in-comes of $100,000 or more. These findings take on added importance as the wealth gap in the United States progressively widens.

Similarly, the rates of various types of difficulties in physical functioning are strongly associ-ated with income (**Table 10.2**).[11,16] The lower the family income, the higher the proportion of

DISEASE OR ILLNESS	HOUSEHOLD INCOME				
	<$35,000	$35,000–49,999	$50,000–74,999	$75,000–99,999	$100,000 OR MORE
Coronary heart disease	8.1	6.5	6.3	5.3	4.9
Stroke	3.9	2.5	2.3	1.8	1.6
Emphysema	3.2	2.5	1.4	1.0	0.8
Chronic bronchitis	6.3	4.0	4.4	2.2	2.4
Diabetes	11.0	10.4	8.3	5.6	5.9
Ulcers	8.7	6.7	6.5	4.7	4.4
Kidney disease	3.0	1.9	1.3	0.9	0.9
Liver disease	2.0	1.6	1.0	0.6	0.7
Chronic arthritis	33.4	30.3	27.9	27.4	24.4
Hearing trouble	17.2	16.0	16.0	16.2	12.4
Vision trouble	12.7	9.8	7.5	5.7	6.6
No teeth	11.6	7.8	5.5	4.2	4.1

TABLE 10.1 Prevalence of Diseases by Income: Percentage of Adults, United States, 2011

Source: Adapted from Woolf SH, Aron LY, Dubay L, et al. *How Are Income and Wealth Linked to Health and Longevity?* Urban Institute; 2015. https://www.urban.org/research/publication/how-are-income-and-wealth-linked-health-and-longevity; National Center for Health Statistics. *Vital and Health Statistics Report.* U.S. Department of Health and Human Services, Centers for Disease Control and Prevention; 2012. https://www.cdc.gov/nchs/data/series/sr_10/sr10_256.pdf

persons who experience significant difficulty performing a range of physical and motor skills that are important for independent activities of daily living. Rates of physical difficulties are two to four times higher among those with incomes below $35,000 as compared to those with incomes of $100,000 or more.

Income and wealth are key determinants of individual and population health. Several mechanisms influence this relationship. First, persons with lower income are much less able to access and pay for quality health services or establish an ongoing long-term relationship with a primary care provider. Second, many do not have health insurance and those who do may lack comprehensive coverage. By default, many rely on using the local ED in lieu of seeking primary care consultations. Third, persons living in poverty are much less likely to receive preventive care, including prenatal care for expectant mothers during pregnancy. Fourth, persons in lower SES strata face a range of health-compromising hardships and barriers, and their home and neighborhood environments are often hazardous to health.[11]

TABLE 10.2 Prevalence of Difficulties in Physical Functioning by Income: Percentage of Adults, United States, 2011

ACTIVITIES THAT ARE VERY DIFFICULT OR IMPOSSIBLE TO PERFORM	HOUSEHOLD INCOME				
	<$35,000	$35,000–49,999	$50,000–74,999	$75,000–99,999	$100,000 OR MORE
Any physical activity	24.5	16.6	12.6	9.6	8.7
Walking one-quarter mile	12.5	7.0	5.5	4.1	3.9
Climbing 10 steps	9.6	4.9	3.7	2.7	2.8
Standing for 2 hours	15.7	9.6	7.1	4.9	5.0
Sitting for 2 hours	6.2	3.3	2.0	1.6	1.1
Stooping, bending, kneeling	14.4	9.5	7.4	5.1	4.7
Grasping/handling small objects	3.1	1.7	1.5	1.2	0.9
Lifting/carrying 10 pounds	8.4	3.8	2.6	2.2	2.1
Pushing/pulling large objects	11.8	6.4	4.5	3.6	3.5

Source: Adapted from Woolf SH, Aron LY, Dubay L, et al. *How Are Income and Wealth Linked to Health and Longevity?* Urban Institute; 2015. https://www.urban.org/research/publication/how-are-income-and-wealth-linked-health-and -longevity; National Center for Health Statistics. *Vital and Health Statistics Report.* U.S. Department of Health and Human Services, Centers for Disease Control and Prevention; 2012. https://www.cdc.gov/nchs/data/series/sr_10/sr10_256.pdf

Meanwhile, persons who enjoy a comfortable level of income and wealth have the financial wherewithal to afford healthy lifestyles. They live in home and neighborhood environments that are conducive to health.

Income and Habitual Diet

Eating a healthy, nutritious diet is foundational for achieving peak health and longevity. However, persons living in low-income settings have minimal access to healthy foods. Poor neighborhoods often lack supermarkets with an affordable and varied selection of fresh fruits and vegetables, lean protein sources, and high-fiber foods. By default, residents in low-SES neighborhoods are forced to patronize food outlets that are available nearby. They typically face a limited food selection characterized by processed foods that are overpriced, calorie-rich, and nutrient-poor.

Income and Physical Activity

The contrast in available health-promoting options extends to physical activity. Persons with lower income are geographically constrained to live in places that are both unhealthy and unsafe. Those with higher incomes can afford health club memberships and live in neighborhoods with safe outdoor green spaces that are well-suited to recreation, walking, cycling, exercise, and sports. Moreover, those with higher incomes are able to afford stable, well-constructed housing in safer neighborhoods with lower levels of pollution, wastes, physical hazards, and crime.

Income and Access to Education

Education provides a potential escape route from poverty and can be an equalizer for future opportunities, with life course implications for health. Educational attainment is itself a strong predictor of health and well-being, even apart from income.[17] Yet, here too there are major inequities in educational opportunities and achievement related to the incomes of the adult generation.[18] The major distinction based on SES is the ability of adults with higher income to send their children to higher quality, college-oriented schools where there is a healthy social environment and minimal student exposure to violence. These schools often have well-prepared and experienced faculty and offer a wide range of elective classes. Many student peers are high-achieving, motivated, and on the path toward higher education. A healthy school environment potentiates academic success which, in turn, tends to shield youth from engaging in substance abuse and other problem behaviors.

As a powerful lesson from the life course perspective that speaks volumes about health inequities, productive, economically successful adults are able to provide advantageous opportunities for their children and transmit health to the next generation. Conversely, adults with lower incomes are less able to produce viable options for their children to generate health. The interconnectedness of income and education provides a compelling illustration of the complex nature of the health-shaping nature of the SDOH.

CHALLENGES AND THREATS TO HEALTH DURING ADULTHOOD

ADULTS WITH FAMILY RESPONSIBILITIES: HEALTH IMPLICATIONS

Adulthood is the period for pairing and parenting and child-rearing. Individuals differ considerably on giving priority to forming long-term, exclusive relationships. During emerging adulthood, many individuals continue to form a range of friendships. School and work environments are particularly well-suited for enlarging social networks.

Many emerging adults begin or continue to explore their sexuality, often without forming committed relationships. During their 20s and 30s, and beyond, many adults move through a series of dating situations. These vary in duration, seriousness, commitment, and stability. This is a life phase that is notable for elevated risks for sexually transmitted infections (STIs) and unplanned pregnancies. Sexual risk relates to having encounters with multiple partners, experimenting with risky sexual behaviors, using protection inconsistently, and failing to negotiate effectively for safer practices. Many adults who know they are HIV-positive or currently infected with another transmissible STI do not disclose this critical information to a prospective sexual partner.

Ultimately, many adults do find a partner with whom they create a long-term exclusive relationship that may be formalized by marriage or another recognized union. A high proportion of these coupled individuals will move on to starting a family, assuming parenting roles, and raising children.

In the child-rearing role, adults are the primary caregivers, ideally delivering the nurturing care for the next generation of young children and later providing guidance to optimize healthy and wise decision-making for their adolescent children. Therefore, the parents who populate the current adult generation are chronologically situated to launch and foster the developmental, educational, and career paths of their children. These adult parenting roles and responsibilities, if fulfilled capably, will favorably influence the health of the generation that follows.

GRAPPLING WITH THE BURDEN OF STRESS DURING ADULTHOOD

It is important to realize that the tasks that mark the first years of adulthood, taking on and filling occupational and parental roles, are not just milestones in the life course, they are also imperative for species survival. Passing on these responsibilities to each successive generation is how life and health are maintained for populations and cultures. Adult years can be exhilarating and also highly stressful.

The responsibilities of adulthood require the current cohort of working adults to pull the financial weight for three generations including those who come before (aging parents) and those who come after (children). The responsibilities of child-rearing are daunting. Achieving "work-life balance" is elusive for most adults. Here we discuss one of the most strongly health-connected consequences of adults' enormous load of responsibilities, specifically, the challenge and threat to well-being posed by life stressors.

Stress is a continuous part of the terrain throughout the entire life course. However, distinguishing features of adulthood, particularly the burden of responsibilities, are stress-provoking. Stress is a product of mind–body interaction. The brain is in dynamic communication with the cardiovascular, immune, and other systems using endocrine and neural pathways for multiway messaging. Daily stressors trigger physiological systems, keeping them teetering on high alert status and disrupting sleep. Stress contributes to unhealthy dietary patterns, elevated blood pressure, and a range of substance use and other health-compromising behaviors. These physiological states are often precursors to clinical disease, operating through what McEwen[19] describes as "allostatic load" on the body. This is stress-induced wear and tear. The adult years represent a prime period for lifelong risks to transform into disease, and stress acts on both sides of this equation. Stress contributes to disease. Disease contributes to stress.

Scientific stress research has been underway now for more than a half century, and Thoits[20] provides a concise summary of five things we know. First, stressors cause significant harm to human health, both physical and mental. Second, exposures to stress are not equally distributed, contributing to physical and mental health disparities and inequities by gender, race, ethnicity, marital status, and social class. This also explains the disproportionate stress exposure for individuals just entering their adult years as they juggle multiple buckets of responsibilities. Third, discrimination is an added stressor for persons of lower SES, or minority race/ethnicity, or other disadvantaged group status. Fourth, and most relevant to this chapter, so we quote directly, "stressors proliferate over the life course and across generations, widening health gaps between advantaged and disadvantaged group members."[20] Fifth, stress effects are lessened for persons who gain mastery in their key life roles, most especially during their adult years. Such mastery often comes with such bonuses as high self-esteem and considerable social support.

During the later years of adulthood, chronic stress translates into disease states. For example, chronic stress burden was definitively related to increased rates of coronary heart disease, hypertension, and type 2 diabetes in a multisite community study.[21] In this study, chronic stress burden was evaluated in a manner that ties directly to the effects of adult roles and responsibilities. Investigators catalogued an extensive array of "current ongoing problems." The life problem stressors that were enumerated were categorized into financial, occupational, interpersonal (stress within significant relationships), caregiving, and health domains.

Stress is a ubiquitous, defining feature of 21st-century living.[22] In a recent study, more than half of respondents reported experiencing a "major stressful event" in the past year. Most reported stressful events specifically related to health, job demands, financial worries, family situations, and "responsibility in general."

CASE STUDY 10.1: THE ESCALATING HOUSING INSECURITY CRISIS FOR EMERGING ADULTS

Emerging adults, and notably, U.S. college students, face a mounting housing insecurity crisis that has been acutely exacerbated by the COVID-19 pandemic and continues to worsen over time. Supply and demand are squeezing college students in the vise of decreasing housing units and increasing rents. Student housing options are simultaneously less available and less affordable. Universities are not helping matters as they have upcharged for their owned residential buildings post-pandemic.

Housing insecurity takes many forms, ranging from the inability of students to pay rent or utilities to loss of housing, forced eviction, and homelessness. Some students are living in a veritable barracks with many roommates, exceeding the capacity of the housing unit. Some are sleeping in friends' homes—couch surfing—living on the good graces and generosity of others but always subject to having that charitable arrangement end abruptly. Some students are living far from campus, sometimes in the next county, because rent is cheaper, but their savings on housing are negatively offset by long commute times, car maintenance expenses, and rising fuel prices. Paying for room and board may come at the expense of decreasing the food allowance and being unable to afford a healthful, nutritious diet, or living in areas that are not conducive to safely engaging in physical activity. Some students live in abjectly substandard housing in dangerous neighborhoods. Some are living out of their cars. Many students need to dedicate time and expense to moving frequently as housing arrangements quickly appear, or dissolve. Depending on the day and the situation, studying at "home" or attending classes online may not be possible.

While no consensus definition for housing insecurity exists, what is nearly universal is students facing multiple hardships as they search for a safe, sustainable housing environment, one that supports rather than interferers with their successful pursuit of higher education and attainment of their academic and career goals. The college experience is replete with expectable stressors across academic, social, financial, and interpersonal domains. Recent years have witnessed an escalating housing dilemma that now adds an overlay of existential stress to the mix.

One of the most cited studies[23] that puts housing insecurity into a data-based perspective is the Hope Center for College, Community and Justice's Basic Needs Survey,[24] based at Temple University. The scale of the survey is impressive. During the prepandemic to midpandemic time period, 2015 to 2021, The Hope Center fielded the #RealCollegeSurvey, described as "the nation's largest, most well-established assessment of students' basic needs." During this time interval, more than 500,000 students from more than 500 institutions of higher education participated.

Housing was a focal point of the survey. However, housing questions were embedded with other items dealing with access to food, mental health, caregiving, employment, and actual use of these supports. Importantly for making insightful comparisons, participant demographics were collected.

The most recent report dates from March 2021, 1 year into the pandemic when COVID-19 variants were just emerging, vaccines were becoming available, and

(continued)

many students were attending classes online. Almost all respondents reported that their classes moved to a virtual format and their campuses closed—creating an acute housing shortage as dorms and on-campus housing units became scarce. Two-thirds of respondents reported difficulty concentrating during online classes. Variable internet connectivity was a constant concern. One-half of the student respondents were living in situations where they needed to care for a household member or help younger siblings in the home with their studies, as they attempted to maintain focus and achieve success in their own studies.

Fully 58% reported one or more "basic needs insecurities" (BNIs), including 48% reporting housing insecurity and 34% reporting food insecurity. Housing insecurity was reported by 52% of those enrolled in 2-year colleges and 43% of students in 4-year institutions. In rank order, the housing items most commonly endorsed included the following did not pay full utilities, did not pay full rent, experienced a rent increase, had an account default and go to collections, moved in with others, lived in an over-capacity housing situation, and left a household that felt unsafe. Fourteen percent endorsed one or more "homelessness" issues, with most indicating that they were staying at the home of a friend or relative.

The survey found stark demographic inequities in self-reported BNIs, including housing. One or more BNIs were reported by 75% of Indigenous students, 70% of African American/Black students, and 70% of American Indian/Alaska Native students, and 65% of LGBTQ students, compared to a still-alarming rate of 54% among White students. Across all races and ethnicities combined, 7% more female students reported BNIs compared to male students. BNIs are also disproportionately high for first-generation students and non-native English speakers.

These disparities in self-reported BNIs, between college men and women, and across races and ethnicities, also had ramifications regarding risks for airborne transmission of the COVID-19 virus in crowded and unhygienic living conditions. Students of color were more likely to be living in home environments with more people and elevated infection risks. Furthermore, many students—and disproportionately students of color—were supporting their rent and tuition costs by working in "essential" job roles where they had to be on the job in person, often in crowded work settings.

Social distancing was generally not possible. In some instances, COVID-19 infection risks were further heightened by inadequate ventilation and unavailability of protective gear and antiseptic hygiene products.

Students living with housing insecurity tend to self-rate their health as poor, and they experience higher rates of depression and anxiety. In the context of students pursuing their higher education to be able to advance educationally, professionally, and economically, housing insecurity is an impediment for achieving these goals. Students facing housing insecurity perform worse in their studies and tend to get lower marks, including lower GPAs, than their counterparts who live in more secure housing. This extends to the point where housing-insecure students and homeless students have diminished "persistence" in school, earn fewer credits over time, and have lower college completion rates.

A summary of key findings[25] that individually and collectively amplified the housing crisis for college students during the height of the pandemic includes several points.

(continued)

First, the COVID-19 pandemic prompted abrupt campus closures, and many schools summarily shut down their residence halls. With almost no warning to allow students to adapt, campus closures created an acute depletion of safe and available housing units designated for student occupancy.

Second, when closures occurred mid-semester, some schools refused to refund students for room and board costs.

Third, college financial aid packages often focus on reducing tuition costs but they are wholly inadequate for covering the full range of real costs incurred, including room and board; public transportation fares; costs for vehicle purchases, fuel, maintenance, and parking; utilities and internet charges; and computer purchase and maintenance costs. Students with children also must pay for childcare.

Faced with these sobering statistics, a set of recommendations was proposed just before fall semester 2021,[26] at a time when COVID-19 was still surging and the highly virulent Delta variant was predominant. Schools were advised to

- create a single point of contact for housing issues,
- identify at-risk students earlier,
- build alliances with local agencies to seek viable housing solutions,
- create awareness of federal aid across campus, and
- inform students and administrators in all academic departments about the housing crisis.

One year later, the pandemic appeared to ebb during fall 2022. In-person education resumed. On-campus housing units reopened. So, was this—the pandemic shifting to "endemic" patterning—the long-awaited solution? What happened to housing and other BNIs? Did reopening cause these dilemmas to diminish and disappear? Did a declining pandemic at least partially solve these debilitating BNIs?

Although more time is needed to assess trends, the immediate answer is an emphatic "No"!

Instead, several compounding, untoward outcomes occurred.

First, after pandemic-imposed moratoriums on rent increases and evictions, landlords steeply increased rents in many cities nationwide. Rents jumped 40% to 60% or more in many areas. Housing costs, historically a major percentage of the monthly budget of students, suddenly soared off the charts.

Second, many colleges and universities that had lost revenues during the pandemic imposed jolting tuition increases. In some cases, on-campus housing prices rose sharply also.

Third, the year 2022 was marked by staggering inflation. In tandem with rent increases, food prices skyrocketed, gasoline prices escalated, and clothing prices went up sharply. Overall inflation rates were the highest in decades, and several of the critical financial sectors for college students saw the highest increases.

Innovative approaches to making college education more affordable are urgently needed. The value of education is so extraordinary that students will sacrifice their physical and mental health and safety to strive toward their education goals. Ominously, housing and basic needs expenses are becoming so prohibitively expensive that they are jeopardizing opportunities for highly motivated students to leverage themselves out of poverty and structural disadvantage by succeeding in their educational endeavors.

HOW HEALTH IS GENERATED DURING ADULTHOOD

Health in adulthood is a product of what has occurred in earlier life phases, during childhood and adolescence, and what occurs in an ongoing manner during the prolonged adult phase of the life course. The adult years represent the period when lifelong risks and exposures reach a critical mass, a veritable tipping point, and disease emerges. The following three examples illustrate the progression of health through the life course, manifesting as health and disease in adulthood.

> **Health in adulthood is a product of what has occurred in earlier life phases, during childhood and adolescence, and what occurs in an ongoing manner during the prolonged adult phase of the life course.**

ADVERSE CHILDHOOD EXPERIENCES AND TOXIC STRESS

As the first example, making the point for the lingering and potentially amplifying effects of early childhood exposures, Shonkoff and associates highlighted the effects of adverse childhood experiences (ACEs) and toxic stress in the first years of life on brain development and ultimately on emerging patterns of health and disease throughout adulthood.[27] The authors operate from an "eco-biodevelopmental" framework and they present an intriguing viewpoint that relates to our life course dimension. They suggest that "many adult diseases should be viewed as developmental disorders that begin early in life." They also propose that early life interventions to alleviate childhood adversity and toxic stress could help diminish health disparities that persist into adulthood, in various forms such as learning impairments, behavioral deficits, psychological distress progressing to psychiatric disorders, physical debility and disease, and diminished well-being.

WEIGHT GAIN IN EARLY ADULTHOOD

As a second example, some risks do not start in childhood but rather have their origins during the adult years. Making the point for the importance of risks that develop within the adult years, detailed analyses of data from very large cohorts of male and female health professionals showed that weight gain that started during the early years of adulthood and continued into middle adulthood strongly predicted both increased risks for major chronic diseases and decreased chances of healthy aging.[28] Moderate weight gain during the adult years was associated with significantly increased incidence of newly diagnosed type 2 diabetes, hypertension, cardiovascular disease (CVD), and obesity-related cancers (**Table 10.3**). Further, an upward stair-step (dose–response) relationship was evident whereby "higher amounts of weight gain were associated with greater risks of major chronic diseases and lower likelihood of healthy aging."[28]

DRUG USE OVER THE LIFE COURSE

As a third example, drug use often begins in adolescence. However, the primary burden of drug use is experienced during the adult years. Regardless of the individual pathway from experimentation to addiction, there is an extremely high risk for periodic relapse. Hser and colleagues examined some of the key elements necessary for intervening with drug use and abuse across the life course, punctuated by these expected and anticipated episodes of relapse.[29] These authors emphasized the need to approach drug use as a chronic condition and to build treatment systems to deliver disease management and provide continuity of care. Equally critical is the ability to create cross-linkages and coordination across various settings where drug users may need to receive their treatment depending on life circumstances, including such diverse systems as criminal justice, mental health, welfare, and healthcare.

TABLE 10.3 Weight Gain from Early to Middle Adulthood and Major Health Outcomes in Older Adult Years: Multivariable-Adjusted IRR for Selected Health Outcomes, Nurses' Health Study ($n = 92,837$)

WEIGHT GAIN IN EARLY TO MIDDLE ADULTHOOD	WEIGHT LOSS >2.5 KG	WEIGHT LOSS <2.5 KG OR WEIGHT GAIN >2.5 KG	WEIGHT GAIN >2.5 KG AND <10.0 KG	WEIGHT GAIN >10.0 KG AND <20.0 KG	WEIGHT GAIN >20.0 KG
Study population	6,363	10,649	26,402	28,479	20,944
HEALTH OUTCOME:	**IRR**	**IRR**	**IRR**	**IRR**	**IRR**
Type 2 diabetes	0.73	1 (reference)	1.89	4.50	10.51
Hypertension	0.90	1 (reference)	1.24	1.58	2.10
Cardiovascular disease	1.08	1 (reference)	1.25	1.35	1.87
Obesity-related cancer	0.92	1 (reference)	1.09	1.29	1.52
Obesity-related cancer in never-smokers	0.92	1 (reference)	1.14	1.38	1.69
Gallstones	0.77	1 (reference)	1.38	2.03	2.76
Severe osteoarthritis	0.94	1 (reference)	1.20	1.31	1.40
Cataract extraction	0.96	1 (reference)	1.01	1.02	1.05
Mortality	1.06	1 (reference)	1.02	1.08	1.14
Mortality in never-smokers	0.99	1 (reference)	1.07	1.17	1.52
Healthy aging outcome	1.22	1 (reference)	0.78	0.56	0.28

IRR, incident rate ratio.
Source: Data from Zheng Y, Manson JE, Yuan C, et al. Associations of weight gain from early to middle adulthood with major health outcomes later in life. *JAMA.* 2017;318(3):255-269. doi:10.1001/jama.2017.7092

HOW DISEASE RISKS EVOLVE OVER THE COURSE OF ADULTHOOD

Adulthood is the life course period when NCD risk factors exert their cumulative, and often multiplicative, effects. These risk factors, including some that originated in childhood or adolescence, ultimately produce subclinical (not yet detectable) target-organ damage in the middle adult years. In time, these underlying physiological changes give rise to detectable symptoms as disease states become outwardly apparent and medically diagnosable. On a population basis, during later years of adulthood, especially for adults in their 50s and 60s, these trends evolve into escalating rates of NCDs. Worldwide, NCDs predominate as the primary causes of disability and premature death. The most common are CVDs (both heart disease and stroke), cancers, and chronic lower respiratory diseases.

RISK FACTORS THAT RISE TO PROMINENCE DURING THE ADULT YEARS

During the adult years, a broad constellation of primary risk factors for a spectrum of NCDs and substance use and mental health disorders are prominent and increasing in frequency and severity. Some of these risk factors peak during the adult years.

For example, the proportion of the population that is overweight and obese increases with age, most notably during the adult years. This is a risk that relentlessly saturates the U.S. adult population as adults age so that by the later adult decades, more than two in three individuals are either overweight or obese. In contrast to most risk factors, this population-wide pattern of increasing body weight is outwardly visible. Weight gain is overtly observable to the individual; their family members, friends, and coworkers; and the surrounding community.

Many adults, despite repeated attempts at maintaining normal weight, sequentially surpass a series of body mass thresholds that signify increasing risk and more severe disease. Quite early in their adult years, many individuals exceed a body mass index (BMI) of 25, the criterion for being overweight. A few years later, they reach a BMI of 30, the cutoff for obesity. Thereafter, many continue their upward progression, with substantial numbers of adults increasing their body mass to a BMI of 40 or higher, a marker of such extreme obesity that these individuals may be eligible for, and encouraged to consider, bariatric surgery (e.g., placement of a gastric band, removal of a portion of the stomach). Worldwide, the rates of obesity increase through the adult years. In some countries with very high obesity rates, the proportion of overweight women is higher at each age than the corresponding proportion of men.[30] Obesity is especially concentrated in the adult decades of life. In fact, BMIs begin to taper in the later adult years and the older adult age range. So, obesity is one risk factor that tends to peak during the adult years of the life course.

For many risk factors other than obesity, the underlying physiological and structural changes are less outwardly noticeable and often unobservable. As one example carrying global significance, systolic and diastolic blood pressures routinely rise with age, especially during the adult years. Yet, unlike obesity, hypertension remains a largely undetected "silent killer."[31] As another example, the proportion of the population with elevated blood glucose increases with age, often a harbinger of type 2 diabetes yet to be diagnosed. Indeed, the onset and occurrence of diagnosed type 2 diabetes rises with age throughout the adult years and through the first decade of older adulthood until about the age of 80.[32] Although it is not possible to "eyeball" individuals whose blood glucose level is rising or to visually "detect" individuals recently diagnosed with type 2 diabetes, there is a telltale, outward clue. Individuals who are obese (which can be outwardly seen) are prime candidates for blood glucose elevations and the development of type 2 diabetes.

This brief list—overweight, obesity, increased blood glucose level, diabetes, and high blood pressure—represents a partial litany of important CVD risk factors. The proportion of people living with each of these risk factors increases with age during adult life. Also, as we illustrate in detail with CVD, these risk factors aggregate and interact in a manner that the health impact of multiple elevated risk factors exceeds that of the sum of the effects of the individual risk factors. As we explain, these risk factors act in concert to amplify risks for early-onset heart attacks and strokes that occur at alarming rates during the later decades of adulthood and well into older adult years.

This brief list—overweight, obesity, increased blood glucose level, diabetes, and high blood pressure—represents a partial litany of important CVD risk factors.

CARDIOVASCULAR DISEASE AS AN ILLUSTRATION OF THE DYNAMICS OF LIFESTYLE RISK FACTORS

CVD—the leading cause of death worldwide and the end result of many of these life course exposures—provides a potent example of how lifestyle behaviors shape patterns of health and disease over the 40 years of adulthood (the focus of this chapter) and beyond. In the international classifications of diseases, CVD is primarily composed of coronary (or ischemic) heart disease and stroke. In 2021, mid-pandemic, heart disease remained the leading cause of death in the United States and stroke ranked fifth, below COVID-19 deaths in third place (**Figure 10.1**).[33]

CVD is also a major contributor to disability. The proportion of U.S. persons currently living with diagnosed CVD increases throughout the adult years. This pattern extends into the older ages. CVD mortality in the United States increases steeply with age during the adult and older adult years.

These now-pervasive and normative patterns were not always the case. In fact, they represent recent phenomena in human history. The 20th and early 21st centuries have witnessed a quantum transformation from the earlier prominence of infectious diseases to the current dominance of NCDs. To be clear, COVID-19's sudden, jarring appearance and rapid circumnavigation of the planet in early 2020 was a harsh reminder that communicable diseases are not vanquished. We must anticipate continuous introductions of emerging infectious diseases. Some will generate initial pandemic surges and remain present and problematic (HIV/AIDS, ever-present influenza risks, COVID-19 and related coronaviruses, other zoonoses). Nevertheless, NCDs are the major killers and disablers.

Among NCDs, CVD has led the way. CVD provides a supremely well-documented example of the interaction among unhealthy behaviors and the onset and progression of disease, not only across the life course of individuals, but on a population basis over periods of decades. A case in point, **Figure 10.2** illustrates the rise in U.S. heart disease mortality over the past century. Observe the exceedingly low numbers of heart disease deaths at the beginning of the 1900s. Heart disease and stroke were the fourth and fifth leading causes of death in the United States in 1900, with three infectious disease causes topping the list. From our current 21st-century vantage point, it is startling to contemplate that heart disease, the current leading cause of death in the United States and worldwide, was only a nominal contributor to mortality as recently as the beginning of the 20th century.

The rise in numbers of CVD deaths in the past century is nothing short of stunning. Indeed, heart disease and stroke emerged during the 1900s as primary contributors to population-wide

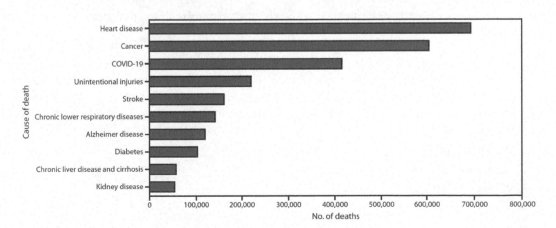

FIGURE 10.1 Provisional leading causes of death, United States, 2021.
Source: Ahmad FA, Cisewski JA, Anderson RN. Provisional mortality data—United States, 2021. *MMWR Morb Mortal Wkly Rep.* 2022;71(17):597-600.

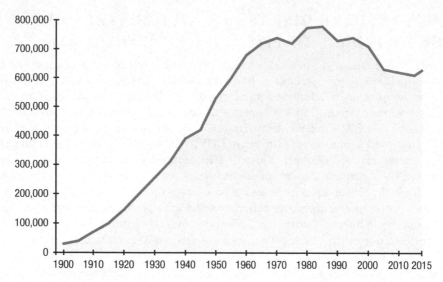

FIGURE 10.2 Deaths attributable to diseases of the heart, United States, 1900 to 2015.
Source: Data from Benjamin EJ, Virani SS, Callaway CW, et al. Heart disease and stroke statistics—2018 update: a report from the American Heart Association. *Circulation.* 2018;137(12). doi:10.1161/CIR.0000000000000558

patterns of disease and death. This was not merely the result of the conquest of infectious diseases. This represented a seismic change in human risk profiles. As one example, the industrial age, especially the 1900s, and the current postindustrial times represent the first era in human history when survival was possible without needing to engage in regular, sometimes strenuous, physical activity. This is also the epoch where diseases of undernutrition were supplanted by diseases of overnutrition.

Identifying Lifestyle Risk Factors for Cardiovascular Disease

Unhealthy lifestyle patterns are the primary drivers of risk for both coronary heart disease and stroke, emerging, as we note throughout this chapter, across the life course. More than any other community-based research endeavor, the Framingham Heart Study has been instrumental for delineating the principal risk factors for heart disease and stroke—and clarifying their rich and complex interplay. The Framingham Heart Study has been ongoing for multiple generations, since its inception in 1948.

One way to simplify the discussion around the key lifestyle risk factors for CVD has been provided courtesy of the American Heart Association (AHA). One of the primary goals of the AHA is helping Americans decrease their risks for CVD. AHA's public education materials present these risk-reducing, health-producing lifestyle behaviors in the clearest terms possible: a blueprint for healthy living called, "Life's Simple 7."[34] Life's Simple 7 consists of a set of action steps for cardiovascular health, condensed into seven statements, together totaling just 16 words:

1. Manage blood pressure
2. Control cholesterol
3. Reduce blood sugar
4. Get active
5. Eat better
6. Lose weight
7. Stop smoking

These action statements sound deceptively simple. Yet the guidance contained here reflects decades of sophisticated research that has demonstrated the causal linkages between seven lifestyle risks and CVD disability and death.

Here are the point-by-point connections between the action step and the corresponding risk-elevating factors that are present among large segments of the U.S. population:

1. Manage blood pressure   Risk factor: elevated systolic and diastolic blood pressure
2. Control cholesterol   Risk factor: elevated blood lipids
3. Reduce blood sugar   Risk factor: elevated blood glucose leading to type 2 diabetes
4. Get active   Risk factor: sedentary lifestyle, physical inactivity
5. Eat better   Risk factor: high-sugar, high-fat, high-sodium, lower-fiber diet
6. Lose weight   Risk factor: overweight and obesity
7. Stop smoking   Risk factor: cigarette smoking, using other nicotine products

Understanding the Dynamics of Lifestyle Risk Factors for Cardiovascular Disease

Focusing especially on these seven risk factors, it is time to take a tour of how risk factors operate individually and in concert. Here is what we know from Framingham and a myriad of research investigations over three-quarters of a century.

First, each of these seven specific risk factors is potentially modifiable. That is why the AHA selected them. The Life's Simple 7 statements present the actions that will favorably modify these risks. There are effective lifestyle interventions and medical treatment options that can reduce elevated blood pressure, lipids, glucose, and body weight; assist smokers to quit; encourage those who are inactive to exercise; and favorably modify diet. In addition to this set of seven malleable risks, there are also important nonmodifiable CVD risk factors that also contribute to, and complicate, the risk equation. Nonmodifiable risks include age, biological sex, family history of CVD, and genetic makeup.

Second, each of these seven risk factors, in isolation, increases the risk for CVD. This is the essence of a risk-elevating factor.

Third, the effect of each individual risk factor is cumulative over time. For example, CVD risk increases with the amount of time a person has lived with uncontrolled blood pressure or obesity.

Fourth, the effect of an individual risk factor may become worse—or riskier—over time. For example, as discussed, for many individuals, the degree of obesity, measured by the BMI, increases over time during the adult years. This is not a static risk but instead one that becomes more severe as the BMI rises. In parallel, blood pressure levels, blood glucose levels, and blood lipid levels may rise throughout the adult years, conferring higher risk with higher values of the risk indicator. The specific risk factor is unchanged but becomes more hazardous as values rise.

Fifth, almost all adult Americans, and in fact, almost all adult world citizens have *at least one* of these seven risk factors.

Sixth, these lifestyle risks tend to cluster, meaning that a person with one risk factor has a high likelihood of having two or more risk factors. Some associations are self-evident. People who eat high-fat diets and are physically inactive often become overweight and eventually obese. Obesity is itself a verifiable risk for diabetes. Less self-evident is the relationship between elevated lipids and elevated blood pressure.

Seventh, the presence of two or more (multiple) risk factors increases CVD risk not just additively but "synergistically." This means that the combined effects of two or more risk factors together amplify CVD risks more than the simple sum of the risks of each individual risk factor (**Figure 10.3**).

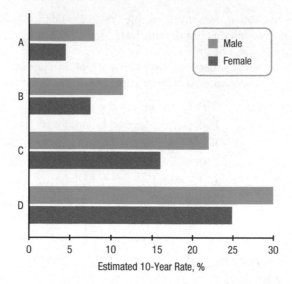

	A	B	C	D
Age	50–54	50–54	50–54	50–54
HDL Cholesterol, mg/dL	45–49	45–49	35–44	35–44
Total Cholesterol, mg/dL	160–199	200–239	200–239	200–239
Systolic BP mmHg, No Treatment	120–129	130–139	130–139	130–139
Smoker	No	No	No	Yes
Diabetes	No	No	Yes	Yes

FIGURE 10.3 Estimated 10-year cardiovascular disease risk in adults 50 to 54 years of age according to levels of various risk factors. BP, blood pressure; HDL, high-density lipoprotein.
Source: Reproduced with permission from Benjamin EJ, Virani SS, Callaway CW, et al. Heart disease and stroke statistics—2018 update: a report from the American Heart Association. *Circulation.* 2018;137(12):e67-e492. doi:10.1161/CIR.0000000000000558

Eighth, almost all adult Americans, and in fact, vast numbers of adult world citizens except those in the lowest income countries, have *at least two* of these seven risk factors. Most adults living in high-income countries worldwide have more than two risk factors.

Ninth, several of the seven AHA-specified risk factors—diabetes, obesity, and hypertension—are diseases themselves, in their own right. So, interventions for these upstream diagnosable medical conditions may have preventive effects on the later onset of CVD as a downstream condition.

Tenth, as a major population health concept that relates to the social ecological dimension, individuals are nested within families, neighborhoods, and communities. The habitual dietary, physical activity, smoking, and healthcare-seeking patterns of populations influence the health of many individuals within that population. For example, entire populations that habitually consume diets high in saturated fats experience elevated CVD risks when compared with populations that observe lean diets. The U.S. Department of Agriculture (USDA) has developed the USDA Food Access Research Atlas to clearly demarcate food deserts nationwide. Researchers identified food deserts in the Atlanta area—defined as areas with both low income and poor access to healthy food—and found a 44% higher rate of myocardial infarction among residents of these areas compared to their counterparts who did not live in food deserts. Interestingly, the analyses indicated that "low area income"—rather than poor access to healthy food—was the primary determinant of the elevated risk for heart attack.

Intervening on Lifestyle Risk Factors for Cardiovascular Disease

The AHA is able to track progress in terms of population adoption of Life's Simple 7 and documented decreases in some population risk factors over time.[34]

The good news is that dramatic progress has been made to reverse the detrimental effects of CVD on population health. This has been accomplished largely through modification of population patterns of risk behaviors. Granted, progress on risk factor modification is slow, incremental, and inconsistent. Nevertheless, over a period of decades, important population-level behavioral changes have occurred, individually and collectively, and contributed to decreases in CVD onset, disability, and death.

First, there have been marked reductions in smoking rates that have been achieved in the United States and in many high-income countries. Second, population mean cholesterol levels have declined significantly. Third, the proportion of persons whose high blood pressure has been detected, treated, and controlled has risen. Not all have reached their ideal target thresholds for lower blood pressures, but most have achieved important reductions in blood pressures.

However, not all seven risk factors—and their corresponding AHA Life's Simple 7 action steps—are moving in the desired direction. These favorable risk changes in the realm of smoking, blood lipids, and blood pressure are somewhat offset by continuing rises in rates of overweight, obesity, elevated blood glucose (related to overweight), and diabetes. Progress on measures of increased physical activity is mixed.

Nevertheless, the death rates per 100,000 from coronary heart disease have declined steeply for both men and women over the period 1950 to 2015 (**Figure 10.4**). The declines in stroke deaths are even more pronounced. This is remarkable progress.

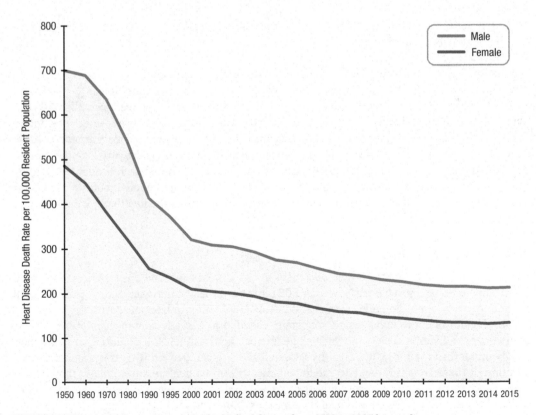

FIGURE 10.4 Deaths by heart disease in the United States from 1950 to 2015 by gender.
Source: Data from Deaths by heart diseases in the U.S. from 1950 to 2015, by gender per 100,000 resident population (2018). Statista, Inc.

HOW PUBLIC HEALTH CAN MITIGATE THESE THREATS TO HEALTH DURING ADULTHOOD

THE HEALTHY PEOPLE APPROACH

We have just discussed CVD and a subset of seven lifestyle-related behavioral risks. How these risk factors interrelate and exert their influence is impressively complicated, and we are talking about just one, albeit major, disease. How then do we address the adult health and disease landscape for an entire nation, considering the multitude of health threats these individuals will encounter along their 40-year path through the adult years? Certainly, the complexity is quite daunting, but consider the Healthy People approach.

Healthy People's First 50 Years

In the late 1900s, the U.S. Department of Health and Human Services (HHS) recognized the need for evidence-based tracking of patterns of health and disease throughout the United States in the present and over future generations. There was a compelling need to identify health promotion and disease prevention strategies that could move the nation steadily forward toward improved health status.

To handle something so multifaceted as health and disease for an entire nation, a new office was established within the hierarchy of HHS and tasked with leading this ambitious initiative. In 1976, the U.S. Congress created the Office of Disease Prevention and Health Promotion (ODPHP) within the Office of the Assistant Secretary of Health inside HHS. The ODPHP, as its name implies, is charged with spearheading disease prevention and health promotion initiatives for the nation.

The practical outcome was a monumental application called Healthy People, an iterative and continuously improving approach that takes on U.S. health, one decade at a time. Healthy People is one of the most comprehensive approaches to improving health and mitigating disease threats through action. The ODPHP is best known as the home base for Healthy People. In fact, almost no one knows ODPHP by name, but Healthy People is known to millions.

For 50 years, since the last decades of the 1900s, Healthy People has been providing 10-year, evidence-based objectives for promoting health and preventing disease for all Americans, focusing in particular on health among adult Americans. The latest iteration is Healthy People 2030. Chapter 4, "At the Heart of Public Health: Social Determinants of Health and Health Equity," presents the Healthy People 2030 goals for the five domains of the SDOH in detail. Providing objectives is coupled with something far more important; Healthy People creates a means for ongoing surveillance to track how the nation is doing in relation to the health objectives that are set for each decade.

Healthy People 2030

Planning for the upcoming 10-year objectives starts almost a decade earlier. Healthy People 2030 came on board just before New Year 2021 and serves as the national guide for the next full decade. Already, the vision and mission statements for 2030 have been prepared.[35]

The Healthy People 2030 vision statement, distilled to a single sentence, references a life course perspective: "A society in which all people can achieve their full potential for health and well-being across the lifespan." Healthy People 2030 is grounded on five "overarching goals," and one of these speaks directly to the life course: "Promote healthy development, healthy behaviors and well-being across all life stages." The mission statement addresses the priority of inclusivity and the elimination of health disparities: "To promote, strengthen and evaluate the Nation's efforts to improve the health and well-being of all people."

Healthy People 2030 is much more expansive and broadly encompassing than its predecessor. So, to figure out how U.S. health is progressing in the ongoing 2020s—up to the end of the year 2030—it is being monitored using the Healthy People 2030 framework. Here is the roster of action steps that the ODPHP is using to guide the process:

- Set national goals and measurable objectives to guide evidence-based policies, programs, and other actions to improve health and well-being.
- Provide data that is accurate, timely, accessible, and can drive targeted actions to address regions and populations with poor health or at high risk for poor health in the future.
- Foster impact through public and private efforts to improve health and well-being for people of all ages and the communities in which they live.
- Provide tools for the public, programs, policy makers, and others to evaluate progress toward improving health and well-being.
- Share and support the implementation of evidence-based programs and policies that are replicable, scalable, and sustainable.
- Report biennially on progress throughout the decade from 2020 to 2030.
- Stimulate research and innovation toward meeting Healthy People 2030 goals and highlight critical research, data, and evaluation needs.
- Facilitate development and availability of affordable means of health promotion, disease prevention, and treatment.

With each new 10-year iteration, Healthy People takes on an additional layer of sophistication. Healthy People has a proven track record of developing consensus-guided goals for the nation and successfully monitoring a burgeoning range of health indicators in a manner that provides information for action. With the input from public health professionals representing a spectrum of research and policy expertise, these goals dovetail with the programmatic and funding priorities across the HHS. So, Healthy People helps to shape the creation and continuation of initiatives that move the United States in the direction of achieving the 10-year goals.

With each new 10-year iteration, Healthy People takes on an additional layer of sophistication.

Healthy People is a valued resource sought out by public health professionals in a variety of roles.

Healthy People is also sufficiently nimble and adept to be able to accommodate emerging health threats whether these are new or newly resistant infectious diseases, climate impacts on national health, natural disasters, or perpetrated acts of violence. As one example, one dimension of the Healthy People violence prevention focus is on intimate partner violence which is both a national and a global public health issue.

CASE STUDY 10.2: EVIDENCE-BASED INTERVENTIONS FOR INTIMATE PARTNER VIOLENCE

Globally, intimate partner violence (IPV), a particularly common form of gender-based violence, is a public health crisis that creates lasting physical and psychological consequences for victims who are predominantly women. The World Health Organization (WHO) created evidence-based clinical recommendations for effective interventions.[36] Elements of a comprehensive strategy include

(continued)

woman-centered care for IPV victims, screening and identification for survivors of IPV, and clinical care for survivors of sexual assault. This direct care for victims is coupled with training of healthcare professionals regarding IPV and other forms of sexual violence. Other components include prioritization of IPV in healthcare policy formulation and mandatory reporting for IPV.

The World Bank commissioned a systematic review of interventions to prevent or reduce violence against women and girls.[37] Specific to IPV, the review distinguished between primary and secondary prevention approaches. Primary interventions aim to reduce new episodes of IPV by intervening before violence occurs. This includes group training for men, and for men and women together. The focus is on "fostering societies, communities, organizations, and relationships in which violence is less likely to occur."

Secondary prevention approaches aim to support and provide services for already-abused women and prevent recurrence of IPV. Approaches here include batterer intervention programs, screening, and survivor services that include both psychosocial interventions and advocacy interventions.

Much remains to be done in terms of advancing efficacious interventions. Most of the established evidence for interventions for IPV to date come from high-income countries, and response to completed acts of IPV are much more common than prevention approaches.[38] Interventions in high-income countries have been shown to improve physical and mental health outcomes for IPV survivors and to increase service utilization. There is little evidence to suggest that these programs reduce the risk for revictimization. Further, there is minimal evidence for the effectiveness of interventions with perpetrators. Actually, interventions introduced for low-income and middle-income countries have shown promise for achieving some degree of IPV and other violence prevention. Programs that are proving to be successful engage stakeholders in multiple ways and take aim at underlying social norms that have traditionally condoned violence and gender inequality.

We describe major depressive disorder, a primary contributor to population-wide disability and debility that primarily centers on the adult years of life (Case Study 10.3; you can access the podcast accompanying Case Study 10.3 by following this link to Springer Publishing Company Connect™: http://connect.springerpub.com/content/book/978-0-8261-8043-8/part/part03/chapter/ch10).

 ## CASE STUDY 10.3: DEPRESSION IN ADULTHOOD

The primary impact of depression, or major depressive disorder, is concentrated in the adult years of life. Depression is a serious mood disorder that can affect the way that individuals think and feel, disrupt sleep patterns, affect relationships, diminish productivity and output, and decrease an individual's capacity for experiencing pleasure and satisfaction in life.[39]

Although one hallmark of depression is persistent sad mood, to be formally diagnosed with depression requires that the individual experience multiple signs and symptoms nearly every day, and during most of the day, for a period of 2 weeks or longer.[39] The following symptoms are assessed to determine whether

(continued)

an individual is depressed (generally a total of five or more must be present to confirm the diagnosis):

- sad, anxious, "down" or "empty" mood
- loss of interest in activities that were previously enjoyed and pleasurable
- feeling hopeless and/or helpless
- feeling guilty or worthless
- irritability
- decreased energy or fatigue
- decreased concentration and difficulty making decisions
- moving or talking more slowly or alternatively, feeling restless or having trouble sitting still
- difficulty falling asleep or staying asleep, waking early, or oversleeping
- change in appetite (increase or decrease) and/or weight (gain or loss)
- thoughts of death or suicide, or suicide attempts

Depressive disorders are leading contributors to the global burden of disease, as assessed by disability-adjusted life years (DALYs),[40] and in particular, the component of DALYs called years lived with disability (YLDs).[41] Depression is less associated with dying early than with living disabled during portions of the adult years owing to depression's impacts on feelings and behavior. Depression saps an individual's ability to live productively and contribute fully in family, occupational, and life roles.

The burden of DALYs caused by mental disorders increased, in the Americas alone, from a total of 16.9 million years in 2000 to, in 2019, a total of 20.6 million years.[42] Depression alone accounted for 29% of the global burden of DALYs caused by mental and behavioral disorders in 2019.[43] In the United States, the situation is still more concerning with 6.56% of DALYs due to mental and behavioral disorders.[43] Once again, in the United States, as also seen globally, depression contributes more DALYs than any other mental health diagnosis. Not surprising therefore, on nationwide surveys, the Centers for Disease Control and Prevention (CDC) documented a rising proportion of persons, aged 55 to 64, reporting that they experience "mentally unhealthy days" because of stress or depression.[44] Further, on the flip side, survey research documented that one of the strongest predictors of being currently gainfully employed is being depression-free.[45]

What is particularly notable is that, in the United States, throughout the entire adult age span, ages 25 to 64 years, mental and behavioral disorders contribute more DALYs than any other disease category (**Figure 10.5**).[46] Once again, depression is the leading diagnosis within the category of mental and behavioral disorders.

Depression is a risk factor for multiple chronic diseases, a comorbidity with other psychiatric disorders, and a definitive risk factor for suicide. In the United States, the proportion of people living with depression increases from late adolescence through middle age and peaks in late middle age—and this proportion is consistently higher in women (**Figure 10.6**).[47] For example, in the adult age range, 40 to 59 years, before the COVID-19 pandemic, there was a prevalence of 8.5% depressive symptoms, while during the pandemic it drastically increased to 26.8%.[48]

(*continued*)

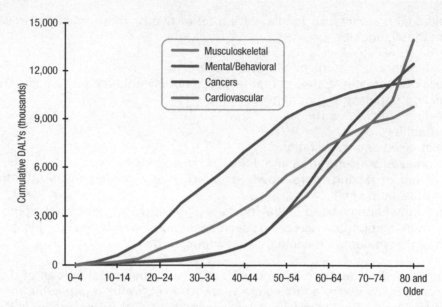

FIGURE 10.5 **Cumulative U.S. DALYs for leading disease/disorder categories by age (2010). DALYs, disability-adjusted life years.**
Source: The National Institute of Mental Health. *U.S. leading disease/disorder categories by age.* Wayback Machine website. http://web.archive.org/web/20210205112437/http://www.nimh.nih.gov:80/health/statistics/disability/us-leading-disease-disorder-categories-by-age.shtml

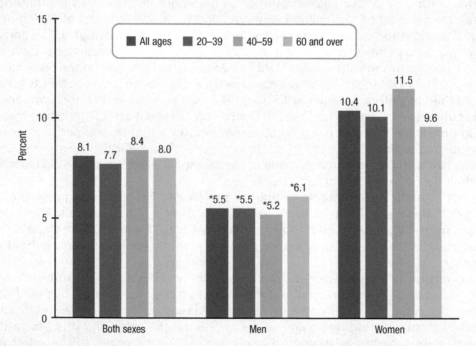

FIGURE 10.6 **Percentage of persons, age 12 and older, with depression, by age and sex, United States, 2013 to 2016. Significantly different from females in same age group.**
Notes: Depression was defined as a score greater than or equal to 10 on the Patient Health Questionnaire.
Source: Pratt LA, Brody DJ. Prevalence of depression among adults aged 20 and over: United States, 2013–2016. https://www.cdc.gov/nchs/products/databriefs/db303.htm

(continued)

Global studies have shown that the prevalence of major depression and subthreshold depression has been progressively increasing in recent decades for older middle age cohorts related to the concomitant increase in multiple types of noncommunicable diseases and the age-related progressive physical limitations.[49] As one indicator, longitudinal studies demonstrate that newly diagnosed depression is related to a long-term decline in cardiorespiratory fitness with age.[50] Also, interrelated declines in physical and mental health across later middle age co-occur and are predicted by a concentration of disadvantages,[51] including socioeconomic risks, across the life course.[52]

Given the population health impacts of depression and the trend data showing that the burden of depression on adult populations is worsening, one important approach is to conduct population screening for this disease. Indeed, as an overture toward achieving long-overdue public health/mental health integration, the CDC now recommends depression screening. For those who screen positive for probable depression, CDC advises home- or clinic-based follow-up that incorporates depression care management (DCM) and cognitive behavioral therapy (CBT), an evidence-based intervention with proven efficacy for the treatment of depression, as needed.[44] As one encouraging outcome of this public health outreach approach, a study in Japan effectively employed a community-based screening intervention to detect suicide risks in middle-aged persons (risks that are strongly tied to depression). In this study, suicide rates declined significantly in the intervention group.[53]

Just as helpful guidance on depression screening for adults and initial encouraging intervention findings were emerging, COVID-19 enveloped the planet and depression rates soared. In March 2022, the WHO released a news brief indicating that COVID-19 had led to a 25% increase in anxiety and depression symptoms worldwide. WHO Director-General, Dr. Tedros Adhanom Ghebreyesus declared, "This is a wake-up call to all countries to pay more attention to mental health and do a better job of supporting their populations' mental health."[54]

As if this quantum increase in disease burden was not enough, the patterns of depression produced by COVID-19 shifted radically toward younger adults, particularly "emerging adults" in the age range 18 to 29 years, and also to youth. Studies conducted by Ettman and team and by the CDC showed a tripling of depression symptoms in young adults during the earliest months of the pandemic, and elevated depression rates tended to persist throughout the early years of the pandemic rather than reverting to baseline.[48,55,56] These troubling trends are now under active surveillance with implications for the mental health of adults in the United States and globally.

In summary, major depressive disorder is particularly focalized in the adult ages both in the United States and globally. Apart from the elevated risk for suicide, most people live with depression rather than die from depression. They live miserably and unproductively with what is actually a very treatable disorder. The debilitating burden of depression can be effectively addressed if individuals are screened, diagnosed, and managed with effective treatments.

The often-repeated expression, "there is no health without mental health,"[57] rings powerfully true in the case of depression because there is, in fact, considerable promise for intervening effectively and restoring function, health, and vibrancy to many individuals and whole populations suffering from this disorder.

EXAMPLES OF PUBLIC HEALTH ACTIONS TO IMPROVE ADULT HEALTH

To promote health in adulthood, public health interventions are often targeted at prevention of NCDs. Action can be taken at various levels of our social ecological framework to target risks for disease. Take, for example, cardiovascular disease and stroke, which are major causes of death and disability globally. Heart diseases are the leading cause of death in the United States, with someone experiencing a heart attack every 40 seconds.[58]

INDIVIDUAL BEHAVIORS AND PRIMARY PREVENTION

Individual behaviors can be risk-elevating or risk-reducing. Shifting to risk-reducing behaviors in early adulthood can prevent the development of cardiovascular disease later on. For example, behavioral counseling related to healthful diets and physical activity among adults can be essential to reduce risk of cardiovascular disease, hypertension, high cholesterol, obesity, and diabetes mellitus.[59] An important marker for a healthful diet for CVD prevention is low sodium intake, with a recommendation of no more than 1,500 mg/day.[60] Engagement in regular physical activity is also a component of CVD prevention, with a recommendation of at least 7,000 steps daily.[61]

COMMUNITY LEVEL INITIATIVES

Community level prevention efforts can be effective in reaching greater numbers of individuals within the population. The AHA outlines the many levels/dimensions that influence cardiovascular disease risk factors and burden (**Figure 10.7**). Their framework identifies specific settings

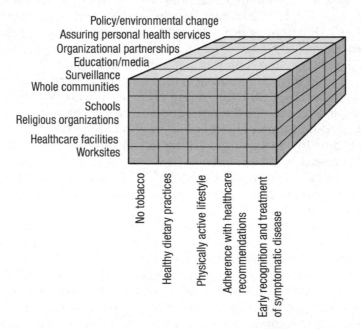

FIGURE 10.7 Conceptual framework for population-wide cardiovascular risk behaviors change.
Source: Pearson TA, Palaniappan LP, Artinian NT, et al. American Heart Association Guide for Improving Cardiovascular Health at the Community Level, 2013 update: a scientific statement for public health practitioners, healthcare providers, and health policy makers. *Circulation.* 2013;127(16):1730-1753. doi:10.1161/CIR.0b013e31828f8a94

for community-based interventions including schools, youth organizations, religious organizations, healthcare facilities, and workplaces.

The AHA supports the CDC's individual- and community-based prevention programs including Million Hearts 2027 and WISEWOMAN.[62] These prevention programs take an approach of reducing individual risk factors, increasing surveillance, conducting research to inform policies and practices that promote prevention, and minimizing health disparities.

Million Hearts 2027[63] emphasizes continual use of the "ABCs" of heart disease, a set of prevention guidelines to optimize care: aspirin as appropriate, blood pressure control, cholesterol management, and smoking cessation. Additionally, the priorities include building healthy communities through (a) decreased tobacco use, (b) increased physical activity, and (c) decreased particulate pollution exposure. The goal of Million Hearts 2027 is to prevent 1 million heart attacks over the course of 5 years, from January 2022 to December 2026. The program takes a health equity approach and focuses efforts on promoting strategies across various platforms for a wider reach.

The AHA and CDC also support the Well-Integrated Screening and Evaluation for Women Across the Nation (WISEWOMAN) program.[64] Serving women aged 40 to 64 years, WISEWOMAN conducts annual prevention screenings for heart disease and stroke. Screenings are conducted for blood pressure, total cholesterol, high-density lipoprotein cholesterol, blood glucose, and BMI. WISEWOMAN partners with the National Diabetes Prevention program, the YMCA, and other organizations to promote and support risk-reducing behaviors to prevent CVD. As exemplified by Million Hearts 2027 and WISEWOMAN, both individual and community-based approaches are needed to address CVD prevention, and each has advantages and challenges as presented in **Table 10.4**.

TABLE 10.4 Comparison of Individual and Community Approaches for Cardiovascular Disease Prevention

INDIVIDUAL: CLINICAL PRACTICE	COMMUNITY: POPULATION APPROACHES AND HEALTH PROMOTION
The standards are randomized, controlled trials	Standards are outcome and process evaluation, using quantitative and qualitative methods
Patients are individuals	The client is the community
Less than therapeutic dose is unacceptable	Preventive dose is rarely applied
Easier to treat an individual	Difficult to scale up health promotion programs that reach the whole population
Outcomes of interventions are individual change	Outcomes are to change the social norms, environments, and behavior of the entire populations
Interventions can focus on most factors relevant to the outcome	Interventions rarely take on social determinants external to the community

Source: Pearson TA. Public policy approaches to the prevention of heart disease and stroke. Circulation. 2011;124(23):2560-2571. doi:10.1161/CIRCULATIONAHA.110.968743

USING POLICIES FOR CHANGE

When enacting policy change, there are four policy approaches to reduce risk behaviors in the community—financial, legal, regulatory, and trade policy.[65] A financial policy might include a financial disincentive to curb harmful behaviors such as a tax on tobacco products, or an incentive to promote healthful behaviors such as a lower cost for healthful food such as fruits and vegetables. A legal policy might take the approach of imposing penalties on those who engage in harmful behaviors, such as smoking in a restricted area. Regulatory policies promote better outcomes (e.g., lower incidence of cardiovascular disease) through regulations and laws that restrict certain activities. An example would be the use of food labels to disclose added sugars, trans fats, and other harmful ingredients on food items. Lastly, trade and marketing policies address the production, purchase, sale, and movement of products that affect risk behaviors, for instance a policy encouraging and supporting fruit production.

SUMMARY

The production of health and disease throughout the expansive 40-year range of the adult phase of the life course strongly relates to three defining roles and responsibilities: (a) generating income and contributing productively to one's community, (b) partnering and parenting the next generation, and (c) engaging in lifestyle behaviors—including diet, physical activity, substance use, sexual behaviors, supportive versus abusive or harmful interpersonal relationships, and safety-minded behaviors versus injury-prone behaviors—that largely determine individual—and generational—health and disease status throughout the adult years.

Educational attainment and productive employment and income generation predict improved health status for the adults themselves, and for the generations that depend on their output: their children and, sometimes, their aging and dependent parents. This can create a daunting challenge for adults who occupy the "sandwich generation" role during a portion of their adult years as they support three generations simultaneously.

The adult years likewise focus energy and attention on parenting the children who will ultimately become the next adult generation. Today's adults are supplying the vital nurturing care for their young children and providing practical guidance and encouragement for their adolescents who are on the cusp of matriculating at institutions of higher education or entering the workforce.

The adult years also represent the life period when the cumulative effects of individuals' lifestyle choices either produce vibrant health and vitality or, alternatively, progressive deterioration and onset of disease states, sometimes leading to premature death in later adult years. Life expectancies in most high-income countries now exceed 65 years, so death during the adult period should be regarded as untimely.

Fortunately, the four decades of adult life provide sufficient time for healthful behavioral choices to offset some of the early life deficits for those who endured ACEs or experimented with unhealthful behavioral choices during adolescence.

End-of-Chapter Resources

 Access additional case study podcasts online at http://connect.springerpub.com/ content/book/978-0-8261-8043-8/

DISCUSSION QUESTIONS

1. Physical inactivity—living a sedentary lifestyle—is a major risk factor for heart disease. However, sitting for most hours of the day is an independent risk factor for heart disease even for those adults who do achieve the days-per-week and minutes-per-day physical activity guidelines. How can adults build-in frequent brief bursts of activity into their daily work schedules?

2. How can adults with children and economically dependent parents (the true "sandwich generation" folks) achieve a healthy "work–life balance" that is critical for their own health?

3. One of the dilemmas in some high-income countries, including the United States—but excluding Japan—is the tendency for a high proportion of working adults to not exercise the discipline of putting a reasonable portion of their earnings into savings. This creates compounding demands on the adult generation: (a) to work industriously all through their adult years (because they are "paying as they go") and (b) to take on the burden of supporting their aging parents who did not save adequately for their own retirement. Is it possible to motivate individuals—and entire generations—to save money in a planful way? What are the health implications?

 A robust set of instructor resources designed to supplement this text is located at **http://connect.springerpub.com/content/book/978-0-8261-8043-8**. Qualifying instructors may request access by emailing **textbook@springerpub.com**.

REFERENCES

1. Phillips M. *Russia is quite literally drinking itself to death*. Quartz. Published May 13, 2015. https://qz.com/403307/russia-is-quite-literally-drinking-itself-to-death

2. Zaridze D, Lewington S, Boroda A, et al. Alcohol and mortality in Russia: prospective observational study of 151,000 adults. *Lancet*. 2014;383(9927):1465-1473. doi:10.1016/S0140-6736(13)62247-3

3. Hartley R. Adulthood: the time you get serious about the rest of your life. *Fam Matters*. 1991;30. https://aifs.gov.au/publications/family-matters/issue-30/adulthood-time-you-get-serious-about-rest-your-life

4. Arnett JJ, Žukauskienė R, Sugimura K. The new life stage of emerging adulthood at ages 18–29 years: implications for mental health. *Lancet Psychiatry*. 2014;1(7):569-576. doi:10.1016/S2215-0366(14)00080-7

5. Arnett JJ, ed. *Emerging Adulthood*. 2nd ed. Oxford University Press; 2015. doi:10.1093/oxfordhb/9780199795574.013.9

6. Arnett JJ. Learning to stand alone: the contemporary American transition to adulthood in cultural and historical context. *Hum Dev*. 1998;41(5-6):295-315. doi:10.1159/000022591

7. Marmot M. Social determinants of health inequalities. *Lancet*. 2005;365(9464):1099-1104. doi:10.1016/S0140-6736(05)71146-6

8. Marmot M. The health gap: the challenge of an unequal world. *Lancet*. 2015;386:2442-2444. doi:10.1016/S0140-6736(15)00150-6

9. Kelly Y, Sacker A, Del Bono E, et al. What role for the home learning environment and parenting in reducing the socioeconomic gradient in child development? Findings from the millennium cohort study. *Arch Dis Child*. 2011;96(9):832-837. doi:10.1136/adc.2010.195917

10. Shah R, Sobotka SA, Chen YF, Msall ME. Positive parenting practices, health disparities, and developmental progress. *Pediatrics*. 2015;136(2):318-326. doi:10.1542/peds.2014-3390

11. Woolf SH, Aron LY, Dubay L, et al. *How Are Income and Wealth Linked to Health and Longevity?* Urban Institute; 2015. https://www.urban.org/research/publication/how-are-income-and-wealth-linked-health-and-longevity

12. National Center for Health Statistics. *Health, United States, 2011*. U.S. Department of Health and Human Services, Centers for Disease Control and Prevention; 2011. https://www.cdc.gov/nchs/data/hus/hus11.pdf

13. Braveman PA, Cubbin C, Egerter S, et al. Socioeconomic disparities in health in the United States: what the patterns tell us. *Am J Public Health*. 2010;100(suppl 1):S186-S196. doi:10.2105/AJPH.2009.166082

14. Pollack CE, Cubbin C, Sania A, et al. Do wealth disparities contribute to health disparities within racial/ethnic groups? *J Epidemiol Community Health*. 2013;67(5):439-445. doi:10.1136/jech-2012-200999

15. Nandi A, Glymour MM, Subramanian SV. Association among socioeconomic status, health behaviors, and all-cause mortality in the United States. *Epidemiology*. 2014;25(2):170-177. doi:10.1097/EDE.0000000000000038

16. National Center for Health Statistics. *Summary health statistics for U.S. adults: National Health Interview Survey, 2011*. U.S. Department of Health and Human Services, Centers for Disease Control and Prevention; 2012. https://www.cdc.gov/nchs/data/series/sr_10/sr10_256.pdf

17. Cutler DM, Lleras-Muney A. *Education and Health: Evaluating Theories and Evidence*. NBER Working Papers 12352. National Bureau of Economic Research; 2006. https://ideas.repec.org/p/nbr/nberwo/12352.html

18. Kawachi I, Adler NE, Dow WH. Money, schooling, and health: mechanisms and causal evidence. *Ann N Y Acad Sci*. 2010;1186(1):56-68. doi:10.1111/j.1749-6632.2009.05340.x

19. McEwen BS. Stressed or stressed out: what is the difference?. *J Psychiatry Neurosci*. 2005;30(5):315-318.

20. Thoits PA. Stress and health: major findings and policy implications. *J Health Soc Behav*. 2010;51 (1 suppl):S41-S53. doi:10.1177/0022146510383499

21. Gallo LC, Roesch SC, Fortmann AL, et al. Associations of chronic stress burden, perceived stress, and traumatic stress with cardiovascular disease prevalence and risk factors in the Hispanic Community Health Study/Study of Latinos Sociocultural Ancillary Study. *Psychosom Med*. 2014;76(6):468-475. doi:10.1097/PSY.0000000000000069

22. Galea S. *Mental Health is Public Health*. Psychology Today. Published October 10, 2019. https://www.psychologytoday.com/us/blog/talking-about-health/201910/mental-health-is-public-health

23. Wood S. *Resources for students facing housing insecurity*. U.S. News World Report. Published April 6, 2022. https://www.usnews.com/education/articles/resources-for-college-students-facing-housing-insecurity

24. Temple University. The Hope Center for College, Community, and Justice. *The hope center basic needs survey*. https://hope.temple.edu/research/hope-center-basic-needs-survey

25. Graham C. *COVID-19 Worsens housing insecurity for college students*. Best Colleges. Published May 6, 2022. https://www.bestcolleges.com/blog/covid-19-housing-insecurity-college-students/

26. Laman B. *The impact of housing insecurity on college students*. TimelyCare. Published August 7, 2021. https://timely.md/blog/housing-insecurity-college-students/

27. Shonkoff JP, Garner AS, Siegel BS, et al. The lifelong effects of early childhood adversity and toxic stress. *Pediatrics*. 2012;129(1):e232-e246. doi:10.1542/peds.2011-2663

28. Zheng Y, Manson JE, Yuan C, et al. Associations of weight gain from early to middle adulthood with major health outcomes later in life. *JAMA*. 2017;318(3):255-269. doi:10.1001/jama.2017.7092

29. Hser YI, Hamilton A, Niv N. Understanding drug use over the life course: past, present, and future. *J Drug Issues*. 2009;39(1):231-236. doi:10.1177/002204260903900119

30. Lobstein T, Jackson Leach R. *Foresight tackling obesities: future choices–international comparisons of obesity trends, determinants and responses–evidence review*. Published October 2007. https://assets.publishing.service.gov.uk/government/uploads/system/uploads/attachment_data/file/295684/07-926A2-obesity-international.pdf

31. World Health Organization. *A Global Brief on Hypertension: Silent Killer, Global Public Health Crisis*. Author; 2013. https://www.who.int/publications/i/item/a-global-brief-on-hypertension-silent-killer-global-public-health-crisis-world-health-day-2013

32. Public Health Agency of Canada. *Diabetes in Canada: facts and figures from a public health perspective*. Government of Canada. Author; 2011:13-25. https://www.canada.ca/en/public-health/services/chronic-diseases/reports-publications/diabetes/diabetes-canada-facts-figures-a-public-health-perspective.html

33. Benjamin EJ, Virani SS, Callaway CW, et al. Heart disease and stroke statistics—2018 update: a report from the American Heart Association. *Circulation*. 2018;137(12):e67-e492. doi:10.1161/CIR.0000000000000558

34. The American Heart Association. *Life's simple 7*. 2017. https://playbook.heart.org/lifes-simple-7/

35. Healthy People 2030. *Healthy People 2030 framework*. https://health.gov/healthypeople/about/healthy-people-2030-framework

36. Shetty P, Howe P, eds. *Responding to Intimate Partner Violence and Sexual Violence Against Women*. World Health Organization; 2013. https://apps.who.int/iris/bitstream/handle/10665/85240/9789241548595_eng.pdf?sequence=1

37. Arango DJ, Morton M, Gennari F, et al. *Interventions to Prevent or Reduce Violence Against Women and Girls: A Systematic Review of Reviews*. World Bank Group; 2014:1-61. http://documents.worldbank.org/curated/en/700731468149970518/Interventions-to-prevent-or-reduce-violence-against-women-and-girls-a-systematic-review-of-reviews

38. Ellsberg M, Arango DJ, Morton M, et al. Prevention of violence against women and girls: what does the evidence say? *Lancet*. 2015;385(9977):1555-1566. doi:10.1016/S0140-6736(14)61703-7

39. The National Institute of Mental Health. *Depression.* https://www.nimh.nih.gov/health/topics/depression/index.shtml

40. Murray CJL, Atkinson C, Bhalla K, et al. The state of US health, 1990-2010. *JAMA.* 2013;*310*(6):591. doi:10.1001/jama.2013.13805

41. Ferrari AJ, Charlson FJ, Norman RE, et al. Burden of depressive disorders by country, sex, age, and year: findings from the global burden of disease study 2010. *PLoS Med.* 2013;*10*(11):e1001547. doi:10.1371/journal.pmed.1001547

42. Pan American Health Organization. *The Burden of Mental Disorders.* https://www.paho.org/en/enlace/burden-mental-disorders

43. Institute for Health Metrics and Evaluation. *Global burden of disease compare tool.* https://vizhub.healthdata.org/gbd-compare/

44. Aldrich N. *CDC Promotes Public Health Approach to Address Depression Among Older Adults.* Centers for Disease Control and Prevention; 2019. https://www.cdc.gov/aging/pdf/cib_mental_health.pdf

45. Brown A, McGreeney K. *In U.S., employment most linked to being depression-free.* Gallup. Published August 23, 2013. https://news.gallup.com/poll/164090/employment-linked-depression-free.aspx

46. The National Institute of Mental Health. *U.S. leading disease/disorder categories by age.* Wayback Machine website. http://web.archive.org/web/20210205112437/http://www.nimh.nih.gov:80/health/statistics/disability/us-leading-disease-disorder-categories-by-age.shtml

47. Pratt LA, Brody DJ. Depression in the U.S. household population, 2009-2012. *NCHS Data Brief.* 2014;172:1-8. https://www.cdc.gov/nchs/products/databriefs/db172.htm

48. Ettman CK, Abdalla SM, Cohen GH, Sampson L, Vivier PM, Galea S. Prevalence of depression symptoms in US adults before and during the COVID-19 pandemic. *JAMA Netw Open.* 2020;3(9):e2019686. doi:10.1001/jamanetworkopen.2020.19686

49. Jeuring HW, Comijs HC, Deeg DJH, et al. Secular trends in the prevalence of major and subthreshold depression among 55–64-year olds over 20 years. *Psychol Med.* 2018;*48*(11):1824-1834. doi:10.1017/S0033291717003324

50. Dishman RK, Sui X, Church TS, et al. Decline in cardiorespiratory fitness and odds of incident depression. *Am J Prev Med.* 2012;*43*(4):361-368. doi:10.1016/j.amepre.2012.06.011

51. Kwon E, Park S. Heterogeneous trajectories of physical and mental health in late middle age: importance of life-course socioeconomic positions. *Int J Environ Res Public Health.* 2017;*14*(6):582. doi:10.3390/ijerph14060582

52. Kwon E, Kim B, Lee H, Park S. Heterogeneous trajectories of depressive symptoms in late middle age: critical period, accumulation, and social mobility life course perspectives. *J Aging Health.* 2018;*30*(7):1011-1041. doi:10.1177/0898264317704540

53. Oyama H, Sakashita T. Community-based screening intervention for depression affects suicide rates among middle-aged Japanese adults. *Psychol Med.* 2017;47(08):1500-1509. doi:10.1017/S0033291717000204

54. World Health Organization. *COVID-19 pandemic triggers 25% increase in prevalence of anxiety and depression worldwide.* Published March 2, 2022. https://www.who.int/news/item/02-03-2022-covid-19-pandemic-triggers-25-increase-in-prevalence-of-anxiety-and-depression-worldwide

55. Ettman CK, Cohen GH, Abdalla SM, et al. Persistent depressive symptoms during COVID-19: a national, population-representative, longitudinal study of U.S. adults. *Lancet Reg Health Am.* 2022;5:100091. doi:10.1016/j.lana.2021.100091

56. Vahratian A, Blumberg SJ, Terlizzi EP, Schiller JS. Symptoms of anxiety or depressive disorder and use of mental health care among adults during the COVID-19 Pandemic—United States, August 2020-February 2021. *MMWR Morb Mortal Wkly Rep.* 2021;*70*(13):490-494. Published April 2, 2021. doi:10.15585/mmwr.mm7013e2

57. Kolappa K, Henderson DC, Kishore SP. No physical health without mental health: lessons unlearned? *Bull World Health Organ.* 2013;*91*(1):3-3A. doi:10.2471/BLT.12.115063

58. Virani SS, Alonso A, Aparicio HJ, et al. Heart disease and stroke statistics—2021 update: a report from the American Heart Association. *Circulation.* 2021;*143*:e254-e743.

59. U.S. Preventive Services Task Force. *Healthy diet and physical activity for cardiovascular disease prevention in adults with cardiovascular risk factors: behavioral counseling interventions.* Published November 24, 2020. https://www.uspreventiveservicestaskforce.org/uspstf/recommendation/healthy-diet-and-physical-activity-counseling-adults-with-high-risk-of-cvd

60. Weintraub WS, Daniels SR, Burke LE, et al. Value of primordial and primary prevention for cardiovascular disease: a policy statement from the American Heart Association. *Circulation.* 2011;*124*(8):967-990. doi:10.1161/CIR.0b013e3182285a81

61. Tudor-Locke C, Leonardi C, Johnson WD, Katzmarzyk PT, Church TS. Accelerometer steps/day translation of moderate-to-vigorous activity. *Prev Med.* 2011;*53*(1-2):31-33. doi:10.1016/j.ypmed.2011.01.014

62. Centers for Disease Control and Prevention. *A Public Health Action Plan to Prevent Heart Disease and Stroke.* https://www.cdc.gov/dhdsp/action_plan/pdfs/action_plan_full.pdf

63. Centers for Disease Control and Prevention. *About Million Hearts® 2027: Million Hearts®.* https://millionhearts.hhs.gov/about-million-hearts/index.html

64. American Heart Association. *CDC prevention programs.* Published May 18, 2018. https://www.heart.org/en/get-involved/advocate/federal-priorities/cdc-prevention-programs

65. Pearson TA. Public policy approaches to the prevention of heart disease and stroke. *Circulation.* 2011;*124*(23):2560-2571. doi:10.1161/CIRCULATIONAHA.110.968743

11

OLDER AGE

LEARNING OBJECTIVES

- Explain the current and ongoing trends as older adults become an increasing proportion of the population and relate this to the demographic transition of decreasing death rates and decreasing birth rates.

- Differentiate "living longer" from "living healthier, longer."

- Describe how risk factors operate dynamically to accelerate the occurrence of disease with increasing age.

- Break down the contributions of accumulating lifetime risks, coupled with diseases of aging, in producing patterns of "multimorbidity" in older age groups.

- Identify promising public health programs to bring generations together for mutual benefit and to create health reciprocally across generations.

OVERVIEW: THE AGING DEMOGRAPHIC TRANSITION

We are living in a progressively aging world.[1] The global population will inevitably age over the coming decades, and the proportion of older adults will continue to increase. This trend is in motion and accelerating, with consequential implications for population health. At the moment when the global population crossed the 7 billion mark in 2012, 562 million were older adults, aged 65 years and beyond, representing 8% of global citizens.[2] Just 7 years later, in 2019, the number of older adults had risen by 141 million persons, to 703 million, and the proportion of older adults had ticked up to 9.13%. So, this aging process is gaining momentum.

At heart, population aging is one of the greatest good news stories of our time—it reflects healthier populations and more of us living longer lives. And, as this happens, our increasing life expectancy is boosting the numbers of older adults and the proportion of older adults in the global population. As the population ages, it creates an enormous set of new opportunities for us to generate health at all stages of the life course, but also, of course, creates challenges for us to ensure that we do what we can to keep populations healthy at all ages.

At heart, population aging is one of the greatest good news stories of our time—it reflects healthier populations and more of us living longer lives.

In this chapter, we examine (a) demographic trends toward aging populations worldwide, (b) the health challenges associated with older populations, (c) how public health can mitigate these threats, and (d) successful examples of public health efforts to improve health through action in older age.

EVOLVING POPULATION PATTERNS IN AN AGING WORLD

According to the World Bank, from 1960 to 2020, in a little over half a century, the proportion of older adults in the global population increased nearly 80%, from 5% to 9% (**Figure 11.1**).[3] This is just the beginning. By the year 2050, there will be 1.6 billion world citizens aged 65 years and older—equivalent to one of every six persons on the planet (17%). This estimate projects a 150% increase in absolute numbers of older adults by 2050 and a near-doubling of their population proportion.

In the United States, the distribution of older adults, aged 65 and over, is anticipated to rise across all racial subgroups from 2020 to 2060, with a projection for a greater increase among Latinx than among non-Latinx citizens (**Table 11.1**).

What is behind this upsurge in numbers of older adults? The progressive aging of our planet's population is partially an outgrowth of the first demographic transition.[4,5] Beginning with European countries in the 18th century, and gaining speed throughout the period of industrialization, historical declines have been observed in deaths, and somewhat more recently, in births. With plummeting mortality, the world's population has increased eightfold since 1800 (**Figure 11.2**).

As a counterpoint, there has been a sudden, and joltingly abrupt, decline in the population growth rate over the past half-century. One of the primary drivers of this downshift in population growth is the precipitous decline in birth rates. The timing of decreasing death rates,

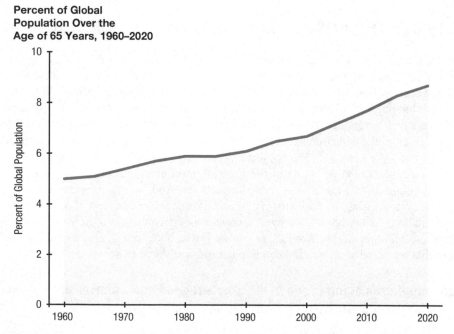

Percent of Global
Population Over the
Age of 65 Years, 1960–2020

FIGURE 11.1 Older adults (ages 65 and above) as a percentage of the global population, 1960 to 2020.
Source: Data from The World Bank Group. Population ages 65 and above (% of total). https://data.worldbank.org/indicator/SP.POP.65UP.TO.ZS

TABLE 11.1   Projections and Distribution of Older Adults, Ages 65 and Older by Race and Latinx Origin, United States, 2020 to 2060

RACE/LATINX STATUS	POPULATION PROJECTIONS (AGES 65 AND OLDER, IN THOUSANDS)				
	2020	2030	2040	2050	2060
Total population	55,969	72,774	79,719	83,739	92,033
Racial Status					
Single race specified					
White	47,166	59,837	63,683	64,760	68,723
Black	5,406	7,810	9,190	10,283	12,374
Asian	2,398	3,525	4,725	5,955	7,274
American Indian/ Alaska Native	416	657	834	996	1,195
Native Hawaiian/Other Pacific Islander	70	119	164	220	274
Multiple races specified	513	828	1,122	1,524	2,192
Latinx Status					
Latinx	4,831	8,023	11,695	15,421	19,516
Non-Latinx	51,138	64,751	68,025	68,318	72,517
Non-Latinx White	42,761	52,594	53,180	51,033	51,440
Non-Latinx Non-White	8,377	12,157	14,845	17,285	21,077

Source: Data from Ortman JM, Velkoff VA, Hogan H. *An Aging Nation: The Older Population in the United States: Population Estimates and Projections* [Current Population Reports]. U.S. Census Bureau; 2014.

followed later by decreasing birth rates, is portrayed in relation to the five stages of the demographic transition (**Figure 11.3**), resulting in a modestly growing global population and a more rapidly growing older population.

Massive numbers of persons born during the population boom in the mid-1900s are now entering their older adult years. However, the generations that follow them are comparatively smaller in size. At the same time, gains in life expectancy are adding years to life. So, on net, increasing proportions of persons alive today are older adults.

Distant future patterns are more difficult to predict. Remarkable cultural changes, marking the "second demographic transition,"[5] are already underway, modifying how we populate the world in rather complicated ways. This includes such phenomena as the post–baby-boom "baby bust," diverse types of couplings and partnerships, and postponement of partnering and parenthood, among other changes. But, for the immediate future decades, expect more older adults.

It is particularly notable that the increase in numbers and proportions of older adults is not uniform worldwide. This is because individual nations, and entire continental regions, are currently at different points along the (first) demographic transition.

World Population Growth, 1760–2100

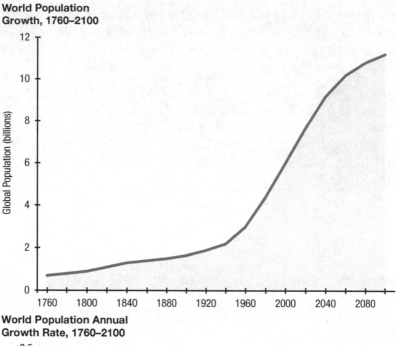

World Population Annual Growth Rate, 1760–2100

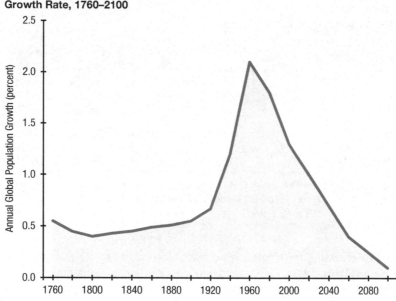

FIGURE 11.2 World population growth, 1760 to 2100.
Source: Data from Roser M, Ortiz–Ospina E. World population growth. 2017. https://ourworldindata.org/world -population-growth

Industrialization, wealth generation, and socioeconomic status (SES) vary by geographical region. The differential pace of aging and the speed of movement along the demographic transition are strongly influenced by the continuum of affluence versus poverty.

Currently, one in six of the world's citizens live in high-income countries. These countries have been at the front end of the demographic transitions, and they have been aging for decades. Consequently, high-income countries already have high population proportions of older adults. Worldwide, one in three adults aged 65 and older and one in two adults aged 85 and older reside in these high-income countries.

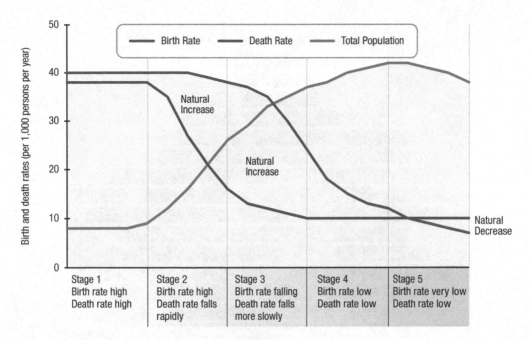

FIGURE 11.3 The five stages of the demographic transition.
Source: Data from Roser M, Ortiz-Ospina E. World population growth. 2017. https://ourworldindata.org/world
-population-growth

However, this pattern is already changing rapidly and dramatically. Lower income countries are swept up in a sharp acceleration toward aging. They may be lagging behind their higher income neighbors, but they are catching up quickly. This is so much so that, by 2050, less than one-fifth of older adults will still be found in high-income nations.

When comparing continental regions, Europe has progressed farthest along the demographic transition over a period of centuries and continuing into recent times. During the upcoming three decades, Asia and Latin America are poised to undergo very rapid aging of their populations. When considering the upper echelons of age, the oldest-old, projections call for a quadrupling of the over-80 population in many countries in Asia and Latin America between 2015 and 2050.

Asia will experience the most expedited aging from now until 2050, at which time it will decisively emerge as the global region with the world's largest over-65 population. By contrast, Africa will remain the relative youngster. The fertility rate for Africa will continue to exceed the replacement rate (the rate required to maintain the current population factoring in deaths and immigrations). This will lead to net population growth and an overall population structure that is younger than any other region.

One of the most compelling population forecasts is how the paths of the world's two "population billionaires," China and India, will diverge conspicuously. In April, 2023, the population of India exceeded 1,425,000,000, surpassing China and assuming the top spot as the world's most populous nation.

China instituted a strict one-child policy in 1979. The effects of this policy on the Chinese population structure will reverberate for generations. The projected change in the population pyramid for China is truly extraordinary (**Figure 11.4**). By the year 2050, the population distribution will appear top-heavy and unwieldy as a hefty proportion of older adults totters on a narrow, shrunken base composed of fewer children, youth, and young adults.

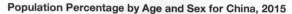

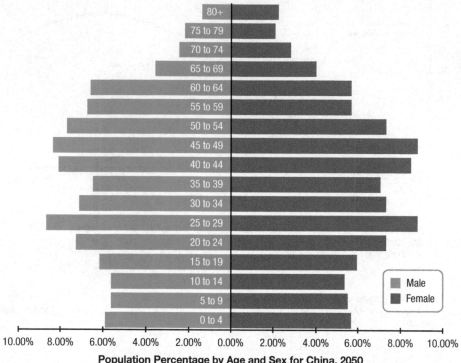

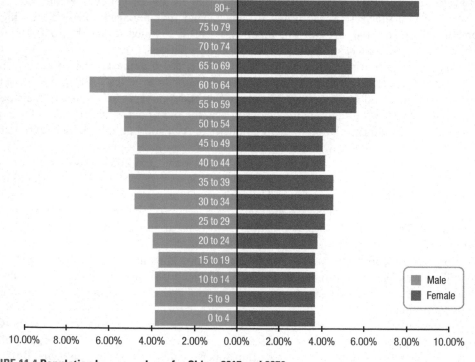

FIGURE 11.4 Population by age and sex for China: 2015 and 2050.
Source: He W, Goodkind D, Kowal P. *An Aging World: 2015. International Population Reports.* 2016. https://www.census
.gov/content/dam/Census/library/publications/2016/demo/p95-16-1.pdf

One of the most compelling population forecasts is how the paths of the world's two "population billionaires," China and India, will diverge conspicuously.

The population of India is projected to surge upward to 1.67 billion by 2050 while the population of China is expected to contract to 1.31 billion by that year.[166] Yet paradoxically, China will still have 100 million more older adults than India at midcentury.

THE CAUSES OF HEALTH IN OLDER AGE

One of the most obvious, yet profound, questions to ask is what causes health in older age? As we contemplate the causes of health in older age, we are buoyed by the preceding discussion that tells us we are living longer. We first reflect on the remarkable upsurge in life expectancy. We then look at whether living longer also means living healthier longer. What is healthy life expectancy? Then we look on the flip side. We drill down to explore the major threats to health in older ages. We indeed live longer, but not because we outrun risks. In fact, we discuss how the lifelong accumulation of risk factors and risk behaviors poses risks to the health of older adults, increases disability, and shortens the years remaining.

LIVING LONGER AND REDUCING RISKS

In less than 50 years, since 1970, the mean age at death has surged forward by 35 years![6] There is simply no precedent for this in all human history. Decreasing death rates have been observed for all age categories, including the oldest old.[7] What this means is that at any attained age, the average remaining life expectancy has increased. As a case in point, in just over a century, comparing the years 1900 and 2009, life expectancy at age 65 leapt from 11.9 to 19.1 years; at age 80, the jump was from 5.3 to 9.1 years.[8]

When we consider the countries with the highest and lowest, male and female, after-65 life expectancies, three patterns are clear. First, women everywhere have an after-65 life expectancy advantage over men. Second, higher income and SES are associated with longer life expectancy. Third, the after-65 life expectancy will increase for men and women, regardless of SES, from now up to 2050 and beyond.

What is responsible for elevating even older age life expectancies upward? Using a slightly different age cut point, age 60, investigators showed how changes in disease patterns contributed to increased life expectancy between 1980 and 2011.[7] In high-income nations, reductions in cardiovascular disease and diabetes deaths were the most important contributors to increased life years for men and women. For men, a further increment in life expectancy was associated with reductions in smoking-attributable deaths. Middle-income countries in Latin America and the Caribbean showed similar patterns of mortality reductions, but the net effect was lower than in high-income countries.

Older adults in low-income countries continue to experience a substantial proportion of illness and death from infectious diseases, and these countries have experienced a more modest advance in life expectancy for the oldest old.[9]

LIVING HEALTHIER LONGER

Marked gains in life expectancy for older adults partially reflect living healthier into advanced years of life. However, being alive longer is not the same as being alive and healthy. The ideal, of course, is to live healthier longer. This implies relative freedom from disease and disability. This also implies a high degree of functionality, both physical and mental. Older adults aspire to live with independence. They desire to perform activities of daily living (ADLs) with ease, strength, mobility, and freedom from debilitating pain and discomfort.

Fries introduced the concept of the "compression of morbidity."[10,11] First, this expression directly describes the ratcheting down of the number of years of ill-health or major activity limitations to as few as possible within the total life span. Second, this expression—compression of morbidity—implies the result of maximally expanding the number of years of robust, disease-free, healthy life. The ideal would be to compress ill-health down to a speck in time. We would all desire to experience a bucketful of healthy life with only a droplet of infirmity at the end of the lifetime.

How do we quantify this concept? Health-adjusted life expectancy (HALE) is a useful summary measure that takes into consideration an individual's functional capacity and the presence of disease or disability. The World Health Organization (WHO) describes the HALE measure as the average number of years that a person can expect to live in full health, offset by the years lived in less than full health due to disease or injury.[12]

The HALE indicator can be calculated from birth or, more relevant to this discussion, from the age of 60 or 65 forward. HALE is usually reported as a population health measure, adding together the HALE values for the individuals making up the population. The HALE metric increased demonstrably across all WHO regions worldwide during the early years of the 2000s. HALE increased for men, women, and both sexes combined both for the entire life span and for older ages. Not surprisingly, HALE is highest for the economically wealthiest regions.

The European Commission maintains a data set for updated computations of many health indictors, including the HALE measure.[13] **Figure 11.5** shows a subset of European nations, in rank order based on post-65 life expectancy for women.

At age 65, French women can expect to live more than 23 additional years on average, the highest among all European nations surveyed. However, for French women, somewhat less than half of their remaining life, about 11 years, would be lived in full health. The average remaining life expectancy for Norwegian women is a bit shorter than for French women, slightly less than 22 years. However, on average, Norwegian women will live more than 16 of these years in full health.

The ratio of HALE to remaining life expectancy represents the proportion of remaining life lived in full health. At the high end, Norwegian men can expect that 80% of their remaining years will be free from activity limitations. Norwegian women can anticipate that 75% of their ongoing life span will be lived in health. In sharp contrast, in Slovakia, not only is remaining life expectancy shorter, but for men only 23% of remaining years of life will be healthy years, and for women, just 16%.

HEALTH THREATS AND CHALLENGES DURING OLDER AGE

One of the defining features of older adult ages is the piling up of long-duration risk factors for noncommunicable diseases (NCDs). Risk factors accumulate and cluster as age advances.[14,15] This concentration of multiple NCD risk factors has implications for disability as well as mortality.

Data from the Global Burden of Diseases, Injuries, and Risk Factors Study (GBD) make the case.[16] A key summary measure used in the GBD study is disability-adjusted life years (DALYs). Each DALY represents 1 year of healthy life lost due to premature death or to disability and activity limitation. Summing the DALYs across all of the members of a population provides a measure of the population burden of disease. DALYs effectively measure the gap between the ideal of full health for all members of a population and the current reality. Unfortunately, many population members are hobbled by disabilities related to chronic diseases and physical limitations.

What are the major contributors to DALYs? In terms of global DALYs, leading risk factors are high blood pressure (9.3% of DALYs), particulate matter pollution (8.3%), and tobacco smoking (7.9%).[16] Further, the combination of physical inactivity and several related dietary risk factors account for an additional 10% of global DALYs.

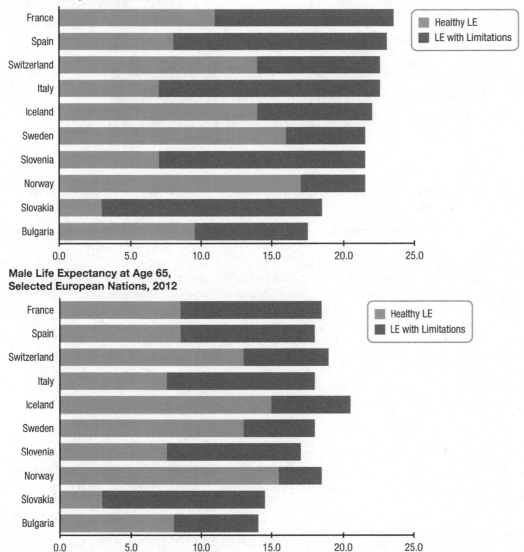

Female Life Expectancy at Age 65,
Selected European Nations, 2012

Male Life Expectancy at Age 65,
Selected European Nations, 2012

FIGURE 11.5 LE and HALE at age 65 by sex for selected European countries, 2012. LE, life expectancy; HALE, health-adjusted life expectancy.

Note: HALE is the average number of years that a person can expect to live in full health by taking into account years lived in less than full health due to disease and/or injury.

Source: He W, Goodkind D, Kowal P. *An Aging World: 2015. International Population Reports.* 2016. https://www.census .gov/content/dam/Census/library/publications/2016/demo/p95-16-1.pdf

A multicountry analysis of 38,000 respondents, aged 50 years and older, across six diverse nations, examined the propensity for risk factors to accumulate.[17] Six NCD risk factors were assessed: current daily tobacco use, frequent heavy drinking, hypertension, insufficient vegetable and fruit intake, low level of physical activity, and obesity. The study found vanishingly small fractions of persons with no risk factors at all, in any of the populations. Two or more concurrent NCD risks were present in 68% to 90% of respondents; and three or more risks were found for 33% to 68% (**Figure 11.6**).

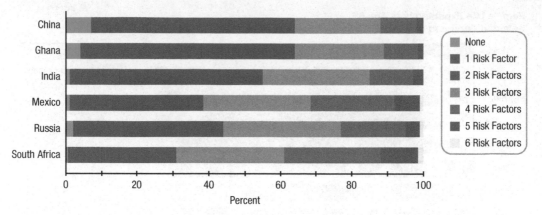

FIGURE 11.6 Percentage distribution of cumulative risk factors among people aged 50 and over for six countries: 2007 to 2010.
Source: He W, Goodkind D, Kowal P. *An Aging World: 2015. International Population Reports.* 2016. https://www.census .gov/content/dam/Census/library/publications/2016/demo/p95-16-1.pdf

The U.S. experience shows that health threats in older age are not uniform throughout a nation. This partly explains the American wealth–health paradox. The United States is indisputably the wealthiest large country in the world, but it is far from the top in life expectancy at age 65 (or at birth) compared with most other high-income countries and even some middle-income countries.[18] The National Research Council flags this incongruous U.S. experience in its bluntly titled comparative analysis, "U.S. Health in International Perspective: Shorter Lives, Poorer Health."[19]

Wealth does not guarantee well-being. One of the reasons for the poor showing of the United States on life expectancy is the existence of marked demographic and geographic health disparities that influence the longevity of older adults.[20] Poorer states, especially those concentrated in the southern United States, had lower "healthy life expectancy" at age 65 than other regions.[21] Dishearteningly, these regional health inequalities are becoming more pronounced over time.[22] Clusters of preventable NCD risk factors—notably hypertension, smoking, obesity, and elevated blood glucose—played a role in creating differential mortality rates and life expectancies by sex, race, and U.S. county of residence over a period of decades.[23,24]

INCREASING DISEASE INCIDENCE AND PREVALENCE OF DISEASES OF AGING

Here is what we know. As just discussed, risk factors accumulate with age. Risk factors cluster, interact, synergize, and elevate risks for disease and disease complications. Incidence and prevalence rates of NCDs are rising with age. The proportions of the population suffering from functional impairments, including mobility limitations and sensory impairments, are rising with age. The proportions of older adults developing progressively worsening cognitive impairment are rising with age. The prevalent medical and psychiatric conditions of the older adult population are placing economic burdens on family budgets and employee health plans. Compared with those who are younger, older persons require more healthcare services, social support systems, and assisted living facilities.

International patterns of disability and death are changing rapidly. In less than a quarter century, from 1990 to 2019, there was a 58% increase in mortality from NCDs.[25] The proliferation and concentration of deaths in older ages is clearly apparent in vital statistics data. Worldwide, 43% of deaths occur in persons 70 years of age and older, and in fact, 23% of deaths occur in persons 80 years and older.[26] At first glance, this may seem alarming that NCDs are becoming more deadly, but it actually points to the opposite scenario.

The higher proportion of NCD deaths in older ages, especially from such causes as heart disease, stroke, chronic lung diseases, and cancers, is actually associated with people living longer prior to dying. Age-standardized death rates (i.e., rates of death applied to a standard age distribution to allow for fair comparison) for these leading NCDs have actually decreased over time.

However, there are marked disparities among countries and entire continental regions when examined by SES. Compared with high-income countries, low- and middle-income countries are experiencing more rapid increases in NCD morbidity and mortality rates.[27] Some of the world's poorest nations are simultaneously dealing with rising death rates from three sources: NCDs, infectious diseases, and injuries. These patterns translate into relatively shorter life expectancies and more disease and disability for older persons living in poor countries. The good news is that gains in life expectancy are anticipated worldwide by 2050 for nations across all income categories. The largest predicted increases will occur for the poorest nations. So, lower income nations will partially catch up.

MULTIMORBIDITY

One outcome of living longer is that there is more of a chronological lifetime during which NCDs can develop. As described in the discussion of cardiovascular disease during the adult years (Chapter 10, "Adulthood"), risk factors for NCDs tend to cluster and interact synergistically, amplifying the effects of the individual risks. Here we find that clinically manifest and diagnosable NCDs frequently co-occur, especially during the older adult years. Multimorbidity describes the situation in which individuals, or subpopulations within a community, are diagnosed with two or more concurrent NCDs.[28-30]

Age, specifically advancing age, is itself a well-documented risk factor for multimorbidity. Studies worldwide, ranging from low- to high-income countries, have demonstrated the risk-elevating contribution of increasing age to multimorbidity. Such studies have been reported from Bangladesh,[31] India,[32] Spain,[33] Scotland,[34] and Germany.[35] In addition to the primary contribution of older age as a risk factor, other contributors to multimorbidity are low income, unemployment, and low levels of education.[36]

It is well known that older adults use healthcare services at high rates, and multimorbidity is a major reason for this. Older adults are routinely treated for more severe and clinically advanced conditions with a high risk for complications. Understandably, management of multiple concurrent diseases is complex and costly. Living with multimorbidity negatively affects well-being and quality of life in a manner that may, in turn, exacerbate these health conditions.[37-39]

Multimorbidity is certainly one hallmark of older age. However, there is also a difference in the mix and blend of common diseases. Older age involves age-specific conditions in addition to a larger array of illnesses that started earlier in the life course.

When thinking of diseases that are tightly concentrated in older age groups, consider the examples of Alzheimer's disease and other dementias, Parkinson disease, stroke, and a wide realm of musculoskeletal and joint conditions, including osteoporosis, hip and limb fractures, and lower back pain. To this litany would be added the complications of low mobility including urinary incontinence and pressure sores.

Owing to a combination of (a) the clustering of risk factors, (b) multimorbidity, and (c) the overlay of more recently acquired diseases of aging, many older adults are being treated simultaneously for a range of concurrent conditions. This adds significantly to the complexity of care both across medical conditions and across a spectrum of providers and care settings.[40] Treatments and medications prescribed for these conditions may themselves set off drug interactions or other exacerbating consequences. Therefore, coordination of care, including social services, is a major issue when designing comprehensive treatment plans for older patients.[41]

ACTIVITIES OF DAILY LIVING

As another point of view on disability, a study conducted in 12 European countries, the United Kingdom, and the United States found that limitations in ADLs rose consistently, steeply, and steadily with age in all countries studied.

ADLs were introduced by Sidney Katz in the 1950s as one of his major contributions to the quantification of the functional assessment of older adults and persons with chronic conditions.[42] ADLs serve as a standardized measure of functional independence—or dependence—for performing such tasks as bathing, dressing, toileting and continence, transferring, and feeding/eating.

One of the contributors to ADL limitations and progressive disability is the gradual replacement of time spent on moderate-to-vigorous physical activity during earlier years by more time spent in seated or reclining postures in later years. Daily sedentary time is an independent risk factor for ADL limitations, independent of physical inactivity.[43]

FRAILTY

Frailty, a characteristic typically ascribed to a subset of older adults, has been described as "a predisabled state."[44] Although the concepts are related, frailty is not identical to disability. What characterizes frailty is vulnerability and fragility as a result of a progressive loss of reserves. Rockwood and colleagues conceive of frailty as a syndrome with multiple dimensions.[45] These investigators quantify frailty using a seven-point Clinical Frailty Scale. The scale begins at the pole of peak fitness, "1—very fit," defined as "robust, active, energetic, well-motivated and fit; these people commonly exercise regularly and are in the most fit group for their age." So, 1 is the antithesis of frail. At the other extreme is "7—severely frail," defined as "completely dependent on others for the ADLs, or terminally ill."

A key distinction is that it is possible to be frail without specific diagnosed disabilities. However, many frail individuals have a combination of multimorbidity and disability. An international study of frailty, based on community-dwelling adults, aged 50 and older, found increasing rates of frailty with age, and also associations with lower levels of education, lower levels of wealth, and female sex.[46]

HEALTHCARE FOR OLDER ADULTS

The nature of health and disease patterns in older ages creates the need for additional types of care settings. Disease symptoms and disability progress and worsen over time while older adults are simultaneously aging. Therefore, a range of options is needed for providing both healthcare and old age care. Most self-evident is the increasing need for long-term care as the population ages. While there are mixed findings regarding whether health costs will necessarily rise with more older adults, there is no such debate regarding the costs of long-term care: The needs and the attendant costs will rise.[47]

What constitutes long-term care? Generally, the term describes services for persons with chronic, prolonged dependencies on assistance with their health or functional needs. Advancing age and diagnosable disability are the strongest predictors of the need for long-term care and the resulting expenditures.[48-52] At present, unpaid caregiving on the part of family and household members and friends continues to be the mainstay for providing long-term care to older adults throughout the world.[53] This dedication of effort, taking on the role of informal caregivers, affects the health and well-being of those who provide the care. A U.S. study attempted to quantify the economic value of informal caregiving, concluding that this care, if compensated, would have a market value of $522 billion.[54] For dementia alone, a condition that is increasing in prevalence and prominence, the value of unpaid caregiving in the United States was estimated at $305 billion in 2020, with an expected increase to $1.5 trillion by 2050.[55,56]

A broadening spectrum of care environments is being designed for persons whose care needs exceed the resources for informal, in-home care. For example, following a health shock, older adults need rehabilitative care both for recuperation and to avoid the alternative of diminishing functionality and increasing dependence. During episodes of serious illness later in life, care options are now broadening to include rehabilitative care. For those who are facing their final life period, various options are being devised to provide palliative, respite, or end-of-life care.

GLOBAL HEALTH NEEDS IN AN AGING WORLD

As the world ages, a key issue will be how to provide healthcare for a large number of older adults who, based on age, will need more health services for more complicated and costly health conditions. As the population ages, it stands to reason that populations will experience progressively more severe health complications of chronic conditions, primarily NCDs. In addition, as the population ages and older adults rely on their younger family members and caregivers, this will create stresses and burdens on multiple generations who share in the care of an aging population.

Longer life spans will lead to significantly larger older populations. There will be increasing numbers of older and sicker people to accommodate. This will necessarily challenge the ability of societies to continuously update healthcare systems and provide sustainable healthcare services.[57-60] Healthcare financing and insurance options will need to be redesigned. Providing health coverage for as many older adults as possible is a current, and looming, global priority. Predictable and exponentially growing health needs align with global imperatives around making universal health coverage (UHC) universally available.

UNIVERSAL HEALTHCARE

Governments and international organizations alike advocate for healthcare and social support systems for older adults.[61-64] They also strongly champion healthcare equity and equality for seniors worldwide. These are policy priorities whose time has come. UHC plays an important role in making this a reality.[65]

The international goal for achieving UHC, as defined by the WHO, is to guarantee that people worldwide can access the health services they need and receive these services at an affordable cost.[66] The motivation behind the promotion of UHC is to extend healthy life expectancy, functional capacities, and well-being throughout the life span. UHC is geared toward providing health services without imposing a crippling financial burden on the consumers.

UHC revolves around three key elements: (a) essential health services, (b) access to health services, and (c) healthcare affordability.[67] Currently, access to health services differs sharply by country and continental region.[68]

Providing UHC is an explicitly stated objective within the Sustainable Development Goals (SDGs).[69] The overarching health goal (SDG 3) is about ensuring healthy lives and promoting well-being for all ages. SDG health objective 3.8 specifically addresses UHC: "achieve universal health coverage, including financial risk protection, access to quality essential healthcare services and access to safe, effective, quality and affordable essential medicines and vaccines for all."[70]

SOCIAL SAFETY NETS

Many high-income countries provide social safety nets that help support living expenses and specific coverage for healthcare during the retirement years. As one example, the United States provides Social Security benefits for retired persons who, along with their employers, have paid into the system during their working years. Likewise, Medicare is a financing mechanism that is available to help cover a range of healthcare expenditures for U.S. citizens over the age of 65. One exception is dental costs, which rely on out-of-pocket or other sources of payment. The United States is an interesting case in that, lacking UHC to cover healthcare expenses during younger ages, some older citizens actually experience improved healthcare access when they turn age 65 and become eligible to receive Medicare benefits.

Many high-income countries provide social safety nets that help support living expenses and specific coverage for healthcare during the retirement years.

Social safety nets and forms of "financial risk protection" are broadly or completely lacking in many low- and middle-income countries. This absence of health insurance or payment support often translates into health-threatening delays in seeking care.[71] One compelling dimension of the financial burdens placed on poor families was elucidated in a scoping analysis of data for 3.66 billion world citizens in 40 low- and middle-income countries. Investigators found that 26% relied on either borrowing money or selling assets, or both, in order to receive health services.[72]

AGING AND THE UNEXPECTED POSSIBILITY OF REALIZING A TRIPLE DIVIDEND

Does aging contribute in a major way to increasing healthcare costs? This may seem like a naïve question, easily answered with a reflexive and emphatic "yes" response. However, evidence is accruing that rebuts this commonly held notion. If healthcare systems and community public health infrastructure make adaptive adjustments to the predictable needs for both healthcare and long-term care of an aging population, they may realize a trio of benefits that seems counterintuitive. This so-called "triple dividend" has been described by the phrase "thriving lives, costing less, contributing more."[73]

Best available data suggest that aging does not necessarily trigger escalating healthcare costs.[74-76] Several studies have shown that, at the population level, a longer life span does not inevitably translate into higher healthcare expenditures, especially when controlling for the higher healthcare costs in the final phase of life.[77-79]

Such analyses are hopeful, with the caveat that the status quo will not sustain healthcare for an enlarging aging population. Timely action on healthcare for older adults must be advocated and advanced.[80] Reanalysis of the true contributors to rising healthcare costs has led to some key realizations. For example, the sharp increase in healthcare utilization and costs frequently comes in the final 1 or 2 years immediately preceding death. This is the case regardless of whether the death occurs in childhood or in the upper reaches of advanced age.[81] Across the population, these final illness costs are equivalent to about one-fourth of total lifetime healthcare costs.

Strategic redirection of funding to prioritize disease prevention,[75,82] along with health promotion and health maintenance for older adults, may offset some of the anticipated cost run-ups for older adults.[83] NCDs in older adults have largely taken the place of infectious diseases, so the healthcare system needs to be redirected away from acute care and toward primary care.[84] It is also the primary care system that can best support the informal caregivers as older adults age and progressively need more constant care, often in home settings.

On the primary and secondary prevention fronts, it should be possible to lessen the burden of illness and infirmity in older ages. Fruitful targets for preventive interventions include smoking cessation, immunization programs for vaccine-preventable diseases stemming from human papillomavirus and influenza and pneumococcal-related infections,[85] and in another realm, cognitive training. The promotion of healthy, socially active aging holds considerable promise for reducing lifetime healthcare expenditures.[86,87]

CHANGING ENVIRONMENTS TO CREATE HEALTH IN OLDER AGE

There are a number of trial programs and policies that are experimenting with how to best integrate older adults into settings where they can contribute and be supported. Reciprocity is built into the design. Older adults have much to offer younger members of the community. Yet the aging process makes it more difficult to find opportunities, transportation, and appropriate venues to make these contributions. Case Study 11.1 provides illustrations of planful changes to social and physical environments that clearly support improved health in older age. These program examples demonstrate outlets for seniors to participate actively and to share their skills.

> **There are a number of trial programs and policies that are experimenting with how to best integrate older adults into settings where they can contribute and be supported.**

On one hand, these programs break new ground. After all, the planet has never had such a large number and high proportion of older citizens who represent a resource to be tapped. On the other hand, there is a curious sense of familiarity about certain aspects of these programs. This is because they harken back to the era of big, sprawling, multigenerational families and neighborly activities.

CASE STUDY 11.1: HOW HEALTHY OLDER ADULTS CAN HELP CREATE HEALTH IN YOUNGER AGES

The U.S. Experience Corps facilitates volunteer participation on the part of older adults working with children in public elementary schools. Each school receives a complement of 7 to 10 senior citizen volunteers who dedicate 15 hours per week throughout the school year, working with children across all grade levels. The program focuses on five learner outcomes: increasing school attendance, stimulating interest in reading, increasing literacy, improving children's problem-solving abilities, and teaching children how to play constructively and nonviolently.

Simultaneously, these structured volunteer activities provide the older adult volunteers with opportunities to apply and even refine a broad repertoire of social, physical, and cognitive skills while leading these educational activities. The volunteers meet as a group and participate in lesson planning. Delivering the curriculum requires them to engage their mental, visual–spatial, and problem-solving faculties. In the process, they are actively socializing with same-age peers, teachers throughout the school, and students. Teaching the students requires the volunteers to be both verbally and physically active.

Controlled trials have demonstrated favorable health outcomes for the older adults who volunteer. Compared with control subjects, the Experience Corps volunteers increased physical strength and capacity,[88] walking speed, and cognitive activity, while also reporting fewer depressive symptoms.[89] The volunteer role increased the richness of the social networks for these older adults and provided a sense of purpose. Volunteers reported that they made meaningful contributions to the academic and social success of the students they mentored. Fully 98% of volunteers rated their satisfaction with the program as high and 80% came back to serve again during the subsequent school year.[90]

HOW PUBLIC HEALTH CAN MITIGATE THREATS TO HEALTH DURING OLDER AGE

The WHO has identified five interrelated strategies to optimize health for older adults: (a) meet basic needs, (b) learn and make decisions, (c) be mobile, (d) build relationships, and (e) contribute.[91] These approaches serve as preventive interventions that together contribute to mitigating threats to health during older age.

MEET BASIC NEEDS

Health at any stage in the life course depends fundamentally on meeting the vital survival needs and ideally, creating a cushion of well-being that exceeds that basic level. In the specific context of health, older adults certainly need access to quality healthcare services and, later in life, to old age care. However, just as foundational is the imperative to meet the underlying needs for adequate housing and economic security.[92,93]

As discussed, the social and economic environment is a primary driver of health. The WHO's report on closing the gap in a generation addresses this forthrightly. "Poor social policies, unfair economic arrangements—through which the already well-off and healthy become even richer and the poor who are already more likely to be ill become even poorer—and bad politics"[94] interfere with the ability of older persons to successfully meet their basic needs and contribute to their own well-being and that of their family and community.

LEARN AND MAKE DECISIONS

It is intriguing to consider older adult years as another stage of development. Older adults retain the capacities to learn, to expand knowledge and skills, to make life decisions, and to make healthy choices.[95] Part of the lifelong learning process relates to making decisions for maintaining health with advancing age. The learning process extends into new roles that come with aging including living in retirement, providing care for a functionally limited spouse or family member, and grappling with the loss of a life partner and other loved ones. Maintaining interest and engagement in life is itself a learning process. Older age should be a time of ongoing personal growth and demonstrable resilience, and for those with more time available, a chance for doing activities of value for self and others.[96]

Frequently, the reflexive appraisal of older age is to assume that this is a time of cognitive deterioration (see Case Study 11.3: Alzheimer's Disease). There are certainly demonstrable declines in mental processing speed, working memory, attention, and executive functions. However, there is considerable stability for intuitive cognitive processes. Moreover, there are considerable opportunities for maintained growth in social and emotional domains. These opportunities are grounded in lifelong learning and the relative stability of social relationships into older years.[97,98] Lifelong learning is expansive in scope and does not stop with aging, covering formal, informal, and educational experiences that address individual and community needs.[99]

BE MOBILE

Mobility is a prominent issue in older age that sets critical limits on capabilities to perform in-home ADLs and to participate in out-of-home work, shopping for necessities, socialization, and volunteerism. Mobility includes activities that are self-powered or rely on assistive devices.[100] To maintain the physical capacities to be freely and safely mobile requires attention to physical activity. With aging comes decline in flexibility, loss of muscle mass, and not infrequently, problems with gait, balance, and coordination. The WHO therefore takes a population-based approach that matches physical activity recommendations for older adults to various levels of capacity.[101]

Social and community environments factor strongly into the ability of older adults to participate in physical activity.[102-104] Available safe spaces, including park areas and footpaths, are highly conducive to walking and socializing for older adults.[105,106] Relatively minor modifications to time management and daily behavior patterns can facilitate older adults maintaining their mobility.[107,108] The benefits of regular moderate-intensity physical activity are well known to maintain aerobic capacity, muscular strength, and flexibility. Not only is aerobic activity recommended to optimize cardiovascular health, but resistance training also takes on increased importance in older ages.

The WHO makes a series of evidence-based recommendations for physical activity in older adults. These include following the age-specific physical activity and dietary guidelines,[109] tempered to the individual's health conditions. The WHO makes the interesting connection that motor vehicle safety and driving performance of older adults are also improved by participating in certain types of physical activity.[110] Exercise behaviors that improve executive functions, coordination, visual attention, and limb flexibility, as well as speed of movement, may help to prevent motor vehicle accidents.[111]

Elderly population health can be supported through redesigning and modifying the built environment. Especially effective are efforts that promote safe outdoor and indoor spaces for walking and physical activity.[112] For example, even in the heavily congested urban environment of Bogotá, Colombia, home to more than 11 million residents, each Sunday, a network of major thoroughfares is closed to motor vehicles. Bogotá citizens can cycle (the program name is "Ciclovia"), walk, run, and rollerblade for long distances, safeguarded by police and volunteers who monitor the routes. This is a citywide event that brings out people of all ages, including many seniors, who participate along with members of their extended families.[113]

Not all older citizens are able to maintain independent mobility without assistance. Also, disability tends to progress with age even when efforts are made to slow that progression. Therefore, many older adults are dependent on various forms of assistive technologies.[114] Some of these individuals are dealing with lifelong vestiges of congenital deformities. More often, these older adults are experiencing later-in-life joint, orthopedic, or arthritic conditions or physical disabilities related to injury or disease such as stroke. Some have a temporary need for these devices during rehabilitation following joint or limb surgery. Regardless of the origin of the condition, the provision of mobility devices for older adults who need them broadly expands the opportunities for these individuals to retain their abilities to live independently and engage actively. Some assistive devices like canes, walkers, and white canes for people with serious visual impairment have been used for centuries and are quite rudimentary. Yet, they make a major difference in helping older adults get around. Assistive devices become increasingly important for the frail and oldest old.[115]

Universal design also factors into mobility for older adults (Case Study 11.2).

CASE STUDY 11.2: UNIVERSAL DESIGN

Universal design is a global movement that integrates health, safety, and social participation into the development and operation of systems and environments that have utility for all citizens.[116] Universal design was introduced by the North Carolina State University College of Design and has special applicability for people with disabilities who are overrepresented among older adults. Its implementation fits closely with the United Nations (UN) convention on the rights of persons with disabilities.[117] Universal design requires both multidisciplinary expertise and high-level political commitment. Universal design is grounded in seven principles as outlined in **Table 11.2**.

(continued)

TABLE 11.2 Seven Principles of Universal Design

Principle 1: Equitable Use
The design is useful and marketable to people with diverse abilities.

Guidelines	
1a.	Provide the same means of use for all users: identical whenever possible; equivalent when not.
1b.	Avoid segregating or stigmatizing any users.
1c.	Provisions for privacy, security, and safety should be equally available to all users.
1d.	Make the design appealing to all users.

Principle 2: Flexibility in Use
The design accommodates a wide range of individual preferences and abilities.

Guidelines	
2a.	Provide choice in methods of use.
2b.	Accommodate right- or left-handed access and use.
2c.	Facilitate the user's accuracy and precision.
2d.	Provide adaptability to the user's pace.

Principle 3: Simple and Intuitive Use
The design is easy to understand, regardless of the user's experience, knowledge, language skills, or current concentration level.

Guidelines	
3a.	Eliminate unnecessary complexity.
3b.	Be consistent with user expectations and intuition.
3c.	Accommodate a wide range of literacy and language skills.
3d.	Arrange information consistent with its importance.
3e.	Provide effective prompting and feedback during and after task completion.

Principle 4: Perceptible Information
The design communicates necessary information effectively to the user, regardless of ambient conditions or the user's sensory abilities.

Guidelines	
4a.	Use different modes (pictorial, verbal, tactile) for redundant presentation of essential information.
4b.	Provide adequate contrast between essential information and its surroundings.
4c.	Maximize "legibility" of essential information.
4d.	Differentiate elements in ways that can be described (i.e., make it easy to give instructions or directions).
4e.	Provide compatibility with a variety of techniques or devices used by people with sensory limitations.

Principle 5: Tolerance for Error
The design minimizes hazards and the adverse consequences of accidental or unintended actions.

Guidelines	
5a.	Arrange elements to minimize hazards and errors: most used elements, most accessible; hazardous elements eliminated, isolated, or shielded.
5b.	Provide warnings of hazards and errors.
5c.	Provide fail-safe features.
5d.	Discourage unconscious action in tasks that require vigilance.

(continued)

TABLE 11.2 Seven Principles of Universal Design (*continued*)	
Principle 6: Low Physical Effort *The design can be used efficiently and comfortably and with a minimum of fatigue.*	
Guidelines	6a. Allow user to maintain a neutral body position. 6b. Use reasonable operating forces. 6c. Minimize repetitive actions. 6d. Minimize sustained physical effort.
Principle 7: Size and Space for Approach and Use *The design provides appropriate size and space for approach, reach, manipulation, and use regardless of user's body size, posture, or mobility.*	
Guidelines	7a. Provide a clear line of sight to important elements for any seated or standing user. 7b. Make reach to all components comfortable for any seated or standing user. 7c. Accommodate variations in hand and grip size. 7d. Provide adequate space for the use of assistive devices or personal assistance.

A number of countries have made the commitment to implementing universal design. For example, Norway is striving to implement universal design nationwide by 2025.[118] Universal design projects are also under way to achieve accessibility in the built environment for older adults in Singapore.[119] From a health educational and advocacy perspective, the WHO has established an "Age-Friendly World" portal that showcases these programs and related resources.[120]

BUILD RELATIONSHIPS

Relationships are crucial to health and well-being in older years of the life span.[121] Referring back to the social ecological model, remember that older adults depend on family and social networks as they age and become increasingly dependent. Older adults also have time and ability to give back to the generations that follow them, as noted in descriptions of Germany's multigenerational centers and the U.S. Experience Corps.

Throughout much of the life course, the anticipatory sense of future time and potential for accomplishment is a major motivator. Many dream of good things yet to come. In older ages, this viewpoint begins to be replaced with a sense of "time left" to contribute and leave a legacy as a strong driver of function and actions. There is an increasing sense that time is finite and counting down. These existential issues have overtones for psychological health and make relationships with aging as well as younger loved ones exquisitely important and sometimes poignant.

Older adults are networked through a generationally expanding range of relationships. With aging, increasing proportions of connections are to younger generations, especially to their children and extended family members. Over time, older adults experience the loss of their parents and then, progressively, the losses of more of their same-age siblings, friends, neighbors, and acquaintances. Meanwhile, they may observe and actively participate, often with great satisfaction, as their children's families grow. Grandchildren are born, grow up, establish relationships, and launch another generation of great-grandchildren. For older adults whose family connections remain healthy and intact, losses are at least partially counterbalanced by this succession of new additions.

The other critical dimension is that over time, more of the responsibilities for care and support for older adults are transferred to their children and community caregivers. In many cultures, family relationships extending into older ages are exemplified by solidarity but may also include elements of ambivalence.[122]

Families differ in their geographic and social closeness, and some older adults are more closely associated with friends and neighbors. Older adults derive direct benefits from positive and supportive connections within their social networks. Residing in cohesive communities with opportunities for active participation by older adults adds an additional element of social capital.[123-125] Together, these direct and indirect social networks promote longer survival and higher quality of life throughout older ages.[126]

The chronology of this stage of the life course imposes increasing limits on social support. With advancing age, more same-age family members and peers pass away, so some of the closest sources of support, including a spouse or life partner, may no longer be available. These losses may not only provoke strong grief and loss reactions but also change the equation in terms of independence. This is especially the case if the caregiving partner passes before the partner who is more dependent on care. Also, with age comes physical and cognitive decline, both of which will diminish the personally experienced availability and quality of social support.

One approach to stimulating constructive relationships among older adults is typified by Cité Seniors in Geneva, Switzerland.[127] Cité Seniors provides a space for seniors to come together, socialize, and enjoy a varied selection of educational seminars, training courses, participatory workshops, and skills classes (e.g., creative arts, computer skills). Cité Seniors also provides a neighborhood venue for senior advocacy and support organizations to meet and convene. Finally, Cité Seniors connects to a broader infrastructure of community-based senior centers.

CONTRIBUTE

This section overlaps with other discussions regarding older adults as resources for the community based on lifelong skill acquisition, accumulated wisdom, and time available to provide care, assistance, mentoring, and community volunteerism. Increasingly over time, as long as age 65 is regarded as the gateway to older adulthood, a higher proportion of older adults will still be in the full-time or at least part-time workforce. In many cases, this is due to financial necessity. It also reflects the fact that many older adults retain their physical prowess, mental acuity, and desire to stay economically and productively engaged. "Work" can be construed as paid employment in a formal or informal economy, unpaid activity to support a home or family enterprise, or self-employment.[128] An interesting finding is that gains in well-being are proportional to the time invested in productive activities.[129]

In addition to working, volunteering is another means to finding fulfillment in older years of life. Volunteering by older adults can be considered to be uncompensated effort that takes place outside the household on behalf of the community.[130] Both work and volunteering by older adults confer health benefits.[131] Among these are reductions in the age-related declines in physical and cognitive capabilities because these faculties are actively engaged in work and volunteer activities.[132]

The WHO notes that "health and volunteering have a reciprocal relationship."[91] On the one hand, healthy older adults are more able and likely to volunteer. On the other, volunteerism bestows health and happiness for older adults who engage.[133,134] Beneficial health effects appear to be related, in part, to the altruism inherent in volunteering,[135] benefits that can even offset the profound impact of losing a spouse.[136]

Volunteering is qualitatively different from the obligatory nature of work or caregiving duties. Volunteering is socially valued and, as such, may produce even more positive health benefits than activities that do not make a social contribution.[137,138] For example, caregiving for a family member is extremely helpful, and may be done with dedication and affection, but also imposes a significant and potentially health-compromising burden on the caregiver.

Volunteering has been shown to produce a plethora of quantifiable health benefits. Volunteers positively self-rate their physical health status.[139-141] Volunteering is associated with lower hypertension risk in older ages.[142] Volunteering, again citing findings from The Experience Corps, is associated with increased physical strength and walking speed.[92,143] Volunteering lowers depressive symptoms.[144-146] Further, even for those over 80 years of age, volunteering enhances physical and mental health.[140] Cattan and coauthors[147] found that volunteerism also improves quality of life. According to these authors, subjective appraisals of the value of volunteerism include having an increased sense of control, being appreciated by the organizers and recipients of the volunteer activities, having a sense of purpose, and having the opportunity to learn while also giving something back.

EXAMPLES OF PUBLIC HEALTH ACTIONS TO IMPROVE HEALTH IN OLDER AGE

Public health actions to promote health in older age address a range of issues, with most focusing on the most common health concerns for older age adults, including dementia and Alzheimer's disease. Dementia does not characterize a single disease, rather it serves as an overall term for loss of memory and other capacities that impede one's daily life.[148] Alzheimer's disease is the most common type of dementia, affecting memory, thinking, and behavior that can reach a level that hinders daily life. The most prevalent, known risk factor for Alzheimer's disease is older age. The proportion of individuals living with Alzheimer's disease increases with age. For example, in 2022, 5.0% of those ages 65 to 74 years, 13.1% of those ages 75 to 84 years, and 33.2% of those ages 85 years and older are living with Alzheimer's disease.[55] Dementia has no currently known cure; however, there are medications and nondrug interventions that may improve quality of life in individuals living with dementia. Case Study 11.3 provides a detailed, data-based discussion of Alzheimer's disease. (You can access the podcast accompanying Case Study 11.3 by following this link to Springer Publishing Company Connect™: http://connect.springerpub.com/content/book/978-0-8261-8043-8/part/part03/chapter/ch11).

CASE STUDY 11.3: ALZHEIMER'S DISEASE

The Alzheimer's Association reports that in the United States in 2022, 6.5 million Americans were living with Alzheimer's disease, with a new case developing every 65 seconds.[149] These upward trends will continue; projections for 2050 indicate that 14 million Americans will be living with Alzheimer's disease at an annual cost of $1.1 trillion (**Table 11.3**).

Direct healthcare costs related to the disease were projected to reach $321 billion in 2022. More than 11 million Americans act in the role of unpaid caregivers for their family members with Alzheimer's disease. In the process, they dedicate 16 billion uncompensated hours to caring for loved ones each year, with an equivalent market value estimated at $272 billion.

Meanwhile, Alzheimer's deaths and mortality rates have risen steadily. Alzheimer's disease was only recently added to the leading causes of death statistics and

TABLE 11.3 Predicted Number of People in the United States with Alzheimer's Disease (in Millions) by Age Group and Percentage of the Group Affected

		AGE 65–74 YEARS		AGE 75–84 YEARS		AGE >85 YEARS	
YEAR	TOTAL NO.	NO.	PERCENTAGE	NO.	PERCENTAGE	NO.	PERCENTAGE
2010	4.7	0.7	3.0	2.3	17.6	1.8	32.3
2011	4.8	0.7	3.0	2.3	17.5	1.9	32.1
2012	4.9	0.7	2.9	2.3	17.4	1.9	32.1
2013	5.0	0.7	2.9	2.3	17.3	2.0	32.1
2014	5.0	0.8	2.9	2.3	17.2	2.0	32.1
2015	5.1	0.8	2.9	2.3	17.1	2.0	32.1
2016	5.2	0.8	3.0	2.4	17.0	2.0	32.1
2017	5.3	0.9	3.0	2.4	16.9	2.1	32.1
2018	5.5	0.9	3.0	2.5	16.7	2.1	32.2
2019	5.6	0.9	3.1	2.6	16.7	2.1	32.2
2020	5.8	1.0	3.1	2.7	16.7	2.1	32.2
2030	8.4	1.3	3.3	4.2	17.2	2.9	32.9
2040	11.6	1.3	3.4	5.4	18.0	4.9	34.6
2050	13.8	1.3	3.3	5.4	18.5	7.0	36.6

Source: Reproduced with permission from Herbert LE, Weuve J, Scherr PA, Evans DA. Alzheimer's disease in the United States (2010–2050) estimated using the 2010 census. *Neurology.* 2013;80:1778-1783. doi:10.1212/wnl.0b013e31828726f5

(*continued*)

ranked seventh as a contributor to U.S. mortality in 2021. Alzheimer's deaths have more than doubled during the first two decades of the millennium.

The U.S. experience is embedded in the broader global patterning of dementias in older adults. The 2020 World Alzheimer's Report indicated that 55 million people were living with dementia worldwide, a figure that is expected to surpass 130 million by 2050.[150] The associated global price tag was predicted to reach $1 trillion in 2018. There is a range of treatment settings that must be made available for the care of this complex disease, including primary care, acute hospital care, and palliative care, among others. Further, care coordination, case management, and support for unpaid family caregivers are additional essentials to address the burden of dementias.

Currently, no cure exists and there are few interventions available to prevent, delay, or slow progression of Alzheimer's disease. However, there is one notable bright spot. Regular physical activity has been described as a "practical, economical, and accessible intervention" for Alzheimer's disease.[151] Research indicates that regular engagement in moderate-intensity cardiovascular and resistance exercise can reduce the risk for developing Alzheimer's disease, and also mitigate and potentially improve the physical and cognitive symptoms of Alzheimer's disease for patients currently diagnosed with the disease.

Interventions include the application of evidence-based practice guidelines to promote physical activity throughout the life course. While Alzheimer's disease is a disease of aging, optimal prevention through physical activity starts much earlier in life. One important step is the formulation of evidence-based messaging on physical activity as a measure to prevent Alzheimer's disease.[152] For example, the Seattle Protocols—which include interventions based on social-learning and gerontological theories—have been devised for Alzheimer's patients and their caregivers.[153] These protocols focus on making regular exercise pleasant and successfully establishing and maintaining attainable exercise goals.

Beyond the prominent needs for receiving effective healthcare, patients with Alzheimer's disease and related dementias, and their caregivers, benefit from a supportive community environment. This is the idea behind the Dementia Friendly America (DFA) Initiative.[154] DFA was inaugurated in 2015 as an expansion of Minnesota's ACT on Alzheimer's program. DFA describes itself as a national network of communities, organizations, and individuals who work to develop community-level support for people living with dementia and their caregivers. The goal of dementia-friendly communities is to allow persons with dementia to "remain in community and engage and thrive in day to day living."[155] DFA is grounded in the principles of equity, inclusion, access, and awareness.

DFA has developed a multiphase program that includes a community toolkit. Each member community is advised to convene a multisector team that includes representatives from healthcare, government, and community-based organizations. DFA purposefully includes people living in the community with dementia and their care partners on the teams. The community adopts dementia-friendly practices and change goals and then disseminates these throughout the area. Many DFA communities identify a specific "champion" organization that coordinates and, in some cases, provides some financial sponsorship for DFA activities. For quality assurance, DFA communities monitor and report on their program progress and accomplishments.

DISEASE PREVENTION AND INDIVIDUAL APPROACHES TO IMPROVE QUALITY OF LIFE

Research is ongoing to identify effective interventions to prevent onset of dementia and Alzheimer's disease, with some of the most promising studies highlighting risk factor modifications that delay onset. The National Academies of Sciences, Engineering, and Medicine reviewed evidence on individual interventions for the reduction of Alzheimer's disease and dementia risk, and found that increased physical activity, blood pressure control, and cognitive training (i.e., activities devised to enhance memory, reasoning, and processing time) were all associated with lower risk of Alzheimer's disease and dementia.[156]

Individuals with Alzheimer's disease also report a disproportionately higher percentage of depressive symptoms, compared to older age persons with intact cognition.[157] Behavioral therapy interventions in this population have shown promise in targeting depressive symptoms which, in turn, increases quality of life. A randomized clinical trial evaluated the administration of behavioral therapy as compared to routine medical care. Those receiving behavioral therapy had a significantly better quality of life compared to those receiving routine medical care.[158] The behavioral therapy group received eight weekly home visits and four monthly phone calls by consultants trained in behavior management. Other programs with demonstrated improvements in quality of life incorporate environmental skill-building programs, occupational therapy for caregivers, cognitive stimulation, and sleep improvement programs.[151]

COMMUNITY-LEVEL INTERVENTIONS

Having community resources for those diagnosed with dementia can provide much-needed support and enhanced quality of life for individuals living with Alzheimer's disease and dementia. The Centers for Disease Control and Prevention (CDC) outlines important community roles to support those living with dementia including assessing burden, risk reduction, care services from support services to healthcare, and public and private resources (i.e., assistance with transportation, dementia-friendly grocery stores, places of worship, and law enforcement). Not all people living with dementia are able to operate vehicles or travel alone with ease. Providing reliable and safe means of transport including buses, railways, caregiver accompaniment, and accessible travel can provide a sense of independence. Grocery stores that are dementia-friendly include staff who are trained to assist those living with dementia as needed (e.g., if choices become overwhelming in the store), to answer questions related to payment machines, and to make adjustments to lighting or signage, if possible.[159] To support a sustained quality of life and familiarity, those who partake in places of worship may continue to do so through dementia-friendly faith communities as in Massachusetts, where some faith organizations host special events such as Memory Sundays and events to raise awareness for those living with dementia in their community.[160] Law enforcement can be a great help for those living with dementia and their families, as law enforcement officials often play a large role in helping to reunite individuals who become separated from loved ones. The Alzheimer's Association Safe Return program[161] is a 24-hour nationwide program that works with law enforcement to identify and return a person living with Alzheimer's disease or related dementia back home in the event they have wandered away.

Taken together, these create a dementia-friendly community. Supporting such a vision is the Administration of Aging (AoA), sitting under the Administration for Community Living (ACL), which provides funding to states and community-based organizations to develop services and supports unique to the needs of people living with dementia and their caregivers.[162]

POLICY ACTIONS FOR ALZHEIMER'S DISEASE AND RELATED DEMENTIAS

Policy actions have the potential to benefit more individuals in the population, including through increased funding for research, and increases in the quality and number of services available for people living with dementia and Alzheimer's disease. In January 2011, the National Alzheimer's Project Act (NAPA) was signed into law. The purpose of the act for Alzheimer's disease and related dementias is to:

(1) be responsible for the creation and maintenance of an integrated national plan to overcome Alzheimer's (2) provide information and coordination of Alzheimer's research and services across all Federal agencies (3) accelerate the development of treatments that would prevent, halt, or reverse the course of Alzheimer's (4) improve the early diagnosis of Alzheimer's disease and coordination of the care and treatment of citizens with Alzheimer's (5) ensure the inclusion of ethnic and racial populations at higher risk for Alzheimer's or least likely to receive care, in clinical, research, and service efforts with the purpose of decreasing health disparities in Alzheimer's (6) coordinate with international bodies to integrate and inform the fight against Alzheimer's globally.[163]

NAPA directs a national plan that incorporates recommendations for actions of importance on programs. There are five goals that guide the national actions to eliminate the burden of Alzheimer's disease and related dementias: (a) prevent and effectively treat Alzheimer's disease by 2025, (b) optimize care quality and efficiency, (c) expand supports for people with Alzheimer's disease and their families, (d) enhance public awareness and engagement, and (e) track progress and drive improvement.[164] Additionally, healthcare reform policies, including the Affordable Care Act and Medicaid Expansion, help those living with Alzheimer's disease and related dementias.[165] The expansion of health insurance coverage helps cover care costs and provides subsidies for those with early-onset dementias with low to moderate income. Furthermore, Medicaid payments allow for an increase in the number of states that offer home and community-based services, which thereby offers more options for care of people living with dementias. Actions at multiple levels of the social ecological framework are essential to support the growing population of persons living with dementia.

SUMMARY

The world has been aging dramatically over a period of less than one century, triggered by a plummeting mortality rate, followed several decades later by a precipitous drop in the birth rate. The ability to support an increasing proportion of older adults, given their diminished output and productivity, and the rising cost and complexity of their health needs, represents a global challenge that nevertheless plays out uniquely for each country.

What produces health in older ages is a combination of the accumulation of lifetime disease risks compounded with the emergence of diseases of aging such as Alzheimer's disease. Together this produces a pattern of multimorbidity. Many older adults are dealing with several significant disease diagnoses simultaneously. For those who have healthcare access, the frequency of medical visits, therapeutic treatments, and medication prescriptions increases with age. Likewise, healthcare costs are often concentrated in older ages.

Nevertheless, there is an optimistic counterpoint in that older adults represent a largely untapped resource of available skills, wisdom, and talents, coupled with an eagerness, readiness, and ability to contribute to their communities. Recruiting older adults to take on volunteer roles provides reciprocal benefits. Participating in community activities actively promotes physical and mental health capabilities for older adults, while the community receives the fruits of their active participation, often performed on a voluntary basis. In fact, there is a prevailing belief that the older population may capably generate a "triple dividend" through the contributions its members are able to make. This dividend has been described vividly: "thriving lives, costing less, contributing more."

End-of-Chapter Resources

Access additional case study podcasts online at http://connect.springerpub.com/ content/book/978-0-8261-8043-8/

DISCUSSION QUESTIONS

1. Discuss strategies to actually achieve the "triple dividend" from our older population as described by the phrase "thriving lives, costing less, contributing more."

2. Contrast the future challenges facing the world's two "population billionaires"—China and India. By 2050, China will have decreased in population size to 1.3 billion but will have the largest older adult population on the planet—with a greatly reduced proportion of adults to support them. What will China do? Meanwhile, India will be the most populous nation, with 1.6 billion citizens. Given this burgeoning population, how will India support older adults?

3. What strategies do you propose to support the growing number of older adults with Alzheimer's disease and their caregivers who experience economic and social stressors as they attempt to care for their loved ones? Workable solutions will require considerable innovation.

SPRINGER PUBLISHING
C⊙NNECT™

A robust set of instructor resources designed to supplement this text is located at http://connect.springerpub.com/content/book/978-0-8261-8043-8. Qualifying instructors may request access by emailing **textbook@springerpub.com.**

REFERENCES

1. He W, Goodkind D, Kowal P. *An Aging World: 2015. International Population Reports.* U.S. Government Printing Office; 2016. https://www.census.gov/content/dam/Census/library/publications/2016/demo/p95-16-1.pdf
2. World Health Organization. *Multisectoral action for a life course approach to healthy ageing: draft global strategy and plan of action on ageing and health.* Published 2016. https://apps.who.int/iris/handle/10665/252671
3. World Bank. *Population ages 65 and above (% of total population).* https://data.worldbank.org/indicator/SP.POP.65UP.TO.ZS
4. Kirk D. Demographic transition theory. *Popul Stud (Camb).* 1996;50(3):361-387. doi: 10.1080/0032472031000149536

5. Lesthaeghe R. The second demographic transition: a concise overview of its development. *Proc Natl Acad Sci U S A*. 2014;*111*(51):18112-18115. doi:10.1073/pnas.1420441111

6. Leach-Kemon K. *The Global Burden of Disease: Generating Evidence, Guiding Policy*. Institute for Health Metrics and Evaluation; 2013. https://www.healthdata.org/sites/default/files/files/policy_report/2013/WB_EuropeCentralAsia/IHME_GBD_WorldBank_EuropeCentralAsia_Overview.pdf

7. Mathers CD, Stevens GA, Boerma T, et al. Causes of international increases in older age life expectancy. *Lancet*. 2015;*385*(9967):540-548. doi:10.1016/S0140-6736(14)60569-9

8. Arias E. United States life tables, 2009. *Natl Vital Stat Rep*. 2014;*62*(7):1-63. https://pubmed.ncbi.nlm.nih.gov/24393483/

9. Salomon JA, Wang H, Freeman MK, et al. Healthy life expectancy for 187 countries, 1990–2010: a systematic analysis for the Global Burden Disease Study 2010. *Lancet*. 2012;*380*(9859):2144-2162. doi:10.1016/S0140-6736(12)61690-0

10. Fries JF. Aging, natural death, and the compression of morbidity. *N Engl J Med*. 1980;*303*(3):130-135. doi:10.1056/NEJM198007173030304

11. Fries JF. The compression of morbidity. *Milbank Q*. 2005;*83*(4):801-823. doi:10.1111/j.1468-0009.2005.00401.x

12. Global Health Observatory Data Repository. *Healthy Life Expectancy (HALE)–Data by WHO Region*. World Health Organization; 2019. http://apps.who.int/gho/data/view.main.HALEXREGv?lang=en

13. Eurostat. *Healthy life years at age 65 by sex*. Published 2016. https://ec.europa.eu/eurostat/web/products-datasets/-/tepsr_sp320

14. Negin J, Cumming R, de Ramirez SS, et al. Risk factors for non-communicable diseases among older adults in rural Africa. *Trop Med Int Health*. 2011;*16*(5):640-646. doi:10.1111/j.1365-3156.2011.02739.x

15. Teo K, Lear S, Islam S, et al. Prevalence of a healthy lifestyle among individuals with cardiovascular disease in high-, middle- and low-income countries. *JAMA*. 2013;*309*(15):1613. doi:10.1001/jama.2013.3519

16. Institute for Health Metrics and Evaluation. *GBD compare*. https://vizhub.healthdata.org/gbd-compare/

17. Wu F, Guo Y, Chatterji S, et al. Common risk factors for chronic non-communicable diseases among older adults in China, Ghana, Mexico, India, Russia and South Africa: the study on global AGEing and adult health (SAGE) wave 1. *BMC Public Health*. 2015;*15*(1):88. doi:10.1186/s12889-015-1407-0

18. Wilmoth JR, Boe C, Barbieri M. Geographic differences in life expectancy at age 50 in the United States compared with other high-income countries. In: Crimmins EM, Preston SH, Cohen B, eds. *International Differences in Mortality at Older Ages: Dimensions and Sources*. National Academies Press; 2010:333-366. https://www.ncbi.nlm.nih.gov/books/NBK62591

19. Woolf SH, Aron L, eds. *U.S. Health in International Perspective*. National Academies Press; 2013. doi:10.17226/13497

20. Murray CJL, Kulkarni SC, Michaud C, et al. Eight Americas: investigating mortality disparities across races, counties, and race-counties in the United States. *PLoS Med*. 2006;*3*(9):e260. doi:10.1371/journal.pmed.0030260

21. Centers for Disease Control and Prevention. State-specific healthy life expectancy at age 65 years—United States, 2007–2009. *MMWR Morb Mortal Wkly Rep*. 2013;*62*(28);561-566. https://www.cdc.gov/mmwr/preview/mmwrhtml/mm6228a1.htm?s_cid=mm6228a1_w

22. Olshansky SJ, Antonucci T, Berkman L, et al. Differences in life expectancy due to race and educational differences are widening, and many may not catch up. *Health Aff*. 2012;*31*(8):1803-1813. doi:10.1377/hlthaff.2011.0746

23. Ezzati M, Friedman AB, Kulkarni SC, Murray CJL. The reversal of fortunes: trends in county mortality and cross-county mortality disparities in the United States. *PLoS Med*. 2008;*5*(4):e66. doi:10.1371/journal.pmed.0050066

24. Danaei G, Rimm EB, Oza S, et al. The promise of prevention: the effects of four preventable risk factors on national life expectancy and life expectancy disparities by race and county in the United States. *PLoS Med*. 2010;*7*(3):e1000248. doi:10.1371/journal.pmed.1000248

25. Institute for Health Metrics and Evaluation. *GBD compare*. https://vizhub.healthdata.org/gbd-compare/

26. Wang H, Dwyer-Lindgren L, Lofgren KT, et al. Age-specific and sex-specific mortality in 187 countries, 1970–2010: a systematic analysis for the global burden of disease study 2010. *Lancet*. 2012;*380*(9859):2071-2094. doi:10.1016/S0140-6736(12)61719-X

27. Daniels ME, Donilon TE, Bollyky TJ. *The emerging global health crisis noncommunicable diseases in low-and middle-income countries*. [Council on Foreign Relations Independent Task Force Report No. 72.]. Published January 9, 2016. doi:10.2139/ssrn.2685111

28. Boyd CM, Ritchie CS, Tipton EF, et al. From bedside to bench: summary from the American geriatrics society/national institute on aging research conference on comorbidity and multiple morbidity in older adults. *Aging Clin Exp Res*. 2008;*20*(3):181-188. doi:10.1007/BF03324775

29. Diederichs C, Berger K, Bartels DB. The measurement of multiple chronic diseases—a systematic review on existing multimorbidity indices. *J Gerontol Ser A.* 2011;*66A*(3):301-311. doi:10.1093/gerona/glq208

30. Fortin M, Hudon C, Haggerty J, et al. Prevalence estimates of multimorbidity: a comparative study of two sources. *BMC Health Serv Res.* 2010;*10*:111. doi:10.1186/1472-6963-10-111

31. Khanam MA, Streatfield PK, Kabir ZN, et al. Prevalence and patterns of multimorbidity among elderly people in rural Bangladesh: a cross-sectional study. *J Health Popul Nutr.* 2011;*29*(4):406-414. doi:10.3329/jhpn .v29i4.8458

32. Pati S, Agrawal S, Swain S, et al. Noncommunicable disease multimorbidity and associated health care utilization and expenditures in India: cross-sectional study. *BMC Health Serv Res.* 2014;*14*(1):451. doi:10.1186/1472-6963-14-451

33. Garin N, Olaya B, Perales J, et al. Multimorbidity patterns in a national representative sample of the Spanish adult population. *PLoS One.* 2014;*9*(1):e84794. doi:10.1371/journal.pone.0084794

34. McLean G, Gunn J, Wyke S, et al. The influence of socioeconomic deprivation on multimorbidity at different ages: a cross-sectional study. *Br J Gen Pract.* 2014;*64*(624):e440-e447. doi:10.3399/bjgp14X680545

35. Kirchberger I, Meisinger C, Heier M, et al. Patterns of multimorbidity in the aged population: results from the KORA-age study. *PLoS One.* 2012;*7*(1):e30556. doi:10.1371/journal.pone.0030556

36. Boutayeb A, Boutayeb S, Boutayeb W. Multi-morbidity of noncommunicable diseases and equity in WHO eastern mediterranean countries. *Int J Equity Health.* 2013;*12*:60. doi:10.1186/1475-9276-12-60

37. Barnett K, Mercer SW, Norbury M, et al. Epidemiology of multimorbidity and implications for health care, research, and medical education: a cross-sectional study. *Lancet.* 2012;*380*(9836):37-43. doi:10.1016/ S0140-6736(12)60240-2

38. Lehnert T, Heider D, Leicht H, et al. Review: health care utilization and costs of elderly persons with multiple chronic conditions. *Med Care Res Rev.* 2011;*68*(4):387-420. doi:10.1177/1077558711399580

39. Schoenberg NE, Kim H, Edwards W, Fleming ST. Burden of common multiple-morbidity constellations on out-of-pocket medical expenditures among older adults. *Gerontologist.* 2007;*47*(4):423-437. doi:10.1093/ geront/47.4.423

40. Boyd CM, Fortin M. Future of multimorbidity research: how should understanding of multimorbidity inform health system design? *Public Health Rev.* 2010;*32*(2):451-474. doi:10.1007/BF03391611

41. Dubois C-A, McKee M, Nolte E. Analysing trends, opportunities and challenges. In: Dubois C-A, McKee M, Nolte E, eds. *Human Resources for Health in Europe.* Open University Press; 2006:15-40. https://www .researchgate.net/publication/242082402_Analysing_trends_opportunities_and_challenges

42. Noelker LS, Browdie R. Sidney Katz, MD: a new paradigm for chronic illness and long-term care. *Gerontologist.* 2014;*54*(1):13-20. doi:10.1093/geront/gnt086

43. Dunlop DD, Song J, Arntson EK, et al. Sedentary time in US older adults associated with disability in activities of daily living independent of physical activity. *J Phys Act Health.* 2015;*12*(1):93-101. doi:10.1123/ jpah.2013-0311

44. He W, Goodkind D, Kowal P. *An Aging World: 2015.* U.S. Government Printing Office; 2016. https://www .census.gov/library/publications/2016/demo/P95-16-1.html

45. Rockwood K, Song X, MacKnight C, et al. A global clinical measure of fitness and frailty in elderly people. *Can Med Assoc J.* 2005;*173*(5):489-495. doi:10.1503/cmaj.050051

46. Harttgen K, Kowal P, Strulik H, et al. Patterns of frailty in older adults: comparing results from higher and lower income countries using the Survey of Health, Ageing and Retirement in Europe (SHARE) and the Study on Global AGEing and Adult Health (SAGE). *PLoS One.* 2013;*8*(10):e75847. doi:10.1371/journal.pone .0075847

47. Rechel B, Doyle Y, Grundy E, McKee M. *How Can Health Systems Respond to Population Ageing?* World Health Organization, Regional Office for Europe; 2009. https://apps.who.int/iris/handle/10665/107941

48. Giovannetti ER, Wolff JL. Cross-survey differences in national estimates of numbers of caregivers of disabled older adults. *Milbank Q.* 2010;*88*(3):310-349. doi:10.1111/j.1468-0009.2010.00602.x

49. Olivares-Tirado P, Tamiya N, Kashiwagi M, Kashiwagi K. Predictors of the highest long-term care expenditures in Japan. *BMC Health Serv Res.* 2011;*11*:103. doi:10.1186/1472-6963-11-103

50. de Meijer C, Wouterse B, Polder J, Koopmanschap M. The effect of population aging on health expenditure growth: a critical review. *Eur J Ageing.* 2013;*10*(4):353-361. doi:10.1007/s10433-013-0280-x

51. Organisation for Economic Cooperation and Development. *Health at a Glance 2013: OECD Indicators.* OECD Publishing; 2013. doi:10.1787/health_glance-2013-en

52. Organisation for Economic Cooperation and Development. Recipients of long-term care. *Health at a Glance 2019: OECD Indicators.* OECD Publishing; 2019. doi:10.1787/c149d939-en

53. Fernández J-L, Forder J, Trukeschitz B, et al. *How Can European States Design Efficient, Equitable and Sustainable Funding Systems for Long-Term Care for Older People?* World Health Organization, Regional Office for Europe; 2009. https://apps.who.int/iris/handle/10665/107942

54. Chari AV, Engberg J, Ray KN, Mehrotra A. The opportunity costs of informal elder-care in the United States: new estimates from the American Time Use Survey. *Health Serv Res.* 2015;*50*(3):871-882. doi:10.1111/1475-6773.12238

55. Alzheimer's Association. 2022 Alzheimer's disease facts and figures. *Alzheimers Dement*. 2022;*18*(4). doi:10.1002/alz.12638

56. Zissimopoulos J, Crimmins E, St Clair P. The value of delaying Alzheimer's disease onset. *Forum Health Econ Policy*. 2014;*18*(1):25-39. doi:10.1515/fhep-2014-0013

57. Lutz W, Sanderson W, Scherbov S. The coming acceleration of global population ageing. *Nature*. 2008;*451*(7179):716-719. doi:10.1038/nature06516

58. Bloom D, Canning D, Fink G. Implications of population aging for economic growth. *Oxford Rev Econ Policy*. 2011;*26*(4):583-612. doi:10.3386/w16705

59. Lee R, Mason A. The price of maturity: aging populations mean countries have to find new ways to support their elderly. *Finance Dev*. 2011;*48*(2):6-11. http://www.ncbi.nlm.nih.gov/pubmed/22822263

60. National Research Council. *Aging and the Macroeconomy: Long-Term Implications of an Older Population*. National Academies Press; 2012. doi:10.17226/13465

61. Krueger AB, Kahneman D, Schkade D, et al. National time accounting: the currency of life. In: Krueger AB, ed. *Measuring the Subjective Well-Being of Nations: National Accounts of Time Use and Well-Being*. University of Chicago Press; 2009:1-79.

62. Stiglitz JE, Sen A, Fitoussi J-P. *Report by the commission on the measurement of economic performance and social progress*. https://ec.europa.eu/eurostat/documents/8131721/8131772/Stiglitz-Sen-Fitoussi-Commission -report.pdf

63. Marmot M, Goldblatt P, Allen J, et al. *Fair Society, Healthy Lives the Marmot Review*. University College; 2010. https://www.instituteofhealthequity.org/resources-reports/fair-society-healthy-lives-the-marmot-review

64. Chatterji S, Byles J, Cutler D, et al. Health, functioning, and disability in older adults—present status and future implications. *Lancet*. 2015;*385*(9967):563-575. doi:10.1016/S0140-6736(14)61462-8

65. Kruk ME. Universal health coverage: a policy whose time has come. *BMJ*. 2013;*347*:f6360. doi:10.1136/bmj .f6360

66. World Health Organization. *Health Systems Financing: The Path to Universal Coverage*. Author; 2016. https:// apps.who.int/iris/handle/10665/44371

67. World Health Organization. *Research for Universal Health Coverage: World Health Report 2013*. Author; 2013.

68. Scheil-Adlung X. ed. *Global Evidence on Inequities in Rural Health Protection: New Data on Rural Deficits in Health Coverage for 174 Countries*. International Labour Office; 2015. https://www.ilo.org/secsoc/information -resources/publications-and-tools/Workingpapers/WCMS_383890/lang–en/index.htm

69. United Nations. *United Nations sustainable development*. Take action for the sustainable development goals. https://www.un.org/sustainabledevelopment/sustainable-development-goals

70. World Health Organization. *Targets of sustainable development goal 3*. Author; 2017. https://www.who.int/ europe/about-us/our-work/sustainable-development-goals/targets-of-sustainable-development-goal-3

71. Saksena P, Hsu J, Evans DB. Financial risk protection and universal health coverage: evidence and measurement challenges. *PLoS Med*. 2014;*11*(9):e1001701. doi:10.1371/journal.pmed.1001701

72. Kruk ME, Goldmann E, Galea S. Borrowing and selling to pay for health care in low–and middle-income countries. *Health Aff*. 2009;*28*(4):1056-1066. doi:10.1377/hlthaff.28.4.1056

73. Early Action Task Force. *Looking Forward to Later Life: Taking an Early Action Approach to Our Ageing Society*. Community Links; 2014. https://www.bl.uk/collection-items/looking-forward-to-later-life-taking-an-early-action -approach-to-our-ageing-society

74. Geue C, Briggs A, Lewsey J, Lorgelly P. Population ageing and healthcare expenditure projections: new evidence from a time to death approach. *Eur J Health Econ*. 2014;*15*(8):885-896. doi:10.1007/ s10198-013-0543-7

75. Bloom DE, Chatterji S, Kowal P, et al. Macroeconomic implications of population ageing and selected policy responses. *Lancet*. 2015;*385*(9968):649-657. doi:10.1016/S0140-6736(14)61464-1

76. Yu TH-K, Wang DH-M, Wu K-L. Reexamining the red herring effect on healthcare expenditures. *J Bus Res*. 2015;*68*(4):783-787. doi:10.1016/J.JBUSRES.2014.11.028

77. Felder S, Zweifel P, Werblow A. Population ageing and health care expenditure: is long-term care different? *Swiss J Econ Stat*. 2006;*142*(V):43-48. https://ideas.repec.org/a/ses/arsjes/2006-v-7.html

78. Felder S, Werblow A, Zweifel P. Do red herrings swim in circles? Controlling for the endogeneity of time to death. *J Health Econ*. 2010;*29*(2):205-212. doi:10.1016/J.JHEALECO.2009.11.014

79. Seshamani M, Gray AM. A longitudinal study of the effects of age and time to death on hospital costs. *J Health Econ*. 2004;*23*(2):217-235. doi:10.1016/j.jhealeco.2003.08.004

80. Boerma T, Eozenou P, Evans D, et al. Monitoring progress towards universal health coverage at country and global levels. *PLoS Med*. 2014;*11*(9):e1001731. doi:10.1371/journal.pmed.1001731

81. Economist Intelligence Unit. *Healthcare Strategies for an Ageing Society*. Philips; 2009. http://graphics.eiu.com/ upload/eb/philips_healthcare_ageing_3011web.pdf

82. Cutler D, Landrum MB, Stewart K. *Intensive Medical Care and Cardiovascular Disease Disability Reductions*. National Bureau of Economic Research; 2006. doi:10.3386/w12184

83. McKee M, Suhrcke M, Nolte E, et al. Health systems, health, and wealth: a European perspective. *Lancet*. 2009;*373*:349-351. doi:10.1016/S0140-6736(09)60098-2

84. Tinetti ME, Fried TR, Boyd CM. Designing health care for the most common chronic condition–multimorbidity. *JAMA*. 2012;*307*(23):2493-2494. doi:10.1001/jama.2012.5265

85. Esposito S, Durando P, Bosis S, et al. Vaccine-preventable diseases: from paediatric to adult targets. *Eur J Intern Med*. 2014;*25*(3):203-212. doi:10.1016/j.ejim.2013.12.004

86. Fried LP. Longevity and aging: the success of global public health. In: Parker R, Sommer M, eds. *Routledge Handbook on Global Public Health*. Routledge; 2011:208-226.

87. Suhrcke M, Arce RS, McKee M, Rocco L. Economic costs of ill health in the European region. In: Figueras J, McKee M, eds. *Health Systems, Health, Wealth and Societal Well-Being*. European Observatory on Health Systems and Policies; 2012. https://eurohealthobservatory.who.int/docs/librariesprovider3/studies—external/health-wealth-social-wellbeing.pdf

88. Fried LP, Carlson MC, Freedman M, et al. A social model for health promotion for an aging population: initial evidence on the experience corps model. *J Urban Health*. 2004;*81*(1):64-78. doi:10.1093/jurban/jth094

89. Hong SI, Morrow-Howell N. Health outcomes of experience corps: a high-commitment volunteer program. *Soc Sci Med*. 2010;*71*(2):414-420. doi:10.1016/j.socscimed.2010.04.009

90. Rebok GW, Carlson MC, Glass TA, et al. Short-term impact of experience corps participation on children and schools: results from a pilot randomized trial. *J Urban Health*. 2004;*81*(1):79-93. doi:10.1093/JURBAN/JTH095

91. Beard J, Officer A, Cassels A, eds. *World Report on Ageing and Health*. World Health Organization; 2015.

92. Blazer DG, Sachs-Ericsson N, Hybels CF. Perception of unmet basic needs as a predictor of mortality among community-dwelling older adults. *Am J Public Health*. 2005;*95*(2):299-304. doi:10.2105/AJPH.2003.035576

93. The World Bank. *World Development Report 2000/2001: Attacking Poverty*. Oxford University Press; 2001. doi:10.1596/0-1952-1129-4

94. Commission on Social Determinants of Health. *Closing the Gap in a Generation: Health Equity Through Action on the Social Determinants of Health*. World Health Organization; 2008.

95. Boulton-Lewis GM. Education and learning for the elderly: why, how, what. *Educ Gerontol*. 2010;*36*(3):213-228. doi:10.1080/03601270903182877

96. Stephens C, Breheny M, Mansvelt J. Healthy ageing from the perspective of older people: a capability approach to resilience. *Psychol Health*. 2015;*30*(6):715-731. doi:10.1080/08870446.2014.904862

97. Carstensen LL, Hartel CR, eds. *When I'm 64*. National Academies Press; 2006. doi:10.17226/11474

98. McKenna A. *The Lifelong Learning Needs of Older People in Ireland: A Discussion Paper*. AONTAS; 2007. https://www.aontas.com/assets/resources/AONTAS-Research/olderpeopleresearch_ppr_2007.pdf

99. Laal M. Lifelong learning: what does it mean? *Procedia Soc Behav Sci*. 2011;*28*:470-474. doi:10.1016/J.SBSPRO.2011.11.090

100. Satariano WA, Guralnik JM, Jackson RJ, et al. Mobility and aging: new directions for public health action. *Am J Public Health*. 2012;*102*(8):1508-1515. doi:10.2105/AJPH.2011.300631

101. Armstrong T, Bull F, Magnussen C, Persson A. *A Guide for Population-Based Approaches to Increasing Levels of Physical Activity: Implementation of the WHO Global Strategy on Diet, Physical Activity and Health*. World Health Organization; 2007.

102. Frank LD, Schmid TL, Sallis JF, et al. Linking objectively measured physical activity with objectively measured urban form. *Am J Prev Med*. 2005;*28*(2):117-125. doi:10.1016/j.amepre.2004.11.001

103. Chad KE, Reeder BA, Harrison EL, et al. Profile of physical activity levels in community-dwelling older adults. *Med Sci Sports Exerc*. 2005;*37*(10):1774-1784. http://www.ncbi.nlm.nih.gov/pubmed/16260980

104. Giles-Corti B, Donovan RJ. Relative influences of individual, social environmental, and physical environmental correlates of walking. *Am J Public Health*. 2003;*93*(9):1583-1589. doi:10.2105/AJPH.93.9.1583

105. Prohaska T, Belansky E, Belza B, et al. Physical activity, public health, and aging: critical issues and research priorities. *J Gerontol Ser B*. 2006;*61*(5):S267-S273. doi:10.1093/geronb/61.5.S267

106. Anderson LA, Slonim A, Yen IH, et al. Developing a framework and priorities to promote mobility among older adults. *Health Educ Behav*. 2014;*41*(1 suppl):10S-18S. doi:10.1177/1090198114537492

107. Bauman A, Merom D, Bull FC, et al. Updating the evidence for physical activity: summative reviews of the epidemiological evidence, prevalence, and interventions to promote "active aging." *Gerontologist*. 2016;*56*(suppl 2):S268-S280. doi:10.1093/geront/gnw031

108. Berensson K, Winfridsson G, Junström, M, eds. *Healthy Ageing-A Challenge for Europe*. The Swedish National Institute of Public Health; 2006.

109. World Health Organization. *Global Recommendations on Physical Activity for Health*. Author; 2015. https://www.who.int/publications/i/item/9789241599979

110. Marottoli RA, Allore H, Araujo KLB, et al. A randomized trial of a physical conditioning program to enhance the driving performance of older persons. *J Gen Intern Med*. 2007;*22*(5):590-597. doi:10.1007/s11606-007-0134-3

111. Marmeleira JF, Godinho MB, Fernandes OM. The effects of an exercise program on several abilities associated with driving performance in older adults. *Accid Anal Prev*. 2009;*41*(1):90-97. doi:10.1016/J.AAP.2008.09.008

112. Garin N, Olaya B, Miret M, et al. Built environment and elderly population health: a comprehensive literature review. *Clin Pract Epidemiol Ment Health.* 2014;*10*(1):103-115. doi:10.2174/1745017901410010103
113. Hernandez JC. *Car-free streets, a Colombian export, inspire debate.* New York Times. June 24, 2008: B6.
114. Rosso AL, Auchincloss AH, Michael YL. The urban built environment and mobility in older adults: a comprehensive review. *J Aging Res.* 2011;*2011*:816106. doi:10.4061/2011/816106
115. Löfqvist C, Nygren C, Széman Z, Iwarsson S. Assistive devices among very old people in five European countries. *Scand J Occup Ther.* 2005;*12*(4):181-192. doi:10.1080/11038120500210652
116. The Center for Universal Design. *Center for universal design.* About UD. https://design.ncsu.edu/research/center-for-universal-design/#:~:text=The%20Center%20for%20Universal%20Design%20was%20established%20in%201989%20under,including%20disabilities%20that%20result%20from
117. United Nations. *Convention on the Rights of Persons with Disabilities and Optional Protocol.* Author; 2007. http://www.un.org/disabilities/documents/convention/convoptprot-e.pdf
118. WHO Age-Friendly World. *The common principles of universal design: the city of Oslo.* https://extranet.who.int/agefriendlyworld/wp-content/uploads/2015/06/The-Common-Principles-of-Universal-design-City-of-Oslo.pdf
119. Building & Construction Authority. *Code on accessibility in the built environment.* Updated November 11, 2018. https://www1.bca.gov.sg/regulatory-info/building-control/universal-design-and-friendly-buildings/code-on-accessibility-in-the-built-environment
120. World Health Organization. *Age-friendly world.* https://extranet.who.int/agefriendlyworld
121. Carstensen LL. The influence of a sense of time on human development. *Science.* 2006;*312*(5782):1913-1915. doi:10.1126/SCIENCE.1127488
122. Silverstein M, Giarrusso R. Aging and family life: a decade review. *J Marriage Fam.* 2010;*72*(5):1039-1058. doi:10.1111/j.1741-3737.2010.00749.x
123. Nyqvist F, Forsman AK, Giuntoli G, Cattan M. Social capital as a resource for mental well-being in older people: a systematic review. *Aging Ment Health.* 2013;*17*(4):394-410. doi:10.1080/13607863.2012.742490
124. Murayama H, Fujiwara Y, Kawachi I. Social capital and health: a review of prospective multilevel studies. *J Epidemiol.* 2012;*22*(3):179-187. doi:10.2188/jea.JE20110128
125. Nyqvist F, Cattan M, Andersson L, et al. Social capital and loneliness among the very old living at home and in institutional settings: a comparative study. *J Aging Health.* 2013;*25*(6):1013-1035. doi:10.1177/0898264313497508
126. Holt-Lunstad J, Smith TB, Layton JB. Social relationships and mortality risk: a meta-analytic review. *PLoS Med.* 2010;*7*(7):e1000316. doi:10.1371/journal.pmed.1000316
127. Ville de Genève Site Officiel. *Cité seniors.* Updated May 8, 2019. https://www.geneve.ch/en/cite-seniors
128. World Health Organization, World Bank. *World Report on Disability.* Author; 2011. https://www.who.int/teams/noncommunicable-diseases/sensory-functions-disability-and-rehabilitation/world-report-on-disability
129. Baker LA, Cahalin LP, Gerst K, Burr JA. Productive activities and subjective well-being among older adults: the influence of number of activities and time commitment. *Soc Indic Res.* 2005;*73*(3):431-458. doi:10.1007/s11205-005-0805-6
130. Miranda V. *Cooking, Caring and Volunteering: Unpaid Work Around the World.* OECD Social, Employment, and Migration Working Papers, No. 116. OECD Publishing; 2011. doi:10.1787/5kghrjm8s142-en
131. Maimaris W, Hogan H, Lock K. The impact of working beyond traditional retirement ages on mental health: implications for public health and welfare policy. *Public Health Rev.* 2010;*32*(2):532-548. doi:10.1007/BF03391615
132. Crawford JO, Graveling RA, Cowie HA, Dixon K. The health safety and health promotion needs of older workers. *Occup Med (Lond).* 2010;*60*(3):184-192. doi:10.1093/occmed/kqq028
133. Thoits PA, Hewitt LN. Volunteer work and well-being. *J Health Soc Behav.* 2001;*42*(2):115. doi:10.2307/3090173
134. Hao Y. Productive activities and psychological well-being among older adults. *J Gerontol Ser B.* 2008;*63*(2):S64-S72. doi:10.1093/geronb/63.2.S64
135. Greenfield EA. Felt obligation to help others as a protective factor against losses in psychological well-being following functional decline in middle and later life. *J Gerontol Ser B.* 2009;*64B*(6):723-732. doi:10.1093/geronb/gbp074
136. Brown SL, Brown RM, House JS, Smith DM. Coping with spousal loss: potential buffering effects of self-reported helping behavior. *Personal Soc Psychol Bull.* 2008;*34*(6):849-861. doi:10.1177/0146167208314972
137. Piliavin JA, Siegl E. Health benefits of volunteering in the Wisconsin longitudinal study. *J Health Soc Behav.* 2007;*48*(4):450-464. doi:10.1177/002214650704800408
138. Morrow-Howell N. Volunteering in later life: research frontiers. *J Gerontol Ser B Psychol Sci Soc Sci.* 2010;*65B*(4):461-469. doi:10.1093/geronb/gbq024
139. Morrow-Howell N. Civic service across the life course. *Generations.* 2007;*30*:37-42. https://www.ingentaconnect.com/content/asag/gen/2006/00000030/00000004/art00007

140. Luoh M-C, Herzog AR. Individual consequences of volunteer and paid work in old age: health and mortality. *J Health Soc Behav.* 2002;*43*(4):490-509. doi:10.2307/3090239

141. Kumar S, Calvo R, Avendano M, et al. Social support, volunteering and health around the world: cross-national evidence from 139 countries. *Soc Sci Med.* 2012;*74*(5):696-706. doi:10.1016/J.SOCSCIMED.2011.11.017

142. Burr JA, Tavares J, Mutchler JE. Volunteering and hypertension risk in later life. *J Aging Health.* 2011;*23*(1):24-51. doi:10.1177/0898264310388272

143. Carlson MC, Helms MJ, Steffens DC, et al. Midlife activity predicts risk of dementia in older male twin pairs. *Alzheimer's Dement.* 2008;*4*(5):324-331. doi:10.1016/j.jalz.2008.07.002

144. McDonnall MC. The effect of productive activities on depressive symptoms among older adults with dual sensory loss. *Res Aging.* 2011;*33*(3):234-255. doi:10.1177/0164027511399106

145. Kim J, Pai M. Volunteering and trajectories of depression. *J Aging Health.* 2010;*22*(1):84-105. doi:10.1177/0898264309351310

146. Kahana E, Bhatta T, Lovegreen LD, et al. Altruism, helping, and volunteering. *J Aging Health.* 2013;*25*(1):159-187. doi:10.1177/0898264312469665

147. Cattan M, Hogg E, Hardill I. Improving quality of life in ageing populations: what can volunteering do? *Maturitas.* 2011;*70*(4):328-332. doi:10.1016/j.maturitas.2011.08.010

148. Alzheimer's Association. *What is dementia?* https://www.alz.org/alzheimers-dementia/what-is-dementia

149. Alzheimer's Association. *2022 Alzheimer's disease facts and figures.* 2022. https://www.alz.org/alzheimers-dementia/facts-figures

150. Prince M, Comas-Herrera A, Knapp M, et al. *World Alzheimer Report 2020: Design, Dignity, Dementia: Dementia-Related Design and the Built Environment.* Alzheimer's Disease International; 2020. https://www.alz.co.uk/research/WorldAlzheimerReport2020.pdf

151. Ginis KAM, Heisz J, Spence JC, et al. Formulation of evidence-based messages to promote the use of physical activity to prevent and manage Alzheimer's disease. *BMC Public Health.* 2017;*17*(1):209. doi:10.1186/s12889-017-4090-5

152. *Dementia Friendly America.* https://www.dfamerica.org/

153. Teri L, Logsdon RG, McCurry SM. Exercise interventions for dementia and cognitive impairment: the Seattle protocols. *J Nutr Health Aging.* 2008;*12*(6):391-394. doi:10.1007/BF02982672

154. Frist B. *Making dementia friendly communities the new normal. Forbes.* July 31, 2015. https://www.forbes.com/sites/billfrist/2015/07/31/making-dementia-friendly-communities-the-new-normal/?sh=1fec65a116b0

155. Dementia Friendly America. *What is Dementia Friendly America (DFA)?* https://www.dfamerica.org/what-is-dfa

156. Leshner AI, Landis S, Stroud C, Downey A. *Preventing Cognitive Decline and Dementia: A Way Forward.* The National Academies Press; 2017.

157. Hsiao JJ, Teng E. Depressive symptoms in clinical and incipient Alzheimer's disease. *Neurodegener Dis Manag.* 2013;*3*(2):147-155. doi:10.2217/nmt.13.10

158. Logsdon RG, McCurry SM, Teri L. Evidence-based interventions to improve quality of life for individuals with dementia. *Alzheimers Care Today.* 2007;*8*(4):309-318.

159. Wisconsin Department of Health Services. *Dementia-friendly grocery stores.* Published May 2016. https://www.dhs.wisconsin.gov/publications/p01269c.pdf

160. Dementia Friendly America Massachusetts. *Faith communities.* https://dfmassachusetts.org/tools/df-training-resources-by-sector/faith-communities/

161. Alzheimer's Association. *Safe return: Alzheimer's disease guide for law enforcement.* 2006. https://www.alz.org/national/documents/safereturn_lawenforcement.pdf

162. ACL Administration for Community Living. *Support for people with dementia, including Alzheimer's disease.* https://acl.gov/programs/support-people-alzheimers-disease/support-people-dementia-including-alzheimers-disease

163. congress.gov. *National Alzheimer's project act.* Published January 4, 2011. https://www.congress.gov/111/plaws/publ375/PLAW-111publ375.pdf

164. ASPE Office of the Assistant Secretary for Planning and Evaluation. *National plan to address Alzheimer's disease.* https://aspe.hhs.gov/national-plan-address-alzheimers-disease

165. Alzheimer's Association. *Improving care.* https://www.alz.org/get-involved-now/advocate/improving-care

166. United Nations. UN DESA policy brief no. 153: India overtakes China as the world's most populous country. 2023. https://www.un.org/development/desa/dpad/publication/un-desa-policy-brief-no-153-india-overtakes-china-as-the-worlds-most-populous-country/

THE METHODS OF PUBLIC HEALTH

12

ANALYTIC APPROACHES AND THE EVIDENCE BASE FOR PUBLIC HEALTH

LEARNING OBJECTIVES

- Outline five actionable steps to advance population health science.
- Select appropriate study designs for specific research questions and investigations.
- Define and differentiate quantitative and qualitative analysis methods.
- Summarize techniques to quantify associations between potential causes of health outcomes.
- Define criteria to select targets for public health interventions.

OVERVIEW: THE GOALS OF POPULATION HEALTH SCIENCE

The ultimate goal of population health science is to track progress toward our goal of promoting health and preventing disease. To promote health and prevent disease on a population scale, we first need to describe the distribution of health in a population. Only then might we be able to judge whether the health of that population is good or bad, acceptable or not acceptable. And how might we make these judgments? What is good health? What is acceptable health? If we observe suboptimal health in a population or differences among populations in terms of health, what might explain them? Our goal is to understand determinants, or causes, of population health, thinking very broadly about determinants, and then ideally to intervene to make improvements.

Causes of health outcomes, as we discuss throughout the book, emerge across the life course and across levels of determinants from a social ecological perspective. As such, causes include individual behaviors (e.g., exposure to maternal smoking in pregnancy, exposure to secondhand smoke in adolescence, smoking as an adult), characteristics and behaviors of family and social networks (e.g., genetic risks for disease, patterns of physical activity, social support), attributes of neighborhoods and cities (e.g., access to green space and healthy food choices, exposure to noise and air pollution), and policies that affect causes of health and health outcomes or both (e.g., seat-belt legislation, tobacco-control policies). The challenge is in disentangling these multilevel factors and the complex relationships among them to best understand where and how we might intervene to improve the health of a population.

In this chapter, we (a) discuss the foundations of qualitative approaches in population health science, (b) examine the foundations of quantitative approaches in population health science, and (c) provide examples that illustrate how each of these approaches guide public health action.

THE ANALYTIC APPROACH TO POPULATION HEALTH SCIENCE

An analytic approach is a process that breaks a problem into more manageable, solvable pieces. Problems are solved when the right analytic approach is applied in the right circumstance. Given the population health science goal to promote health and prevent disease on a population scale and to track progress toward an outcome, how might we break this problem into more manageable pieces, particularly given the complexities of factors that bring about population health?

> **An analytic approach is a process that breaks a problem into more manageable, solvable pieces. Problems are solved when the right analytic approach is applied in the right circumstance.**

Epidemiology and biostatistics are the basic sciences of public health. These disciplines provide the tools and techniques to assess and understand the causes of population health so that we may improve health in populations. Epidemiology is the study of the distribution and determinants of disease and is critically important in population health science. Biostatistics is a related science focused on understanding variability in potential causes and outcomes in order to infer associations and relationships among them.

Keyes and Galea[1] articulate seven steps for what they call the "epidemiology of consequence." Here we adapt these slightly into five actionable steps for population health science:

1. Define the population.
2. Define and measure the health outcome and potential causes of health.
3. Take a sample from the population for analysis.
4. Evaluate potential causes of population health.
5. Identify targets for public health action.

In the following sections, we describe each of these steps in detail.

DEFINE THE POPULATION

Populations are groups of individuals, often defined by specific attributes of person (e.g., people of a specific age or with other attributes in common), place (e.g., a geographic region), and time (e.g., a particular year or season of the year). In statistics, a population is the universe of all participants we concern ourselves with and about whom we would like to make inferences.

To identify what can be done to improve health, we first must understand health. Specifically, what is the extent of disease, or the distribution of the health outcome, in the population of interest? To understand this, we need data.

There are multiple techniques, resources, and repositories to access data. We can of course collect it, going to all members of the population to gather or assess their health information. However, there are also a number of publicly available data sources that can offer insights into health issues across many different populations, although they may not be as specific, locally relevant, or timely as we might need.

For example, the National Center for Health Statistics is one "center" within the Centers for Disease Control and Prevention (CDC) charged with collecting, organizing, and disseminating data to support policies aimed at improving the health of the U.S. population.[2] They collect data from public and private partners and produce data reports summarizing births, deaths, health outcomes, and utilization of healthcare services by region, state, sex, race/ethnicity, and so on. Researchers within the World Health Organization (WHO) perform a similar function, collecting and organizing data on over 1,000 health outcomes globally.[3]

As one type of health indicator that summarizes a critical aspect of health in a population, the CDC and the WHO regularly report mortality rates. Mortality rates are numbers of deaths scaled by population size per unit time. What this means, practically speaking, is that mortality rates are expressed as the number of deaths per 1,000 or per 100,000 people in a population per year. The mortality rate is computed for the population of interest, specified in terms of place (e.g., national mortality rate for Uganda, state mortality rate for Utah) and person characteristics (e.g., mortality rate for U.S. women over the age of 65 years).

For example, the WHO calculated the annual global adult mortality rate for persons aged 15 to 60 years for 2016. The result was 142 deaths per 1,000 persons aged 15 to 60 per year. This could also be presented as a probability of death of 0.142 (14.2%) per person per year. The WHO also reported adult mortality rates in each of six WHO regions (**Table 12.1**).

Note that the adult mortality rate in Africa is more than three times higher than that in the Western Pacific region and more than double that in the WHO Americas regions. These data provide evidence of a problem that needs addressing.

DEFINE AND MEASURE HEALTH OUTCOMES AND POTENTIAL CAUSES OF HEALTH

In order to improve health, we must define the relevant health outcome and determine the best approach to measuring that outcome. We must also define potential causes of health, which, building on the life course and social ecological frameworks, might range from demographic characteristics of the individual, such as age, biological sex, socioeconomic status, education, or income; or characteristics of the neighborhood, city, state, or country.

TABLE 12.1 Annual Mortality Rate per 1,000 Persons, Ages 15 to 60 Years, and Probability of Death Globally and for WHO Regions, 2016

WHO REGION	DEATHS PER 1,000 PERSONS	PROBABILITY OF DEATH (PERCENTAGE)
Africa	277	0.277 (27.7%)
Southeast Asia	171	0.171 (17.1%)
Eastern Mediterranean	150	0.150 (15.0%)
Americas	126	0.126 (12.6%)
Europe	113	0.113 (11.3%)
Western Pacific	87	0.087 (8.7%)
Total global	**142**	**0.142 (14.2%)**

WHO, World Health Organization.
Source: Data from World Health Organization. Adult mortality data by WHO region. Updated May 7, 2018. http://apps
.who.int/gho/data/view.main.1340?lang=en

There is no one measure that captures an individual's health. There is rather a range of health outcomes that are often used to describe different aspects of health. These include, but are not limited to, measures of disease, longevity, and quality of life.

Mortality, described earlier, is just one of a number of important health outcomes. Additional quantifiable measures of disease include prevalence (the number of existing cases) and incidence (the number of new cases) of specific conditions such as cardiovascular disease, dementia, pneumonia, influenza, and so on.

Longevity is generally measured by life expectancy. The most common measure of life expectancy is life expectancy at birth, which is the average number of years that a person can expect to live, or the average age at death.

There are a number of measures of quality of life. A popular measure is the Quality of Life Scale (QOLS), which consists of 16 items that address such areas as well-being, relationships with others, engagement in social and community activities, participation in recreational activities, and independence.[4] Participants completing a QOLS report their level of satisfaction in each of a series of life domains using an ordinal scale (e.g., a one-to-five or one-to-seven scale). Responses are summed to produce an overall quality-of-life score. There are many other health-related quality-of-life assessment measures that examine specific aspects of quality of life including physical health, mental health, and social functioning. Some of these scales (measures) are targeted to specific diseases and disorders and others are more generic.

Consider the example of diabetes as a disease outcome. Diabetes is a serious condition shown to cause cardiovascular disease, blindness, and lower leg amputations. Diabetes currently affects more than 400 million people, and the prevalence is increasing worldwide, particularly in low- and middle-income countries. The WHO produces diabetes fact sheets for each country, detailing the prevalence and mortality rates for men and women.[5] For example, in 2016, the prevalence of diabetes in the United States was 9.8% for men and 8.3% for women. During the same year, the sex-specific prevalence was lower in Switzerland (6.9% for men and 4.4% for women) and higher in Egypt (14.2% for men and 18.2% for women).

What might explain these differences in prevalence of diabetes across countries? Are there specific causes of diabetes that could be addressed to prevent diabetes and therefore reduce these differences? Two important individual risk factors for diabetes are obesity and an unhealthy diet. Might there be differences among countries in social, political, and cultural factors that affect obesity, diet, and diabetes? How do we identify these factors and perhaps, more importantly, determine what impact we might have on diabetes or other health outcomes if we could intervene?

Identification and measurement of potential causes of any disease can also be challenging. For example, suppose we focus on cardiovascular disease as our health outcome and consider hypertension (high blood pressure) as a potential cause. Measuring hypertension sounds straightforward enough. According to the American Heart Association, hypertension is defined as a systolic blood pressure (SBP) equal to or greater than 130 mmHg and/or diastolic blood pressure (DBP) equal to or greater than 80 mmHg.[6] However, these criteria were recently changed, and other sources, including the CDC, still cite previous cutoff points of SBP equal to or greater than 140 mmHg and/or DBP equal to or greater than 90 mmHg.[7] This inconsistency in the definition of hypertension, from respected sources, is raised here to illustrate how even measures that are based on objective criteria require careful definition. Diagnostic criteria change as new information becomes available bearing on levels of population risk. In every investigation, it is very important for the investigators to clarify their definitions of the key measurement variables to ensure that fair and accurate comparisons and interpretations are made when they present their data and results.

Another example further illustrates the complexity of measurement. Suppose we are interested in understanding and evaluating causes of autism in populations. Autism is a developmental disorder that is increasingly prevalent (**Table 12.2**). Today, approximately 1% of

TABLE 12.2   Prevalence of Autism Spectrum Disorder in 8-Year-Old Children, United States, 2000–2010

SURVEILLANCE YEAR	BIRTH YEAR	AUTISM SPECTRUM DISORDER PREVALENCE PER 1,000 CHILDREN	CASES OF AUTISM PER NUMBER OF CHILDREN
2000	1992	6.7	1 in 149
2002	1994	6.6	1 in 152
2004	1996	8.0	1 in 125
2006	1998	9.0	1 in 111
2008	2000	11.3	1 in 88
2010	2002	14.7	1 in 68

Source: Data from Centers for Disease Control and Prevention's Autism and Developmental Disabilities Monitoring Network. https://www.ncbi.nlm.nih.gov/books/NBK332896

the world's population has autism. In the United States, more than 3.5 million people have autism.[8] There is no blood test or other medical tests to diagnose autism. Instead, an autism diagnosis is based on the clinical judgment of a trained medical professional and is far more subjective than the diagnosis of hypertension. Although there have been discredited theories as to what might cause autism, including the much-publicized assertion that autism might be caused by the childhood measles, mumps, and rubella vaccine (an assertion that has been soundly refuted), to date there are no documented causes of autism. What might then explain the uptick in autism? Causes are factors that precede the diagnosis, and autism is usually diagnosed early in childhood. In considering potential causes, we must think broadly. Are there individual, social, or cultural experiences in utero or in very early childhood that could cause autism?

Once we have identified and measured health and potential causes of population health, we then evaluate whether, and to what extent, these potential causes are associated with the health outcome of interest. Note that in the scientific literature, causes are also known as exposures, determinants, or risk factors. There are very specific techniques for assessing associations and causality that quantify the nature or direction of associations and also the strength of associations. Once we find an association, it is then critical to evaluate whether the same association would apply to all populations or whether the nature and strength of associations vary across populations. Because there are almost always multiple causes to consider, we need to understand how these multiple causes interact with one another to produce health. We discuss these technicalities in some detail in the following sections.

TAKE A SAMPLE FROM THE POPULATION FOR ANALYSIS

In an ideal world, we would like to gather data from every member of the population. But populations are usually large. In most situations, it is not possible to measure health outcomes, and potential causes of health, for every member of the population to determine associations. Instead, we take a sample of participants from the population. By definition, the sample is smaller than the population from which it is selected. The sample should, insofar as possible, be representative of the population so that whatever associations that are observed in the sample are likely to exist in the population itself.

The sample is the subset of the population on which we perform our analyses. The exact size of the sample needed to ensure precision in statistical results depends on the situation. Generally speaking, a larger sample provides more precise statistical results. There is a point, however, where increasing the size of the sample does not offer much gain in precision. Determining the size of a sample is key for any study. We should not conduct any study with too small a sample (as results will not be meaningful) or too large a sample (there is no justification for involving more participants when fewer participants would yield the same precision).

There are many ways in which we collect data for research studies and evaluations. The study design is the process whereby participants are selected for a study or evaluation and data are collected to address the particular question of interest. While more and more data are generated every day, the need for carefully designed studies and analysis has never been more important. As a caution, more data (big data) can be misleadingly reassuring. There are many different study designs, and the optimal design for a given situation depends on a number of factors including what is known about the topic under study and the prevalence of the health outcome and the potential causes. The choice of study design also hinges on ethical, logistical, and financial issues.

Observational and Experimental Study Designs

Before describing a few popular study designs, we first outline design types. Study designs can be classified as observational or experimental. As the label implies, in observational studies we observe what is happening in a population (or a sample of the population) in terms of the prevalence or development (incidence) of risk factors and the prevalence or development (incidence) of health outcomes—without manipulating groups or assigning individuals to conditions. We observe. We watch. In contrast, in experimental studies we intervene and create comparison groups, often by randomization, that ideally differ only in terms of one particular risk factor or exposure and we then follow all participants to see how health outcomes develop, or progress, and compare these health outcomes between groups.

Individual-Level and Population-Level Study Designs

Study designs are also classified as individual level or population level. In individual-level observational and experimental studies, risk factors and health outcomes are measured for each individual participant in the study. In population-level observational studies, risk factors and health outcomes are measured in the aggregate, for example, at the community or country level. In population-level experimental studies, groups or communities are randomized, rather than individuals, to receive specific treatments or services. The latter are sometimes called cluster-randomized studies. Outcomes are also measured in the aggregate, at the group or community level, and compared.

Popular Study Designs

We now outline popular study designs that are used in public and population health research and evaluation (**Table 12.3**). We describe three types of observational studies—cross-sectional, cohort, and case–control studies—and one type of experimental study, the randomized controlled trial. Each study design can theoretically be conducted at the individual or population level.[9]

Observational: Cross-Sectional Study

When analyses are focused on describing populations, for example, estimating the extent of disease or the extent of exposure to a risk factor or a potential cause of disease, cross-sectional studies are appropriate. A cross-sectional study is conducted at a point in time, and the participants in the analysis sample are representative of the population defined by person, place, and time.

TABLE 12.3   General Features of Popular Study Designs

DESIGN TYPE	DESIGN	GENERAL FEATURES
Observational	Cross-sectional study	Participants are representative of the population defined by person, place, and time.
		Prevalence of potential causes, prevalence of the health outcome, and the association between potential causes and prevalence of the outcome are estimated at a point in time.
	Cohort study	Participants are free of the outcome of interest and followed over time for the development of that outcome.
		Prevalence of potential causes, incidence of the health outcome, and the association between potential causes and incidence of the outcome are estimated.
	Case–control study	Cases are participants with the health outcome of interest and controls are a random sample of participants from the same population that produced the cases but are free of the outcome.
		Prevalence of potential causes and the association between potential causes and the outcome are estimated.
Experimental	Randomized controlled trial	Participants are randomized to receive the intervention (e.g., new treatment, new program) or not (e.g., placebo, standard care) and followed for incidence of the health outcome or disease progression.
		The effect of the intervention on the health outcome (or disease progression) is estimated.

Exposure and disease are measured in each participant, and the association between exposure and disease at a particular point in time is estimated.

Cross-sectional studies can also be conducted at the population level and are sometimes called ecological or correlation studies, and the unit of analysis is not the individual but a higher-level unit such as city, state, or country. Exposure and disease at the unit level (e.g., city, state) are again measured at a point in time. Although cross-sectional studies might be the easiest to conduct, they have limitations. First, because they are conducted at a particular point in time, it is not possible to establish temporality and therefore we cannot be sure that a potential cause preceded disease. Second, we can only estimate prevalence of risk factors or exposures and disease at a point in time; we can say nothing of incidence of disease, which is often of greater interest. Third, when conducting a cross-sectional study at the population level, there is potential for what is called the ecological fallacy, which occurs when there is an association at the higher level but not at the individual level. For example, there may be an association observed between exposure and disease at the country level, yet the same association does not persist within individuals. This is not always the case with ecological studies, but it is possible and often difficult to assess.

Observational: Cohort Study

A second popular observational study design is the cohort study. Cohort studies involve a group of participants (a cohort) who are free of the health outcome of interest (e.g., disease) and are followed for the development of that outcome or disease over time. Some participants are exposed to the risk factor of interest and some are not, and the goal is to draw an association between the risk factor and the health outcome. Cohort studies can be conducted at the individual level (e.g., to evaluate the association between hypertension and cardiovascular disease) or at the population level (e.g., to evaluate the association between state-level policies on minimum wage and mental health). Cohort studies can be prospective (participants are enrolled before the outcome occurs) or retrospective (the study is initiated after the outcome occurs), but again both exposed and unexposed participants are enrolled and tracked (e.g., using electronic medical records) for the development of disease or outcome.

In designing cohort studies, attention must be paid to the prevalence of disease as cohort studies are not optimal for rare diseases because they require too many participants to ensure adequate precision in results. Attention must also be paid to the timing of disease. That is, prospective cohort studies are not optimal for diseases that take years to develop as it can be difficult to retain participants in studies with long durations. Also, attention must be paid to the nature of the exposure. If exposures are rare, investigators may need to oversample those who are exposed rather than taking all comers to ensure sufficient numbers of exposed participants for analysis.

Observational: Case–Control Study

A third popular observational study is the case–control study. In a case–control study, participants are identified based on their outcome status. Cases are those with the outcome or disease of interest, and controls are those free of the outcome or disease of interest. Controls are a random sample from the same population that produced the cases and are used to estimate the distribution of the exposure or risk factor in the population. Exposure status is determined for each case and for each control, and then the association between exposure and outcome status is estimated. Case–control studies are very efficient for rare diseases or diseases that take years to develop, and for situations in which it is difficult or expensive to measure exposure status (e.g., if exposure is based on an expensive medical test).

Observational: Confounding as a Limitation

All observational studies are prone to issues of confounding—specifically other variables or attributes that mask or enhance the association between the risk factor of interest and the outcome. For example, a prospective cohort study might be designed to investigate the association between hypertension and the development of cardiovascular disease. It is possible that people with hypertension are older, more likely to have high cholesterol, and more likely to have a family history of cardiovascular disease than those without hypertension, as risk factors tend to cluster. Individuals with hypertension may also have experienced more stressful life experiences or live in unsafe neighborhoods. All of these other factors may confound the primary focus of the study, which is to quantify the possible association between hypertension and cardiovascular disease.

Experimental: Randomized Controlled Trial

A popular experimental study is the randomized controlled trial, also called a clinical trial or an intervention study. Clinical trials are one approach to controlling for confounding because participants (or communities) are randomized to the exposure or intervention of interest (e.g., a new drug versus placebo, a behavioral intervention versus standard practice) and then followed for disease occurrence or progression. The randomization component is unique to these designs and has substantial benefits. In theory, randomization ensures that the comparison groups are well balanced and thus, any observed differences in health outcome can be attributed to the exposure or intervention. Despite this benefit, not all investigations are suitable to be studied using a clinical trial. Could we, for example, study the effects of obesity or poverty on health outcomes using a clinical trial? Such studies would never be possible as we could not randomize participants to be obese or not, or to live in poverty or not.

The optimal study design for any investigation depends on the nature of the risk factors and health outcomes, ethics, politics, and finances. Once a study design is determined, participants are sampled from the population and data are collected for analysis. In the next section, we describe quantitative and qualitative methods of analysis and how they are used in population health science to evaluate causes of population health.

> The optimal study design for any investigation depends on the nature of the risk factors and health outcomes, ethics, politics, and finances.

EVALUATE POTENTIAL CAUSES OF POPULATION HEALTH

Causes are necessary conditions for an outcome to occur. We must identify causes and understand the ways in which they affect health outcomes in order to design interventions to promote better health. The approach to identifying causes of population health must be systematic and comprehensive, and in considering potential causes, we must be aware of our own biases and preconceptions. Causes must be considered at multiple social ecological levels (individual; family and social network; neighborhood and city; and country) and across the life course (perinatal, childhood, and adolescence; adulthood; and older age). Once we have identified potential causes of health, we determine how best to measure them and then judge whether and in what ways they are associated with health.

There are a number of measures of association that quantify the nature and strength of associations between exposures or risk factors and health outcomes. Once an association is observed, the next question is whether that observed association is causal or not. This is a key and quite complicated step in any analysis. Establishing cause requires that there is an observed association, that the cause precedes the health outcome, and that there is no other explanation— despite thinking very broadly about other factors across multiple social ecological levels and over the life course—that could account for the observed association.

For example, there is a statistically significant and positive association between ice-cream sales and rates of drowning (higher rates of ice-cream sales are associated with higher rates of drowning). Despite this strong positive association, this relationship is not necessarily causal— ice-cream sales are higher in summer months as is the number of people who swim in pools, lakes, and oceans; thus, the observed association might be entirely explained by seasonality.

To evaluate potential causes of population health, we need data or evidence and measures of association and causation. Quantitative and qualitative analyses are approaches whereby we collect and analyze data and evaluate whether they support or refute hypotheses, ideas, and positions about potential causes of population health. Although we cannot cover each area comprehensively, in the next section we provide a summary of both approaches to help refine our intuition regarding statistical thinking.

Quantitative Methods

Quantitative analysis begins with identifying key variables. These are the exposures (potential causes) and health outcomes. Although both exposures and outcomes can take many forms, to simplify things, we focus on continuous (also called quantitative or measurement variables) and categorical variables with two response categories, which are also called binary or indicator variables. The analytic techniques we outline in our example can be generalized, with some modifications, to apply to other variable types.

Let us consider an example. Suppose we are interested in understanding the health of youth between the ages of 12 and 16 years. We consider two outcome variables, quality of life and diagnosis of asthma. Quality of life is a continuous variable measured on a scale from zero to 100 with higher scores indicating a better quality of life. Diagnosis of asthma is a binary variable (yes/no).

We also consider two potential causes of quality of life and diagnosis of asthma, the number of cigarettes smoked in the past 100 days and whether or not the adolescent lives in a state where tobacco products are regulated in schools. There are many more potential causes of quality of life and diagnosis of asthma; we consider just two here to illustrate concepts and computations.

Suppose, in this example, we use a prospective cohort study and enroll a sample of 500 adolescents living across the United States who are between the ages of 12 and 16 years and free of asthma in January 2020. At the time of recruitment, each adolescent reports the number of cigarettes smoked in the past 100 days. We also record the state in which they reside so that we can determine the smoking regulations that apply. Each participant is followed for 1 year at which time they complete a QOLS and are tested for asthma.

The key variables in this study are continuous and categorical (binary) measures of exposure and health, as summarized in **Table 12.4**.

The first step in any analysis is to generate summary statistics on key variables in the study sample. For continuous variables (exposures or outcomes), means and standard deviations are usually reported. The mean represents a typical value and the standard deviation is a measure of variability around the mean (interpreted as the average deviation from the mean). When the distribution of a continuous variable is subject to extremes (very high values or very low values relative to the others), we instead report the median as a measure of a typical value as it is not influenced by extremes. For binary variables, it is sufficient to report the number and percentage of respondents in the category of interest (e.g., those who live in states where smoking is regulated in schools, those with a diagnosis of asthma). Summary statistics for the study variables are summarized in **Table 12.5**.

The mean quality-of-life score is 75.2 with a standard deviation of 6.8 units, suggesting that there might be room for improvement in quality of life as the score ranges from 0 to 100. At 1 year, 36 (7.2%) of the participants develop asthma. Recall that no participants had a diagnosis of asthma at enrollment, so these are new, or incident, cases of asthma. The mean number of cigarettes smoked is 4.9 with a standard deviation of 5.1. This variable is one that is likely subject

TABLE 12.4   Examples of Exposure and Health Outcomes by Variable Type

VARIABLE TYPE	EXPOSURE	HEALTH OUTCOME
Continuous	**Number of cigarettes smoked** • In the past 100 days • Self-reported measure	**Self-reported QOL** • Measured on a scale of 0–100 • Higher scores indicate higher QOL
Categorical	**State: school tobacco regulation** • Reside in a state where it is unlawful for any student to use tobacco products on school grounds during school hours • Response options: Yes/No	**Diagnosis of asthma** • Response options: Yes/No

QOL, quality of life.

TABLE 12.5 Summary Statistics on Study Variables ($n = 500$)

VARIABLE TYPE	EXPOSURE	HEALTH OUTCOME
Continuous	**Number of cigarettes smoked** Mean (standard deviation): **4.9 (5.1)**	**Self-reported QOL** Mean (standard deviation): **75.2 (6.8)**
Categorical	**State: school tobacco regulation** Number (percentage): **420 (84.0%)**	**Diagnosis of asthma** Number (percentage): **36 (7.2%)**

QOL, quality of life.

to extremes—suppose in our analysis sample that 40% of the participants did not smoke while those who did smoked between 100 and 1,000 cigarettes over the past 100 days. Here we might instead report the median of 1.8 cigarettes smoked in the past 100 days. And last, 420 (84%) of 500 participants live in states where tobacco products are regulated in schools.

Once we describe the exposures and health outcomes, we proceed to evaluate associations between them. Depending on the study design used and the variable types, different measures of association are appropriate. Associations between one exposure and one outcome are called crude or unadjusted measures of association. It is almost always the case that multiple exposures or causes work together to produce health, in which case we often then generate adjusted measures of association (i.e., measures of association adjusted for other variables that might play a role). Consider first our binary outcome—diagnosis of asthma. Because all of the participants were free of asthma at enrollment, we observe new or incident cases and thus could generalize from our sample that the annual incidence of asthma is 7.2% (assuming that our analysis sample is representative of the population of young people free of asthma).

Next, we want to evaluate whether living in states where smoking is regulated in schools is associated with the incidence of asthma. **Table 12.6** summarizes the association between state regulation and incidence of asthma.

Among young people living in states where smoking is regulated in schools ($n = 420$), there were 26 new cases of asthma as compared to 10 new cases among youth living in states where smoking is not regulated in schools ($n = 80$). The incidence of asthma among those living in states where smoking is regulated in schools is $26/420 = 0.062$, or 6.2%. The incidence of asthma among those living in states where smoking is not regulated in schools is $10/80 = 0.125 = 12.5\%$. Is there an association between the regulation and incidence of asthma?

TABLE 12.6 New Cases of Asthma in Relation to State-Level Tobacco Regulation in Schools

TOBACCO REGULATION	ASTHMA DIAGNOSIS		
	ASTHMA DIAGNOSED	ASTHMA-FREE	TOTAL
Tobacco regulated in schools	26	394	420
Tobacco not regulated in schools	10	70	80
Total	**36**	**464**	**500**

A popular measure of association between two binary variables (a binary exposure and a binary outcome) is the risk ratio (RR, also called the relative risk). It is computed here by taking the ratio of the incidence of asthma among those living in states where smoking is regulated in schools ($26/420 = 0.062$) to the incidence of asthma among those living in states where smoking is not regulated in schools ($10/80 = 0.125$). Usually the numerator of the RR is the experimental or intervention group, but the groups can be reversed as long as the reader is clear on how the measure is constructed. Here, $RR = 0.062/0.125 = 0.495$, and it is interpreted as follows. Adolescents living in states where smoking is regulated in schools have about half the incidence of asthma compared to those living in states where smoking is not regulated in schools. It is also fair to say that the incidence of asthma is approximately double ($1/0.495 = 2.02$) among young people living in states where smoking is not regulated in schools when compared to those living in states where smoking is regulated in schools.

Next, we want to evaluate whether living in states where smoking is regulated in schools is associated with quality of life. **Table 12.7** summarizes the means and standard deviations of the quality-of-life measure according to whether adolescents live in states where smoking is regulated in schools.

Is there an association between the regulation and self-reported quality of life? Because quality of life is a continuous outcome variable, we no longer focus on proportions but on means. To evaluate associations, we compare mean quality of life between adolescents living in states where smoking is and is not regulated in schools. Among adolescents living in states where smoking is regulated in schools ($n = 420$), the mean quality of life is 77.1 as compared to a mean of 65.2 among those living in states where smoking is not regulated in schools ($n = 80$). The difference in means is 11.9 scale points, with young people living in states where smoking is regulated in schools having a higher quality of life by 11.9 scale points.

The relative risk and difference in means quantify the association between a binary exposure and binary and continuous outcomes, respectively. The important questions are whether a 50% reduction in incidence of asthma and a difference of 11.9 scale points on the QOLS are important and impactful. This can be judged by practical importance and also by statistical significance. Practical importance is judged by someone with expertise in a particular area who can interpret whether a RR or difference in means translates to a real difference in health. A 50% reduction in the incidence of asthma in states where there are regulations about smoking in schools would seem to be an important reduction. If that reduction holds across populations, that could translate to thousands of young adults being spared of asthma. However, the latter is only true if we can attribute the 50% reduction to the school regulation. The difference in mean quality-of-life scores is a bit harder to judge. Higher quality-of-life scores are better, but is a difference of almost 12 scale points a meaningful difference in quality of life? We may need more information on the scale and its scoring to judge.

TABLE 12.7   QOL in Relation to State-Level Tobacco Regulation in Schools

TOBACCO REGULATION	QOL		
	NUMBER OF PARTICIPANTS	QOL MEAN	QOL STANDARD DEVIATION
Tobacco regulated in schools	420	77.1	6.5
Tobacco not regulated in schools	80	65.2	8.2
Total	**500**	**75.2**	**6.8**

QOL, quality of life.

Statistical significance is another approach to judge the importance of our findings. When we estimate a RR, a difference in means, or any other measure of association, we do so based on one analytic sample. We hope that the sample is representative of the population and that the same association holds in the population. The fact is, we have only one sample, and associations might vary in other samples selected from the same population. Because in statistical inference we generate estimates about populations based on a single sample, we must recognize that there might be some sampling variability. Rather than inferring that the observed RR or difference in means applies directly to the population, we often generate confidence interval estimates, which incorporate sampling variability and represent a range of plausible values for the association in the population. Confidence intervals are constructed by starting with the estimate of association from our sample and building in what is called a margin of error. The margin of error includes an estimate of the variability of the statistic (called the standard error) and a probability component reflecting the level of confidence we choose (the most typical level of confidence is 95%).

In our sample, we estimate the RR to be 0.495 and suppose that we compute a 95% confidence interval estimate of 0.375 to 0.729. Any of the values in the confidence interval are possible estimates of the RR. Because the confidence interval does not include the null (or no difference) value of 1.0 (the RR is computed by taking the ratio of two proportions; the RR is 1.0 when the two proportions or risks are equal), we say that there is a statistically significant difference in incidence of asthma between groups. Suppose that our sample size was a bit smaller and we estimate a RR of 0.495 with a 95% confidence interval of 0.04 to 1.02. In this case, we would conclude that there was a reduction in incidence in the sample, but it is not statistically significant because the 95% confidence interval includes the null value of 1.0.

We can follow a similar approach for the difference in means. We estimated the difference in mean quality-of-life scores of 11.9 units. A 95% confidence interval for the difference in mean quality-of-life scores is 10.2 to 13.5. The interpretation is that we are 95% confident that the true difference (i.e., the difference in the population means) is anywhere between 10.2 and 13.5 scale points. We conclude that the difference in means is statistically significant because the confidence interval does not include the null value of 0. Note that the null value for a difference is 0 whereas the null value for a ratio is 1.0.

Confidence interval estimates are one way to judge statistical significance based on whether the null value is included in the interval. Another option is based on p values, which summarize statistical significance in tests of hypothesis. In tests of hypothesis, we formulate a research hypothesis (usually that there is an association) and test it against what we call the null hypothesis (that there is no difference or no association). We examine the sample data to determine if the data support the research hypothesis or not. Statistical computing packages are often used to make this assessment and they produce p values, which allow us to judge statistical significance. p values represent the incompatibility of the data with the assumed statistical model. Usually, people claim statistical significance if the p value is .05 or smaller (this criterion is generally applied, but a more or less stringent criterion can also be applied).

In our example, we observe a RR of 0.495. We could run a test of hypothesis to determine if this estimate provides statistically significant evidence of an association, that is, a statistical difference in incidence of asthma between youth living in states where smoking is regulated in schools as compared to those who do not. Suppose the test of hypothesis produces a p value = .0231. Because the p value = .0231 is less than .05, we conclude that there is a statistically significant difference in incidence of asthma between adolescents living in states where smoking is regulated in schools and those who do not. Note that both the confidence interval approach and the test of hypothesis approach produce similar conclusions—that there is a statistically significant association. Both approaches, however, are based on the crude association between school regulations and incidence of asthma.[10]

In the crude analysis, incidence of asthma is lower in youth living in states where tobacco products are regulated in schools. But what if the young people who live in those states reported smoking fewer cigarettes in the past 100 days, or live in homes where they are less exposed to secondhand smoke, or live in neighborhoods where there is very little air pollution and so on? Is it appropriate to attribute the reduction in incidence of asthma to school regulations, given these other factors and the ways in which they may be related to incidence of asthma? When reviewing and interpreting data, it is important to be skeptical and to ask, could anything else explain this?

There are epidemiological and statistical techniques to control or adjust for other factors in an attempt to disentangle the impact of multiple potential causes of health outcomes. In determining causes of population health and targets for interventions to promote health, we must isolate, insofar as possible, the impact of each potential cause. Although none of the causes work independently or in isolation, the work is to determine where we might intervene to have the greatest impact on health.

Qualitative Methods

Qualitative methods are used to understand context, people, and relationships. For example, in population health, we need to understand how social, political, economic, and environmental factors affect health (context); how people understand, process, and experience potential causes of health and health outcomes (people); and how all of these factors interact to produce health (relationships).

Qualitative methods give different insights into research questions that are not possible with quantitative assessments. In many areas, both qualitative and quantitative methods are applied. The two approaches should be seen as complementary, and not in opposition, as each approach offers unique advantages. Quantitative methods might be optimal to capture incidence of disease (e.g., asthma, diabetes, dementia, influenza) in populations, but qualitative methods might be best to capture barriers to practicing preventive measures (e.g., What barriers prevent inactive people from taking up regular exercise programs? When a treatment is proved to be effective for a particular condition, why are patients not adherent in taking it?). In fact, many investigators use both quantitative and qualitative analyses in a single investigation, which is called a mixed methods analysis.

Qualitative analysis is a field unto itself; here we briefly introduce some of the popular qualitative methods used in population health science. Two popular methods of data collection for qualitative research are interviews and focus groups. Interviews are used to gather data from individuals regarding their beliefs, experiences, and positions on issues. Interviews can be structured, semistructured, or unstructured. As the names suggest, structured interviews are very prescriptive, essentially interviewer-administered questionnaires, which include a series of predetermined questions that generally do not allow for elaboration or much additional discussion. Semistructured interviews include a few questions that address the main topics of interest but allow for discussion and elaboration on issues that may not have been previously identified. Unstructured interviews are the least prescriptive and are generally used when not much is known on a specific topic, and thus unstructured interviews are useful for discovery.

Focus groups are another method of data collection and are group discussions on a particular issue. They are usually overseen by a moderator or facilitator who raises topics and questions and guides the discussion through structured questions and prompts. Focus groups might include participants with similar backgrounds and positions or might be purposefully organized to include participants with varied backgrounds and positions, depending on the issue. Focus groups tend to work well with six to eight participants, and discussions often work best when questions start at a more general level and move to the specific level.

Qualitative analysis involves, among other things, coding of qualitative data that are captured by interviews or focus groups into themes that provide some explanation and interpretation of the phenomenon under study. These data are not easily converted into numbers that can be summarized. Instead, text in transcripts from interviews and focus groups are analyzed, organized, and summarized. Qualitative data analysis can be iterative. Often the data collection and analysis occur simultaneously.

There are popular software systems available for qualitative data analysis to assist the investigator in transcribing, translating, labeling, coding, and structuring the data for analysis. Regardless of the software system used, the investigator drives the process of analysis, whereas the system facilitates organization, management, and summarization of large amounts of data into reports and figures.

A qualitative analysis might be largely descriptive where the range of responses to a particular question is articulated and the frequency with which each is reported is summarized. The analysis can go further to identify clusters or patterns of responses among specific participant groups. The interpretative, and more challenging, aspect of the analysis is in understanding what the data mean with regard to health. This leads to generalizations in the form of explanations to key questions about social and other factors.

A qualitative data analysis report includes the details of the process used to collect, manage, and organize data; the methodology used for transcribing and coding themes; and the interpretation and implications for new policies or practices.

IDENTIFY TARGETS FOR PUBLIC HEALTH ACTION

Once we identify potential causes of population health, we then need to determine which potential causes are modifiable and what effect or impact modifications might have on population health. If we intervene in some way, can we shift population health? Age, for example, is a cause of many health outcomes but there is nothing we can do to slow aging. On the other hand, individual behaviors such as smoking or lack of physical activity are potentially modifiable. It is important to focus on individual healthy behaviors, but perhaps even more important are the social, political, and environmental factors that influence these behaviors and, in many ways, have greater impact on population health.

Public health programs and policies are often aimed at the community, state, or national levels and are designed to shift the distributions of causes of health and, in turn, health outcomes. For example, the top 10 public health achievements of the first decade of the 21st century in the United States include substantial reductions in vaccine-preventable diseases, prevention and control of the spread of infectious diseases, tobacco control, improvements in infant health, reductions in traffic fatalities, prevention of cardiovascular disease and cancer, improvements in occupational safety, prevention of childhood lead poisoning, and increases in public health preparedness.[11] These achievements can be attributed to policies and interventions by federal, state, and local public health agencies.

The top 10 public health achievements of the 21st century worldwide are reductions in child mortality; reductions in vaccine-preventable diseases; increased access to safe drinking water and sanitation; prevention and control of the spread of malaria, HIV/AIDS, and tuberculosis; tobacco control; improvements in road safety; and increases in preparedness and response to global health threats.[12] These achievements too can be attributed to investments in infrastructure and systems, and new private, community, and political partnerships. It is important to keep in mind, however, that despite these achievements, inequities persist.

HOW ANALYTIC APPROACHES GENERATE EVIDENCE AND GUIDE PUBLIC HEALTH ACTION

Improvements in population health depend on good research, policies, and practice. Public Health 3.0 is an initiative led by the U.S. Department of Health and Human Services (HHS) and a call to action to "engage multiple sectors and community partners to generate collective impact" to improve population health.[13] Public Health 3.0 identifies five critical dimensions needed to improve health, one of which is "timely and locally relevant data, metrics, and analytics." Accurate and timely data are essential for evidence-based decision-making; there are more and more data available every day, and these data must be turned into actionable information through carefully designed and implemented analyses.

Improvements in population health depend on good research, policies, and practice.

Public health action includes interventions, policies, and programs that promote health. Qualitative and quantitative methods allow us to gather data or scientific evidence in support of interventions, policies, and programs that might positively affect health. Quantitative analyses allow us to estimate potential causes of health outcomes and in particular, assess the strength of associations so that we might direct resources toward programs that have the potential for greatest impact. Qualitative analysis gives insights into how interventions, policies, and programs work best and what challenges might be present in implementation or sustainability. Once interventions, policies, and programs are implemented, they should continue to be thoroughly evaluated to ensure that they remain effective.

We observe how both qualitative and quantitative methods can be applied in tandem to document traumatic exposures and to evaluate the effectiveness of psychological interventions for women victims of the prolonged armed conflict in Colombia, South America (Case Study 12.1; you can access the podcast accompanying Case Study 12.1 by following this link to Springer Publishing Company Connect™: http://connect.springerpub.com/content/book/978-0-8261-8043-8/part/part04/chapter/ch12).

CASE STUDY 12.1: ANALYZING FORCED DISPLACEMENT AS A PUBLIC HEALTH ISSUE USING MIXED METHODS

According to the Office of the United Nations High Commissioner for Refugees (UNHCR), the United Nations refugee agency, in 2021 there were 89.3 million forcibly displaced persons worldwide.[14] These individuals have had to flee from their homes, and their home communities, because of armed conflict or generalized violence. This rising tally of conflict-displaced individuals includes 53.2 million internally displaced persons (IDPs) still residing within the borders of their countries of origin, 27.1 million refugees who are seeking a safe haven in another country, and 4.6 million asylum seekers. As the UNHCR website proclaims, 31 people are newly displaced every minute.[15] The 2022 Russian invasion of Ukraine increased that number by more than 10 million, bringing total numbers of forced migrants due to violence to almost 100 million.

Given the diverse international spectrum of humanitarian emergencies, and conflict-induced migration, how can analytical methods be used to characterize this global public health crisis, identifying the causes of health in these populations, targeting public health actions, and intervening to diminish the negative health impacts? The answer is, there are multiple ways.

First, it is important to quantify the numbers of individuals affected, enumerating refugees and IDPs. In addition to UNHCR, the Internal Displacement Monitoring Centre (IDMC) works tirelessly to create up-to-date tabulations of IDPs throughout the world.[16] This is daunting work, but critically important, as each new conflict erupts and dislocates lives and livelihoods.

(continued)

Second, it is critical to elucidate the types of exposures, or risk factors that can lead to health consequences, experienced by those who are displaced. This often starts with qualitative studies that are conducted with small groups of refugees or IDPs to elicit and create an inventory of what they have experienced. In the case of forced displacement, there is a powerfully memorable instant in time when individuals depart their homes and communities, often never to return. Based on this pivotal point in life, researchers can ground their qualitative inquiries, and their quantitative data collection, in relation to what happened before, during, and after the life-changing moment of displacement.

Third, careful studies are able to assess current physical and mental health status, in some cases supported by data from medical examinations and interviews. In the case of forced displacement, health consequences feature combinations of physical and psychological harm.

We illustrate these points using the case example of IDPs in Colombia, South America. In 2016, Colombia officially shifted to "postconflict" status following 52 years of continuous civil war. The IDMC estimated numbers of Colombian IDPs, and the Colombian government and various nongovernmental organizations (NGOs) also produced their own figures. In 2021, Colombia had 5.2 million IDPs according to IDMC. The Colombian government had officially designated these individuals as "victims of the armed conflict" who are now eligible for services and protection. Colombia accounts for 84% of IDPs throughout the Americas and 9% of the worldwide census. Seventy percent of Colombian IDPs are women and children. Most Colombian IDPs were originally poor rural residents who were forced to relocate to large urban centers.

As mentioned, conflict-induced internal displacement is a multiphase process. Let us examine the exposures during each phase: before, during, and after displacement. The commonality is that all phases are psychologically stressful and collectively increase the risks for psychological distress and diagnosable psychiatric disorders. Some exposures involve forms of physical harm, and all involve the potential for psychological impact.

The predisplacement period is marked by a series of traumatic exposures, often over a period of years, as armed actors (Colombia had multiple groups of guerrilla and paramilitary combatants) infiltrate rural areas, gradually seizing control and imposing new codes of conduct. These infiltrators initially enforced their power with threats, but threats were often followed by assassinations, massacres, forced recruitment of local youth into their ranks, and other atrocities. As different armed groups came in, or when the Colombian Army or National Police became involved, many local residents were directly exposed to military combat, bombings, land mines, and munitions. So, the period before displacement was most notable for potentially traumatizing exposures including many forms of threatened or actual violence and physical harm.

The moment of displacement ("la salida"—the departure) was characterized by the totality and finality of losses. IDPs left their homes and all forms of personal possessions, family heirlooms, photographs, and sentimental objects. Just as profoundly, from the social ecological perspective, they walked away from their family members who remained, and they walked away from their friends, neighbors, social networks, and communities. They gave up their livelihoods including their land, crops, animals, and tools. These occupations had also served as the basis for

(continued)

their personal identity, their community status, their reputation for their crafts and skills, and their self-esteem. All of this was lost in an instant.

Postdisplacement relocation to city centers was extremely disorienting, and the initial transition, lasting months or years, was fraught with great hardship including homelessness, unemployment, poverty, and lack of urban job and survival skills.

Summarizing then, this litany of exposures could be simplified as predisplacement traumas, displacement phase losses, and postdisplacement relocation life changes. From an analytic perspective, these exposures can be documented and examined in relation to measures of current psychological health. This was done in Colombia with IDP women who had relocated to the capital city of Bogotá. Given this tangled complexity of displacement exposures, it was not surprising to find that almost two-thirds of the women had clinically significant symptom elevations for posttraumatic stress disorder (PTSD), depression, and/ or anxiety disorders at the time of study, typically years after the moment of displacement.

Given this burden of psychological distress and disorder, what analytical approaches could be helpful? Even at the level of an early feasibility/acceptability study, the following steps were implemented involving both qualitative and quantitative elements—a "mixed methods" approach. First, by hosting multiple focus groups of IDP women (the population targeted for psychosocial intervention), and representatives of governmental and community-based organizations working with IDPs and program staff, qualitative analyses explored the spectrum of pre-, peri-, and postdisplacement exposures and stressors. Second, once the participants were recruited and enrolled, and baseline data collection was conducted, quantitative epidemiological analyses were used to assess the extent of exposure to stressors, by phase, for each participant and to assess current symptom levels of common mental disorders using validated, Spanish language versions of internationally standardized assessment instruments. Third, biostatistical methods were used to identify the stressors most strongly predictive of current mental health status. Fourth, these findings were then used to guide the application of an evidence-based, WHO-sanctioned, intervention. The intervention, "interpersonal counseling" (the brief version of interpersonal psychotherapy) appeared to successfully lower psychiatric symptom levels during an initial pilot study.

There were a few more components to the study, but in short, the project aimed at examining the feasibility of (a) recruiting sufficient numbers of participants; (b) screening for trauma/loss exposures and for symptoms of PTSD, major depressive disorder, and generalized anxiety disorder; (c) intervening using a locally adapted version of an evidence-based treatment (interpersonal counseling); (d) referring women with elevated symptom levels to specialized services; (e) retaining study participants in the intervention until symptom resolution was achieved; and (f) conducting follow-up assessments of study participants. This case clearly argues for strong analytic methods as useful tools for examining what produces health in complex real-world environments.

We conclude with a case study that reports findings from a data analytic study regarding extreme and expanding disparities in wealth by race/ethnicity that contribute powerfully to health inequity (Case Study 12.2).

CASE STUDY 12.2: THE ESCALATING WEALTH GAP AS A DRIVER OF HEALTH INEQUITY

In the United States, extraordinary racial disparities in wealth have persisted for centuries and have worsened sharply during the COVID-19 pandemic. The wealth gap is deeply embedded in structural racism,[17] and solutions to redress these inequities are dauntingly complex.

According to the U.S. Department of Treasury,[18] wealth is defined as assets minus liabilities. Assets reflect the total financial value of a household. Assets include the home, physical possessions (e.g., automobiles, equipment, appliances, furnishings, artwork, heirlooms, jewelry, artifacts), savings, retirement accounts, financial investments, and cash. Liabilities are debts—all things owed—in such forms as home mortgages, personal loans, credit card balances, student loan debt, or other financial obligations. Wealth comes from multiple sources and is not the same as income. However, income can contribute to, and be transformed into, wealth through saving or investing a portion of earnings.

Racial inequities are apparent at the level of the paycheck. The U.S. Federal Reserve states,[19] "in the United States, the average African American/Black and Hispanic/Latinx households earn about half as much as the average White household." However, the wealth gap far exceeds the income gap. A prepandemic study conducted in 2019 found that the median wealth of White families ($184,000) was five times the wealth of Hispanic families ($38,000) and eight times the wealth of African American/Black families. Then, in a 2-year interval, the COVID-19 pandemic expanded the gap for African Americans/Black families to 10-fold.[20] The historical record has demonstrated that the wealth gap rarely shrinks and over the long term widens and worsens. The COVID-19 pandemic injected additional inequality. These trends bode badly for future generations of persons targeted for marginalization.

The roots of the wealth gap are multifactorial and multiplicative.[21] Researchers at Brandeis University compared wealth generation for White and African American/Black families over a 25-year span and found a tripling of the wealth gap during those two and one-half decades.

These investigators identified five factors that interact synergistically to limit the accumulation of wealth for non-White families generally, and for African American/Black families specifically. The single most potent predictor of wealth inequality was the number of years of home ownership, accounting for 27% of the differential in relative wealth. Post–World War II, African American/Black citzens were barred from participation in government-sponsored programs that created incentives for home ownership. Racial segregation and redlining of poor neighborhoods relegated African American/Black homeownership to residential areas with lower property values, slower rates of real estate appreciation, and lower resale prices, while making it extremely difficult for African American/Black borrowers to qualify for a mortgage. The continuing inability to build wealth by investing in quality real estate in prime neighborhoods places a severe limitation on wealth generation through the vehicle of home equity, the major contributor to the wealth differentials. The historical legacy of total dispossession during slavery, followed by exclusion from housing incentive programs, racial segregation in housing options, and overt discrimination in lending practices created a situation where wealth accumulation for African American/Black citizens through home ownership was late in starting and remains meager compared with White citzens.

(continued)

Three additional components that place persons of color at financial disadvantage compared to White populations are among the most recognized and prominent social determinants of health: lower levels of educational attainment, lower income, and higher rates of unemployment.

The final factor that capped growth in individual and household wealth was the dearth of outside financial support and inheritance. This represents a completely understandable and multigenerational consequence of reduced educational, occupational, and income-earning opportunities.

Let's flip this upside down. Wealth itself is a driver of health.[22]

Wealth effectively, and quite literally, buys health, both directly and indirectly. Directly, wealth buys quality health insurance coverage, access to preventive care, and readily available referrals for consultation with highly trained specialists. Indirectly, wealth supports a stable, salutary lifestyle. Persons with wealth can live in safe neighborhoods with outdoor green spaces for recreation and fitness activities. Persons with wealth have easy access to nutritious foods and a healthy diet. Persons with wealth can send their children to quality public or private schools where college-bound youth receive first-rate education from dedicated teachers in well-equipped facilities. Persons with wealth often launch their children into personally fulfilling, wealth-producing careers where they will become self-supporting and productive wealth generators themselves.

Wealth offers protection against unexpected adversities as has become starkly apparent during the COVID-19 pandemic. The wealthiest are emerging wealthier, while the poorest have become both relatively and absolutely poorer by comparison.

By almost all health metrics, people with wealth live healthier lives. Wealth is a safeguard against chronic stress. Wealth is associated with fewer chronic disease risk factors plus earlier detection and improved control of identified risk factors. Wealth is associated with improved functional status, higher levels of independence with aging, and reduced rates of premature mortality.

So, wealth is desirable for many reasons and confers better health.

Importantly, this is not a zero-sum game where some must be poor in order for others to be wealthy. There is no incentive for maintaining the egregious wealth gap. None other than the Assistant Secretary for Economic Policy Benjamin Harris and Economist Sydney Schreiner Wertz lay this out plainly,[18] stating, "Wealth is essential for economic security because it can be used for consumption, which is directly connected to well-being…. Wealth gives households the ability to pursue an education, take employment or investment risks, move to new neighborhoods, buy a home, and start a business." Recall that lack of wealth deprives individuals, and entire race/ethnic subgroups of our population, from sharing the health and goodness that wealth can bring. The authors' bottom line is summed up as, "…wealth is necessary for individual economic mobility and growth of the economy as a whole." By having individuals, households, and entire segments of the U.S. population "left behind," the whole of American society is diminished economically and socially.

Yet, intervening to stop and reverse the damaging and disparaging course of the runaway wealth gap is challenging and will require moral and political will. Derenoncourt and colleagues[23] state forthrightly, "In the absence of policy interventions or other forces leading to improvements in the relative wealth-accumulating conditions of Black Americans, wealth convergence is not only a distant scenario, but an impossible one."

(continued)

Furthermore, the wealth gap has lifelong, and indeed, multigenerational conse-quences. Darrick Hamilton states,[24] "The wealth position a child is born into will shape opportunity, outcomes, and health throughout life."

The wealth gap originated in the institution of slavery. In a National Public Radio (NPR) interview,[25] Derenoncourt presented the harsh reality of this fact:

> Let's start back in 1860. This was before Emancipation, when about 4 million of the 4.4 million Black people in America were enslaved. Slavery robbed the vast majority of Black Americans of the ability to amass wealth and pass it on to their children. They themselves were a form of wealth—other people's wealth. In this barbaric world, the ratio of white-to-Black wealth was 56 to 1. Said in a different way, for every dollar the average white person had, the average Black person had only about 2 cents.

With an underpinning grounded on structural racism, structural solutions will be necessary to dismantle these entrenched racial disparities in economic secu-rity. Political will and effective policy formulation are needed to diminish hous-ing discrimination, create safety nets for households in financial jeopardy, open educational doors and occupational pathways, and create equitable avenues for savings, investment, and wealth accumulation.

SUMMARY

In population health science, we aim to promote health and prevent disease based on timely and relevant evidence or data. We propose five actionable steps. First, we define the population of interest or the group of individuals with whom we are concerned. Second, we define and measure the health outcome of interest (e.g., mortality, longevity, prevalence or incidence of a specific disease) and the potential causes of that health outcome, thinking broadly about causes across social ecological levels and over the life course. Third, we select a sample for analysis. The sample is a representative subset of the population selected based on a specific study design. The optimal study design for any investigation depends on a number of factors such as the prevalence and incidence of the health outcome and its potential causes, logistical issues, and ethical con-cerns. Fourth, we evaluate the potential causes of health. In particular, we assess the strength of association between each potential cause and the health outcome of interest. This involves the application of quantitative and qualitative analysis methods to determine meaningful, import-ant, and statistically significant associations between potential causes and the health outcome. Fifth, we identify targets, or modifiable causes, for public health action. And once we implement interventions or actions to promote health, we again gather and analyze data to ensure that they are working as intended.

End-of-Chapter Resources

Access additional case study podcasts online at http://connect.springerpub.com/ content/book/978-0-8261-8043-8/

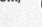

DISCUSSION QUESTIONS

1. Think of a health measure whose definition (criteria) has changed over time. What impact would this have on the use of the measure in public health research and practice?

2. What study design would you use to study whether a particular drug to treat maternal hypertension in pregnancy was associated with adverse pregnancy outcomes? Discuss the advantages and disadvantages of your choice.

3. Suppose we implement a media campaign to educate youth about the risks of opioid addiction. What data would be important to collect and analyze to determine if the campaign is effective?

A robust set of instructor resources designed to supplement this text is located at **http://connect.springerpub.com/content/book/978-0-8261-8043-8**. Qualifying instructors may request access by emailing **textbook@springerpub.com**.

REFERENCES

1. Keyes KM, Galea S. *Epidemiology Matters: A New Introduction to Methodological Foundations.* Oxford University Press; 2014.
2. Centers for Disease Control and Prevention. *The NCHS mission.* https://www.cdc.gov/nchs/about/mission.htm
3. World Health Organization. *Global health observatory data repository.* http://apps.who.int/gho/data/node.home
4. Burckhardt CS, Anderson KL. The Quality of Life Scale (QOLS): reliability, validity, and utilization. *Health Qual Life Outcomes.* 2003;*1*:60. doi:10.1186/1477-7525-1-60
5. World Health Organization. *Diabetes.* https://www.who.int/diabetes/en
6. American Heart Association. *The facts about high blood pressure.* https://www.heart.org/en/health-topics/high-blood-pressure/the-facts-about-high-blood-pressure
7. Centers for Disease Control and Prevention. *Facts about hypertension.* https://www.cdc.gov/bloodpressure/facts.htm
8. Autism Society of Southwest Louisiana. Facts and Statistics. https://autismsocietyofswla.com/facts-%26-statistics
9. Aschengrau A, Seage GR. *Essentials of Epidemiology in Public Health.* 3rd ed. Jones & Bartlett; 2014.
10. Sullivan LM. *Essentials of Biostatistics in Public Health.* 3rd ed. Jones & Bartlett; 2017.
11. Centers for Disease Control and Prevention. Ten great public health achievements—United States, 2001–2010. *MMWR Morb Mortal Wkly Rep.* 2011;*60*(19):619-623. https://www.cdc.gov/mmwr/preview/mmwrhtml/mm6019a5.htm?s_cid=fb2423
12. Centers for Disease Control and Prevention. *CDC identifies top global public health achievements in first decade of 21st century [Press release].* Published June 23, 2011. https://www.cdc.gov/media/releases/2011/p0623_publichealth.html
13. DeSalvo KB, Wang YC, Harris A, et al. Public health 3.0: a call to action for public health to meet the challenges of the 21st century. *Prev Chronic Dis.* 2017;*14*:E78. doi:10.5888/pcd14.170017
14. The United Nations High Commissioner for Refugees. *Global trends: forced displacement in 2021.* 2022. https://www.unhcr.org/publications/global-trends-2021
15. United Nations High Commissioner for Refugees. *Global trends: forced displacement in 2017.* https://www.unhcr.org/statistics/unhcrstats/5b27be547/unhcr-global-trends-2017.html
16. The Internal Displacement Monitoring Centre. *About us.* https://www.internal-displacement.org/about-us
17. Lynch EE, Malcoe LH, Laurent SE, Richardson J, Mitchell BC, Meier HCS. The legacy of structural racism: associations between historic redlining, current mortgage lending, and health. *SSM Popul Health.* 2021;*14*(100793). doi:10.1016/j.ssmph.2021.100793
18. Harris B, Wertz SS. *Racial differences in economic security: the racial wealth gap.* U.S. Department of the Treasury. Published September 15, 2022. https://home.treasury.gov/news/featured-stories/racial-differences-economic-security-racial-wealth-gap

19. Aladangady A, Forde A. *Wealth inequality and the racial wealth gap.* Board of Governors of the Federal Reserve System. Published October 22, 2021. https://www.federalreserve.gov/econres/notes/feds-notes/wealth-inequality-and-the-racial-wealth-gap-20211022.html

20. Mineo L. *Racial wealth gap may be a key to other inequities.* The Harvard Gazette. Published June 3, 2021. https://news.harvard.edu/gazette/story/2021/06/racial-wealth-gap-may-be-a-key-to-other-inequities/

21. Shapiro T, Meschede T, Osoro S. *The roots of the widening racial wealth gap: explaining the black-white economic divide.* Brandeis University Institute on Assets and Social Policy. Published February 2013. https://heller.brandeis.edu/iere/pdfs/racial-wealth-equity/racial-wealth-gap/roots-widening-racial-wealth-gap.pdf

22. South E, Venkataramani A, Dalembert G. Building black wealth–the role of health systems in closing the gap. *N Engl J Med.* 2022;387(9):844-849. doi:10.1056/NEJMms2209521

23. Derenoncourt E, Kim CH, Kuhn M, Schularick M. *Wealth of two nations: the U.S. racial wealth gap, 1860-2020.* NBER Working Paper 30101. 2022.

24. Ahmad N. *Why building black wealth is key to health equity.* Robert Wood Johnson. Published September 9, 2021. https://www.rwjf.org/en/blog/2021/09/why-building-black-wealth-is-key-to-health-equity.html

25. Rosalsky G. *Why the racial wealth gap is so hard to close.* NPR. Published June 14, 2022. https://www.npr.org/sections/money/2022/06/14/1104660659/why-the-racial-wealth-gap-is-so-hard-to-close

13

THE PRACTICE
OF PUBLIC HEALTH

LEARNING OBJECTIVES

- Summarize the three core functions of public health.
- Compare and contrast active versus passive surveillance.
- Discuss the structure, goals, and functions of global and U.S. public health systems.
- Identify the key components of policy development.
- Differentiate efficacy and effectiveness, and explain the importance of each in translating research into practice.

OVERVIEW: THE SCOPE OF PUBLIC HEALTH PRACTICE

Public health practice involves all that is done to improve health, including activities, programs, infrastructure, interventions, services, and processes that prevent disease and promote health for all people, everywhere. Public health practice involves the delivery of public health services at the global, national, state, and local levels—everything done to prevent disease and promote health. Government agencies, nongovernmental organizations (NGOs), nonprofit organizations, private organizations, academic institutions, community-based organizations, policy advocates, and individuals all engage in public health practice.

> Public health practice involves all that is done to improve health, including activities, programs, infrastructure, interventions, services, and processes that prevent disease and promote health for all people, everywhere.

Public health practitioners work with individuals to promote healthy behaviors such as quitting smoking and eating healthier foods. They work in community agencies to implement screening, injury prevention, and teen pregnancy prevention programs. They work in governmental organizations to educate communities, to increase and enforce motor vehicle safety regulations, to respond to natural disasters, and to ensure that restaurants are inspected and drinking water is safe. Public health practice affects all of our lives, from birth to death. Before we describe the three essential functions of public health practice—assessment, policy development, and assurance—and how they work together to promote health, we first outline the structure of the public health systems in the United States and abroad, recognizing that some of these systems are very loosely defined.

In this chapter, we (a) discuss the structure of public health today, from global to local levels, (b) differentiate the role of public health practitioners at each of these levels, (c) explore the challenges faced by the practice of public health, and (d) describe the careers possible within public health and how the learnings from this book can inform those careers.

PUBLIC HEALTH SYSTEMS

GLOBAL TO LOCAL PUBLIC HEALTH

Global and U.S. public health systems include public and private organizations, state and local health agencies and departments, law enforcement agencies, emergency medical services, hospitals, drug treatment centers, churches, community coalitions, schools, and many other organizations. There are several public health organizations that operate on a global level, including the World Health Organization (WHO) and the World Bank. The WHO is engaged in data collection and monitoring of health indicators across the globe and also in setting global health policies and procedures. The World Bank funds public health projects including workforce training, healthcare delivery, public health systems, infrastructure projects, and public health interventions.

In the United States, the public health infrastructure operates at the federal, state, and local levels. The U.S. Department of Health and Human Services (HHS) is the lead federal agency charged with enhancing and protecting the health of all Americans.[1] HHS is headed by the Secretary of Health and Human Services, a member of the president's cabinet. The HHS ensures that all levels of government have the capacity to provide public health services. HHS supports state and local agencies through trainings and grants, acts in a coordination capacity when health issues span more than one state, provides additional public health response capacity when states are unable to fully handle the demands posed by emergencies or disasters, and establishes public health goals in concert with state and local stakeholders.[2]

> **In the United States, the public health infrastructure operates at the federal, state, and local levels.**

Within the overarching and expansive structure of HHS, there are several agencies whose functions are generally known to the public. The Centers for Disease Control and Prevention (CDC) is the primary organization charged with protecting and promoting the people's health in the United States. The National Institutes of Health (NIH) includes 17 distinct institutes that provide research funding for a range of medical, public health, and population health issues. The Food and Drug Administration (FDA) is responsible for ensuring food safety and monitoring the safety and efficacy of drugs, medical devices, and vaccines. The Indian Health Service oversees healthcare and public health programs for federally recognized tribes of American Indian/Alaska Native (AI/AN) peoples throughout the United States.

State health departments offer a broad spectrum of services. A brief sampling includes asthma prevention and control, addiction services, family nutrition programs, and suicide and youth violence prevention programs. In concert with the CDC, state health departments collect data on health indicators for monitoring and evaluation purposes (e.g., Behavioral Risk Factor

Surveillance System, Youth Risk Behavior Surveillance System) and identify disadvantaged populations that might need intervention.

Local health departments (LHDs) vary in terms of their structure and independence. Some LHDs are subunits of their state health department, while others are run by local governments. LHDs offer services such as child and adult immunizations. LHDs detect and investigate local infectious disease outbreaks. LHDs routinely conduct sanitation inspections of local restaurants and monitor the health and safety of local daycare and preschool programs.[3] AI/AN public health is overseen by tribal health departments under the jurisdiction of the Indian Health Service.

Regardless of their specific structures, the goals of public health systems around the world are comparable. Many countries have ministries of health that organize and oversee efforts to promote health, prevent disease, and offer resources and services to support the health of their citizens. Some ministries of health operate at a national level while others have subsidiary units that offer services regionally. Departments of public health and ministries of health offer services to promote the health of their populations and collect and organize data to monitor health conditions and trends. In some countries, public health systems directly deliver healthcare to the public as part of a national health service.

Many NGOs are also active in public health practice (**Figure 13.1**). NGOs frequently partner with governmental agencies to promote health. It is important to recognize, however, that regardless of the commitment of NGOs to public health, it is the governmental agencies that have the mandate, authority, and legal responsibility to protect the health of the public. In the United States, LHDs provide some clinic services but are just one element of a much more complex and diverse healthcare delivery system. The operations of almost all public health systems worldwide, regardless of jurisdictional level, incorporate the same three core functions of public health practice, which we now discuss.

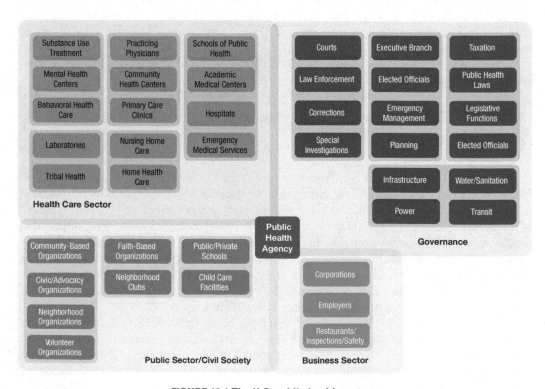

FIGURE 13.1 The U.S. public health system.

THREE CORE FUNCTIONS OF PUBLIC HEALTH PRACTICE

The three core functions of public health are assessment, policy development, and assurance (**Table 13.1**).[4] Assessment involves collecting and analyzing data from populations that address health outcomes of interest and identifying emerging health issues that need attention or improvement. Policy development involves the development and implementation of policies, plans, and laws that address the health problems that have been identified for the

TABLE 13.1 Continuous Cycle of Public Health Core Functions and Essential Services

3 CORE FUNCTIONS		10 ESSENTIAL PUBLIC HEALTH SERVICES		EXAMPLES OF PUBLIC HEALTH PRACTIONERS PROVIDING THESE SERVICES
1	Assessment	1	Assess and monitor population health status, factors that influence health, and community needs and assets	Disease surveillance specialist; Infectious disease epidemiologist; Biostatistician
		2	Investigate, diagnose, and address health problems and hazards affecting the population	Disease outbreak epidemiologist; Environmental health specialist/ investigator
2	Policy development	3	Communicate effectively to inform and educate people about health, factors that influence it, and how to improve it	Health communications specialist; Public information officer; Health educator
		4	Strengthen, support, and mobilize communities and partnerships to improve health	Community organizer; Community health educator
		5	Create, champion, and implement policies, plans, and laws that impact health	Health policy analyst; Government relations specialist
		6	Utilize legal and regulatory actions designed to improve and protect the public's health	Legislative aide; Health policy analyst; Public health inspector
3	Assurance	7	Assure an effective system that enables equitable access to the individual services and care needed to be healthy	Diversity, equity, inclusion specialist; Community health worker; Health system specialist; Healthcare administrator
		8	Build and support a diverse and skilled public health workforce	Public health trainer/educator; Diversity, equity, inclusion specialist
		9	Improve and innovate public health functions through ongoing evaluation, research, and continuous quality improvement	Quality improvement specialist; Program evaluator
		10	Build and maintain a strong organizational infrastructure for public health	Organizational behavior specialist; Information technology officer; Program evaluator

Source: Adapted from Centers for Disease Control and Prevention. Public health system and the 10 essential public health services. https://www.cdc.gov/publichealthgateway/publichealthservices/essentialhealthservices.html

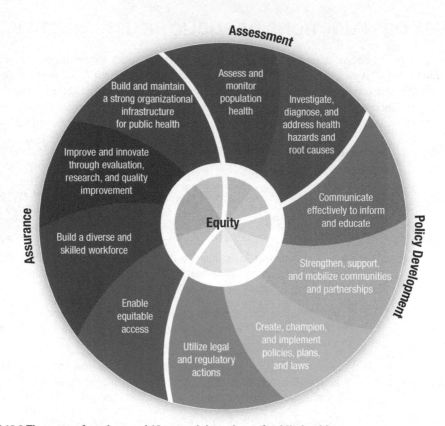

FIGURE 13.2 Three core functions and 10 essential services of public health.
Source: From Centers for Disease Control and Prevention. Public health system and the 10 essential public health services. 2020. https://www.cdc.gov/publichealthgateway/publichealthservices/essentialhealthservices.html

population of the jurisdiction served. Assurance involves equitable access to resources and programs; evaluation of how well interventions, programs, and policies are working to promote health; and creation and maintenance of a strong infrastructure for public health.

> **The three core functions of public health are assessment, policy development, and assurance.**

These three functions do not represent discrete steps that are performed in sequence, but rather they work together continuously to create a cycle that is ongoing (**Figure 13.2**). For example, monitoring activities might reveal a public health issue that needs addressing. A program might then be launched to address this issue. While the program is in progress, and as part of ongoing program evaluation, data may reveal a barrier to accessing program services that urgently needs to be redressed. Once the program is adjusted to overcome the identified access barrier, ongoing monitoring evaluates whether the problem has been resolved. This is an iterative process, a cycle. Appropriately, Figure 13.2 depicts the three core functions and the corresponding 10 essential services of public health in a manner that clearly highlights the cyclical nature of this process.

ASSESSMENT

Public health assessment, the first of the three core functions, involves the systematic collection and analysis of data to assess and monitor the health of populations. Assessment data are useful to identify infectious disease outbreaks such as influenza or Ebola, to monitor trends in chronic conditions and noncommunicable diseases (NCDs), such as diabetes and to evaluate public health impacts of natural disasters such as hurricanes or wildfires. The most useful assessments offer insights into the magnitude of health problems, who they affect most, why, and how. These data can be used to understand the natural history of health conditions and how these conditions change over time.

Assessment is critical for detecting and monitoring disease outbreaks and epidemic patterns. Surveillance data, which we describe in detail in what follows, are data that are captured over time that allow us to rapidly identify unexpected and potentially epidemic increases in disease occurrence above the baseline (endemic) level. Increases that exceed the expected levels need attention. With these data in hand, we can then investigate causes of health and take actions to address them.

> **Assessment is critical for detecting and monitoring disease outbreaks and epidemic patterns.**

Passive and Active Surveillance of Health Conditions

Surveillance is the ongoing systematic collection and analysis of health data to assess the extent of health problems or disease in populations. Surveillance data are used to design, monitor, and evaluate effectiveness of interventions, programs, and policies that are implemented to address health problems in populations. Surveillance data are generally organized by person (age, sex, race/ethnicity of participants), place (geographic region), and time (week, month, year).

Public health surveillance data are not limited to disease outbreaks. They may include vital statistics such as birth and death certificates. Birth and death records are required by law in many places and thus are very complete. Death records are extremely useful for defining leading causes of mortality. For example, in 1900, the top five causes of death in the United States were pneumonia and influenza, tuberculosis, gastrointestinal infections, heart disease, and cerebrovascular disease. This contrasts sharply with present day patterns where, in 2021, heart disease, cancer, COVID-19, unintentional injuries, and cerebrovascular disease (stroke) topped the list.[5] It is important for us to examine causes of death because these data help us to understand health of populations and determine public health actions and interventions that might ultimately prevent disease and death. Some countries have less sophisticated and comprehensive vital statistics data systems, thus requiring that these countries apply estimation techniques to develop data that are comparable to other nations.[6]

In addition to birth and death certificates, other aspects of health are regularly monitored using different types of surveillance. Passive surveillance is often dictated by laws that include requirements for practitioners to report certain health conditions as they arise. Specifically, passive surveillance involves reporting of diseases as they are diagnosed by healthcare providers or by laboratories based on specific diagnostic tests. Reports are sent from EDs, clinics, hospitals, or laboratories to local, state, or national health departments, or to ministries of health. These data are compiled and analyzed to determine whether there is an impending disease outbreak or another public health problem requiring timely attention and response.

In the state of Massachusetts, for example, healthcare professionals, hospitals, and laboratories are required by law to report certain communicable and infectious diseases within 24 hours to their local boards of health; these local boards immediately forward this information to the Massachusetts Department of Public Health.[7] Among the mandatorily reportable diseases are suspected and confirmed cases of measles, mumps, rabies, tuberculosis, chickenpox, influenza, Lyme disease, Zika, and multiple forms of sexually transmitted infections, including chlamydia infection, gonorrhea, and HIV infection.

A Weekly Influenza Surveillance Report Prepared by the Influenza Division

Outpatient Respiratory Illness Activity Map Determined by Data Reported to ILINet

This system monitors visits for respiratory illness that includes fever plus a cough or sore throat, also referred to as ILI, not laboratory confirmed influenza, and may capture patient visits due to other respiratory pathogens that cause similar symptoms.

2022–23 Influenza Season Week 51 ending Dec 24, 2022

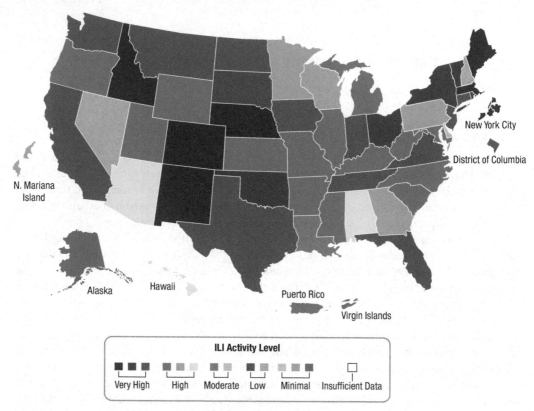

FIGURE 13.3 Influenza activity in the United States, week ending December 24, 2022.
Note: This map indicates geographic spread and does not measure the severity of influenza activity.
Source: From Centers for Disease Control and Prevention. Weekly US map: influenza summary update. 2022. https://www.cdc.gov/flu/weekly/usmap.htm

At the national level in the United States, the CDC has a Surveillance Resource Center that offers toolkits and guidance on best practices for surveillance; information on regulatory, legal, ethical, and policy issues related to surveillance; and perhaps most importantly, open access to interactive databases with real-time data across a range of health topics.[8] Data are available on birth defects, indicators of child and adolescent health, chronic and infectious diseases, occupational safety, and vaccinations. Users can query these databases for specific statistics or monitor disease occurrence by state. For example, **Figure 13.3** shows the extent of influenza activity by state for the week ending December 24, 2022; showing very high activity in states spread throughout the entire nation.

Globally, the WHO also offers guidance on standards for surveillance. The WHO gathers and organizes data from around the globe on selected diseases including diphtheria, hepatitis B, mumps, pertussis, tetanus, and yellow fever.[9]

Users may query the WHO databases for statistics on any country or region, which include the number of cases of each disease reported or estimated per year as well as data on percentages of the population vaccinated with specific antigens per year. For example, **Figure 13.4** shows immunization coverage around the world for HepB3 in infants in 2019.

Active surveillance works differently from, but can complement, passive surveillance. Active surveillance is underway when the public health agency is directly and actively engaged in collecting data about a certain threat to health. For example, if a case of chickenpox is reported to a local board of health, an active surveillance protocol may be initiated to reach out to hospitals and healthcare providers in the area to inquire about other potential cases. Active surveillance also refers to regularly scheduled data collection in the form of interviews, surveys, and reviews of medical records used to gather systematic data on a variety of health conditions. Active surveillance is more purposeful than passive surveillance and generally results in more complete and accurate reporting of the extent of disease in populations. The CDC, for example, conducts regular surveys of U.S. adults and children to gather extensive data through surveys and physical examinations on multiple measures of health.[10]

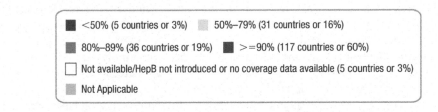

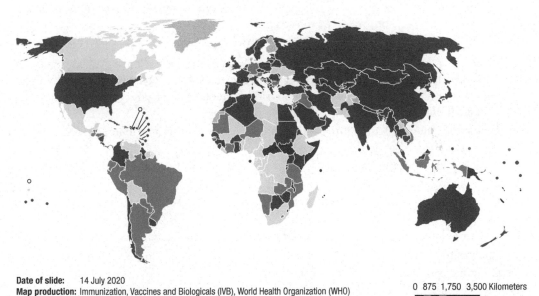

Date of slide: 14 July 2020
Map production: Immunization, Vaccines and Biologicals (IVB), World Health Organization (WHO)
Data source: WHO/UNICEF coverage estimates 2019 revision, July 2020.
194 WHO Member States.

0 875 1,750 3,500 Kilometers

FIGURE 13.4 Immunization coverage with HepB3 in infants, 2019.
Source: https://cdn.who.int/media/docs/default-source/immunization/global_monitoring/slidesglobalimmunization.pdf

By way of example, suppose you eat at a fast-food restaurant (we will not name the restaurant!) and 12 hours later you have extreme stomach cramps and begin sweating and vomiting. Your first thought may not be to call the local board of health to report your condition. However, it is extremely important that the report is made. This report is an example of passive surveillance. Once the report is made, your local public health professionals may begin to investigate—active surveillance kicks in. They gather data from you on your recent whereabouts and where you might have eaten to identify the potential cause. They develop a case definition, based on your symptoms, so that they can then search for other similar cases in the immediate vicinity and surrounding areas. If other cases are identified, interviews are conducted with those individuals to find commonalities that could reveal the potential culprit. Testing is done to determine the site and source of the contamination, and once identified, the source can be controlled.

These steps for monitoring health to identify health problems may sound straightforward—one step leads to another and soon enough the problem is solved. In the next section, we discuss in more depth how investigations are conducted and just how challenging it can be to investigate causes of health.

Investigation of Causes of Health Issues

Potential causes of health issues must be investigated across multiple sectors by public health professionals, community organizations, and industry partners all working together. In the case of an outbreak, the source must be identified as quickly as possible so that it can be contained and eliminated. This often requires the engagement and collaboration of people and organizations across multiple sectors. Ongoing or emerging health issues require prevention strategies to mitigate future health problems. For these strategies to be effective, they must be targeted at the right conditions or circumstances that produce health, which occur at multiple levels and across sectors. And importantly, alongside any investigative process is a well-designed communication strategy to address concerns of the public and other key stakeholders.

Tracking down an outbreak may require both epidemiologic analyses of individuals who meet the case definition in terms of signs and symptoms, and environmental investigations involving gathering and testing of food, water, or soil samples.

The following is a typical sequence of steps involved in a disease outbreak investigation:

- Identify the appropriate investigators who have the requisite experience to tackle the problem and other available human resources such as professionals in local, state, and national agencies or ministries of health and professionals in other non-health-related industries or organizations.
- Define the issue. (Is it an outbreak and how do we know? Or is it an emerging or persistent issue?)
- Validate the report of the health issue with laboratory tests or medical procedures as necessary.
- Create a case definition to ensure that any further surveillance efforts capture the same health condition.
- Gather data using appropriate surveillance and monitoring techniques.
- Analyze the data.
- Generate hypotheses about potential causes.
- Collect more data to test these hypotheses about potential causes.
- Define appropriate control measures or prevention strategies.
- Implement control measures and prevention strategies.
- Communicate results.
- Continue to monitor to ensure that the issue has been contained or that prevention strategies are effective.

Each phase of the investigation has its challenges. Consider an example that illustrates the importance of communication in the investigative process and the challenging issues that arise that may affect different constituencies. Suppose that three different people independently seek medical attention at three different EDs within a 100-mile radius for severe stomach cramps and diarrhea. Each person is interviewed and reports eating local shellfish within the past 24 hours. Each case is reported to the local board of health, which initiates an investigation.

While the investigation is taking place, and these are always done as expeditiously as possible but do take time, should the public be notified? And if so, how should the public be notified? Is it the most responsible course of action to push out an alert that local shellfish might be contaminated? Suppose that the region where the reports are made is a low-income area but a popular summer vacation destination, and most residents' livelihoods depend on shell fishing or the restaurant business. What are the implications of communicating too early or too late? The human, practical, and political repercussions are complicated!

POLICY DEVELOPMENT

Policy development is the second of the three core functions (Table 13.1 and Figure 13.2). Health policies, plans, and laws are designed to promote health or to support health goals in populations. In 2013, the American Public Health Association, in collaboration with the Public Health Institute and the California Department of Public Health, released "Health in All Policies: A Guide for State and Local Governments," which offered guidance for collaboration on policies and activities across sectors to address social, economic, and environmental determinants of health (across the life course from a social ecological perspective).[11]

> **Health policies are designed to promote health or to support health goals in populations.**

Policy development, as a core function of public health, includes communicating, informing, educating, and empowering people with the resources they need to understand health issues and to address factors that affect health. Policy development also involves engaging and supporting formal and informal community organizations and partnerships to address health problems. And most literally, policy development entails developing policies that promote health.

Informing, educating, and empowering people around health issues requires that relevant information and resources are available, accessible, and understandable. Engaging community organizations to address health issues requires collaboration among organizations that are health related and those that are not (i.e., collaboration across different sectors). Faith-based organizations, schools, recreational facilities, social clubs, corporations, law enforcement agencies, and special interest groups can affect positive changes that promote health for individuals, neighborhoods, cities, states, and political and social structures. By working together, recommendations for programs and policies to address salient local needs and issues can be developed in a manner that garners community support and is sustainable over time.

For example, suppose a community determines a need to address childhood obesity. Local data show an upward trend in numbers of children who meet the criteria for obesity, and emerging research findings link childhood obesity to future health problems. A simple solution might address individual behavior changes such as encouraging youth to engage in more physical activity and supporting families to prioritize healthier diets for their children. But are these realistic, effective, and sustainable solutions? Likely not.

A better approach is to consider root causes, maybe even causes not previously thought to be directly related to childhood obesity or other health issues. These require addressing policies related to housing, access to green space, availability of healthy versus processed foods in homes and at school, nutrition assistance programs, and policies on mass production of low-cost, calorie-dense foods, just to name but a few. Given the range and complexity of possible causes, how do public health professionals determine the best course of action when there appear to be so many different potential pathways? Evidence-based decisions and ongoing evaluation are the key. Policies must be developed based on data and continuously evaluated to ensure that they not only prevent disease but also promote health over time.

Applying Scientific Knowledge Generated by Public Health Science

Public health and population health scientists design and conduct analyses to identify determinants of health. Once these determinants are identified, tested, and supported by data, this knowledge can then be used to develop interventions, programs, and policies. Because most causes of health operate on multiple social ecological levels and across the life course, these interventions, programs, and policies must address the complex interplay of individual behaviors, social networks, community norms, and political and environmental factors.

The translation of research into practice in public health is challenging. Brownson et al.[12] suggest a framework for translating research into public health action that includes four phases:

1. Discovery: finding the determinants or causes of disease
2. Translation: converting research findings into actionable, scalable plans
3. Dissemination: communicating research and action steps in culturally sensitive ways
4. Change: adopting new programs and policies

The successful implementation of this or any other comparable framework requires engagement, support, ongoing training, and collaboration.

Research studies determine the efficacy of interventions and programs, while the translation of research findings into practice determines effectiveness of interventions and programs (see **Box 13.1**). Efficacy refers to how well interventions and programs work under ideal or controlled conditions, and effectiveness refers to how well interventions and programs

---

BOX 13.1 TRANSLATING SCIENCE, EFFICACY, AND EFFECTIVENESS

Research studies of efficacy examine the effect of a new intervention or program under ideal and highly controlled conditions, whereas effectiveness studies examine the effect of a new intervention or program accounting for participant-, provider-, and system-level factors that are generally more important for practitioners and policy makers.[13]

EFFICACY STUDIES

Question: Does the intervention or program work under ideal or controlled conditions?
Intervention/program: standardized, strictly monitored, no other concurrent interventions
Participants: highly selected (as per eligibility criteria) and homogeneous
Providers/practitioners: highly trained (as per study protocol)

EFFECTIVENESS STUDIES

Question: Does the intervention or program work in real-world settings?
Intervention/program: applied as per standard practice, other concurrent interventions
Participants: unselected and heterogeneous
Providers/practitioners: representative of all providers/practitioners (variable experience and training)

work in more typical, realistic settings. In experimental research studies (e.g., randomized controlled trials), participants are often highly selected and managed throughout the trial as the new intervention is evaluated for efficacy. When research results are translated into practice, we are concerned with how well the new intervention works when applied more broadly (effectiveness).

Consider an example evaluating a new drug to treat hypertension (high blood pressure). The WHO indicates that one in three adults worldwide has hypertension, which contributes to nearly 9 million deaths worldwide, and accounts for half of all deaths due to cardiovascular disease and stroke.[14] A randomized controlled trial is designed to evaluate a new lower cost medication for hypertension. Suppose the trial is designed to include participants with high blood pressure who also have regular primary care physicians and insurance coverage provided by their employers. They also have cell phones and stable housing. These eligibility criteria might be put into place to ensure that researchers can follow the participants in the trial to gather data necessary to fully evaluate the drug.

The trial is run and finds that the new lower cost medication significantly reduces blood pressure in participants, and the results are judged to be valid. What impact might this drug have on the millions of people affected by hypertension if made available to all people with hypertension? The drug was shown to be efficacious in the randomized controlled trial, but is it effective in practice? Would participants who lack stable housing or who do not have insurance experience the same results?

Ensuring access to beneficial treatments is an important part of addressing a problem like hypertension. A more effective approach, however, involves thinking about how we might prevent people from developing hypertension in the first place. Research also tells us that hypertension disproportionately affects African American/Black populations in the United States. Hypertension also affects those who are obese and less physically active. A comprehensive approach to addressing hypertension must address the underlying factors. Translating research results into policy and public health practice means working with communities to develop, evaluate, and implement community changes that prevent and control diseases. Strategies to promote health are most effective when community members are active and engaged in addressing the root causes of disease, and these causes vary by community and depend heavily on local culture. Thus, public health professionals must collaborate with community members to appropriately translate research findings into locally relevant practices that promote health and prevent disease.

Explicating the Role of Public Health in Informing and Developing Evidence-Based Policy

The American Public Health Association states that "Society must create and maintain the conditions under which members of the community can be healthy. The responsibility for maintaining and improving the public's health lies with all sectors of society."[15] This policy statement captures well the essence of the shared collective responsibility to generate health in populations.

Even though it takes all sectors to make a difference, it is the responsibility and authority of public health to ensure the health of the public. The role of public health is to provide leadership in developing policies that affect population health. The responsibility and authority for developing and implementing these policies lies with public health agencies. These agencies are responsible for assessing and ensuring individual, community, and environmental health, which includes access to affordable and safe housing, sanitation, access to affordable healthy foods, and access to safe water and clean air. Public health agencies cultivate partnerships with other organizations that provide services and ensure that policies are in place to address those most at risk and vulnerable in communities. Public health agencies educate and inform the public, special interest groups, and policy makers based on evidence or data that they collect. They explain the implications of these data and put forth their recommendations for programs, policies, and interventions that promote positive change. Last, public health agencies provide technical assistance to communities, as needed, to ensure that public health services, programs, interventions, and policies are successful.

In 2017, the HHS published "Public Health 3.0. A Call to Action to Create a 21st Century Public Health Infrastructure."[16] The report calls for a new framework for public health practice to build on prior successes but also to engage in new and different approaches to tackle a broader range of determinants of health across the life course and social ecological system. The report makes five recommendations:

1. Public health practitioners should take a lead role in defining strategies to address social determinants of health.
2. Public health agencies should collaborate with a wider range of community stakeholders.
3. Accreditation criteria for public health agencies should be modified to ensure that public health professionals are trained to address social determinants of health.
4. Locally relevant and timely data should be collected, analyzed, and shared with communities to monitor and evaluate public health practices.
5. More funding should be secured to support these new initiatives.

ASSURANCE, MONITORING, AND EVALUATION

Assurance is the third core function of public health (Figures 13.2 and 13.3). Once interventions, programs, and policies are implemented, it is important to ensure that they are working as intended. This requires ongoing monitoring and evaluation or regular gathering of data and other information to address whether interventions, programs, and policies are working well, and are accessible to all. The follow-up questions of interest are: If programs are working well, why are they working well? If not, why not?

Assurance as a core function of public health includes supporting and enforcing regulations and laws that promote health and safety, making services and programs available to all who need them, delivering services and programs through a competent trained workforce, and evaluating implementation and achievement of services and programs. The regulations and laws that require enforcement include those related to food safety, air quality, sanitation, and wastewater; timely investigation of hazardous and occupational exposures; and transparent reviews of new drugs and devices.

Enforcement of these regulations in the United States falls to different agencies. For example, enforcement of clean air legislation is overseen by the Environmental Protection Agency (EPA). Assurance of food safety is overseen by the FDA, which contracts with state and local public health agencies to conduct inspections. The primary objectives in the enforcement of such regulations and laws are to prevent disease and promote health.

Monitoring and evaluation are processes that involve the collection and analysis of data about an intervention, program, or policy to assess its impact. Well-designed monitoring and evaluation plans offer insights into barriers, ensure equitable access and accountability, and provide evidence to demonstrate the effectiveness or impact of interventions, programs, or policies.

In order to evaluate impact, the goal (what success looks like) of the intervention, program, or policy must be articulated. Once the goal is identified, the activities that will be implemented to achieve that goal are defined in detail. Monitoring and evaluation plans take a specific form, often starting with inputs, which are human, financial, and organizational resources that are available and deployed in specific activities. These result in outputs, or immediate results of activities, that map to objectives or desired outcomes that demonstrate success or impact as defined in the goal. Some monitoring and evaluation plans also include timelines and budgets, which are extremely important from a funder's point of view. Supporting documents would accompany this plan with additional details on specific data elements to be collected and by whom, details on how data will be disseminated, a detailed budget, and a timeline.

In brief summary, components of an evaluation plan include the following:

Goal: what success looks like in measurable terms along a timeline
Inputs: resources needed to implement activities (human, financial, material)
Activities: efforts required to produce outputs along with measurable indicators
Outputs: products or actions needed to produce outcomes
Outcomes: longer term, population-level results

Outputs are more immediate results from activities such as numbers of individuals trained and numbers of services provided. In contrast, outcomes are longer term, population-level results related to changes in knowledge, behavior, and attitudes that indicate whether the program goal is being achieved.

Monitoring and evaluation are most effective when plans are defined with input and engagement from a wide range of stakeholders. Stakeholders include people who will directly benefit from specific interventions, programs, and policies, as well as those who will deliver interventions, programs, and policies, along with community partners, funders, and special interest groups. Empowering and engaging a wide range of stakeholders creates a process that is more likely to lead to successful and impactful interventions, programs, and policies. This is ideal because community partners not only have the information that they need to monitor and improve programs that are important to them, but there is also transparency and accountability toward a shared goal.

Making Services Available

An important part of the evaluation process is ensuring equitable access to interventions, programs, and services that promote health. Optimally, accessible services can be used by all people, and everyone has the same benefit of use regardless of their ability or social standing. Services that prevent disease and promote health must be implemented fairly. All communications about eligibility and access to services must be culturally and linguistically appropriate. There must be assistance for those who need it to ensure that they connect and can take full advantage of interventions, programs, and services. Ensuring fair implementation of any program that effectively prevents disease and promotes health requires partnership and collaboration with multiple agencies and constituencies, as outlined in the next example.

An important part of the evaluation process is ensuring availability and accessibility of interventions, programs, and services that promote health.

The U.S. Department of Agriculture's Food and Nutrition Service offers a Supplemental Nutrition Assistance Program (SNAP) to eligible low-income families across the United States. Eligibility is based on income, accounting for the number of people in the household and their access to other resources. To secure access to SNAP benefits, applicants must apply to their local SNAP office in the state where they reside. The SNAP website has resources to direct applicants to the office nearest them. If the applicant is found to be eligible, SNAP benefits are loaded onto an electronic card, which functions like a debit card. On a monthly basis, the card can be used to purchase groceries at authorized food stores, which can be found using an online locator tool. The SNAP program is extremely valuable for many people, and there are many helpful online tools that offer assistance to those accessing and using the benefit. To use these tools effectively, however, requires awareness of the SNAP program, access to the Internet, and some skill in navigating internet resources. A key component of making public health services available is effective communication and support for engaging end users in a manner that recognizes their abilities and is cognizant of their resources or lack thereof.

Delivering Services to the Public

Delivering services and programs that prevent disease and promote health requires active partnerships between public health agencies with authority and responsibility for the public's health and partners who are competent and trained to deliver programs and services as intended. This is where schools and programs of public health can help to train the next generation of public health professionals with formal training in public health but can also educate professionals in other sectors about the core functions and essential services of public health.

Public health professionals, advocates, and allies can also work to secure continued and expanded funding to support the needed services that prevent disease and promote health, particularly for those who are vulnerable. These efforts, taken together, create a much needed infrastructure to develop, deliver, and sustain programs and services that promote health. Once programs and services are in place, they must continue to be evaluated for effectiveness, accessibility, and quality. Evaluation data should be public and transparent so that programs and services can continue to be enhanced and improved with new ideas and innovation.

We illustrate the operation of the key functions and essential services of public health by examining an innovative approach to safeguarding patients with special medical needs during hurricanes (Case Study 13.1; you can access the podcast accompanying Case Study 13.1 by following this link to Springer Publishing Company Connect™: http://connect.springerpub.com/content/book/978-0-8261-8043-8/part/part04/chapter/ch13).

CASE STUDY 13.1: PUBLIC HEALTH PRACTICE DURING FLORIDA HURRICANE SEASON

Sometimes public health practice is nothing short of lifesaving. Those who are called to serve the public's health both include and extend beyond the public health workforce, but all can be considered in a broad sense to be contributing to public health practice. We examine the State of Florida's special needs hurricane shelter program for electronically dependent individuals as an applied example of the operation of the three core functions and 10 essential services of public health practice.

In times of disaster, the care of populations with special needs requires a tailored response targeted to the nature of the disaster and the needs of the special population.[17,18] The State of Florida has created a sophisticated system for support of a special population of persons on long-term oxygen therapy (LTOT) whose survival is challenged during extended electrical power outages in the aftermath of hurricanes. Florida's statewide system of special needs shelters is structured to care for this unique subgroup of technology-dependent persons. The evolution of this system invoked all three core functions of public health: assessment, policy development, and assurance.

According to Rear Admiral Brian W. Flynn, U.S. federal advisor for disaster behavioral health for more than 20 years, "Special populations are groups of people whose needs may require additional, customized, or specialized approaches in preparedness for, response to, and recovery from extreme events." Persons on LTOT clearly qualify under this definition.

By focusing primarily on persons receiving LTOT and other noninstitutionalized persons with special technology needs who are able to live independently, Florida has created the special needs shelter program. When a hurricane approaches the Florida peninsula and the trajectory is well defined, shelters are activated for the cluster of counties that are in the projected path.

(continued)

The special needs shelter program acts to safeguard persons with special needs from a hurricane's physical forces of harm by providing fortified shelters—with auxiliary electrical power—positioned inland from the coasts. Special shelters sustain persons on LTOT with healthcare and basic needs including food, water, bedding, sanitary facilities, and most importantly, life-sustaining electrical power. Public health nurses and allied staff comfort clients by providing highly competent bedside care and attentive psychosocial support. Shelter accommodation is also provided for one caregiver per special needs client so that clients can connect with their usual sources of support. Personnel in the shelters advise those seeking refuge regarding shelter operations, the status of the storm, and the postimpact transition back to home and community life. Finally, staff encourage the special needs clients and their caregivers to participate in the informal community of shelter residents and care providers.

TECHNOLOGY-DEPENDENT PERSONS WHO ARE ELECTRICALLY DEPENDENT

Oxygen-dependent persons are a subset of special populations of technology-dependent persons that have evolved and continue to expand based on life-extending advances in medical science. Prior to the advent of medical devices capable of increasing survival, these individuals succumbed to their chronic medical conditions at a much earlier stage in the clinical course. Now they are able to survive for additional years of life, with progressively more advanced disease, as long as there is uninterrupted access to life-sustaining technology. However, the reliance of these technologies on electrical power is a vulnerability. LTOT patients are vulnerable to power failures that, if prolonged, may be fatal. Therefore, technology-dependent persons—special populations that have only recently come into existence because of the creation of life-sustaining technologies—have quickly ascended to high-priority status for disaster planning and preparedness, especially in areas at high risk for hurricanes. Clearly, hurricane-caused power outages are life-threatening events for a sizable population of electrically dependent persons. The State of Florida now has a roster of 35,000 registered special needs clients who are eligible for special shelter services statewide.

HUMAN–MACHINE DYADS

The majority of persons receiving LTOT have been diagnosed with chronic obstructive pulmonary disease (COPD). Historically, COPD was a rare disease, but the incidence and prevalence of COPD increased sharply throughout the 1900s because of the mass adoption of the cigarette smoking habit that was popularized early in that century. Cigarette smoking is the predominant risk factor for COPD; about 90% of COPD cases are smoking-attributable. COPD cannot be cured or reversed, but its progression can be slowed by treatments and lifestyle changes.

The prominence of COPD as a leading cause of death in the United States has spurred the development of technologies to extend the life span for those affected. To date, the major breakthrough has been the introduction of the oxygen "concentrator." This device selectively removes nitrogen from ambient air (which consists of 78% nitrogen and 21% oxygen), thereby "concentrating" the oxygen fraction. Some machines can produce air with oxygen concentrations of 95% or higher. In common parlance, patients receiving LTOT commonly refer to their concentrators as "nebulizers."

(*continued*)

Persons on LTOT are tethered to an apparatus. Mobility is restricted because these individuals spend many hours each day connected to their oxygen concentrator. As the disease progresses, so does the dependence on the equipment. The daily routine involves most hours connected by a 10-foot "lifeline" of plastic nasal tubing to a mechanical device, approximately the size of a canister vacuum cleaner, which has a 20-foot-long retractable electrical power cord that is plugged into an electrical outlet. Most units have backup battery support to sustain oxygen flow during short-term power outages that may occur. While survival is extended for COPD patients, sometimes for periods of years, the quality of life is certainly diminished for those who must live as a human–machine dyad.

Constant availability of dependable electrical current is a key to survival for persons on LTOT because electricity is required both to power the in-home concentrators in real time and to recharge the batteries for the portable units. No LTOT apparatus has been designed to maintain function during extended power outages that are characteristic of the post hurricane environment. Power may not be restored for periods of days to weeks in the most devastated or remotely isolated areas.

FLORIDA'S SPECIAL NEEDS SHELTER PROGRAM: CUSTOMIZED SUPPORT FOR PERSONS ON LONG-TERM OXYGEN THERAPY

The special needs shelter program integrates the expertise and person power of many professionals. Because persons on LTOT represent a population with a severe chronic disease, and many patients have multiple diagnoses, such as diabetes, public health professionals form the hub for shelter staffing. Administratively, shelter operations are coordinated by the county's Office of Emergency Management (OEM). Representatives of mass transit, police, fire rescue, emergency medical services (EMS), facility maintenance, and voluntary organizations active in disasters (VOAD) each play an active counterpart role. Public health nurses and allied professionals are central to the care provided, but taking an expanded view of public health practice, all partners are integrated into the effort of maintaining the health and survival of this special needs population.

SHELTER ACTIVATION AND CLIENT TRANSPORT

As the tropical system makes its approach toward land, a hurricane warning is issued by the National Hurricane Center for a stretch of Florida coastline and the decision is made to activate the shelters in counties within the "cone of probability" for a hurricane strike. Registered special needs clients are notified and a schedule for client pickup is created. County mass transit makes house calls to retrieve oxygen-dependent persons who elect to use the transportation option. Registered clients are encouraged to bring a designated caregiver with them. The caregiver, usually the client's spouse or adult child, is typically someone with knowledge of the person's medical treatment needs. Most caregivers also have had practice using and adjusting the client's particular brand of oxygen concentrator.

SPECIAL NEEDS SHELTER OPERATIONS: A COMPLEMENT OF PERSONNEL SERVING A SHELTERING COMMUNITY

The special needs shelter environment becomes a physically and socially isolated community during the hurricane. Planful approaches—guided by Florida's repetitive experience with storms—have helped to define the complement of personnel

(continued)

that needs to be on board when the storm strikes. County OEM administrators open the shelter. The shelter unit leader is a county emergency operations center professional who is accompanied by a small contingent of staff. They operate the shelter according to a well-defined incident management system. Each shelter has a designated public information officer to handle media inquiries and communications staff to maintain contact with the OEM and other key components of the countywide hurricane response.

In the first hours, facility management personnel and volunteers assemble and arrange the cots. Auxiliary power generators are inspected to verify that they are fully operational and fueled. Some shelter sites have an electrical plant specialist available for the duration of shelter activation.

Public health nurses from the county department of health are central to the operation. A respiratory therapist is on staff, bringing intimate knowledge of the workings of many models of oxygen concentrators. Backup concentrators have been stocked along with replacement parts, chemicals, and refills for the major brands of concentrators.

Many persons with COPD have multiple diagnoses. Registered clients are requested to bring their medications with them, but in the event of an extended shelter stay, or emerging medical conditions, a fully stocked pharmacy is provided on premises, with a registered pharmacist on duty.

Some shelter sites have a complete EMS team on board with medical equipment and an advanced life support vehicle inside the shelter. Large shelters also have a crew of firefighters who typically are also trained in emergency medical procedures. A contingent of county Sheriff's Office law enforcement personnel stay in the shelter. Depending on the facility, there may also be private security on the premises.

Three meals—breakfast, lunch, and dinner—are prepared daily by volunteer staff from the American Red Cross, Salvation Army, or other VOADs. Light snack foods are available throughout the day. Oxygen-dependent persons cannot queue up for food because of their physical connection to their oxygen concentrators. Any attempt to do so would result in a tangle of tubing, cords, and equipment. This necessitates the availability of a small corps of additional volunteers who deliver the prepared food to the bedside of each person and dispose of the trash.

SPECIAL NEEDS CLIENTS AND CAREGIVERS: THE SPECIAL NEEDS SHELTER EXPERIENCE

Caregivers are mobile and able to forage for specific care needs, snacks, or other necessities. They are effective client advocates. It is the caregivers who are convened (because of their physical mobility and mental clarity) when shelter staff provide updates and briefings about the status of the storm, shelter operations, postimpact damage assessments, neighborhoods that are deemed safe for return, and plans for shelter discharge and stand-down.

Regarding social support, clusters of clients on LTOT and their caregivers create small enclaves or communities over the course of the shelter stay. Caregivers share responsibilities for watching over the multiple clients in their immediate vicinity, retrieving snacks, getting updates, and seeking out staff for needs that arise. Groupings of clients and caregivers pass the time in conversation, playing cards, or in other forms of casual socialization. Many "buddyships" are forged that may extend over multiple shelter stays across multiple storms.

(continued)

The COVID-19 era required adjustments to the protocols and logistics. These included seeking alternative hotel accommodations where LTOT patients and caregivers could have separate rooms to avoid congregate shelter settings. In the special needs shelters that were activated, protocols were modified to increase spacing, increase ventilation, require masking, and limit movement of caregivers to the minimum necessary. Alcohol wipes, hand sanitizer, and disposable dinnerware were included in the revised guidance for shelter operations.

CONCLUDING COMMENTS

Public health practice must be adaptable to new situations. That is certainly illustrated here. The development of Florida's special needs shelter network is the result of a series of unlikely events, spanning more than a century. Let us connect the dots. The invention, promotion, and widespread addiction to cigarettes throughout the early 1900s led to a dramatic upsurge in the prevalence of smoking and smoking-related diseases. Among these diseases, smoking basically "created" COPD, now the third leading cause of death in the United States. People with COPD suffer greatly, and only a few decades ago they died very prematurely. Their end-of-life struggles with COPD motivated the invention of life-sustaining technologies, specifically the oxygen concentrator, which makes LTOT possible and prolongs life. However, there remains a threat to life; the oxygen concentrators depend on the continuous availability of electrical current. The backup battery life cannot outlast the weeks-long power disruptions in the aftermath of a strong hurricane.

So, Florida's special needs shelter network is the latest innovation in this novel sequence of events.

Public health and other professionals are called upon to staff special needs shelters to ensure the survival of a special subpopulation that, historically speaking, has just come into being. What do we mean? Smoking manufactured cigarettes dates back just over a century. COPD as a prominent cause of disability and death has been recognized only since the mid-1900s. The new LTOT technology that allows former cigarette smokers with advanced COPD to extend their lives goes back only a few decades.

Based on this still-evolving saga, the Florida Department of Health and their community disaster preparedness and response partners employed the three core functions of public health practice. They assessed the situation, developed policy, and constructed an elaborate yet workable system that successfully assures safety and survival for this special needs population.

CAREERS IN PUBLIC HEALTH

Public health professionals are the vanguard for performing the three core functions and the 10 essential services of public health. Public health professionals are involved in assessing community health; creating, implementing, and evaluating public health policies; conducting surveillance of health indicators; educating the community on health threats or prevention initiatives; and so much more. The following is a sample of the many roles played by public health professionals.

EPIDEMIOLOGIST

Public health epidemiologists study diseases in a population. This may involve understanding where and how disease outbreaks began, how diseases are transmitted among individuals, and whether there are effective treatments for disease. An epidemiologist may work in a variety of settings including universities, hospitals, and government organizations. Responsibilities of a public health epidemiologist may include designing studies to gather data, data collection and analysis, and interpretation and reporting of results for public health action. Epidemiologists work in lab settings, in the field, or in an office environment. Epidemiologists have strong quantitative skills and often have a background in biology or medicine. They constantly apply a critical analysis lens to their work as they evaluate scientific information and data they gather and analyze at the local level.

HEALTH EDUCATOR

Health educators work with clients regarding lifestyle changes to meet health goals, focusing on promoting good health and preventing disease. A public health educator assesses the health needs of those they serve, devises programs and materials for health education, obtains and evaluates data to evaluate the effectiveness of educational programs, and advocates for wellness and health promotion in the community. A health educator might work in a community setting, a school, a corporation, or a nonprofit organization. Health educators understand medical terminology and possess strong communication, interpersonal, instructional, and problem-solving skills and capabilities.

BIOSTATISTICIAN

Biostatisticians work to disentangle data received and make valid inferences that can be used to solve problems in public health. A biostatistician collects, analyzes, and summarizes data to evaluate the extent of disease penetration and impact in a particular population, the efficacy of a new drug or intervention, the association between potential risk factors and disease, or the effectiveness of public health campaigns. Biostatisticians work as data managers, data analysts, or statistical programmers in public health departments, academic settings, industry (e.g., pharmaceutical companies), and healthcare organizations. Biostatisticians have a strong mathematical background, interest and skills in data analysis, and good interpersonal skills. Biostatisticians are very attentive to detail.

ENVIRONMENTAL HEALTH SCIENTIST AND SPECIALISTS

Environmental health scientists and specialists investigate natural and manmade resources that impact our planet's health and explore associations between environmental exposures and health. Environmental health specialists collect and analyze samples from soil and water and they inform policies to promote a healthy environment. Environmental health specialists work with organizations and industries to reduce waste, minimize pollution, and conserve natural resources. An environmental health scientist may focus on toxic chemicals, waste management, exposure assessment, climate and health, or other specialized applications. Environmental health scientists often work for state governments, local governments, federal governments, and engineering services. Their work requires a knowledge in natural sciences, deductive and inductive reasoning, critical thinking, and strong communication skills.

HEALTH POLICY ANALYST

Health policy analysts evaluate current health policies to determine how they affect individual and community health, and healthcare quality. They also formulate policies that are patient-centered and improve access to healthcare for all. Health policy analysts gather and analyze data to understand policy impacts, they evaluate how resources are allocated and the associated health outcomes. Analysts typically work in healthcare delivery systems, nonprofit organizations, branches of state and federal government, and private sector consulting firms. Health policy analysts are focused on health equity, and they must communicate findings to diverse audiences. Health policy analysts must have strong communication skills, in addition to skills in data analysis and budgeting.

RESEARCH COORDINATOR

Research coordinators are essential for the success of any research endeavor. Working under the guidance of the principal investigator of the study, research coordinators manage and coordinate all aspects of the study. This often includes ensuring compliance with federal guidelines and institutional policies, training research personnel, overseeing study participant recruitment, ensuring compliance of HIPAA (Health Insurance Portability and Accountability Act) regulations, collecting and managing research data, and ensuring the ethical conduct of research. Research coordinators often work in academic settings, hospitals, laboratories, pharmaceutical companies, or public agency settings. This work requires attention to detail, administrative skills, strong communication skills, and knowledge of study rules and regulations to assure compliance.

COMMUNITY HEALTH WORKER

Community health workers are essential to the communities they serve, as they facilitate access to health and social services through culturally competent practice. These public health professionals serve as trusted liaisons between their community members and public health services and programs. Community health workers enhance health literacy among members of their community through outreach, community education, counseling, social support, and advocacy. They can work in a variety of settings including rural, urban, AI/AN nations, and metropolitan areas. The work of community health workers is often focused in marginalized communities with limited resources and access to healthcare. Thus, community health workers are essential in connecting communities to what they need to achieve good health through strong communication skills, interpersonal skills, system navigation, and cultural responsiveness.

PROGRAM MANAGER

Program managers lead programs that support the missions and goals of their respective organizations. Effective leadership and management of all aspects of these programs are essential to their success, ideally translating to better health outcomes for the intended community. Program managers prioritize resources, manage budgets, create operating plans, train and motivate staff, and direct efforts to improve community health and program performance. The work may take place in private and public sectors. Position titles include program coordinator, program analyst, account manager, associate director, or senior project manager. Program managers have strong leadership and communication skills, conflict resolution skills, knowledge of project management principles, and a risk management mind-set.

The careers we describe here are but a handful of the many public health opportunities that are available to promote and protect the health of populations. The American Public Health

Association (APHA) website lists up-to-date employment options in the field as well as opportunities for internships and fellowships.[19] The Public Health Jobs website, run by the Association of Schools and Programs of Public Health, posts career options available by field and location for those interested in public health work.[20] The CDC website is another resource for aspiring public health professionals that lists fellowship and internship opportunities to engage in meaningful public health work.[21]

FURTHER EDUCATION IN PUBLIC HEALTH

Public health can be studied at a variety of levels in tailored programs suited to various sectors of public health interest. At the undergraduate level, there are both BS and BA degree programs that include foundational training in public health. Bachelors programs are diverse in structure and curriculum, with some designed as preprofessional degrees and others with a liberal arts focus. At the graduate level, there are also a variety of masters programs tailored to public health studies, with the most common being the MPH. Most MPH programs allow students to concentrate or specialize in a particular area of public health including, but not limited to, biostatistics, community health, environmental health, epidemiology, global health, health policy, prevention sciences, and healthcare management. The MPH degree is a professional degree focused on the practice of public health. In comparison, the MSPH is an academic-, or research-focused degree. At the doctoral level, the PhD is a highly specialized degree focusing on preparation for teaching and research in the public health field globally, nationally, or locally. The DrPH degree is a professional degree focused on the highest levels of practice and leadership in public health. Regardless of the level, all educational offerings in public health provide skills and knowledge to approach public health challenges.

CASE STUDY 13.2: RESILIENT SYSTEMS TO SAFEGUARD KIDNEY DIALYSIS SERVICES DURING A CLIMATE-DRIVEN HURRICANE

Public health practice involves all that is done to improve health, including activities, programs, infrastructure, interventions, services, and processes that prevent disease and promote health for all people, everywhere. Considering the social ecological framework, public health practice involves the delivery of public health services at multiple levels to promote health. Government agencies, NGOs, nonprofit organizations, private organizations, academic institutions, community-based organizations, policy advocates, and individuals all engage in public health practice. We examine a life-saving application of public health practice, describing an elaborate and ever-evolving system for maintaining access to hemodialysis for patients with end-stage kidney disease (ESKD). We describe the heroic efforts of kidney dialysis services during Hurricane Ian in 2022.

More than 750,000 patients in the United States are surviving with a diagnosis of ESKD. Race/ethnic disparities are pronounced, with rates of ESKD that are 3.4 and 1.5 times higher among African American/Black and Hispanic populations respectively, compared to the general population [Gupta 2021]. Among ESKD patients, 71% (about 500,000) rely on in-center hemodialysis, the most common dialysis modality.[22] In-center patients usually require hemodialysis three times weekly to adequately manage the complications of ESKD. Disruptions to this care regimen

(continued)

may adversely affect their health and may be life-threatening. Understandably, ESKD patients depend on the lifeline of in-center dialysis and require customized approaches for disaster preparedness.

We illustrate the practicalities and complexities involved in maintaining and reestablishing dialysis services for ESKD patients throughout Florida as they prepared for, and recovered from, their encounter with Hurricane Ian in late September 2022.

Hurricane Ian began as a tropical wave in the Atlantic Ocean just eastward of the Windward Islands. After moving into the Caribbean Sea, the wave began to organize into a rotating system that ultimately became Hurricane Ian as it approached the Cayman Islands. Ian intensified as it moved over western Cuba, knocking out electrical power to the island nation's 11 million citizens, before emerging into the Gulf of Mexico. On September 28, 2022, Hurricane Ian made landfall along Florida's southwest coast, close to Fort Myers, as the fifth strongest storm to impact the United States mainland. Maximum sustained wind speeds reached 155 mph, just 2 mph below the threshold for a Category 5 hurricane. In addition to powerful winds, Hurricane Ian caused a catastrophic storm surge, exceeding 10 feet in some places; produced 1 to 2 feet of rainfall across the central peninsula of Florida; and triggered a multitude of spin-up tornadoes. High ocean heat content was the energy source that powered Ian. Anomalously warm waters extended from the surface to the depths of the Gulf.

Prior to landfall, wind shear conditions were also favorable for intensification. Coupled with these conditions, the forward speed of Hurricane Ian slowed as it made landfall, which caused sustained wind, surge, and rainfall for large areas of the southwestern Gulf Coast of Florida. Studies continue to suggest that anthropogenic climate warming is producing a generation of more intense, wetter tropical cyclones.[23] Research also suggests that climate change may be amplifying rapid intensification events[24] and causing storms to stall near landfall in North America.[24]

Considering the ferocity of this climate-driven hurricane, how were ESKD patients safeguarded from interruptions of their vital hemodialysis sessions? Fortunately, these giant cyclonic systems can be detected days in advance and tracked over time, and timely warnings can be issued for populations likely to be affected. Therefore, some ESKD patients had the opportunity and the wherewithal to evacuate to safer locales and continue their dialysis uninterrupted. This was not a realistic option for most, but they too were safeguarded by the extraordinary efforts of the kidney dialysis services.

Dialysis services corporations, including several with international operations, provide kidney dialysis services and a wide range of resources for ESKD patients in countries around the globe. Major dialysis services corporations have professionals dedicated to disaster preparedness. These companies and their staff members do not self-define as public health practitioners, but the roles they perform when disasters threaten or strike precisely fit the mold of public health practice.

The following account is based on the activities of two major dialysis providers—in Florida during Hurricane Ian. These dialysis services attentively tracked the trajectory of Hurricane Ian for more than a week as the system formed and the path and intensity estimates became better defined. Based on timely, high-quality weather forecast guidance, the providers activated their disaster plans well before

(continued)

Hurricane Ian was moving northward from the Caribbean, crossing Cuba, and approaching Florida's west coast.

One "advantage" that dialysis services have that is unique to this patient population is that they see every patient multiple times weekly. Regular dialysis is critical for survival. Therefore, these dialysis providers were guaranteed to see all patients in the days immediately prior to Ian's landfall. The only exception was the subset of patients who evacuated, and their whereabouts were also tracked.

The dialysis services developed case transition reports for each dialysis client. Once the timing and location of probable impact was better known, the dialysis providers moved their dialysis appointments up by one day, predialyzing their patients on the day before the storm. Hurricane Ian made landfall on a Wednesday, so the providers arranged 3-hour dialysis sessions (rather than the usual 4-hour sessions to accommodate the volume) on Tuesday or, in some cases, in the dawn hours of Wednesday morning. When patients arrived for their appointments, they received a sealed plastic bag with their essential dialysis information, national emergency contact numbers, and emphatic guidance to answer their cell phones when called by dialysis personnel the day after the storm. This admonition—to answer the phone—was based on having providers calling patients using their personal cell phones—because the dialysis centers were closed as the storm moved through the area.

Updated patient contact information was entered into the companies' disaster tracker databases located in states remote from Florida. Reports were generated as tracker information was continuously updated in real time. By knowing the locations of their patients, the dialysis providers were able to guide patients to the nearest operational dialysis facility, even as the situation was constantly changing based on the storm hazards and the postimpact situation regarding the integrity of facilities, electrical power, water, and physical access. By having direct cell phone contact, the providers were able to problem-solve with patients who were unable to reach a dialysis center. In one instance, the provider arranged for the National Guard to rescue a dialysis patient stranded on the roof of his home in a storm-flooded neighborhood.

Prior to the arrival of Hurricane Ian, dialysis centers arranged for solid wastes to be picked up for proper hygienic disposal because of storm surge and flash flooding risks and the dangers of having "sharps" and contaminated fluids in the flood waters.

At the time when Hurricane Ian made landfall on Wednesday, September 28, 232 dialysis centers operated by these major dialysis services were closed. As the storm moved across the central Florida peninsula on Thursday, most centers remained closed. However, by Friday, half of the centers were back in operation. Most centers returned to functionality over the weekend, and by Monday, 230 of the 232 dialysis centers were serving their patients. Most patients were dialyzed within 4 days or less, with a handful waiting 5 days for dialysis. There were no hospitalizations for kidney emergencies among the thousands of dialysis patients served by these 232 centers, and no deaths.

Knowing that power outages can be widespread and prolonged as these massive cyclonic systems disrupt infrastructure, all hemodialysis centers are equipped with high-wattage diesel-powered auxiliary generators—or, in some instances,

(continued)

generators are staged nearby and transported to centers requiring backup power. Dialysis services transported substantial quantities of diesel fuel to the centers in the impact zone to supply the generators for multiple days. Gasoline was also transported to the centers to allow dialysis center employees to fill their cars (power outages make it impossible to pump gas at many stations).

Given the expectation that some employees might sustain damage to homes or encounter impassable roadways leading to the centers, the dialysis providers paid for blocks of hotel rooms or improvised other staff accommodations. Staff members were encouraged to bring their family members so that they could stay safely together in the rooms. This allowed dialysis personnel to report to work in nearby centers to continue dialyzing patients throughout the storm—and be with family during off-duty hours. Box trucks of palletized food were brought to the centers to feed the staff.

Kidney dialysis requires 300 to 400 liters of water per dialysis treatment per patient. Several centers required tankers of water to be brought in to supply the needs of the dialysis process. In several centers, water pressure was insufficient due to power outages, or local water supplies were contaminated.

Security services were provided through long-standing contracts with security professionals comprised of retired police officers who were able to arrive in pairs to work alternating 12-hour shifts at centers in vulnerable locations. The dialysis providers deployed technical support personnel from out of state to their centers that sustained minor damage to make structural repairs to the buildings and verify that dialysis equipment was working properly.

Given the life-sustaining nature of the work they do, dialysis providers are able to use the FirstNet communication systems that give them top priority for available cell services. This is the same system used by fire/rescue, law enforcement, and emergency management professionals.

The dialysis providers continuously monitored Hurricane Ian and the operational status of all centers using their tracker systems. As soon as hurricane Ian passed an area, dialysis center personnel were making cell phone calls to their patients to determine their status and any emergency needs and guide them to available dialysis services. During Ian, the dialysis providers successfully contacted and accounted for 100% of their Florida patients within 72 hours.

Some ESKD patients attempted to receive dialysis at area hospitals, but most hospitals were not equipped to dialyze patients, instead directing these patients to nearby dialysis centers. Because dialysis is a time-sensitive, life-sustaining procedure, dialysis services dialyzed patients who were not on their regular rosters but urgently required treatment.

The experiences of these dialysis services, safeguarding their ESKD patients throughout the ravages of Hurricane Ian, exemplify public health practice at its best and most effective. Public health practice is pragmatic and life-saving at the same time. Lessons are continuously learned, and processes are refined, to better serve the public's health. This includes bringing innovation and dedication to supporting a range of medically vulnerable patient populations, including ESKD patients whose lives depend on access to hemodialysis, blue sky or gray sky.

SUMMARY

Public health practice is the application and implementation of policies, programs, and services at local, state, national, and global levels to promote population health. Public health agencies engage with many other sectors to offer resources and services to promote health and prevent disease and injury. Public health systems, locally and globally, operationalize their efforts around three core functions: assessment, policy development, and assurance. Assessment includes the systematic collection and analysis of data to assess community health needs, investigate health outbreaks, monitor trends, and analyze causes of health issues. Policy development includes engagement of community organizations and other stakeholders to address community needs and to develop polices, in partnership with community organizations and other stakeholders, complete with goals, objectives, and action plans that are responsive to their needs. Assurance involves monitoring and evaluation of policies, programs, and services through systematic collection, analysis, and dissemination of data to community stakeholders. The three core functions aim to educate, engage, and empower individuals and communities to take control of their health. The three core functions are not performed in sequence as discrete steps but rather as a continuous cycle toward improving policies, programs, and services that produce population health.

> **Public health agencies engage with many other sectors to offer resources and services to promote health and prevent disease and injury.**

End-of-Chapter Resources

Access additional case study podcasts online at http://connect.springerpub.com/content/book/978-0-8261-8043-8/

DISCUSSION QUESTIONS

1. Identify a program comparable to the SNAP described in this chapter. How does it function? Do you see any barriers to accessing its services?
2. Consider a recent study where an intervention (e.g., a medical treatment, a behavioral modification) was shown to be effective in promoting health or reducing disease progression or onset. How might these findings be translated into practice? What are the challenges?
3. You are charged to develop a new policy on your campus to reduce the intake of sugar-sweetened beverages. What approach would you take? Who would you engage in developing the policy? What are the potential barriers to its implementation and acceptance?

 A robust set of instructor resources designed to supplement this text is located at **http://connect.springerpub.com/content/book/978-0-8261-8043-8.** Qualifying instructors may request access by emailing **textbook@springerpub.com.**

REFERENCES

1. The U.S. Department of Health & Human Services. *About HHS*. 2019. www.hhs.gov
2. Trust for America's Health. *Public Health Leadership Initiative: An Action Plan for Healthy People in Healthy Communities in the 21st Century*. Author; 2006.
3. NACCHO Voice. *2016 National profile of local health departments*. Published January 25, 2017. https://nacchovoice.naccho.org/2017/01/25/2016-national-profile-of-local-health-departments
4. Institute of Medicine. *The Future of Public Health*. National Academies Press; 1988.
5. Jones DS, Podolsky SH, Greene JA. The burden of disease and the changing task of medicine. *N Engl J Med*. 2012;366(25):2333-2338. doi:10.1056/NEJMp1113569
6. World Health Organization. *Global Health Estimates*. https://www.who.int/data/global-health-estimates#:~: text=They%20are%20produced%20using%20data,Disease%20and%20other%20scientific%20studies
7. Mass.gov. *105 CMR 300.00: reportable diseases, surveillance, and isolation and quarantine requirements*. Published February 3, 2017. https://www.mass.gov/doc/105-cmr-300-reportable-diseases-surveillance-and-isolation-and-quarantine-requirements/download#:~:text=The%20purpose%20of%20105%20CMR, surveillance%2C%20isolation%20and%20quarantine%20requirements
8. Centers for Disease Control and Prevention. *Interactive database systems*. https://www.cdc.gov/surveillancepractice/data.html
9. World Health Organization. *WHO Recommended Surveillance Standards*. Published February 2, 1999. https://www.who.int/publications/i/item/who-recommended-surveillance-standards
10. Centers for Disease Control and Prevention. *About the National Health and Nutrition Examination Survey*. https://www.cdc.gov/nchs/nhanes/about_nhanes.htm
11. Rudolph L, Caplan J, Ben-Moshe K, Dillon L. *Health in All Policies: A Guide for State and Local Governments*. American Public Health Association and Public Health Institute; 2013. http://www.phi.org/uploads/files/Health_in_All_Policies-A_Guide_for_State_and_Local_Governments.pdf
12. Brownson RC, Kreuter MW, Arrington BA, True WR. Translating scientific discoveries into public health action: how can schools of public health move us forward? *Public Health Rep*. 2006;121(1):97-103.
13. Singal AG, Higgins PDR, Waljee AK. A primer on effectiveness and efficacy trials. *Clin Transl Gastroenterol*. 2014;5(1):e45. doi:10.1038/ctg.2013.13
14. World Health Organization. *World Health Day 2013: measure your blood pressure, reduce your risk*. Published April 3, 2013. https://www.who.int/news/item/03-04-2013-world-health-day-2013-measure-your-blood-pressure-reduce-your-risk#:~:text=3%20April%202013%20%7C%20Geneva%20%2D%20To,or%20about%20one%20billion%20people
15. American Public Health Association. *The role of public health in ensuring healthy communities*. Published 2014. https://www.apha.org/policies-and-advocacy/public-health-policy-statements/policy-database/2014/07/30/10/48/the-role-of-public-health-in-ensuring-healthy-communities
16. DeSalvo KB, Wang YC, Harris A, et al. Public health 3.0: a call to action for public health to meet the challenges of the 21st century. *Prev Chronic Dis*. 2017;14:170017. doi:10.5888/pcd14.170017
17. Federal Emergency Management Agency. *Preparing for Disaster for People with Disabilities and Other Special Needs*. Author; 2004. https://www.fema.gov/pdf/library/pfd_all.pdf
18. BCFS Health and Human Services. *Guidance on Planning for Integration of Functional Needs Support Services in General Population Shelters*. Federal Emergency Management Agency; 2010. https://www.fema.gov/pdf/about/odic/fnss_guidance.pdf
19. American Public Health Association. *Professional development*. https://apha.org/professional-development
20. Public Health Jobs. https://publichealthjobs.org/
21. Centers for Disease Control and Prevention. *Fellowships and training opportunities*. https://www.cdc.gov/fellowships/index.html
22. Knutson T, Camargo SJ, Chan JCL, et al. Tropical cyclones and climate change assessment. Part II: projected response to anthropogenic warming. *Bull Am Meteorol Soc*. 2020;101(3):E303-E322. doi:10.1175/BAMS-D-18-0194.1
23. Hall TM, Kossin JP. Hurricane stalling along the North American coast and implications for rainfall. *NPJ Clim Atmos Sci*. 2019;2:17. doi:10.1038/s41612-019-0074-8
24. Bhatia KT, Vecchi GA, Knutson TR, et al. Recent increases in tropical cyclone intensification rates. *Nat Commun*. 2019;10(1):635. doi:10.1038/s41467-019-08471-z

14

COMMUNITY ENGAGEMENT AND ADVOCACY TO PROMOTE AND PROTECT HEALTH

LEARNING OBJECTIVES

- Explain "intersectoral public health" and why it is important to promote population health.
- Summarize why laws are necessary to promote and protect public health.
- Outline how, why, and by whom health impact assessments are conducted.
- Discuss the key components of knowledge translation models.
- Compare the roles and functions of different stakeholders in public health advocacy.

OVERVIEW: PUBLIC HEALTH IS CONCERNED WITH THE CULTURAL AND ECONOMIC CONTEXTS THAT SHAPE HEALTH

Public health action to address the social and economic determinants of health, to improve the conditions of daily life, to address inequities and imbalances in resources and power, and to measure impacts of action must involve governments, communities, and businesses from all sectors including those that are not specifically health related, special interest groups, advocates, and individuals. This is not easy to do.

Public health has enjoyed many triumphs over the past century which have appreciably improved our collective well-being. Highlighting some of these triumphs, scientists at the Centers for Disease Control and Prevention (CDC) regularly create and disseminate lists of the top 10 public health achievements, both for U.S. and global populations. Each of the achievements made these lists based on public health action that addressed policies and politics, and the cultural, social, and economic contexts that shape health. And there is much more work yet to be done.

Public health has enjoyed many triumphs over the past century which have appreciably improved our collective well-being.

In this chapter, we (a) outline the multiple sectors that affect health across the life course, (b) discuss formal models for knowledge translation into action, summarizing how ideas become knowledge that ultimately becomes public health policy and practice, (c) describe the particular role of community engagement as a partner to public health practice, and (d) examine how public health advocates across sectors to generate the cultural, social, and economic conditions that promote health.

THE MULTIPLE SECTORS THAT SHAPE THE HEALTH OF THE PUBLIC

Over a decade ago, the Committee on Assuring the Health of the Public in the 21st Century was formed to create a framework to ensure public health in the United States.[1] Their report called for increased "emphasis on an intersectoral public health system" that included governmental public health agencies, the healthcare system, academic institutions, community organizations, religious groups, employers, and the media. The report suggested a need for clearly articulated systems of accountability and expanded communications to ensure that high-quality public health services are widely available and accessible.

Governmental public health agencies are often stretched in terms of their human and financial resources, resulting from their ever-expanding portfolio of functions and duties. Although governmental agencies have the ultimate responsibility and authority for the public's health, they simply cannot make progress working alone. Academic public health institutions are an important part of the public health infrastructure. As public health issues evolve, the public health workforce needs more training and skills development to be effective, creating a need for partnerships between public health agencies and academia—schools and programs of public health that are training the next generation of public health professionals. Mid-career public health professionals also need skills training, and academic institutions must offer relevant trainings in formats that are flexible and accessible for working professionals.

Governmental public health agencies are often stretched in terms of their human and financial resources, resulting from their ever-expanding portfolio of functions and duties.

Community-based organizations are another critical component of the public health infrastructure as they often best understand the needs of their neighborhoods and the approaches that might be most effective to address them. These partnerships between public health agencies and community organizations, ideally formed at the planning and assessment stages, create opportunities for more effective and sustainable actions that promote health.

Employers play an important role in the public health infrastructure as they affect economic, social, and environmental aspects of health in the communities in which they are based. Employers often offer healthcare benefits to employees and their families. Employer-paid wages and salaries influence access to housing and overall quality of life in communities.

Partnerships between public health agencies and the media are important as public health action requires engagement of many sectors and individuals, with differing backgrounds and interests, who must understand public health issues to engage in solutions successfully and effectively. The media are critical for disseminating accurate and timely information widely in culturally and linguistically appropriate ways about health issues and determinants of health. Case Study 14.1, "Laws and the Health of the Public," highlights the intersection of the legal sector—a sector that might not at first be thought to be considered health-related—and public health.

Partnerships between public health agencies and the media are important as public health action requires engagement of many sectors and individuals, with differing backgrounds and interests, who must understand public health issues to engage in solutions successfully and effectively.

WHY PUBLIC HEALTH MUST EXTEND TO A BROAD RANGE OF ACTORS AND SECTORS

Population health is determined by factors that cross multiple sectors and systems. Health impact assessment (HIA) is an emerging field that presents the scientific evidence on the health effects of new policies, laws, regulations, and programs to those in decision-making positions. The Robert Wood Johnson Foundation and the Pew Charitable Trusts provide support for the Health Impact Project, which is a U.S. initiative to support the use of HIAs with funding, training, technical assistance, and dissemination of findings.[2] The World Health Organization (WHO) also advocates for HIA to help ministries of health and local public health agencies collaborate across sectors to promote health and health equity.[3]

The core of HIA is intersectoral collaboration, which brings together public health, community organizations, political groups, businesses, law, architecture, transportation, agriculture, trade, healthcare, and many others. Together, these groups evaluate data from multiple perspectives considering social, economic, environmental, and cultural determinants of health and how they are affected by new policies and programs. Although these collaborations are critical to improving population health, they have their challenges in terms of differing priorities and constraints among constituents, lack of understanding of the others' goals, systems and processes, and lack of common vocabulary and terminology. Critical elements of successful intersectoral collaboration include openness and flexibility. However, the most critical element is agreement on the goal—promoting health and health equity—and all strategies must be directed toward that goal. Strategies must target institutions, systems, cultures, environments, and behaviors to be impactful. The following example highlights the intersection of politics and public health.

The core of HIA is intersectoral collaboration, which brings together public health, community organizations, political groups, businesses, law, architecture, transportation, agriculture, trade, healthcare, and many others.

CASE STUDY 14.1: LAWS AND THE HEALTH OF THE PUBLIC

Laws play a critical role in protecting and promoting public health. Many public health powers are inherent state powers, also known as the state's "police" and "parens patriae powers."[4] The federal government has authority over health matters granted to it by the U.S. Constitution, primarily through the government's authority over foreign and interstate commerce and national defense and its powers to impose taxes and spend the revenue.

For much of the 20th century, public health practitioners in the United States operated principally on the assumption that states[5] were the primary source of law governing health matters. Until the mid-1900s, public health work was concentrated[6] in local health and environmental departments, where controlling infectious diseases and contaminated food and water in the community were the focus of the profession. Today, however, public health is a far more expansive[7] national and global field,[8] one in which federal legislation and regulatory agencies provide the legal framework and substantial funding for public health programs and services. State and local public health programs still perform valuable core functions in providing services, but many of these (including surveillance, evaluation, the Ryan White HIV treatment act,[9] and family planning services) would not exist in the absence of federal regulation and funding.[10]

Legal frameworks are supportive of, and necessary for, public health achievement. For example, **Table 14.1** shows how the 10 great public health achievements,[11]

TABLE 14.1 Ten Great Public Health Achievements, 1900–1999, and Selected Supportive Laws and Legal Tools, United States

PUBLIC HEALTH ACHIEVEMENTS	SELECTED SUPPORTIVE LAWS AND LEGAL TOOLS		
	LOCAL	STATE	FEDERAL
Control of infectious disease	Sanitary codes and drinking water standards; quarantine and isolation authority; zoning ordinances and building codes; mosquito- and rodent-control programs; inspection of food establishments	Authority to conduct disease surveillance, require disease reports, and investigate outbreaks; regulation of food supplies; licensure of health professionals	Public Health Service Act of 1944; Safe Drinking Water Act of 1974; National Environmental Protection Act of 1976
Motor vehicle safety	Speed limits; limitation on liquor-store hours; penalties for serving inebriated bar patrons	Seat-belt, child-safety-seat, and motorcycle-helmet laws; vehicle inspections; driver licensing and graduated driver licensing systems; authorization to conduct sobriety checkpoints; zero tolerance for alcohol among drivers under age 21 years; prohibition on alcohol	Performance and crash standards for motor vehicles; standards for road and highway construction; safety-belt use in some commercial vehicles; financial assistance to states to promote and enforce highway safety initiatives; airbag warning labels; creation of state

(continued)

TABLE 14.1 Ten Great Public Health Achievements, 1900–1999, and Selected Supportive Laws and Legal Tools, United States (*continued*)

PUBLIC HEALTH ACHIEVEMENTS	SELECTED SUPPORTIVE LAWS AND LEGAL TOOLS		
	LOCAL	STATE	FEDERAL
		sales to minors; 0.08% blood alcohol content per se laws; speed limits	offices of highway safety; federal court ruling upholding motorcycle-helmet use
Fluoridation of drinking water	Ordinances authorizing fluoridation; referendums and initiatives authorizing fluoridation	Legislation authorizing fluoridation; court ruling upholding fluoridation	Federal court rulings upholding fluoridation of public drinking water supplies; Environmental Protection Agency caps on fluoride levels
Recognition of tobacco use as a health hazard	Excise taxes; restrictions on retail sale to minors; clean indoor air laws	Excise taxes; restrictions on retail sale practices; clean indoor air laws; funding for public anti-smoking education; lawsuits leading to the Master Settlement Agreement of 1995	Excise tax; mandated warning labels; prohibition of advertising on radio and television; penalties on states not outlawing sale to persons under age 18 years; financial assistance to state and local tobacco-control programs; Department of Justice lawsuit to recover healthcare costs
Vaccination	School board enforcement of school entry vaccination requirements	Court ruling supporting mandatory vaccination; school entry admission laws	Court ruling supporting mandatory vaccination; licensure of vaccines; financial aid to state vaccination programs
Decline in deaths from coronary heart disease and stroke	Education and information programs	Tobacco-control laws; education and information programs	Food-labeling laws; Department of Transportation funding for bikeways and walking paths; National High Blood Pressure Education Program
Safer and healthier foods	Standards for and inspection of retail food establishments	Mandated niacin enrichment of bread and flour; standards for and inspection of foods at the producer level; limits on chemical contamination of crops	Pure Food and Drug Act of 1906 and later enactments to regulate foods and prescription drugs; mandated folic acid fortification of cereal grain products; limits on chemical contamination of crops; food stamps; the Women, Infants, and Children Program; school meals

(*continued*)

TABLE 14.1 Ten Great Public Health Achievements, 1900–1999, and Selected Supportive Laws and Legal Tools, United States (*continued*)

PUBLIC HEALTH ACHIEVEMENTS	SELECTED SUPPORTIVE LAWS AND LEGAL TOOLS		
	LOCAL	STATE	FEDERAL
Healthier mothers and babies	Sewage and refuse ordinances; drinking water codes; milk pasteurization	Establishment of maternal and child health clinics; licensure of obstetrics healthcare professionals; mandated milk pasteurization; funding for Medicaid services	Drinking water quality standards; creation of the Children's Bureau (1912) with education and service programs; licensure of sulfa drugs and antibiotics; creation of the Medicaid program; the Infant Formula Act of 1980
Family planning	Funding for family planning clinics	Authorization to provide birth control services; authority to provide prenatal and postnatal care to indigent mothers	Family Planning Services and Population Research Act; Supreme Court rulings on contraceptive use
Safer workplaces	Authority to inspect for unsafe conditions; building and fire safety codes	Laws to inspect and regulate workplace safety practices, including toxic exposures; criminal penalties for grossly negligent worker injury or death	Minimum safety standards for federal contractors; inspection and regulation of mine safety; mandates on states to adopt minimum workplace safety standards; Occupational Safety and Health Act of 1970

Source: From Goodman RA, Moulton A, Matthews G, et al. Law and public health at CDC. *MMWR Morb Mortal Wkly Rep.* 2006;55:29-33. https://www.cdc.gov/mmwr/preview/mmwrhtml/su5502a11.htm#tab1

as articulated by the CDC, are all linked to supportive laws at the local, state, and federal levels.[12]

In some respects, the origin of all public health regulation, the British Public Health Act of 1848,[13] provided a prototype for how we may indeed improve public health by working on a range of sectors. It established new laws about improving both urban sanitary conditions and formal public health infrastructure. The act was driven, perhaps idealistically,[14] by the very particular concerns of its era. Coming right around the time of a major cholera outbreak, when acting to improve public health had become a pressing national imperative, the act established a general, central board of health,[15] and in some places, local boards of health. The local boards were then tasked with dealing with issues such as water supplies and the removal of garbage and sewage. The act created positions for persons who were accountable for public health and penalties for noncompliance. In some ways, this measure was visionary in its focus on prevention and in establishing accountability for the health of the public. In reviewing the long-term impact of the act,[16] its approach remains resonant and relevant today, but comparable acts may not be able to achieve traction in our time, given the challenges that assertive legislation[17]

(*continued*)

aiming to improve public health has faced in the country. Perhaps ironically, the central driver for the act was more economic than aspirational toward healthier populations. Edwin Chadwick,[18] the champion and namesake of this piece of legislation, knew that if he could improve the health of the poor, fewer people would seek relief from the government, ultimately saving money centrally.

Global examples[19] also provide some grounding about the scope of public health legislation that may have lessons in the domestic context. The Public Health Act in Northern Ireland[20] was passed in 1967 to deal principally with infectious disease control, and it was amended in 2008 to include the prevention of contamination by means of aircraft. The Quebec Public Health Act[21] in 2002 affirmed the Minister of Health and Social Services' authority to protect health and passed specific legislation on vaccination registries, fluoridation of drinking water, infectious disease, and other crucial matters. Many similar public health acts have been passed around the world with the intention of clarifying the role of public health officials and allowing them to take immediate action for certain health hazards that present threats to the public. These acts take a rather traditional view of public health, targeting primarily infectious disease control. But there are exceptions that perhaps can motivate a more ambitious and proactive approach to the promotion of public health.

The Health in All Policies (HiAP)[22] approach, first proposed in Europe, aspires to make health central to policy making in all sectors of the economy. The approach recognizes that the production of health must arise from the engagement of multiple sectors in order to create conditions for healthy populations. Other examples of HiAP approaches include the Adelaide Statement[23] in South Australia and Act-Now BC[24] in Canada. The HiAP concept is also embedded in the Affordable Care Act, through the establishment of the National Prevention Council,[25] under the direction of the Surgeon General, which has included the articulation of a National Prevention Strategy that lays out a framework for cross-sectoral action on health. The limitation of the latter is that it does not establish legislative ties to these actions, but rather acts to frame action by engaging multiple partners.

Legislative action stands to improve the health of the public. The challenge is that much of our conception of legislative actions for public health has focused on the specific regulation of public health by relevant agencies. Although this is necessary, it is but a small piece of a much larger picture, and the need exists for a broader embrace of the social and structural changes required to promote health and prevent disease. This is a call back to the roots of public health, as exemplified in the British Public Health Act of 1848, echoed in more recent HiAP efforts.

Molly Ivins, the late journalist, argued in a 2004 speech for the central role of politics in our daily lives, saying,

> *The qualifications of the people who prescribe your eyeglasses, whether or not the lady who dyes your hair knows what she's doing, how deep you will be buried when you die . . . the books your children will read in schools . . . all of those are consequences of a political decision.*[26]

Ivins' words reflect that reality that politics is a foundational determinant of health.[27] Politics plays a key role in influencing the conditions—economic, social, environmental—that lay the groundwork for population health. From policies which shape the condition of our currency[28] to whether we have clean air and water,[29] to the legal appointments which intersect with key civil rights issues,[30] politics is at the heart of our collective wellbeing. As we consider politics, it follows that we should also think about a hinge on which our politics turns—the electoral process.

In our history, we see how elections can have profound, long-lasting effects, and that these effects can be the result of very slim margins. This was the case, for example, in the election of 1876. The race was between the Democratic candidate Samuel J. Tilden and the Republican candidate Rutherford B. Hayes.[31] Both men hoped to succeed Ulysses S. Grant, the Civil War commander-turned-president who used the power of the executive branch to help safeguard the rights of slaves who had been freed during the Civil War. Grant upheld civil rights in a number of ways, including working in support of the Fifteenth Amendment and opposing the Ku Klux Klan with military force.[32-37] Hayes was in the same political party as Grant—the Republican party, to which Abraham Lincoln had belonged—and the party at that time was committed to enforcing Reconstruction policies in the South, where the rights of African Americans were under attack. The 1876 election, which was critical to the continuation of these efforts, was, in the end, too close to call. Tilden received 4,284,020 votes and Hayes received 4,036,572 votes. Meanwhile, allegations of fraud kept 20 electoral votes in dispute. Arguments over who won the election dragged on for months before the matter was settled in a backroom deal.[38] The deal stipulated that Democrats would consent to the election of the Republican Hayes if Hayes agreed to pull the military from the South. This meant allowing southern legislatures to adopt segregationist policies, leaving the African American/Black population vulnerable to the injustice of what would become the Jim Crow system of institutional racism.[39] The long-term effect of this historical injustice remains with us in the legacy of racism which continues to undermine health in the present day. Addressing the historical forces that helped create this poor health means reckoning with the political conditions of the 19th century, with the 1876 election acting as a turning point.[40-43]

The election of 1876 reflects how elections can worsen the injustice and institutionalized bigotry that harms health in this country. But elections can also support progress, shaping a healthier, more just nation. This was the case nearly a century after the election of 1876, in the election of 1964, which saw Lyndon Baines Johnson run against Barry Goldwater.[44-46] Johnson's overwhelming victory in that election, in which he carried 44 states and Goldwater carried just six, gave him the political capital to continue his work in support of civil rights. After the assassination of President John F. Kennedy, Johnson worked to pass an historic civil rights bill.[47,48] Following his landslide win, he broadened his focus and worked to pass ambitious domestic legislation. With a two-thirds majority for his party, the Democrats, in the House and Senate, Johnson was able to help pass nearly 200 pieces of significant legislation. Examples include the Voting Rights Act of 1965, Medicare and Medicaid, part of a legislative package Johnson would call the Great Society.[49-52] Though Johnson's presidency would be overtaken by civil disturbances and the war in Vietnam, his legislative achievements after the 1964 election created a legacy which continues to have an effect on American society and on American health. Medicare and Medicaid remain central to Americans' capacity to access healthcare, and the Great Society's engagement with education, poverty, the environment, and conditions within cities reflect how government can address the foundational determinants of health, supporting vulnerable populations and helping to create the conditions for social justice.[53-56] In 1964, the U.S. population used the electoral process to speak in support of such an effort, endorsing Johnson's earlier work to shape a more just society through the Civil Rights Act of 1964. Their unambiguous endorsement gave Johnson the "green light" to move ahead with bold reforms, shaping a model for how the federal government can function as a change agent for advancing social justice.[57]

More recently, we have seen the influence of politics on health in the words and actions of former President Trump, who has echoed the calls of many Republicans to repeal the Affordable Care Act, which he called an "incredible economic burden."[58-60] In reality, the law was in many ways beneficial for the country's health.[61] Even former President Trump seems to have acknowledged the importance of expanded healthcare coverage, as he said he would "broaden healthcare access, make healthcare more affordable and improve the quality of care available to all

Americans." In his case, this meant promising to give vendors permission to sell health insurance across state borders, promising to permit taxpayers to deduct health insurance premiums from their returns, as well as promising to ensure transparency in healthcare pricing from providers. Former President Trump also expressed the belief that providing healthcare to undocumented immigrants represents an $11 million burden on the health system and he has suggested that more stringent immigration laws could "relieve healthcare cost pressures on state and local governments." He has also emphasized the role of economics in shaping health, saying that "the best social program has always been a job—and taking care of our economy will go a long way toward reducing our dependence on public health programs." While this leaves unaddressed the significant challenge economic inequality poses to health, it at least reflects an engagement with the ineluctable role of economics in shaping health and an acknowledgement that a comprehensive health policy should look past treatment alone to address the fundamental drivers of health.

Outside of the U.S., we saw the power of politics in the wake of the 2016 "Brexit" referendum in the United Kingdom. After the referendum, some of the Leave supporters expressed surprise at their side's unexpected victory.[62] One Leave supporter said after the vote, "I'm shocked that we actually voted to leave. I didn't think that was going to happen. My vote, I didn't think, was going to matter too much because I thought we were just going to remain."[63] Some U.S. voters echoed this in 2016, expressing similar skepticism that their vote would do much to shape the outcome of that election. Yet the outcome of elections, and their long-term legacies, reflect our collective responsibility to continue to stay involved with politics as a means of creating a healthier world.

THE ROLE OF COLLECTIVE ACTION IN CREATING THE CONDITIONS THAT MAKE PEOPLE HEALTHY

Public health has a history of collaboration through formal and informal partnerships that promote health. None of the domestic or global achievements in public health would have been possible without effective collaboration across sectors. Without continued sustainable collective and collaborative action to promote population health, programs and activities that have been put into place will be taken up by those who are already advantaged.

Governmental public health agencies are critical in collective action as they have the ultimate responsibility and legal authority over public health. Individual organizations and groups, while well-intentioned, can slow progress or weaken efforts if they are not part of a coordinated strategy. Public health practitioners have the requisite knowledge and skills to lead efforts to promote population-level change, but successful implementation of policies, programs, and services requires participation and collaboration.

Beaglehole et al. argue that modern public health practice requires five essential themes, which are rarely practiced[64]:

- Health systems leadership (they argue that the long-term strategy for health systems should be defined by public health leaders to ensure that focus lies on improving population health rather than individual healthcare)
- Collaborative actions (as led by governmental agencies)
- Multidisciplinary approaches (ensuring that interventions, programs, and policies that are developed based on evidence address the multifactorial determinants of health)
- Political engagement in public health policy (stronger public health leadership is needed to engage politicians in policies that go beyond what has been possible to date)
- Community partnerships (effective programs and policies require engagement and collaboration with the communities being served to ensure commitment, support, and sustainability)

There is growing recognition that the way to address some of our most pressing health inequities requires collaboration of multiple sectors, both public and private, health-related and non-health-related. We have ample evidence (data) to highlight the many inequities in health that exist and persist. In 2006, the Office of Minority Health, an agency within the U.S. Department of Health and Human Services (HHS), released a report, "National Partnership for Action to End Health Disparities,"[65] detailing a strategy that relied heavily on community engagement to address health disparities. The National Partnership for Action (NPA) defines health disparities broadly to include:

> *individuals who have systematically experienced greater obstacles to health based on their racial/ethnic group; religion; socioeconomic status; gender; age; mental health; cognitive, sensory, or physical disability; sexual orientation or gender identity; geographic location; or other characteristics historically linked to discrimination or exclusion.*[64]

There is growing recognition that the way to address some of our most pressing health inequities requires collaboration of multiple sectors, both public and private, health-related and non-health-related.

Their process for addressing health inequities is based on five goals and is illustrated in **Figure 14.1**.[65]

The NPA report focuses on community engagement and collective action, recognizing that determinants of health are complex and cannot be addressed by government agencies, public or private businesses, or special interest groups acting independently, no matter how passionate or committed they might be. Progress will only be made when there is collective, collaborative, and organized engagement across all sectors.

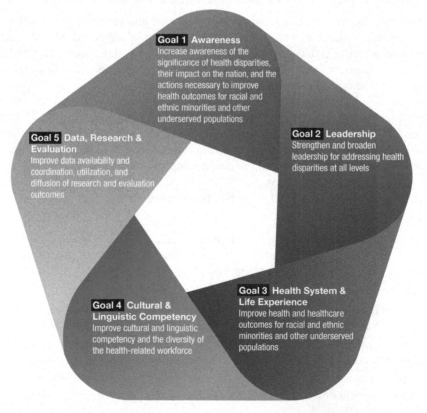

FIGURE 14.1 Goals and strategies of the National Partnership for Action to end health disparities.
Source: Adapted from The Office of Minority Health. About the NPA. Updated February 22, 2018. https://www.nichd.nih .gov/sites/default/files/about/meetings/2011/Documents/rollins_rural_health_120211.pdf

FORMAL MODELS FOR KNOWLEDGE TRANSLATION INTO ACTION

Several terms can be used to describe the process of translating knowledge into action, including *implementation science, dissemination and diffusion, knowledge uptake and transfer,* and *knowledge translation.*[66] We focus here on the term *knowledge translation,* defined by the Canadian Institutes of Health Research (CIHR) in 2000 as

> *the exchange, synthesis, and ethically-sound application of knowledge—within a complex system of interactions among researchers and users—to accelerate the capture of the benefits of research for Canadians through improved health, more effective services and products, and a strengthened health care system.*[67]

Regardless of the specific term used to describe the process, the key aspect is not just dissemination of knowledge but rather use of knowledge—moving knowledge into action to promote health.

For knowledge translation to be successful, the overall goal must be embraced by multiple stakeholders representing different constituencies and sectors. Although the goal may seem narrowly focused on improving population health, the approaches must address social, cultural, economic, political, and environmental determinants that are appropriately tailored to the specific context. To address multilevel determinants requires a broad range of sectors, working together, with all constituents adequately trained to do the work. Ongoing monitoring and evaluation are also necessary for tracking progress, as is communication on short- and long-term outcomes and progress toward the overall goal. Ultimately, programs, policies, and supportive systems must be institutionalized so that new behaviors and action persist and are sustainable.

There are several different models and frameworks for knowledge translation, and all are multipronged (i.e., involving multiple activities by various actors from different sectors), iterative, bidirectional, and focused on adoption of new behaviors, practices, and policies that promote population health. The models and frameworks differ in terms of their specific approaches but have several common elements. Here we define two such elements. The first is creation and synthesis of knowledge to be translated, and the tailoring of this knowledge to local contexts and situations. This might involve the synthesis of research data, focus group data, expert reviews, and stakeholder interviews.

> There are several different models and frameworks for knowledge translation, and all are multipronged (i.e., involving multiple activities by various actors from different sectors), iterative, bidirectional, and focused on adoption of new behaviors, practices, and policies that promote population health.

The second element is a dissemination strategy and accompanying activities, actions, and plans, which are tailored to specific audiences and deployed. A critical component of the dissemination strategy is ongoing monitoring and evaluation, review, revision, and sustainability.

The CDC provides tools and guidance to translate knowledge into action using the Knowledge to Action (K2A) framework[66] (**Figure 14.2**) for public health professionals and others involved in translating evidence-based programs, policies, and interventions into public health action.[68] The CDC's tools focus on planning and include sets of questions for each stage of the K2A process including intervention, administration, implementation, and evaluation around roles, resources, and timing of activities. **Table 14.2** displays an example of one set of questions focused on translating public health interventions into practice.

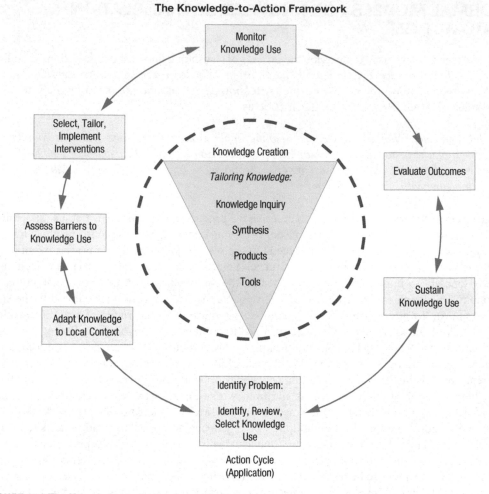

FIGURE 14.2 The Knowledge to Action framework.
Source: Reproduced with permission from Straus SE, Tetroe J, Graham I. Defining knowledge translation. *CMAJ.* 2009;181(3-4):165-168. doi:10.1503/cmaj.081229

ADVOCACY AND COMMUNITY ENGAGEMENT AS CORE COMPONENTS OF PUBLIC HEALTH

Advocacy is "the act or process of supporting a cause or proposal." Dr. Mary Bassett, in a commentary on public health advocacy, notes that, do "The business of improving population health has always been linked to action."[69] She argued that the need for public health advocacy is greater than ever, as what we eat, where we live, and our access to healthcare determine our health. The need for public health data is also more important than ever. With timely and locally relevant public health data in hand (quantitative evidence), coupled with information on what people experience (qualitative data), communities can effectively advocate for their health. The process of advocacy and the data required for successful advocacy are described in detail in the following sections.

TABLE 14.2 Public Health Practice: Performing the Tangible Tasks and Action Steps to Achieve Public Health Objectives

QUESTIONS FOR THOSE PERSONS RESPONSIBLE FOR:			
INTERVENTION DEVELOPING OR TESTING	ADMINISTRATIVE DECISION-MAKING	IMPLEMENTING	EVALUATING

• Have the essential intervention elements (core components) been clearly identified and communicated effectively to the practice community?	• Are the resources and supporting structures available to allow our organization to deliver the intervention with fidelity?
	• Is this intervention scalable for widespread impact?
	• Does the intervention need to be tailored to our community or population? If so, who will do that and how will we ensure fidelity?
		• Are the tools and resources necessary to implement the intervention available?
		• Do we need to tailor the intervention to meet the needs of our target audience? If so, how will we accomplish this?
		• How will we ensure fidelity to the intervention?
		• For practice-based evidence, do we have implementation lessons learned or adaptations that should be further tested with effectiveness and implementation studies or used to inform knowledge into practice?
			• How will we assess:
			
			  o If the intervention was implemented with fidelity?
			  o If the intervention had the desired or expected effect?
			  o If the intervention was delivered in the most efficient and cost-effective way possible?
			  o How satisfied intervention participants or recipients are with the intervention?

THE ACTIVIST ROLE OF PUBLIC HEALTH

There are many ways to advocate for public health action, and every voice counts. The American Public Health Association (APHA) has a wealth of resources openly available on their website to help advocates in developing and running successful advocacy campaigns. They also offer open access to many tools and templates such as draft letters to members of Congress on specific issues, scripts for phone calls to legislators, and fact sheets that can be used to engage others. All of these resources are intended to support advocates in educating and assisting legislators toward making the right policy decisions, based on evidence, that promote health.

Christoffel offers a framework for public health advocacy based on three stages: information, strategy, and action.[70] These stages are not dissimilar to stages employed for successful public health practice. The information stage is focused on collecting and analyzing data or evidence that describes the health issue or problem, how the health issue has evolved over time, and potential determinants or causes of the issue. The strategy stage involves devising a plan to address the determinants or causes of the issue—as always, considering causes over the life course and the multiple sectors that affect health. As part of the strategy stage, a detailed plan is devised with short-, intermediate-, and long-term goals that allow public health professionals to track progress. The action stage is where strategies, activities, and programs are implemented. Successful implementation occurs when there are changes in beliefs, behaviors, policies, and procedures that affect population health. Christoffel efficiently summarizes how various participants, constituents, and sectors engage in advocacy through each of the three stages of this framework (**Table 14.3**).

TABLE 14.3 Public Health Advocacy: Participant Roles

PARTICIPANT	INFORMATION	STRATEGY	ACTION
Coalitions	Request data	Public education	Lobby
		Policy focus identification	Testify
		Bring disparate players together	Get out the vote
		Work with legislators	
		Amplify group efforts	
		Coordinate group efforts	
Community groups	Tap resident knowledge	Public education	Lobby
	Request data	Join coalitions	Testify
		Work with legislators	
		Mobilize residents	
Individual health service providers	Case studies, series	Clinical perspective	Counsel
	Research studies	Public education	Lobby
	Define clinical issues	Build coalitions	Testify
			Vote
Health provider organization	Identify needed data	Policy statements	Lobby
	Some research	Model bills	Testify
		Clinical guidelines	
		Join/support coalitions	
		Public education	
Journal editors	Quality control via peer review	Special issues	Publish papers and editorials
		Choose reviewers	Issue press releases

(continued)

TABLE 14.3 Public Health Advocacy: Participant Roles (*continued*)

PARTICIPANT	INFORMATION	STRATEGY	ACTION
Journalists	Investigative work	Public education	Publish stories
Lawyers and other legal experts	Describe and interpret laws and their implications	Develop and teach options for application of and changes in laws	Bring suits and injunctions, draft rules and laws
Legislators	Request data Authorize data work Fund data work	Hold hearings Draft legislation Draft regulations	Pass laws Fund enforcement
Private sector (sometimes including manufacturers and retailers)	Fund data work Fund research	Funding priorities Fund coalitions Fund public education	Apply safety standards
Researchers and academicians	Conduct research and evaluation	Develop data-based and theoretical concepts to guide prevention planning; educational curricula for students	Publish papers Write editorials Testify Media interviews Determine course and qualifying exam questions Vote
Research funding agencies	Fund research Quality control via peer review	Funding priorities Consensus statements	Testify
Victims	Bear witness Participate in research	Victim perspective Public education Join coalitions	Lobby Testify Vote

Many organizations, governmental offices, social service groups, community-based nonprofits, public health agencies, and advocacy groups play significant roles in ensuring the conditions for healthy populations. Schools of public health also have a role in this public health enterprise. There are at least four areas around which schools of public health (academic public health) can play an activist role in promoting public health, outlined in the following.

> **Many organizations, governmental offices, social service groups, community-based nonprofits, public health agencies, and advocacy groups play significant roles in ensuring the conditions for healthy populations.**

First, academic public health has a responsibility to generate scholarship around issues that are of direct relevance to public health practice. Rigorous scholarship must be aimed at informing the practical needs of public health practice—scholarship that applies the tools of science to inform the day-to-day workings of public health practitioners. Schools and programs must continue to engage their educational communities and those with whom they work and serve to better understand current issues, such as homelessness, gun control, and the opioid crisis. For example, as the public health practice world has grappled with emergency preparedness as part of its sphere of influence, substantial public health scholarship has considered how health system capacity can best be built to inform public health preparedness efforts.[71]

Second, building on the responsibility of academic public health to transmit knowledge, schools must continue to provide academic support for public health practice partners. Schools must build the capacity to effectively educate students across a broad range of sectors, ensure that educational opportunities are readily available and useful to practice partners, and continue to evolve educational offerings informed by the needs of public health practice.

Third, academic public health has a duty to develop innovative approaches to public health practice that can later be adopted by partners in practice communities. Academic institutions are not generally involved in direct service or program delivery. However, schools generate ideas that can serve to transform programs and projects that are then carried forward by practice partners.

The fourth element moves beyond the remit of public health practice to embrace all sectors that have a role in shaping the health of the public. It is now clearly understood that most of the drivers of population health are not within the control of traditional health sectors themselves. Urban planning, tax code structure, healthcare resource allocation, and the packaging of calorie-dense and nutrient-poor food all shape the health of the public. Decisions on these areas are all well outside the scope of public health practice, but they should not be outside academic public health. Schools must engage these areas to inform decisions that influence the health of populations. There is a rich academic scholarship in public health that articulates the centrality of nonhealth actors in influencing health, and schools should consider how to leverage academic assets to effect change.[72]

HOW DATA INFORM ADVOCACY AND ACTION TOWARD IMPROVING HEALTH

Qualitative and quantitative data can be used to generate compelling and powerful messages and stories that motivate others to take action toward improving health. Quantitative data can be used to define the scope of an issue, and qualitative data can be used to describe experiences or context; both types of data are important in strengthening messages and stories.

Incorporating data into messages must be done carefully and thoughtfully.[73,74] Three key questions are worth considering before including data in messaging that aims to engage others:

1. Why do we need data?
2. Are available data timely and relevant?
3. Are data understandable to all audiences?

We explore each question in more detail.

First, it is critical to think through why data are needed and how data can strengthen or make a better case for a health issue, program, or policy. Quantitative data are useful to convey the extent of a health problem or the reach of a health service (e.g., 3.9 million children gained access to healthy food through the Women, Infants, and Children [WIC] program the past year). Qualitative data can bring issues to life with testimonials and experiences from people not unlike those who might engage.

Second, the data used to promote advocacy and sustain public health action must be timely and relevant to the issue at hand. There are a number of public use data sets that can be useful to frame a particular issue. However, sometimes public use data do not exist or do not precisely address the issue; thus, data must be collected on an issue, program, or service. It is important to only include data that are relevant, relatable, and support the case. Although there may be many more data points, facts, and figures available, they should be included only if they are relevant. When data are cited, they should be referenced so that interested readers can find the source data and perhaps learn more about a particular issue.

Third, data inform advocacy and action as long as they are understandable. Data must be explained in culturally and linguistically appropriate ways. Visual presentations of data can be especially powerful, as people process visual data faster than they can digest tables of numbers or text descriptions of issues. However, data visualizations must also be carefully crafted so that they are understandable to all audiences. Basic charts are often the most effective for conveying trends over time, progress toward goals, or differences in achievement among groups.

EXAMPLES OF PUBLIC HEALTH ACTIONS INFORMED BY COLLECTIVE ACTION

An Institute of Medicine's Population Health Improvement Roundtable report points out that "some of the challenges to establishing population health derive from political and social concerns . . . [and] one of the hallmarks of the field is its attention to the social causes of disease and health."[75] This draws on the importance of social causes and roots of public health and, by extension, social movements. The report argues that research and action must go hand in hand in order to facilitate change, and that new technological developments such as electronic medical records or "big data" in the form of social media have the potential to integrate economic or social information into both research and policy change.

There is good academic literature on this issue.[76,77] Here we comment on two compelling case studies that provide useful thoughts looking forward, and an inquiry into how this applies to two issues of tremendous contemporary salience.

Perhaps most iconic in public health is the movement to change tobacco consumption that began in the 1950s and continued for the next several decades. This provides useful insights into the phases of change through broad social movements. Professor Constance Nathanson argued in 1999 that its relative success compared to many other movements had much to do with the persuasive use of information on health risks through grassroots mobilization for nonsmokers' rights[78] as well as with the weakness in the opposition.

The movement can be broken down into three main phases: the first phase, in which the health connection was made between tobacco and lung cancer, primarily in the medical press and including the famous Doll and Hill reports[79] and the 1964 Surgeon General's Report on Smoking and Health[80]; the second phase, the "struggle for regulation" in which Congress excluded tobacco from being regulated under several acts, and loopholes were used to create milder warning labels; and the third phase, the "discovery of innocent victims," in which the nonsmokers' rights movement was born and the Surgeon General urged the addition of a bill of rights for the nonsmokers to include a ban on smoking in all public spaces in 1971. Seen through this lens, restaurant smoking bans may have been due to nonsmokers' rights activism in conjunction with greater consumer sensitivity to health risks and media hyperbole. Nathanson's distillation that "in a society increasingly skeptical of experts and expert knowledge, it is critically important to develop agile institutional mechanisms that link population health science and practice . . . [because] research alone will not produce change" is particularly relevant. However, the work is not done on smoking—arguably public health's greatest achievement over the past century—and there are still many subpopulations with high prevalence of smoking even today,[81] but we have seen great strides over the past half-century, partially due to a social movement.

The story of change around motor vehicle safety is another great public health achievement of the past century. Health behavior change in populations around this issue was inseparable from denormalization of previously accepted behavior.[82,83] In particular, this example provides generalizable lessons about the elements of social norm transformation that can be leveraged toward change. Lawrence Green and Andrea Gielen[82] suggest that three key elements emerged to contribute to these changing norms around seat-belt use. First, public health initiatives provoke less controversy when they involve children compared to similar actions advocated for adults. To this point, child car-seat use was one of the aspects of vehicle safety that was adopted almost seamlessly compared to others. Second, many sectors, including health, transportation, and law enforcement, came together with community advocates to support legislation and education on car seats in the late 1980s. Third, media and social marketing were paramount in promoting vehicle safety. The National Highway Traffic Safety Administration conducted large public education programs that helped to shape public opinion and gather support to policy change. One of the most successful, and highly recognizable, campaigns is the "Click It or Ticket" slogan.[84] In 1984, seat belts were worn by only 15% of drivers, a figure that increased to 82% by 2007,[85] an extraordinary feat.

The story of change around motor vehicle safety is another great public health achievement of the past century.

What are the implications of observations for these two topics of contemporary resonance? What is the relevance for the battles in which population health must engage looking ahead toward creating the conditions that make people healthy?

Evidence of the health consequences of racism,[86] and the unconscionable and persistent health inequities in this country, is incontrovertible.[87] The Black Lives Matter movement has helped bring race relations to the forefront of public discussion[88] with the weight of moral urgency as instances of racism and injustice in the criminal justice system resound across the United States. This movement builds on long-standing racial inequities and has been compared to the civil rights movement.[89] Both movements are arguably predicated on the same core injustice; with the civil rights movement being catalyzed by voting rights and Black Lives Matter forming in response to institutionalized racism and treatment of African American/Black individuals by the justice system. In an echo of the social change paradigm, a group of Black Lives Matter activists published a set of specific policy recommendations called Campaign Zero,[90] which proposed policing changes and compared presidential candidates' positions on related issues with their potential outcomes. This approach aimed to mobilize a diverse organizational constituency and bring about a convergence of political opportunities with target vulnerabilities. In a more up-to-date twist than previous movements, social media and technology have played a key role in this movement thus far,[91] both mobilizing and spreading awareness and news of compelling current events.

Our brief look at two historically successful social movements, the antismoking and the car safety movements, provide lessons for current and future efforts. Success in this regard around the issue of racial inequity could serve to create a better, and indeed healthier, world.

EXAMPLE OF COLLECTIVE ACTION INFORMED BY PUBLIC HEALTH EVIDENCE AND ACTIVITY

Gun violence is among the preeminent public health challenges of our time, a belief shared by many in public health, and, hearteningly, an increasing number of people outside the field.[92] The growing acknowledgment that gun violence is a public health problem opens the door to public health solutions, and a commonsense, data-informed approach to this challenge, as the gun debate continues to unfold.

The extraordinary prevalence of firearm-related violence in the United States stands in harsh contrast with our peer nations. Between the Columbine High School shooting on April 20, 1999, and December 31, 2012, for example, there were 66 school shootings worldwide, of which 50 occurred in the United States. In 2015, the United States had the highest rates of firearm homicide (24.9 times higher than other nations) and firearm suicide (9.8 times higher than other nations) among 23 populous high-income nations.[93] Through 2021, a total of 693 mass shootings occurred across the nation, with 42 incidents being school shootings.[94] As time goes on, the issue prevails among our nation. On May 24, 2022, the third deadliest school shooting took place at Robb Elementary School in Uvalde, Texas, with 21 lives taken as dozens of well-armed responders delayed their entry into the school to confront the lone gunman.[95]

The United States clearly has a long and complicated relationship with firearms, and, constitutional rights aside, there are abundant organizations and large numbers of high-profile arguments on the side of unfettered firearm availability in this country.[96] But it seems worthwhile to set aside the rights argument for the moment and ask a simpler question: What is the role of public health in an issue that has clear public health consequences?

Even though arguments around the rights to gun ownership often center around self-protection from other firearms,[97] the evidence is overwhelmingly clear that this logic is not supported by the data. Extant studies on the risks of firearm availability on firearm deaths have provided clear evidence of an increased risk of both homicide and suicide.[98,99] A recent meta-analysis (meta-analysis is a type of statistical analysis that pools data from multiple smaller studies on a particular topic to build more precise estimates of association) of 16 observational studies,[100] conducted mostly in the United States, estimated that firearm access was associated with a threefold greater risk for suicide and a twofold greater risk for homicide compared to those without access. Women were at higher risk of homicide victimization compared to men.[99] In the case of firearm suicide, adolescents appear to be at particularly high risk, relative to adults. A 2013 study led by Michael Siegel found that U.S. states with higher estimated rates of gun ownership experienced a higher number of firearm-related homicides.[101] That study, covering 30 years (1981–2010), found a robust correlation between estimated levels of gun ownership and actual gun homicides at the state level, even when controlling for factors typically associated with homicides.

Another recent study examined the association between firearm legislation and U.S. firearm deaths by state between 2007 and 2010,[102] creating a "legislative strength score" based on five categories of legislative intent: curbing firearm trafficking, strengthening Brady background checks, improving child safety, banning military-style assault weapons, and restricting guns in public places. Higher legislative strength scores were associated with lower firearm mortality, and statistical models that accounted for sociodemographic and economic differences among states showed that, compared to those in the lowest quartile of legislative strength scores, those in the highest quartile had a lower firearm suicide rate and a lower firearm homicide rate (**Figure 14.3**).[102]

These studies are roundly supportive of causal relationships between firearm availability and firearm mortality and, conversely, of firearm legislation as protective against firearm deaths. Some concern about "reverse causation" explaining the relationship between firearm availability and firearm homicide has been raised, suggesting that gun availability increases as a reaction to rising homicide rates or personal threat. However, although some studies indicate that higher homicide rates may precede higher gun ownership,[98] this bias is unlikely to explain away a majority of the observed effect. In particular, it would likely not account for women and children—those most frequently affected by firearm homicide.[98] Importantly, by contrast, the literature on firearms and firearm-related suicide is not subject to the same potential of reverse causation,[99] but does suffer from a dearth of longitudinal studies.

These studies are roundly supportive of causal relationships between firearm availability and firearm mortality and, conversely, of firearm legislation as protective against firearm deaths.

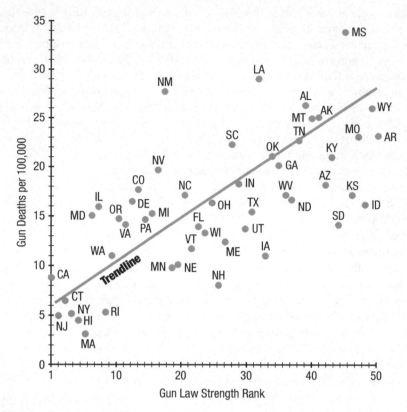

FIGURE 14.3 Firearm legislation and firearm-related fatalities in the United States.
Source: Data from Giffords Law Center to Prevent Gun Violence. https://giffords.org/lawcenter/resources/scorecard/

Despite the clear evidence that guns pose a threat to health, the public health community has been unable to get traction as an effective voice on this issue. While translatable lessons from successful public health campaigns on smoking,[103] unintentional poisonings, and car safety abound, the political will necessary to implement and test them has been absent and under unremitting attack. In Florida in 2011, physicians and other health practitioners were subject to legislation that, in effect, restricts discussion with patients on guns or gun safety (HB 155),[104] legislation that has been challenged but recently upheld in court.[105] Similar efforts have been pushed in other states. Moreover, while manufacturers of a wide range of products including cars, medications, and medical devices are subject to regulation and legal action that hold them accountable for product safety risks, gun manufacturers appear to be immune to such forces. Indeed, perhaps that lack of accountability contributes to the widespread availability of guns like the Bushmaster AR-15 semiautomatic rifle, used in the Sandy Hook massacre, which are designed explicitly to "deliver maximum carnage with extreme efficiency" and have no place in civilian settings.[106]

While acknowledging the broader issues around the balance of rights and privileges, and with a nod to the challenges embedded in thinking about paternalism in public health,[107] public health should be a clear voice against the legal widespread availability of a pathogen, firearms, that other peer nations have long conquered.

Would we tolerate such lapses in our legal response to other prevalent health challenges? Imagine for a moment that, because of emphatically articulated rights-based arguments, the United States remained alone among peer countries in not having automobile seat-belt laws and that our automobile death rate was sevenfold greater than that of Canada. Would that be tolerable?

The ultimate solution to the firearm epidemic does not lie with the doctors who treat firearm victims nor with the community-based providers who try to keep youths away from guns. It lies, rather, with policy makers and legislators. Public health plays a central role in engaging these stakeholders and other constituencies and sectors through clear and compelling data-driven research and scholarship. It is only then that we have any hope of turning the tide on what is truly a preventable epidemic.

We conclude with a case example that powerfully illustrates collective action and community resilience (Case Study 14.2; you can access the podcast accompanying Case Study 14.2 by following this link to Springer Publishing Company Connect™: http://connect.springerpub.com/content/book/978-0-8261-8043-8/part/part04/chapter/ch14).

CASE STUDY 14.2: CITIZEN ACTION FOR DISASTER MITIGATION

Life-saving community engagement represents a highly developed dimension of population health as individual citizens come together collectively with the common cause of ensuring mutual protection for all. This was exemplified by the experience of Fargo, North Dakota (population: 105,000), in 2009 when this city faced its most severe flood threat. Fargo accomplished something rare in the annals of disaster response—disaster prevention. The coordinated actions of tens of thousands of Fargo citizens, supplemented by volunteers from neighboring farming communities, completely prevented floodwaters from entering the city.

Fargo is located along the western flank of the Red River to the north. The Red River is unusual for several reasons. Even though North Dakota is in the far north of the continental United States, the Red River flows farther northward through Manitoba, Canada, and ultimately empties into Lake Winnipeg. Each year, the spring thaw threatens to flood the river cities located close to the headwaters of the Red River, including Fargo. The risk for severe flooding depends on the depth of the winter snow pack and how rapidly the thaw takes place.

The Red River is also geologically young with no deeply carved channel. The floodplain forms a broad shallow basin with virtually no gradient. Spring flooding is like filling a saucer as the slow-moving Red River swells sideways and fills vast expanses of farmland with frigid water.

Having experienced significant—and memorable—inundation during the historic 1997 Red River Flood, Fargo citizens and civic leaders devised communal strategies for protecting the city from future floods with sandbag dikes and levee fortifications. The most extreme challenge occurred in 2009 when the river rose to 24 feet above flood stage. The community activated all able-bodied persons. In local parlance, Fargoans transformed themselves into "flood fighters."

The 2009 flood fight relied on the strong backs and energized efforts of 85,000 individuals. Citizens and neighbors worked nonstop shifts inside the Fargo Dome, a large indoor football stadium that was repurposed for filling sandbags. Dubbed "Sandbag Central," the dome became the center of operations. To add to ranks, all secondary students in grades 8 through 12 were let out of school to take their turns at the sand piles. Through this collective activity, 8.5 million sandbags were filled and placed on pallets inside the dome. This was only the first part of the process.

Simultaneously, with remarkable precision, brigades of citizens were deployed to vulnerable sections of the riverbank, and to isolated homes and structures, where they were met by flatbed trucks hauling pallets of sandbags. Subfreezing temperatures are the norm in March and April, so sandbags had to be stored

(continued)

inside the heated stadium and then transported for a just-in-time rendezvous with the waiting teams. Parka-clad citizens had just minutes to stack the bags, while the sand remained sufficiently warm and malleable to sculpt into tight-packed levees. For weeks, Fargo's flood fighters braved blizzard conditions to construct sandbag fortifications. The levees required continuous monitoring.

Stress was palpable and rising steadily along with the river level. Fargoans knew that a single breech in the barricades would result in widespread flooding.

Fortunately, the levees did not fail, and the icy waters of the engorged Red River of the north were held back. In the end, aerial views showed Fargo appearing like a dry island encircled by a vast liquid landscape of floodwaters. Although the overflow of the Red River ringed the city on all sides for miles, Fargoans remained safely barricaded from the floodwaters.

Fargo achieved what is rarely possible—actual disaster prevention. Fargo was able to accomplish this feat for three reasons. First, it was possible to precisely predict the flood hazard in advance, in terms of time and place. Second, Fargo had devised effective disaster risk-reduction interventions to neutralize the flood threat. Third, Fargo citizens stepped up in a remarkable show of community resilience.

This strategy of community engagement was not viewed by locals in public health terms but rather as a survival strategy that had the desired result of protecting the town from catastrophic flooding. Invoking effective prevention measures can effectively short-circuit a disaster threat. This also averted a cascade of harmful public health consequences. Citizens were spared from exposures to glacially cold waters filling their homes and to the attendant damage, destruction, infrastructure disruption, resource loss, displacement, physical harm, and psychological distress.

Savvy to both stress and psychological distress inherent in the flood operation and the uncertainty of success during a year when the river reached record heights, Fargo developed contingency plans to shelter children, frail older adults, and other subpopulations of persons with special needs, as well as to maintain services and stockpile psychiatric medications for the subpopulation of persons with severe and persistent mental illness. The North Dakota director of medical services, a psychiatrist, was at the table with the mayor of Fargo, civic leaders, and emergency managers. He was frequently broadcasting messages on themes of resilience and positive coping to Fargo and Red River Valley communities via a range of media channels and identifying available resources and support services.

Having experienced widespread flooding in 1997, the citizens of Fargo responded with grit and determination to prevent a recurrence. Beginning in 1998, Fargo had 14 consecutive years when the Red River rose above flood stage, and every year the flood fighters prevented city flooding. The city has not flooded again. This year-over-year success of Fargo's citizens not only supports the public's health in times of disaster threat but has melded into the community's highly resilient and self-sufficient "floodplain identity."

SUMMARY

Public health has experienced a number of achievements over the past century, and none are attributable to any single entity. Public health action requires the engagement of many stakeholders including governmental public health agencies (which have the ultimate authority and responsibility), healthcare systems, community organizations, religious groups, employers, and so many others. Each plays a distinct but critically important role in producing health. Legal frameworks provide the infrastructure and support for public health, and the HiAP approach aims to make health central in policies across all sectors of the economy. HIA, where groups from all sectors collaborate to collect and analyze data on the ways in which new policies, regulations, and programs are effective in promoting health, is critical for ongoing improvements. And as new research emerges, knowledge is translated into action by engaged stakeholders using reciprocal, iterative approaches that are appropriately tailored to specific communities and groups. Yet, despite many achievements, there is much more to be done, and it will continue to require collective, coordinated engagement. Every individual, group, community, and organization can play a role by engaging and advocating for public health action.

End-of-Chapter Resources

Access additional case study podcasts online at http://connect.springerpub.com/ content/book/978-0-8261-8043-8/

DISCUSSION QUESTIONS

1. Consider the phrase "Think globally, act locally" with respect to public health issues. What does it mean to you and how might you apply this to a locally relevant public health issue?
2. Discuss the Black Lives Matter movement or the #MeToo movement through the lens of this chapter. What are the current strategies used by the movement? Are they successful? How can academic public health support this?
3. Consider potential strategies to advocate for gun control. Why do you think your strategy could be successful? What are the potential barriers or challenges?

SPRINGER PUBLISHING CONNECT™

A robust set of instructor resources designed to supplement this text is located at **http://connect.springerpub.com/content/book/978-0-8261-8043-8**. Qualifying instructors may request access by emailing **textbook@springerpub.com**.

REFERENCES

1. Institute of Medicine Committee on Assuring the Health of the Public in the 21st Century. *The Future of the Public's Health in the 21st Century*. National Academies Press; 2002. doi:10.17226/10548
2. The Pew Charitable Trusts. *Health impact project*. https://www.pewtrusts.org/en/projects/archived-projects/health-impact-project
3. World Health Organization. *WHO Kobe*. https://extranet.who.int/kobe_centre/en
4. Feuerstein S, Fortunati F, Morgan CA, Coric V, Temporini H, Southwick S. Civil commitment: a power granted to physicians by society. *Psychiatry (Edgmont)*. 2005;2(8):53-54. http://www.ncbi.nlm.nih.gov/pubmed/21152172
5. Public Health Law Center. *State & local public health: an overview of regulatory authority*. Published April 2015. https://www.publichealthlawcenter.org/resources/state-local-public-health-overview-regulatory-authority
6. Centers for Disease Control and Prevention. Achievements in public health, 1900-1999: changes in the public health system. *MMWR Morb Mortal Wkly Rep*. 1999;48(50):1141-1147. https://www.cdc.gov/mmwr/preview/mmwrhtml/mm4850a1.htm
7. Carter J, Slack M. Public health at the local, state, national, and global levels. In: Carter J, Slack M, eds. *Pharmacy in Public Health: Basics and Beyond*. American Society of Health-System Pharmacists; 2009.
8. Boston University School of Public Health. *Global health*. http://www.bu.edu/sph/about/departments/global-health
9. HIV/AIDS Bureau. *Who was Ryan White?* https://hab.hrsa.gov/about-ryan-white-hivaids-program/about-ryan-white-hivaids-program
10. Centers for Disease Control and Prevention. *Public Health Financing*. Author; 2013. https://www.cdc.gov/publichealthgateway/docs/finance/public_health_financing-6-17-13.pdf

11. Centers for Disease Control and Prevention. Ten great public health achievements—United States, 1900-1999. *MMWR Morb Mortal Wkly Rep.* 1999;*48*(12):241-243. https://www.cdc.gov/mmwr/preview/mmwrhtml/00056796.htm

12. Goodman RA, Moulton A, Matthews G, et al. Law and public health at CDC. *MMWR Suppl.* 2006;*55*:29-33. https://www.cdc.gov/mmwr/preview/mmwrhtml/su5502a11.htm#tab1

13. UK Parliament. *The 1848 Public Health Act.* https://www.parliament.uk/about/living-heritage/transformingsociety/towncountry/towns/tyne-and-wear-case-study/about-the-group/public-administration/the-1848-public-health-act/#:~:text=The%20Act%20established%20a%20Central,removal%20of%20nuisances%20and%20paving

14. Alderslade R. The Public Health Act of 1848. The act's qualities of imagination and determination are still needed today. *BMJ.* 1998;*317*(7158):549-550. doi:10.1136/bmj.317.7158.549

15. Fee E, Brown TM. The Public Health Act of 1848. *Bull World Health Organ.* 2005;*83*(11):866-867. https://apps.who.int/iris/handle/10665/269524

16. Calman K. The 1848 Public Health Act and its relevance to improving public health in England now. *BMJ.* 1998;*317*(7158):596-598. doi:10.1136/BMJ.317.7158.596

17. Grynbaum MM. *New York's ban on big sodas is rejected by final court. New York Times.* Published June 27, 2014. https://www.nytimes.com/2014/06/27/nyregion/city-loses-final-appeal-on-limiting-sales-of-large-sodas.html?_r=2

18. Science Museum Group. *Sir Edwin Chadwick 1800–1890.* https://collection.sciencemuseumgroup.org.uk/people/cp159375/edwin-chadwick

19. Fidler DP. International law and global public health. *Univ Kansas Law Rev.* 1999;*48*(1):652. https://www.repository.law.indiana.edu/cgi/viewcontent.cgi?referer=&httpsredir=1&article=1655&context=facpub

20. legislation.gov.uk. *Public Health Act (Northern Ireland) 1967.* http://www.legislation.gov.uk/apni/1967/36/contents

21. Publications Quebec. *Public Health Act.* http://legisquebec.gouv.qc.ca/en/ShowDoc/cs/S-2.2

22. Rudolph L, Caplan J. *Health in All Policies: A Guide for State and Local Government.* Public Health Institute; 2013. https://www.phi.org/thought-leadership/health-in-all-policies-a-guide-for-state-and-local-government/

23. World Health Organization, Government of South Australia, Adelaide. *Adelaide Statement on Health in All Policies.* 2010. https://apps.who.int/iris/handle/10665/44365

24. Public Health Association of BC. *ActNow BC.* http://www.actnowbc.ca

25. National Prevention Council. *National Prevention Strategy.* Department of Health and Human Services; 2011. https://www.hhs.gov/sites/default/files/disease-prevention-wellness-report.pdf

26. YouTube. *Molly Ivins speaks at Tulane.* https://www.youtube.com/watch?v=alWkzljdv3E

27. Galea S. *Macrosocial Determinants of Population Health.* Springer; 2007. doi:10.1007/978-0-387-70812-6

28. ushistory.org. *Economic policy.* http://www.ushistory.org/gov/11c.asp

29. Rice D. *175 nations sign historic Paris climate deal on Earth Day. USA TODAY.* Published April 22, 2016. https://www.usatoday.com/story/news/world/2016/04/22/paris-climate-agreement-signing-united-nations-new-york/83381218

30. Barnes R. *Supreme Court rules gay couples nationwide have a right to marry. Washington Post.* Published June 25, 2015. https://www.washingtonpost.com/politics/gay-marriage-and-other-major-rulings-at-the-supreme-court/2015/06/25/ef75a120-1b6d-11e5-bd7f-4611a60dd8e5_story.html?utm_term=.4577642c94a0

31. Thirteen/WNET. *Jim Crow stories.* https://www.thirteen.org/wnet/jimcrow/stories_events_election.html

32. History.com. *Reconstruction.* Published October 29, 2009. https://www.history.com/topics/american-civil-war/reconstruction

33. Waugh J. *Ulysses S. Grant: domestic affairs.* Miller Center. https://millercenter.org/president/grant/domestic-affairs

34. *Ulysses S. Grant and civil rights.* Grant Monument Association. https://grantstomb.org

35. History.com. *Ku klux klan.* May 30, 2012. https://www.history.com/topics/reconstruction/ku-klux-klan-video

36. U.S. National Park Service. *Grant and the 15th Amendment.* https://www.nps.gov/articles/ulysses-s-grant-the-15th-amendment.htm#:~:text="While%20strongly%20favoring%20the%20course,ratified%20on%20February%203%2C%201870

37. PBS/WSKG. *Passage of the Fifteenth Amendment.* http://www.pbs.org/wgbh/americanexperience/features/grant-fifteenth

38. History.com. *Compromise of 1877.* https://www.history.com/topics/us-presidents/compromise-of-1877

39. Thirteen/WNET. *The rise and fall of Jim Crow.* https://www.thirteen.org/wnet/jimcrow

40. American Public Health Association. *The impact of racism on the health and well-being of the nation.* https://www.apha.org/events-and-meetings/webinars/racism-and-health

41. Silverstein J. *How racism is bad for our bodies. The Atlantic.* Published March 12, 2013. https://www.theatlantic.com/health/archive/2013/03/how-racism-is-bad-for-our-bodies/273911

42. History.com. *Black codes.* June 1, 2010. https://www.history.com/topics/black-history/black-codes

43. U.S. history.org. *Rebuilding the old order.* http://www.ushistory.org/us/35d.asp

44. Wikipedia. *1964 United States presidential election.* https://en.wikipedia.org/wiki/1964_United_States_presidential_election

45. WhiteHouse.gov. *Lyndon B. Johnson*. https://www.whitehouse.gov/about-the-white-house/presidents/lyndon-b-johnson/

46. Biography.com. *Barry Goldwater biography*. https://www.biography.com/people/barry-goldwater-9314846

47. WhiteHouse.com. *Statement by the Press Secretary on the President John F. Kennedy assassination records*. Published 2017. https://www.presidency.ucsb.edu/documents/statement-the-press-secretary-the-president-john-f-kennedy-assassination-records

48. History. *Civil Rights Act of 1964*. January 4, 2010. https://www.history.com/topics/black-history/civil-rights-act

49. Medicare.gov. *Medicare.gov: the official U.S. government site for Medicare*. https://www.medicare.gov

50. Medicaid.gov. *Medicaid home*. https://www.medicaid.gov

51. The Leadership Conference on Civil and Human Rights. *VRA anniversary letter to House Judiciary Chairman Bob Goodlatte*. Published August 10, 2015. http://civilrights.org/resource/vra-anniversary-letter-to-house-judiciary-chairman-bob-goodlatte

52. Tumulty K. *The great society at 50. Washington Post*. May 17, 2014. https://www.washingtonpost.com/sf/national/2014/05/17/the-great-society-at-50/?utm_term=.d6f3006f79a5

53. Zelizer J. *A 1965 failure that still haunts America*. CNN. Published January 19, 2015. https://www.cnn.com/2015/01/19/opinion/zelizer-lbj-watts-riots

54. PBS/WSKG. *Johnson's war. American experience*. http://www.pbs.org/wgbh/americanexperience/features/lbj-johnsons-war

55. YouTube. *LBJ state of union war on poverty*. https://www.youtube.com/watch?v=qfT03Ihtlds

56. Boston University School of Public Health. *Social justice, public health*. May 15, 2016. https://www.bu.edu/sph/2016/05/15/social-justice-public-health

57. Walsh KT. *The most consequential elections in history: Lyndon Johnson and the election of 1964. US News*. https://www.usnews.com/news/articles/2008/09/17/the-most-consequential-elections-in-history-lyndon-johnson-and-the-election-of-1964

58. MSNBC. *On groundhog day, republicans vote to repeal Obamacare*. February 2, 2016. http://www.msnbc.com/rachel-maddow-show/groundhog-day-republicans-vote-repeal-obamacare

59. *Healthcare reform paper*. https://assets.donaldjtrump.com/HCReformPaper.pdf

60. HHS.gov. *About the Affordable Care Act*. https://www.hhs.gov/healthcare/about-the-aca/index.html

61. Boston University School of Public Health. *The present and future uninsured*. Published October 25, 2015. http://www.bu.edu/sph/2015/10/25/the-present-and-future-uninsured

62. MarketWatch. *The Brexit vote: everything you need to know about the referendum*. Published June 23, 2016. https://www.marketwatch.com/story/the-brexit-vote-everything-you-need-to-know-about-the-referendum-2016-06-07

63. Sundby A. *Brexit result shocks some voters who wanted U.K. to leave European Union*. CBS Interactive. Published June 24, 2016. https://www.cbsnews.com/news/brexit-result-shocks-voters-uk-leave-european-union

64. HealthyPeople.gov. *Disparities*. November 20, 2012. http://www.healthypeople.gov/2020/about/disparitiesAbout.aspx

65. Rollins R. U. S. Department of Health & Human Services. *The National Partnership for Action to End Health Disparities*. Published December 2, 2011. www.nichd.nih.gov/sites/default/files/about/meetings/2011/Documents/rollins_rural_health_120211.pdf

66. Straus SE, Tetroe J, Graham I. Defining knowledge translation. *CMAJ*. 2009;*181*(3-4):165-168. doi:10.1503/cmaj.081229

67. The Canadian Institutes of Health Research. *About us*. http://www.cihr-irsc.gc.ca/e/29418.html

68. Centers for Disease Control and Prevention. *Applying the Knowledge to Action (K2A) Framework: Questions to Guide Planning*. Author; 2014. https://www.cdc.gov/chronicdisease/pdf/k2a-framework-6-2015.pdf

69. Bassett MT. Public health advocacy. *Am J Public Health*. 2003;*93*(8):1204. https://www.ncbi.nlm.nih.gov/pmc/articles/PMC1447936

70. Christoffel KK. Public health advocacy: process and product. *Am J Public Health*. 2000;*90*(5):722-726. http://www.ncbi.nlm.nih.gov/pubmed/10800420

71. Walsh L, Craddock H, Gulley K, et al. Building health care system capacity to respond to disasters: successes and challenges of disaster preparedness health care coalitions. *Prehosp Disaster Med*. 2015;*30*(02):112-122. doi:10.1017/S1049023X14001459

72. Schoeni RF, House JS, Kaplan GA, Pollack HA. *Making Americans Healthier: Social and Economic Policy as Health Policy*. Russell Sage Foundation; 2008.

73. Women, Infants, and Children. U.S. Department of Agriculture Food and Nutrition Service. https://www.fns.usda.gov/wic/women-infants-and-children-wic

74. U.S. Department of Agriculture. *Evidence-based WIC advocacy: using data*. Published March 2018. https://media.nwica.org/2018-wic-evidence-based-wic-advocacy.pdf

75. National Academy of Sciences. *Roundtable on population health improvement*. http://www.nationalacademies.org/hmd/Activities/PublicHealth/PopulationHealthImprovementRT.aspx

76. Nathanson CA. *Disease Prevention as Social Change: The State, Society, and Public Health in the United States, France, Great Britain, and Canada*. Russell Sage Foundation; 2009.

77. Lefebvre RC. *Social Marketing and Social Change: Strategies and Tools for Health, Well-Being, and the Environment*. Jossey-Bass; 2013.

78. Nathanson CA. Social movements as catalysts for policy change: the case of smoking and guns. *J Health Polit Policy Law*. 1999;*24*(3):421-488. doi:10.1215/03616878-24-3-421

79. Doll R, Hill AB. The mortality of doctors in relation to their smoking habits; a preliminary report. *Br Med J*. 1954;*1*(4877):1451-1455. http://www.ncbi.nlm.nih.gov/pubmed/13160495

80. Public Health Service, Office of the Surgeon General. *Smoking and Health*. 1964. https://profiles.nlm.nih.gov/spotlight/nn/catalog/nlm:nlmuid-101584932X202-doc

81. Brown DW. Smoking prevalence among US veterans. *J Gen Intern Med*. 2010;*25*(2):147-149. doi:10.1007/s11606-009-1160-0

82. Kahan S, Gielen AC, Fagan PJ, Green LW. *Health Behavior Change in Populations*. Johns Hopkins University Press; 2014.

83. Boston University School of Public Health. June 14, 2015. *Making the acceptable unacceptable*. http://www.bu.edu/sph/2015/06/14/making-the-acceptable-unacceptable

84. National Highway Traffic Safety Administration. *Seat belts*. https://www.nhtsa.gov/risky-driving/seat-belts

85. Government Accountability Office. *Traffic safety: improved reporting and performance measures would enhance evaluation of high-visibility campaigns*. GAO-08-477. Published April 25, 2008. https://www.gao.gov/products/gao-08-477

86. Boston University School of Public Health. *Racism and the health of the public*. May 3, 2015. http://www.bu.edu/sph/2015/05/03/racism-and-the-health-of-the-public

87. Boston University School of Public Health. *On health inequalities*. June 7, 2015. http://www.bu.edu/sph/2015/06/07/on-health-inequalities

88. John E, Perez-Pena R. *University of Missouri protests spur a day of change*. New York Times. November 10, 2015. https://www.nytimes.com/2015/11/10/us/university-of-missouri-system-president-resigns.html

89. Harris FC. *The next civil rights movement?* Dissent Magazine. Published 2015. https://www.dissentmagazine.org/article/black-lives-matter-new-civil-rights-movement-fredrick-harris/#:~:text=Unlike%20the%20civil%20rights%20movement,insistence%20on%20black%20humanity%20has

90. Campaign Zero. *Our Work*. https://www.joincampaignzero.org/solutions

91. Stephen B. *Social media helps Black Lives Matter fight the power*. Published 2015. https://www.wired.com/2015/10/how-black-lives-matter-uses-social-media-to-fight-the-power

92. Kristof N, Marsh B (Graphics). *New York Times. How to reduce shootings*. November 6, 2017. https://www.nytimes.com/interactive/2017/11/06/opinion/how-to-reduce-shootings.html

93. Grinshteyn E, Hemenway D. Violent death rates in the US compared to those of the other high-income countries, 2015. *Prev Med*. 2019;*123*:20-26. doi:10.1016/j.ypmed.2019.02.026

94. Cox JW, Rich S, Chiu A, et al. *More than 356,000 students have experienced gun violence at school since Columbine*. The Washington Post. Published April 20, 2018. https://www.washingtonpost.com/graphics/2018/local/school-shootings-database/

95. Galea S. *POV: The killing we continue to fail to stop*. BU Today. Published May 25, 2022. https://www.bu.edu/articles/2022/pov-we-continue-to-fail-to-stop-gun-violence/?utm_campaign=bu_today&utm_source=email_20220526&utm_medium=intrograph&utm_content=opinion

96. Second Amendment Foundation. *Second Amendment Foundation*. https://www.saf.org

97. ConstitutionAlly. *ConstitutionAlly Home Page*. https://constitutionalrightspac.com/index

98. Hepburn LM, Hemenway D. Firearm availability and homicide: a review of the literature. *Aggress Violent Behav*. 2004;*9*(4):417-440. doi:10.1016/S1359-1789(03)00044-2

99. Miller M, Hemenway D. The relationship between firearms and suicide: a review of the literature. *Aggress Violent Behav*. 1999;*4*(1):59-75. doi:10.1016/S1359-1789(97)00057-8

100. Anglemyer A, Horvath T, Rutherford G. The accessibility of firearms and risk for suicide and homicide victimization among household members: a systematic review and meta-analysis. *Ann Intern Med*. 2014;*160*(2):101-110. doi:10.7326/M13-1301

101. Siegel M, Ross CS, King C. The relationship between gun ownership and firearm homicide rates in the United States, 1981-2010. *Am J Public Health*. 2013;*103*(11):2098-2105. doi:10.2105/AJPH.2013.301409

102. Fleegler EW, Lee LK, Monuteaux MC, Hemenway D, Mannix R. Firearm legislation and firearm-related fatalities in the United States. *JAMA Intern Med*. 2013;*173*(9):732-740. doi:10.1001/jamainternmed.2013.1286

103. Mozaffarian D, Hemenway D, Ludwig DS. Curbing gun violence: lessons from public health successes. *JAMA*. 2013;*309*(6):551-552. doi:10.1001/jama.2013.38

104. Florida House of Representatives. *CS/CS/HB 155—privacy of firearm owners*. 2011. https://www.myfloridahouse.gov/Sections/Bills/billsdetail.aspx?BillId=44993

105. SphericalXS. *NRA wins over free speech—Florida doctors silenced on guns by court*. Daily KOS. July 30, 2014. https://www.dailykos.com/stories/2014/07/30/1317592/-NRA-Wins-Over-Free-Speech-Florida-Doctors-Silenced-On-Guns-By-Court

106. Boston University School of Public Health. *A hate crime against LGBT communities, with weapons of war*. June 19, 2016. https://www.bu.edu/sph/news/articles/2016/a-hate-crime-against-lgbt-communities-with-weapons-of-war/

107. Jones MM, Bayer R. Paternalism and its discontents: motorcycle helmet laws, libertarian values, and public health. *Am J Public Health*. 2007;*97*(2):208-217. doi:10.2105/AJPH.2005.083204

15

PUBLIC HEALTH IN A COMPLEX WORLD: SYSTEMS THINKING AND IMPLEMENTATION SCIENCE

Salma M. Abdalla also contributed to this chapter

LEARNING OBJECTIVES

- Explain why public health science and practice need to view populations as complex.
- List analysis methods applicable to research on populations as complex systems.
- Discuss the concept of policy resistance in the context of public health interventions.
- Discuss how politics, funding, communication, and logistics determine the success of implementation of public health interventions.
- Explain weak points in the implementation chain.
- Compare and contrast different healthcare systems around the globe.

OVERVIEW: POPULATIONS AS COMPLEX SYSTEMS

The global obesity epidemic is on the rise despite the enormous investment in research and campaigns to combat it. Traditional public health initiatives—the majority of which focus on individual behavior—have yet to successfully reduce the burden of the epidemic. At first glance, factors that lead an individual to becoming obese are simple; your weight is determined by what you eat, how much you eat, and whether you exercise or not. But that is not the full story: many factors influence an individual's weight ranging from genetics and paternal obesity to policies. What you eat and whether you exercise are influenced by your educational level and income, the availability of grocery stories in the neighborhood you live in, and the built environment that promotes or hinders walking and exercise. Moreover, eating behaviors are affected by policies that regulate marketing and taxation of highly processed food or subsidies for certain agricultural products among other factors. A closer examination shows that the health outcome "obesity" is clearly not the product of a linear causal process but rather a complex system of multiple, diverse, and interconnected factors.[1]

Public health is concerned with studying the health outcomes of groups, including the distribution of health outcomes within these groups. Our dominant methodological approach in public health, which reduces systems to their simplest component and applies principally linear methods to understand the relation between potential causal factors and health indicators, has yielded substantial public health success. There is, however, a growing appreciation of the challenges of this approach, particularly as we recognize the need to address multiple factors within complex system frameworks in order to improve health. In this chapter, we (a) discuss what complex systems are and how the work of public health has to be concerned with complex systems, (b) describe how to construct a logic model that can describe the complex problem that requires public health action, (c) present examples of how the application of complex system approaches can help improve the health of the public, (d) outline the core tenets of implementation science and why they are critical to public health action, (e) identify fragile points in the implementation chain where interventions can fail, and (f) analyze how public health systems can be built to create stronger paths to implementation.

> **Public health is concerned with studying the health outcomes of groups, including the distribution of health outcomes within these groups.**

POPULATION CHARACTERISTICS

Generally, the word *population* is used to describe a collection of people, or other organisms, that share a specific location they inhabit. However, populations can also be defined through other organizational characteristics. Populations are more than a random collection of individuals. Keyes and Galea propose two conditions to define a population: (a) a population must have more than one individual and (b) individuals within a population must share at least one common characteristic.[2] Most populations are changeable targets with individuals moving in and out of the defining characteristics (e.g., geographic area, a health condition, or an age group along the life course) of the population. People may also be lost from a population through death. Hence, at any moment in time, the composition of a population is dynamic and changeable.

COMPLEX SYSTEMS

Complexity exists in all levels of nature from the subatomic level to the population level and beyond. Our brains, living cells, immune system, the financial markets, and ecosystems are all complex systems. These systems are complex because they are composed of heterogeneous individual agents with numerous relationships and interactions. The nature of these interactions has an effect on the overall behavior of the system and how the system ultimately self-organizes. Complex systems may exhibit nonlinearity in the behaviors of its agents. Such systems are characterized by feedback loops in which small changes in an individual agent can lead to remarkable system-wide effects that cannot solely be explained by the change in the individual agent. Another key feature of complex systems is that they are adaptive. This means that complex systems do not passively respond to events or interventions but rather reorganize into a new equilibrium following insults, impacts, or interventions. For example, our brains reorganize to learn from experiences, and species evolve to create a new ecosystem in response to climate change. Because of all these features, complex systems are characterized by nonlinearity in their dynamics, randomness, and emergence.[3,4]

POPULATIONS AS COMPLEX SYSTEMS

Populations exhibit properties of complex systems as they are more than the sum of their parts. Individuals within a population do not behave in a linear way; they interact with one another, building relationships and networks. Individuals dynamically self-organize, evolve, and adapt. They respond haphazardly to rules and often create subcultures of their own that can be resilient to imposed changes.[5] Moreover, a multitude of interacting factors (e.g., political, economic, and social) influence the health of a population. These interrelations are temporally dependent and characterized by nonlinearity, feedback loops, and trade-offs.[6]

A COMPLEX SYSTEM APPROACH TO UNDERSTAND THE HEALTH OF POPULATIONS

HOW TO CONSTRUCT A LOGIC MODEL DESCRIBING A COMPLEX PROBLEM THAT REQUIRES PUBLIC HEALTH ACTION

Logic models are simplified visual illustrations of complex problems or interventions. Models explain the logical flow and links that connect different components of an issue. Visual models and diagrams organize our thinking on complex issues and can be used to identify appropriate public health actions. Logic models can range from simple to very complex. All logic models ultimately aim to introduce interested parties to a common language, a point of reference, and a road map of the sequence of events leading to the desired results. Logic models present an understanding of the relationship among different components of an issue, the activities planned to address the issue, and the expected results.

> **Visual models and diagrams organize our thinking on complex issues and can be used to identify appropriate public health actions.**

There are two major components of every logic model: planned work and intended results. Planned work includes (a) resources or inputs—such as human or financial resources—available to be directed toward addressing a problem and (b) activities that refer to what we do with the resources. The intended results component consists of (a) outputs, the direct results of actions; (b) outcomes, the specific short-term or longer-term changes in behavior, knowledge, skills, or level of functioning; and (c) impact, the overarching change in the system, either intended or unintended, over the upcoming decade. Logic models follow the "if . . . then" reasoning and are to be read from top to bottom (**Table 15.1**) or, in other depictions, from left to right (moving forward in time).

EXAMPLES SHOWING THE USE OF COMPLEX SYSTEM APPROACHES TO IMPROVE THE HEALTH OF THE PUBLIC

A complex system approach can enhance public health interventions through accounting for the interconnected elements of a population that both determine, and are determined by, health indicators and can ultimately affect health outcomes.

Adopting a complex system approach to study the spread of infectious diseases was one of the earliest applications of the concept in public health. The course of infectious disease transmission is the result of complex interactions between biology, the environment, and society. Using a complex system approach helped move theories of infectious diseases from simplistic temporal

TABLE 15.1 How to Read a Logic Model

	STEPS	STEP NAME	EXPLANATION
Your planned work	1 ▼	Resources/inputs	Certain resources are needed to operate your program.
	2 ▼	Activities	**IF** you have access to resources and inputs, **THEN** you can use them to accomplish your planned activities.
Your intended results	3 ▼	Outputs	**IF** you accomplish your planned activities, **THEN** you hope to deliver the amount of product and/or service that you intended.
	4 ▼	Outcomes	**IF** you accomplish your planned activities to the extent you intended and generate the desired outputs, **THEN** your participants will benefit in certain ways.
	5	Impact	**IF** these outcomes—in terms of benefits to participants—are achieved, **THEN** certain changes in organizations, communities, or systems might be expected to occur.

Source: Data from W.K. Kellog Foundation Program Staff. *Using Logic Models to Bring Together Planning, Evaluation, and Action: Logic Model Development Guide.* W.K. Kellogg Foundation; 2004. https://www.naccho.org/uploads/down loadable-resources/Programs/Public-Health-Infrastructure/KelloggLogicModelGuide_161122_162808.pdf

models to frameworks that recognized the significance of geography, travel patterns, social interactions, and nonrational behavior in the spread of infectious diseases. Over time, applications of a complex system approach to infectious diseases ranged from describing the dynamics of the spread of diseases to testing the impact of control strategies. For example, using a complex system approach led to identifying the role of social connections in the transmission of HIV. Studies found that social networks and their interactions with other population characteristics largely determine the dominant method of contact that spreads HIV in a population.[7]

The Models of Infectious Disease Agent Study (MIDAS) is one example of a collaborative modeling network to control infectious diseases. MIDAS uses computational, statistical, and mathematical models to understand the dynamics of infectious diseases and ultimately help populations detect, prepare for, and respond to threats of infectious diseases.[8]

The use of a complex system approach in public health is not limited to communicable or infectious diseases. Behaviors driving noncommunicable diseases (NCDs) are increasingly identified as products of complex systems.[9] Picking up from where we started the chapter, there have been multiple attempts to look at the obesity epidemic through a complex system lens. For example, the government of the United Kingdom adopted a complex system approach to respond to rising levels of obesity in the country and initiated the Foresight project.[10] The project included over 300 experts from different disciplines to produce a 40-year plan to combat the epidemic. The final report modeled the "central engine" of obesity as a function of four key variables: primary appetite control, dietary habits, physical activity, and psychological ambivalence. The model (**Figure 15.1**) shows how these four variables and their subcomponents represent a

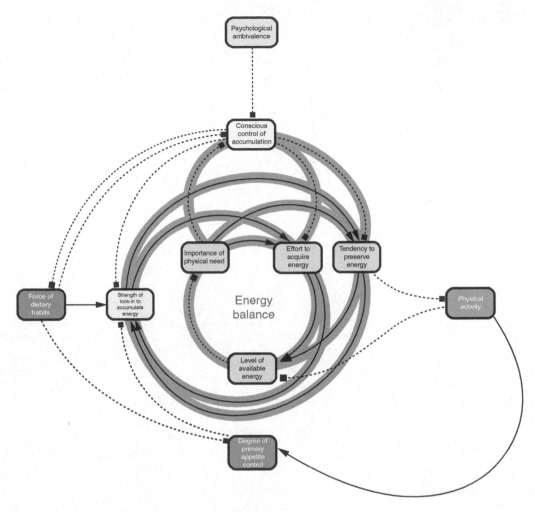

FIGURE 15.1 Four key variables that act as a control engine for obesity.
Source: GOV.UK. Tackling obesities: future choices. Published October 17, 2007. https://www.gov.uk/government/collections/tackling-obesities-future-choices

complex system of causal influences. Importantly, this central engine is a small subset of a much larger complex system (**Figure 15.2**), which includes different domains such as social psychology, activity environment, and food production.

Another example of using a complex system approach in public health is in the realm of tobacco control. Tobacco use is one of the most preventable causes of death, but tobacco control is also one of the biggest success stories of public health addressing complex systems. Even though traditional methods were very successful in identifying a causal chain between tobacco use and disability and death, gradually, scientists began to understand the need for complex system approaches for tobacco control as tobacco use and addiction are shaped by many interacting individual and organizational factors. For example, the National Cancer Institute (NCI) created a causal map to illustrate some of the feedback loops (they identified more than 1,900) among smokers, tobacco growers, the public health field, governments, and the tobacco industry (**Figure 15.3**).

Moreover, it is becoming increasingly clear that tobacco control efforts likely have complicated—and sometimes unintended—consequences on political and economic systems, in

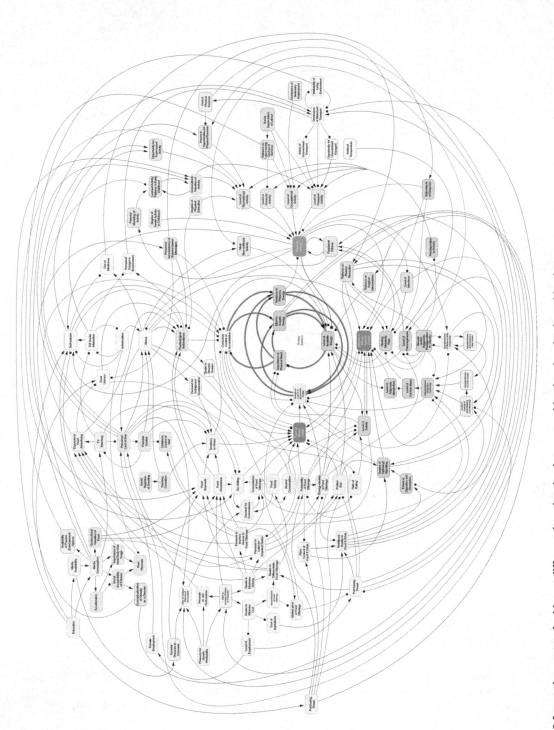

FIGURE 15.2 A complex system looking at different domains that interact and lead to the obesity epidemic.

Source: From Gov.UK. Tackling obesities: future choices. Published October 17, 2007. https://www.gov.uk/government/collections/tackling-obesities-future-choices

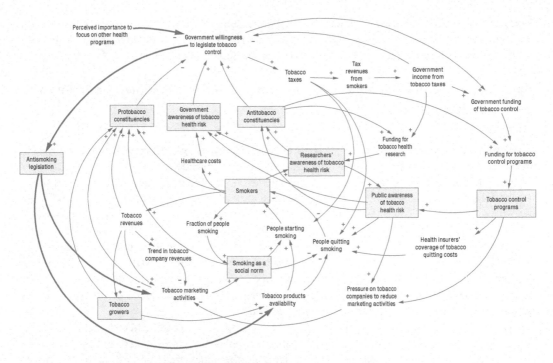

FIGURE 15.3 Feedback loops in a system dynamics model of tobacco control.
Source: Reproduced with permission from Best A, Tenkasi R, Trochim W, et al. Systemic transformational change in tobacco control: an overview of the Initiative for the Study and Implementation of Systems (ISIS). In: Casebeer AL, Harrison A, Mark AL, eds. *Innovations in Health Care: A Reality Check.* Palgrave Macmillan; 2006:189–205.

addition to population health. These consequences include, but are not limited to, changes in healthcare costs, employment, budgets on both state and local levels, and health disparities.[7]

AN OVERVIEW OF THE METHODS OF ANALYSIS APPLICABLE TO COMPLEX SYSTEMS

Many public health analyses apply linear methods to investigate relationships between potential causal factors and health outcomes. These methods treat the pervasive characteristics of populations as additional variables to be controlled for rather than influential properties in their own right.[5] There is no question that these methods have yielded major successes over the past century. Nonetheless, there is a growing appreciation of limitations of these approaches and the need to identify methods that simultaneously investigate multiple causes of health outcomes in a population. There are a number of methods that factor the different levels of characteristics of a population into the analysis of a complex public health issue. We focus on two methods in this chapter: social network analysis and agent-based modeling.

Social network analysis characterizes network structures, or a subset of a network, to understand their effects on behaviors and health outcomes. Social network analysis focuses on the patterns and implications of relationships on social actors. Hence, it is most valuable in studying population-level outcomes when relational characteristics are implicated in the behavior of networked individuals. Social network analysis has been used for understanding the social contagion of obesity, smoking, alcohol use, and back pain, among others.[11] For example, a social network analysis has shown that noticeable clusters of obese persons extend to three degrees of separation; in the analysis, a person's chances of becoming obese increased by 57% if they had a friend who became obese in the time interval. A comparably high percentage increase in obesity was found among siblings over fixed periods of time. Social network analysis can also be used to assess the role of social network structures as a determinant of health inequities on a population level. For example, obesity may spread faster and more comprehensively among ethnic minorities than their White counterparts as they have higher density social networks.[12]

Social network analysis focuses on the patterns and implications of relationships on social actors.

Agent-based models (ABMs) are computer simulations of agents, over simulated time, in simulated space. ABMs have gained traction over the past decade because they present an opportunity to study health determinants at multiple levels of influence that might pair with social interactions to produce population health. Because they allow for feedback, reciprocity between exposures, and interrelation between causes, ABMs can be used for complex system analysis.[11] For example, one review developed an ABM of the influence of social and behavioral factors on obesity and cardiovascular diseases. The review simulated the effect of a policy of investing in healthy food stores in neighborhoods on changes in body mass index (BMI) over time in relation to strength of social network ties. The review found that the policy intervention had a more rapid and greater maximum impact under weak network ties. However, stronger network ties led to more persistent results, which took longer to dissipate.[1]

Other methods compatible with a complex system approach to public health include systems dynamics models and microsimulations. Systems dynamics models represent the real world by dividing the population into categories and using mathematical representations of how these categories interact.[13] A microsimulation model simulates individuals within a population to understand variations in disease-relevant characteristics among individuals and how these characteristics produce a population distribution of health outcomes.[14] While the public health field is starting to use complex system analyses to shape interventions and policies, complex system analysis methods, such as the ones outlined in this chapter, remain underutilized in public health training and practice.[7]

POLICY RESISTANCE AND THE LIMITATIONS OF OUR UNDERSTANDING

Because many of the issues targeted by public health are complex and can sometimes overwhelm our ability to understand them, we often fail to discover the distal impacts of interventions. The limitation of our understanding usually leads to generating unintended consequences, side effects, or "policy resistance" for seemingly well-designed public health policies or programs. Policy resistance refers to the "tendency for interventions to be defeated by the system's response to the intervention itself."[15] Policy resistance often arises from a mismatch between the complexity of systems we aim to study and intervene on, and our capacity to understand these systems. While the world is dynamic, interconnected, and evolving, we continue to use static and reductionist models to intervene. A decision taken on by one actor within a system can have a ripple effect across the entire system. Moreover, on the opposite side, acting on multiple actors may have lesser effect than expected.[15]

There are many examples of policy resistance or unintended consequences of public health interventions attributable to the lack of understanding a system's dimensions when designing a policy or a program. For example, following the widespread use of highly effective antiretroviral treatment that dramatically reduced mortality rate among persons living with HIV infection, there was an increase in risky behaviors and unprotected sex.[16] Moreover, while the widespread use of antibiotics without much regulation created a dramatic shift in medical care and increased life expectancy, we are now faced with the rise of drug-resistant pathogens.[17] The increase in risky driving following the introduction of antilock brakes is another example.[18]

ON THE NEED FOR TRANSDISCIPLINARY APPROACHES TO UNDERSTAND COMPLEX POPULATION HEALTH SYSTEMS

Many of the determinants of population health and the drivers of health inequities have social, economic, and environmental causes that extend beyond the direct influence of the health sector. This means that understanding the complexity of population health systems requires adopting approaches from multiple disciplines and sectors. The health sector alone does not have the needed knowledge, tools, capacity, and budget to address the complex causes of health in a population.[19]

Consider the complexity inherent in bringing transdisciplinary approaches to the protection of special medical needs patients—including safeguarding their life-sustaining care—when confronted by disasters and extreme events. Case Study 15.1 examines the intersection of four elements: (a) climate change making (b) hurricanes more destructive at a time when (c) COVID-19 makes sheltering more dangerous and (d) patients diagnosed with cancer are undergoing active treatment.

CASE STUDY 15.1: A COMPLEXITY TALE—CLIMATE, 'CANES, COVID-19, AND CANCER

The dynamics of public health in a complex world are powerfully illustrated as we examine the nexus of climate, 'canes (hurricanes), COVID-19, and cancer. Let's start by introducing each element in turn and considering the interactions.

First, climate is changing rapidly and alarmingly. In *Climate Change 2022: Impacts, Adaptation, and Vulnerability*, the Intergovernmental Panel on Climate Change updates the current state of "complex, compound, and cascading risks" to planetary health and survival.[20,21] Climate change itself is vastly complex, and its scientific exploration is unequalled in scope and scale.

Second, as one illustration of layered risks influenced by climate change, hurricane activity is increasing over recent decades.[3] These tropical cyclonic systems—variously termed hurricanes, typhoons, and cyclones—are becoming stronger and wetter and decreasing their forward speed as they move over land.[22-26] They also have a propensity to move slowly along coastlines while maintaining their strength over warm waters.[27] Collectively, tropical cyclones are becoming more dangerous, damaging, and traumatizing for human populations in the path. Increasingly destructive storms have the potential to severely damage homes, schools, and businesses; disrupt electrical power and critical infrastructure; and render healthcare systems inoperable.

Third, the ongoing COVID-19 pandemic acts as a threat multiplier.[28] The sporadic emergence of COVID-19 variants of concern (VOCs)—characterized by combinations of high infectivity, increased illness severity, and capability for evading immune protection despite vaccination—increases population risks for airborne transmission leading to COVID-19 illness. The likelihood for COVID-19 spread is greatly amplified in communities with low levels of vaccine coverage.

How does the pandemic intersect with climate-driven hurricane risks to population health? When COVID-19 is circulating in communities that are projected to be in the storm's path, proven mitigation measures for protecting populations from hurricane hazards—specifically, evacuation and sheltering—are transmuted into risk behaviors for airborne transmission of COVID-19.[29-31] Moving and gathering people together in congregate hurricane shelters for their protection increases contagion risks.

(continued)

Fourth, medically vulnerable patients (MedVPs) represent a diverse subset of the population that is particularly susceptible to the harmful effects of climate-potentiated hurricanes in the era of COVID-19. A core set of hurricane disaster preparedness actions is common to the general public and to MedVPs alike: creating a flexible and realistic family disaster plan, knowing the local hazards of primary concern, stockpiling supplies, and developing contingencies for when—and how—to safely evacuate and shelter.

Yet, each MedVP population has distinctive needs related to their specific medical condition. Examples include persons with asthma who must have an ample supply of inhalers; persons with type 1 diabetes who must have adequate quantities and varieties of insulins and glucose monitoring supplies; persons with end-stage kidney disease who require uninterrupted access to renal dialysis; persons living with spinal cord injury/disorder who need electrical power for their mobility devices, inclusive disability access, and ongoing respiratory therapies to keep airways clear; and patients with chronic obstructive pulmonary disease (COPD) who need electrical power for their oxygen concentrators.

Here we consider one MedVP group in more detail: cancer patients who are currently undergoing active treatment (e.g., chemotherapy, radiation therapy) for solid cancers. How can these individuals prepare for an approaching hurricane while actively receiving their treatment sessions and maintaining their schedule of supportive care visits? This is indeed challenging. COVID-19 in the community further compounds risks to health for patients in treatment.

An expanding literature describes how Atlantic hurricanes disrupt therapies for cancer patients receiving active treatment regimens—and worsen survival outcomes.[32-34] As one example, Hurricane Maria's devastating passage through Puerto Rico in 2017 caused widespread and prolonged power outages.[34] Faced with 2- to 3-week interruptions in radiation therapy, interventional radiologists devised strategies on the fly, developing altered fractionation or dose escalation protocols for their patients with lung, head and neck, uterine cervix, breast, and prostate cancers. In the aftermath, these clinicians thoroughly revamped hurricane preparedness procedures to adapt to the complexities they encountered—and yet, Hurricane Maria predated the arrival of COVID-19.[34]

Further improvisations would be required in the pandemic era. During 2020, the first hurricane season of the COVID-19 pandemic, evacuation and sheltering procedures had to be modified. Both the Federal Emergency Management Agency (FEMA) and the Centers for Disease Control and Prevention (CDC) updated their guidance for safer congregate sheltering procedures. These community shelters, perennially considered to be the resource of last resort, now had to contend with airborne COVID-19 infection risks. Historically and more commonly, storm-experienced families living along the U.S. hurricane coast tend to evacuate short distances to shelter—and socialize—in the better-built homes of family and friends who live inland. Masking, social distancing, and observant hygiene have not been part of the process—and often were not observed in 2020.

Unfortunately, 2020 was the busiest Atlantic hurricane season on record with 30 named storms. No COVID-19 vaccines were available. Most of the 11 storms that made landfall in the continental U.S. came ashore just as the entire U.S. hurricane coast was experiencing a steep summer surge of COVID-19 cases. Sheltering procedures were largely improvised, requiring more spacing between shelter occupants when possible, wearing masks, and cleansing hands and surfaces—very crude infection control procedures.

(continued)

COVID-19 transmission risks were higher for cancer patients because of their increased vulnerability to both contracting and dying from severe COVID-19 disease,[35-41] or developing serious "long COVID" sequelae.[42] Susceptibility to COVID-19 was extremely elevated for cancer patients undergoing active treatment, some of whom were immunocompromised.

During hurricane season 2021, effective COVID-19 vaccines were widely available. A high level of vaccine uptake could have altered the risk landscape for COVID-19 transmission dramatically, and especially for persons living with cancer and receiving treatment. Adherence to vaccination could have been the strongest deterrent to the massive Gulf Coast surge of COVID-19 cases caused by the Delta variant that was both highly infectious and highly virulent, leading to increased rates of hospitalization and death. Instead, the Gulf states led the nation in Delta cases during the peak of hurricane season, while the vaccination rates throughout the region were woeful.

In fact, when Hurricane Ida intensified right up to the moment of landfall in New Orleans on August 29, 2022 (ironically, the 16th anniversary of Hurricane Katrina), the two most impacted Gulf states—Louisiana and Mississippi—had the lowest vaccination rates in the nation.

All of the elements came into play simultaneously. Hurricane Ida, the strongest storm of the 2021 season, bore all of the hallmarks of a climate-driven storm. Ida came ashore in New Orleans at Category 4 intensity, complicating care for cancer patients receiving treatment at the Stanley S. Scott Cancer Center and other care facilities. Some care centers were not operable for variable periods of time due to storm damage. Power outages and lack of internet made communications with providers difficult, leading to canceled and missed appointments that affected treatment regimens. Some patients needed to restart their therapies with new providers in locales outside the area of severe storm impact. Many pharmacies in the impact zone lost power, including the capability for refrigeration, forcing them to discard quantities of vital cancer medications and delaying refills.

While no study has documented the extent of COVID-19 infection and illness in cancer patients during and after Ida, the excess vulnerability of cancer patients was notable. What was more observable was that staffing at cancer treatment centers was affected due to a multitude of challenges including providers dealing with their own storm recovery and providers ill with COVID-19—or caring for their family members with COVID-19. In some instances, there was a delay for cancer patients urgently needing inpatient beds because of COVID-19 surge admissions already occupying the beds.

Wrapping up our tale of superimposed risks, we observe:

1. Climate change is evolving and worsening.
2. Climate change is transforming hurricane hazards, making them more dangerous and traumatizing.
3. The overlay of pandemic COVID-19, particularly with the sporadic introduction of new variants, makes hurricane evacuation and sheltering more complicated.
4. Health risks are further magnified for MedVPs, including persons living with cancer.

Taken together, the mission of safeguarding cancer patients from the intertwined threats of hurricane impact and COVID-19 spread is intricate—and complex.

BRIDGING DISCOVERY SCIENCE AND THE DELIVERY OF EVIDENCE-BASED INTERVENTIONS

THE ROLE OF IMPLEMENTATION SCIENCE

In the early days of sea travel, scurvy was responsible for the death of more sailors than war or accidents. A captain suspected that lemon juice might help reduce mortality and recommended that some of the ships he supervised give three teaspoons to sailors daily. The experiment worked; all these sailors remained healthy while onboard other ships, 110 out of 278 sailors who did not receive lemon juice died over the same time period. Despite the clear benefits of citrus fruits and juices in preventing scurvy, it took the British navy more than 250 years to implement this cheap and effective intervention while other innovations such as bringing new ships into the fleet were promptly accepted.[43] This gap from discovery to delivery is not unique; adoption and dissemination of innovation is a challenge across many fields, including public health and healthcare.[44]

Implementation science is "the study of methods to promote the adoption and integration of evidence-based practices (EBPs), interventions, and policies into routine healthcare and public health settings."[45] The field's scope is broader than traditional research and focuses—in addition to patient-level interventions—on provider, organization, and policy levels of healthcare and public health. The field aims to close the gap between discovery and delivery of interventions through the use of theoretical frameworks and transdisciplinary methods. Implementation science originally evolved from practice-based interventions in the 1960s. Accelerated funding by multiple parties has shifted the focus of implementation science toward filling the gap between scientific discoveries and the application of innovations to improve population health.[46]

WHY ROBUST IMPLEMENTATION APPROACHES ARE ESSENTIAL TO PUBLIC HEALTH

Because public health interventions are often context-specific and complex, knowledge about the most effective implementation methods is critical to improving the health of a population and promoting health equity. Ineffective implementation is neither affordable nor sustainable, which is particularly problematic in a resource-scarce field like public health.[47] There is ample evidence of the success of affordable and lifesaving public health interventions. Nevertheless, we often have little understanding of the best methods to deliver those interventions effectively in different settings and health systems.

Implementation science sheds light on the gap between what can be achieved in theory and the real-world factors that govern practice. It is estimated that it takes an average of 17 years to incorporate EBPs into routine general practice in healthcare and public health. Unfortunately, even this disappointing estimate might be overly optimistic. Only about half of EBPs in clinical care ever achieve widespread adoption.[48] The gap between discovery and delivery can also be, in part, due to the lack of guidance in the literature on which interventions truly produce results. This in turn is due to the lack of coherent methodological frameworks to evaluate interventions. This trend is shifting as implementation science gains more ground, especially in global health.

Although both the medical and public health fields have made great advancements over the past century, every day about 830 women die from preventable pregnancy- and childbirth-related complications.[49] In 2020, 5.6 million children under the age of 5 died.[50] More often than not, those deaths were avoidable through proper design, planning, and execution of EBPs that minimize adverse pregnancy outcomes. For example, we know that insecticide-treated bed nets disrupt the malaria transmission cycle and that oral rehydration therapy is effective in reversing the consequences of diarrhea, yet there is a global lag in ensuring that both interventions are used effectively and widely.[51]

THE CORE TENENTS THAT GUIDE EFFECTIVE IMPLEMENTATION

POLITICAL SUPPORT

It is difficult for interventions to succeed without political support. Political support often translates into better access to governmental collaborators as well as funding opportunities. The pivotal role political support plays in advancing or hindering effective implementation could not be clearer than in the case of global efforts to eradicate poliomyelitis. In 1988, the World Health Assembly (WHA) launched the Global Polio Eradication Initiative (GPEI) to work toward the goal of eradicating the disease at a time when 350,000 polio cases occurred annually. This initiative was supported by national governments across the globe. The U.S. government has been a leader in this endeavor and has volunteered support from the CDC and the U.S. Agency for International Development (USAID) in efforts to assist countries to achieve complete eradication.[52] Since the campaign began, poliomyelitis has been eliminated from 120 countries and five of six World Health Organization (WHO) regions. Currently, poliomyelitis remains endemic in only two countries: Afghanistan and Pakistan. In 2021, only six polio cases were detected worldwide. Isolated cases may be detected in other nations.[53] A single case in Malawi in 2022 prompted a mass vaccination program targeted for 2.9 million children.

ADEQUATE FUNDING

Funding is pivotal for effective implementation of interventions. In the case of poliomyelitis, the continuous provision of funding has been instrumental in the advancement toward the global goal of eradicating the disease. For example, in 2019, the United States appropriated $241 million for this effort.[29]

Securing adequate funding is a major challenge for successful implementation of new policies and programs. In almost all implementation proposals, the projected costs—including costs of labor, materials, and technical assistance—are often as important as evidence of program effectiveness in shaping the decisions of interested parties to either adopt or reject an initiative. Conducting an economic evaluation provides communities and policy makers with evidence of the feasibility, scalability, and sustainability of public initiatives and leads to informed decision-making.[54] Yet, cost/benefit analyses of programs remain uncommon in public health.[55]

CLEAR COMMUNICATION

Effective communications operate on several fronts: convincing individuals to change their behaviors, advocating for implementation of public health initiatives within institutions, and increasing political will and commitment in favor of health programs and policies. For example, the Mothers Against Drunk Driving (MADD) campaign transformed societal perceptions on drinking and driving in the United States and ultimately led to increased political support to change the laws in the country.[56] Communication is also important within entities charged with implementing an intervention. For an implementation to be successful, the implementers need to be well-informed of the mission and goals of an intervention.[57]

In the case of poliomyelitis, well-planned communication efforts were instrumental to the success of vaccination efforts and in maintaining communities' trust in vaccines. Successful communication plans about the importance of the polio vaccine included media briefings, collaborator engagement, and social mobilization that were guided by research findings.[58]

EFFECTIVE MANAGEMENT OF LOGISTICS

In addition to funding and communication, successful implementation is contingent upon effective management of logistics. Streamlining logistics increases the impact of an initiative. A reliable supply of commodities creates a culture of confidence and motivates target populations to seek and use services offered. Moreover, effective management of logistics enhances quality of care; well-supplied programs provide better services. Effective management of logistics also creates cost-effectiveness, which in turn translates to lower budgets and more political support.[59]

Streamlining logistics increases the impact of an initiative.

In the case of polio, an effective, globally coordinated vaccine supply chain has been an integral part of the global eradication success story. Throughout the duration of this international initiative, one priority has been continuous planning and evaluation to ensure a reliable supply of poliovirus vaccine year over year.[60]

FRAGILE POINTS IN THE IMPLEMENTATION CHAIN WHERE INTERVENTIONS CAN FAIL

Both individual factors (e.g., ideology) and organizational factors (e.g., improper management of resources and cultural norms) can be barriers to successful implementation of public health initiatives. Barriers to successful implementation often arise when policy makers and implementers do not consider contextual factors that can affect their proposed policies or programs. Interventions can fail if there is a lack of effective communication delivered to community members, other collaborators, and intervention staff and a lack of understanding of the context or culture. Moreover, issues in supply-chain management, open distribution channels, available human resources, and geographic access are critical elements bearing on the success or failure of an intervention.[61] Cultural and social norms can also present challenges for implementation. Norms can influence socioeconomic or gender discrimination or cultural preferences that prevent communities from accessing and benefitting from a particular intervention.[28]

HOW PUBLIC HEALTH SYSTEMS CAN BE BUILT TO CREATE STRONGER PATHS TO IMPLEMENTATION

Public health systems do not operate in a vacuum. As we illustrated earlier, the health of populations is driven by actions of multiple sectors. Public health systems must engage these different sectors to achieve better health outcomes for populations. One step to build public health systems that acknowledge determinants of health that are linked to other sectors is the recent rise of the concept of Health in All Policies (HiAP). HiAP is "an approach to public policies across sectors that systematically takes into account the health implications of decisions, seeks synergies, and avoids harmful health impacts in order to improve population health and health equity. It improves accountability of policymakers for health impacts at all levels of policymaking. It includes an emphasis on the consequences of public policies on health systems, determinants of health, and well-being."[62] The approach requires a recognition that many of the current health challenges, including chronic diseases, climate change, and health inequities, are complex and often linked. This requires building public health systems that work across sectors, advance collaboration, and encourage innovative solutions.[63]

There are examples of initiatives reforming health systems to address social determinants of health and improve program implementation. One is the initiative by the Chilean government to adopt the work of the WHO Commission on Social Determinants of Health. The Ministry of Health created a national strategy for health equity and chose six health programs to reorient in a manner that would address social determinants of health and reduce health inequities among the Chilean population. Other countries that started similar reforms include Spain, Indonesia, and Nepal.[64]

Practical implementation of multisectoral approaches to create healthier populations is currently driven by cities rather than countries. For example, the city of Los Angeles created the Healthy Design Workgroup in 2012. The group was led by the Health Department and included Regional Planning, Parks and Recreation, Internal Services Department, the Fire Department, Community Development Commission, Public Works, Beaches and Harbors, the Arts Commission, the Chief Information Office, and the Chief Executive Office. The group was tasked with developing and implementing policies that encourage access to transit, safe walking, bicycling, and access to outdoor physical activities and to community gardens and farmers' markets. The workgroup was successful in implementing many interdepartmental activities including high-visibility crosswalks at dangerous intersections.[65]

THE INTERSECTION OF PUBLIC HEALTH WITH HEALTHCARE DELIVERY SYSTEMS

THE U.S. HEALTHCARE SYSTEM AND ITS LINK TO POPULATION HEALTH

The United States ranks 138 out of 184 countries in maternal mortality; 46 countries have a lower rate than the United States.[66] The United States ranks 170 out of 225 countries in infant mortality; 55 countries have a lower infant death rate than the United States.[67] The United States ranks 43 out of 224 countries on life expectancy; residents in 42 countries live longer than those in the United States.[68] More than two-thirds of Americans are overweight or obese. Diabetes[69] and cardiovascular diseases are leading causes of disease and death in the United States.

Even though many factors contribute to these numbers, there is no question that the structure of the healthcare system plays an important role in shaping the health of the U.S. population. The United States spends more money on healthcare per capita than any other country with a 50% higher expenditure compared to the second-highest country, Norway. Yet, as the statistics show, spending is not matched by an appropriate return on investment. Unlike the majority of high-income countries, the United States still does not provide a form of universal health coverage (UHC). It is, thus, not surprising that the United States scores lower than most of the high-income countries on many critical health indicators.

The U.S. healthcare system was largely developed through the private sector with little involvement from the government. The majority of Americans continue to receive their coverage through private health insurance, and, unlike the majority of other high-income countries, a substantial number of Americans lack health insurance. The adoption of the Affordable Care Act aimed to move the United States closer toward UHC, but deficiencies and inequalities in access and quality of healthcare persist. In 2019, more than 28.9 million nonelderly Americans remained uninsured.[70] The "uninsured" status is disproportionally high among race/ethnic minorities, persons of lower socioeconomic status, and those with limited education. These groups are already vulnerable to health inequities linked to many diseases. Moreover, while specialty care is relatively strong in the United States, overall, Americans have less access to primary care than people living in other high-income countries. The same applies to continuity of care. To illustrate, Americans with complex illnesses are less likely to keep the same physician for 5 years than their counterparts in other countries.[28,71]

The U.S. healthcare system was largely developed through the private sector with little involvement from the government.

HEALTHCARE SYSTEMS WORLDWIDE

Healthcare systems are complex and perform multiple functions, depending on the country and context. Healthcare systems serve different goals in different settings, and the structure of healthcare systems varies around the world. Most healthcare systems follow one of four models: the Beveridge model, the Bismarck model, the National Health Insurance or Tommy Douglas model, and the out-of-pocket model (**Table 15.2**).

In the Beveridge model, healthcare, similar to the police or public libraries, is financed and provided by the government through taxes. In this model, most, if not all, healthcare facilities are owned by the government. Countries that use this model include Great Britain, New Zealand, and most of the Scandinavian countries.

The Bismarck model is operationalized in many forms, but all mandate an insurance system—usually called "sickness funds"—which is often financed by employers and employees jointly. Like the insurance system in the United States, healthcare provision is often private. However, unlike the insurance system in the United States, the Bismarck model aims to cover all citizens, even if not employed. Countries that use this model include Germany, the Netherlands, and Japan.

The National Health Insurance model is a government-run insurance system that covers all citizens, uses private-sector providers, and is funded by taxpayers. This system runs at a lower cost than the U.S. system but limits the range of covered medical services and has longer waiting periods. Canada is a prime example of such a system.

The out-of-pocket model characterizes most countries around the world. It is used by countries that are too poor to have a national system. In countries that use this model, the rich can pay for healthcare and the poor remain sick or die from disease.[72]

The WHO has championed health as a human right since its inception in 1948. With increasing recognition of the importance of providing access to care for all citizens in order to maintain a healthy population, the WHO advocates strongly for the adoption of a UHC model by all countries. UHC means that "all individuals and communities receive the health services they need without suffering financial hardship. It includes the full spectrum of essential, quality health services, from health promotion to prevention, treatment, rehabilitation, and palliative care."[73] The United Nations (UN) is actively promoting the goal of UHC for all countries by 2030 as part of the Sustainable Development Goals (SDGs).

TABLE 15.2 Different Healthcare System Models Adopted Worldwide

MODEL	STRUCTURE	FINANCING	EXAMPLE
Beveridge model	Most, if not all, healthcare facilities are owned and operated by the government	Financed by the government through taxes	Great Britain
Bismarck model	Most healthcare facilities are privately run	An insurance system that is mostly financed through joint employer–employee payments	Germany and Japan
National Health Insurance	Healthcare facilities are privately run	A government-run insurance system that is taxpayer funded	Canada
Out-of-pocket	No specific structure	No specific financing, and the individual pays for most services out of pocket	Majority of countries

The unanticipated national opioid epidemic in the United States, first detected in middle-aged White Americans, is a product of complex causation that implicates our healthcare delivery systems (Case Study 15.2; you can access the podcast accompanying Case Study 15.2 by following this link to Springer Publishing Company Connect™: http://connect.springerpub.com/content/book/978-0-8261-8043-8/part/part04/chapter/ch15).

CASE STUDY 15.2: MAKING YOUR PAIN GO AWAY/CREATING AN OPIOID EPIDEMIC

A startling reversal of the long-term downturn in mortality was noted as death rates rose steeply for White Americans, aged 45 to 54, over the past decade. This was unexpected, curious, and not amenable to easy explanation. Princeton economists Case and Deaton describe this phenomenon as "deaths of despair" in persons who were grappling with job loss, income stagnation, a sense of being bypassed by the American dream, and polysubstance use leading to suicides and alcohol and drug deaths. Perhaps the major driver specific to this demographic was the spike in overdose deaths largely related to the licit and illicit use of opioid pain relievers (OPRs). Middle-aged White Americans are more likely to die from an opioid overdose than any other racial group.[74] The death rate for non-Whites was in decline while the death rate for Whites was rising.[75] Whites had a higher rate of drug-induced deaths than the overall—all races combined—rate of drug deaths.

Between 2000 and 2014, the death rate from OPRs increased by 200%.[76] Provisional data from the CDC's National Center for Health Statistics indicated there were an estimated 107,622 drug overdose deaths in the United States during 2021, an increase of nearly 15% from the 93,655 deaths estimated in 2020. The 2021 increase was half of what it was one year earlier, when overdose deaths rose 30% from 2019 to 2020. Three in four overdose deaths in 2021 (75% or 80,816 deaths) involved opioids.[77]

The trend in prescribing OPRs appears to follow the trend of OPR-related deaths. Non-White, especially African American/Black patients, are less likely to be prescribed opioids for back pain.[78]

Prescriptions for OPRs surged after strong advocacy to make pain assessment a routine part of primary care in the 1990s; pain is "the fifth vital sign." The other vital signs are temperature, pulse (heart rate), respirations, and blood pressure. Although the frequency and level/severity of pain symptoms reported by Americans have not changed since 1999,[79,80] the quantity of prescribed opioids, such as hydrocodone, oxycodone, and methadone, has quadrupled.[81] As far back as 2008, the United States accounted for 81% of oxycodone (Percocet) and almost 100% of hydrocodone (Vicodin) prescriptions worldwide.[82] Moreover, about 20% of patients with noncancer pain symptoms in the United States receive an opioid prescription.[57]

OPRs carry extremely high addiction potential related to the neurophysiology of these medications that act upon the pain/pleasure dopaminergic neurotransmitter pathways in the brain. Taking OPRs is dually reinforced. Alleviation of pain is a powerful negative reinforcer (take OPR, reduce/eliminate the aversive pain stimulus), while the concomitant stimulation of the addiction circuitry is a strong positive reinforcer (take OPR, experience pleasurable sensations). Habituation develops rapidly, requiring increasing doses of OPRs to achieve the same levels of pain reduction/pleasure sensation.

(continued)

Factors that led to the steep, and uncontrolled, increase in prescriptions for OPRs in the United States are complex and interconnected. Many include the intersection of addiction and profit. First, physicians overprescribing opioids to reduce the pain of their patients is central to the opioid overdose epidemic in the country.[83] Between 1998 and 2008, more than 6% of the U.S. adult population abused prescription drugs, more than all other forms of drug abuse combined. During the same period, hospitals reported a 400% increase in narcotic prescription abuse-related admissions and a 200% rise in narcotic prescription abuse deaths.[84] There does not, however, seem to be a consensus among physicians regarding best practices to prescribe opioids.[57] In California, for example, 3% of prescribing physicians account for 55% of opioid prescriptions.[61]

Second, while physicians' prescription habits are important, the reasons why physicians adopt such habits are as important. Marketing strategies by pharmaceutical companies are an important driver of the trend of overprescriptions by physicians.[85] Since the 1990s, pharmaceutical companies actively pushed to increase the availability of prescription opioids in the marketplace. While companies cannot be faulted for trying to make a profit, the tactics used by pharmaceutical companies to boost the sale of prescription opioids were less than ethical at times.[86] To illustrate, let us examine the practice by pharmaceutical company Purdue Pharma to sell the opioid OxyContin. The company used a combination of marketing to physicians, expanding the medical conditions in which the drug can be used, and mislabeling the drug as "abuse resistant" to get physicians to prefer prescribing OxyContin over other drugs. Over a period of 10 years, the company made a profit of $3.1 billion from the sales of the drug.[87]

The complexity of the opioid epidemic increases when those who were initially treated for pain symptoms become polydrug users and turn to "street" drugs. Once addicted to prescription OPRs, people frequently divert to using heroin as a less expensive alternative that is available throughout the United States in highly pure form. Drug experimentation often leads to drug mixing, for example, heroin with fentanyl, which leads to a much higher probability of overdose. Once OPR users transition to heroin, many further transition to injection. Beyond the initial aversion to injection, users rapidly find the intravenous route of administration to be much more dependable for producing the pain relief/pleasure sensations. With injection came additional public health risks such as elevated rates of HIV, hepatitis C, and other blood-borne infections. Additional injection-related risks include abscesses, infections, and death of tissue (necrosis) at the injection site. Moreover, polydrug addiction is associated with criminal activities, risky sex, or other behaviors to support the drug habit. All the while, the overdose risk continues to loom large.

There are a number of efforts, such as the CDC's new guidelines for prescribing opioids for chronic pain, which aim to address the epidemic. The guidelines recommend that opioids be considered in highly specific situations such as alleviating intractable pain during end-of-life care, but not prescribed as first-line medications for chronic pain.[88] The CDC has provided funding to states to improve safe prescribing practices.[89] These efforts seem to be working, and the number of opioid prescriptions has fallen in recent years in parallel with the realization of the dangers of OPR prescribing practices.[90]

(continued)

The Food and Drug Administration (FDA) also recently limited high-dose for-mulations of opioids. These efforts have led to decreasing methadone-related deaths.[91] There are also multiple state and local efforts that have shown promise in addressing the opioid epidemic through engaging communities. One example is the Angel program developed by the Gloucester Police Department in Massa-chusetts.[92] The program offered a voluntary, no arrest, direct referral for detoxifica-tion and, ultimately, rehabilitation for those who need it.[93] During its first year, the program served hundreds of people.[94] The success of the model encouraged more than 150 police departments in 28 states to adopt and replicate the program.[95]

SUMMARY

Populations are complex systems that are influenced by political, economic, and social factors. A complex systems approach can enhance public health interventions through accounting for the interconnected factors that determine—and are determined by—health indicators. A complex systems approach to public health can extend beyond conceptual understanding of what deter-mines the health of populations (e.g., the interconnected factors driving the obesity and opioid epidemics) to enlighten empirical analyses. A number of methods factor the different levels of characteristics of a population into the analysis of a complex public health issue such as social network analysis and agent-based modeling.

Lack of understanding of the complexity of the factors affecting the health of populations can lead to policy resistance. For example, the widespread use of antibiotics without much reg-ulation led to the rise of drug-resistant pathogens. As such, it is important to take a methodical approach to our public health practice, or what we often refer to as implementation science. Im-plementation science adopts frameworks that aim to close the gap between scientific discovery and the delivery of public health interventions.

Improving the health of populations cannot be achieved without the existence of accessi-ble and well functioning healthcare systems. Healthcare systems vary greatly around the globe, and the WHO has been advocating for the adoption of universal healthcare—which guarantees healthcare access to all—regardless of the healthcare system adopted by a country.

End-of-Chapter Resources

Access additional case study podcasts online at http://connect.springerpub.com/ content/book/978-0-8261-8043-8/

DISCUSSION QUESTIONS

1. What else do you think can be done to eradicate the opioid epidemic in the United States in addition to the efforts discussed in this chapter?

2. Do you know of any other worldwide strategies like the GPEI that have been successful in eradicating a disease on a global scale?

3. You are charged with implementing UHC in your country. Who are the interested parties to consider when developing your implementation plan? What are the potential barriers to its implementation and acceptance?

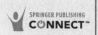 A robust set of instructor resources designed to supplement this text is located at http://connect.springerpub.com/content/book/978-0-8261-8043-8. Qualifying instructors may request access by emailing textbook@springerpub.com.

REFERENCES

1. Galea S, Riddle M, Kaplan GA. Causal thinking and complex system approaches in epidemiology. *Int J Epidemiol.* 2010;39:97-106. doi:10.1093/ije/dyp296
2. Keyes KM, Galea S. *Population Health Science.* Oxford University Press; 2016. https://global.oup.com/academic/product/population-health-science-9780190459376?cc=us&lang=en&
3. Pearce N, Merletti F. Complexity, simplicity, and epidemiology. *Int J Epidemiol.* 2006;35(3):515-519. doi:10.1093/ije/dyi322
4. Cornell CIS. *What is a complex system?* http://www.cs.cornell.edu/rz/ISAT/7March97/ppframe.htm
5. Braithwaite J. Growing inequality: bridging complex systems, population health and health disparities. *Int J Epidemiol.* 2018;47(1):351-353. doi:10.1093/ije/dyy001
6. El-Sayed AM, Galea S. Systems science and population health. In: El-Sayed AM, Galea S, eds. *Systems Science and Population Health.* Oxford University Press; 2017. doi:10.1093/acprof:oso/9780190492397.001.0001
7. Luke DA, Stamatakis KA. Systems science methods in public health: dynamics, networks, and agents. *Annu Rev Public Health.* 2012;33:357-376. doi:10.1146/annurev-publhealth-031210-101222
8. National Institutes of Health. Collaboration Details: Models of Infectious Disease Agent Study (MIDAS). https://crs.od.nih.gov/CRSPublic/View.aspx?Id=5701
9. Roux AVD. Complex systems thinking and current impasses in health disparities research. *Am J Public Health.* 2011;101(9):1627-1634. doi:10.2105/AJPH.2011.300149
10. GOV.UK. *Tackling obesities: future choices.* Published October 17, 2007. https://www.gov.uk/government/collections/tackling-obesities-future-choices
11. El-Sayed AM, Scarborough P, Seemann L, Galea S. Social network analysis and agent-based modeling in social epidemiology. *Epidemiol Perspect Innov.* 2012;9(1):1. doi:10.1186/1742-5573-9-1
12. Christakis NA, Fowler JH. The spread of obesity in a large social network over 32 years. *N Engl J Med.* 2007;357(4):370-379. doi:10.1056/NEJMsa066082
13. Lofgren E. Systems dynamics models. In: El-Sayed AM, Galea S, eds. *Systems Science and Population Health.* Oxford University Press; 2017:77-86.
14. Basu S. Microsimulation. In: El-Sayed AM, Galea S, eds. *Systems Science and Population Health.* Oxford University Press; 2017:99-112.
15. Sterman JD. Learning from evidence in a complex world. *Am J Public Health.* 2006;96(3):505-514. doi:10.2105/AJPH.2005.066043
16. Cassell MM, Halperin DT, Shelton JD, Stanton D. Risk compensation: the Achilles' heel of innovations in HIV prevention? *BMJ.* 2006;332(7541):605-607. doi:10.1136/bmj.332.7541.605
17. Leung E, Weil DE, Raviglione M, Nakatani H. The WHO policy package to combat antimicrobial resistance. *Bull World Health Organ.* 2011;89(5):390-392. doi:10.2471/BLT.11.088435
18. Winston C, Maheshri V, Mannering F. An exploration of the offset hypothesis using disaggregate data: the case of airbags and antilock brakes. *J Risk Uncertain.* 2006;32(2):83-99. doi:10.1007/s11166-006-8288-7
19. De Leeuw E, Peters D. Nine questions to guide development and implementation of health in all policies. *Health Promot Int.* 2015;30(4):987-997. doi:10.1093/heapro/dau034
20. Intergovernmental Panel on Climate Change. *Climate change 2022: impacts, adaptation and vulnerability.* In Pörtner H-O, Roberts DC, Tignor M, Poloczanska ES, Mintenbeck K, Alegría A, Craig M, Langsdorf S, Löschke S, Möller V, Okem A, Rama B, eds. *Contribution of Working Group II to the Sixth Assessment Report of the Intergovernmental Panel on Climate Change.* Cambridge University Press. 2022. https://www.ipcc.ch/report/ar6/wg2/
21. Cutter SL. Compound, cascading, or complex disasters: what's in a name? *Environ Sci Policy.* 2018;60(6):16-25. doi:10.1080/00139157.2018.1517518
22. Elsner JB, Kossin JP, Jagger TH. The increasing intensity of the strongest tropical cyclones. *Nature.* 2008;455(7209):92-95. doi:10.1038/nature07234
23. Kossin JP, Knapp KR, Olander TL, Velden CS. Global increase in major tropical cyclone exceedance probability over the past four decades [published correction appears in *Proc Natl Acad Sci USA.* 2020;117(47):29990]. *Proc Natl Acad Sci USA.* 2020;117(22):11975-11980. doi:10.1073/pnas.1920849117
24. Bhatia KT, Vecchi GA, Knutson TR, et al. Recent increases in tropical cyclone intensification rates [published correction appears in *Nat Commun*]. *Nat Commun.* 2019;10(1):635. doi:10.1038/s41467-019-08471-z

25. Kossin JP. A global slowdown of tropical-cyclone translation speed [published correction appears in *Nature*. 2018;564(7735):E11-E16]. *Nature*. 2018;*558*(7708):104-107. doi:10.1038/s41586-018-0158-3

26. Li L, Chakraborty P. Slower decay of landfalling hurricanes in a warming world [published correction appears in *Nature*. 2021;593(7857):E4-E11]. *Nature*. 2020;*587*(7833):230-234. doi:10.1038/s41586-020-2867-7

27. Wang S, Toumi R. Recent migration of tropical cyclones toward coasts. *Science*. 2021;*371*(6528):514-517. doi:10.1126/science.abb9038

28. Salas RN, Shultz JM, Solomon CG. The climate crisis and COVID-19–A major threat to the pandemic response. *N Engl J Med*. 2020;*383*(11):e70. doi:10.1056/NEJMp2022011

29. Shultz JM, Fugate C, Galea S. Cascading risks of COVID-19 resurgence during an active 2020 Atlantic hurricane season. *JAMA*. 2020;*324*(10):935-936. doi:10.1001/jama.2020.15398

30. Shultz JM, Kossin JP, Ali A, et al. Superimposed threats to population health from tropical cyclones in the prevaccine era of COVID-19. *Lancet Planet Health*. 2020;*4*(11):e506-e508. doi:10.1016/S2542-5196(20)30250-3

31. Shultz JM, Kossin JP, Hertelendy A, et al. Mitigating the twin threats of climate-driven Atlantic hurricanes and COVID-19 transmission. *Disaster Med Public Health Prep*. 2020;*14*(4):494-503. doi:10.1017/dmp.2020.243

32. Man RX, Lack DA, Wyatt CE, Murray V. The effect of natural disasters on cancer care: a systematic review. *Lancet Oncol*. 2018;*19*(9):e482-e499. doi:10.1016/S1470-2045(18)30412-1

33. Nogueira LM, Sahar L, Efstathiou JA, Jemal A, Yabroff KR. Association between declared hurricane disasters and survival of patients with lung cancer undergoing radiation treatment. *JAMA*. 2019;*322*(3):269-271. doi:10.1001/jama.2019.7657

34. Gay HA, Santiago R, Gil B, et al. Lessons learned from Hurricane Maria in Puerto Rico: practical measures to mitigate the impact of a catastrophic natural disaster on radiation oncology patients. *Pract Radiat Oncol*. 2019;*9*(5):305-321. doi:10.1016/j.prro.2019.03.007

35. Lee LY, Cazier JB, Angelis V, et al. COVID-19 mortality in patients with cancer on chemotherapy or other anticancer treatments: a prospective cohort study [published correction appears in *Lancet*. 2020;396(10250):534]. *Lancet*. 2020;*395*(10241):1919-1926. doi:10.1016/S0140-6736(20)31173-9

36. Lee LYW, Cazier JB, Starkey T, et al. COVID-19 prevalence and mortality in patients with cancer and the effect of primary tumour subtype and patient demographics: a prospective cohort study [published correction appears in *Lancet Oncol*. 2020]. *Lancet Oncol*. 2020;*21*(10):1309-1316. doi:10.1016/S1470-2045(20)30442-3

37. Garassino MC, Whisenant JG, Huang LC, et al. COVID-19 in patients with thoracic malignancies (TERAVOLT): first results of an international, registry-based, cohort study. *Lancet Oncol*. 2020;*21*(7):914-922. doi:10.1016/S1470-2045(20)30314-4

38. Pinato DJ, Lee AJX, Biello F, et al. Presenting features and early mortality from SARS-CoV-2 infection in cancer patients during the initial stage of the COVID-19 pandemic in Europe. *Cancers (Basel)*. 2020;*12*(7):1841. doi:10.3390/cancers12071841

39. Kuderer NM, Choueiri TK, Shah DP, et al. Clinical impact of COVID-19 on patients with cancer (CCC19): a cohort study [published correction appears in *Lancet*. 2020;396(10253):758]. *Lancet*. 2020;*395*(10241):1907-1918. doi:10.1016/S0140-6736(20)31187-9

40. Pinato DJ, Zambelli A, Aguilar-Company J, et al. Clinical portrait of the SARS-CoV-2 epidemic in European cancer patients. *Cancer Discov*. 2020;*10*(10):1465-1474. doi:10.1158/2159-8290.CD-20-0773

41. Wilkinson E. COVID-19 pandemic to lead to thousands of additional UK lung cancer deaths. *Lancet Oncol*. 2022;*23*(1):20. doi:10.1016/S1470-2045(21)00699-9

42. Pinato DJ, Tabernero J, Bower M, et al. Prevalence and impact of COVID-19 sequelae on treatment and survival of patients with cancer who recovered from SARS-CoV-2 infection: evidence from the OnCovid retrospective, multicentre registry study. *Lancet Oncol*. 2021;*22*(12):1669-1680. doi:10.1016/S1470-2045(21)00573-8

43. Schmidt NA, Brown JM. *Evidence-Based Practice for Nurses: Appraisal and Application of Research*. 3rd ed. Jones & Bartlett; 2014.

44. Leonard-Barton D, Kraus WA. *Implementing new technology*. *Harvard Business Review*. Published November, 1985. https://hbr.org/1985/11/implementing-new-technology

45. Osanjo GO, Oyugi JO, Kibwage IO, et al. Building capacity in implementation science research training at the University of Nairobi. *Implement Sci*. 2016;*11*(1):30. doi:10.1186/s13012-016-0395-5

46. Lobb R, Colditz GA. Implementation science and its application to population health. *Annu Rev Public Health*. 2013;*34*:235-251. doi:10.1146/annurev-publhealth-031912-114444

47. MacDonald M, Pauly B, Wong G, et al. Supporting successful implementation of public health interventions: protocol for a realist synthesis. *Syst Rev*. 2016;*5*(1):54. doi:10.1186/s13643-016-0229-1

48. Bauer MS, Damschroder L, Hagedorn H, et al. An introduction to implementation science for the non-specialist. *BMC Psychol*. 2015;*3*(1):32. doi:10.1186/s40359-015-0089-9

49. World Health Organization. *Maternal mortality*. Published February 16, 2018. https://www.who.int/news-room/fact-sheets/detail/maternal-mortality

50. World Health Organization. *Child mortality (under 5 years)*. January 28, 2022. https://www.who.int/news-room/fact-sheets/detail/levels-and-trends-in-child-under-5-mortality-in-2020

51. Peters DH, Tran NT, Adam T. *Implementation Research in Health: A Practical Guide*. World Health Organization; 2013.

52. The Henry J. Kaiser Family Foundation. *The U.S. government and global polio efforts.* Published October 3, 2022. https://www.kff.org/global-health-policy/fact-sheet/the-u-s-government-and-global-polio-efforts

53. Thompson KM, Tebbens RJD. Eradication versus control for poliomyelitis: an economic analysis. *Lancet.* 2007;*369*(9570):1363-1371. doi:10.1016/S0140-6736(07)60532-7

54. Rabarison KM, Bish CL, Massoudi MS, Giles WH. Economic evaluation enhances public health decision making. *Front Public Health.* 2015;*3*:164. doi:10.3389/fpubh.2015.00164

55. National Research Council and Institute of Medicine. Implementation and dissemination of prevention programs. In: O'Connell ME, Boat T, Warner KE, eds. *Preventing Mental, Emotional, and Behavioral Disorders Among Young People: Progress and Possibilities.* National Academies Press; 2009. doi:10.1016/S0140-6736(07)60532-7

56. Frieden TR. Six components necessary for effective public health program implementation. *Am J Public Health.* 2014;*104*(1):17-22. doi:10.2105/AJPH.2013.301608

57. Greenhalgh T, Robert G, Macfarlane F, et al. Diffusion of innovations in service organizations: systematic review and recommendations. *Milbank Q.* 2004;*82*(4):581-629. doi:10.1111/j.0887-378X.2004.00325.x

58. Brink S. *Can't Help Falling In Love With A Vaccine: How Polio Campaign Beat Vaccine Hesitancy. NPR.* May 3, 2021. https://www.npr.org/sections/health-shots/2021/05/03/988756973/cant-help-falling-in-love-with-a-vaccine-how-polio-campaign-beat-vaccine-hesitan

59. U.S. Agency for International Development. *The Logistics Handbook a Practical Guide for the Supply Chain Management of Health Commodities.* Author; 2011. https://www.ghsupplychain.org/logistics-handbook

60. UNICEF. *Eradicating polio.* https://www.unicef.org/immunization/polio

61. The Rural Health Information Hub. *Common implementation challenges.* https://www.ruralhealthinfo.org/toolkits/rural-toolkit/3/implementation-challenges

62. World Health Organization. *Health promotion.* https://www.who.int/teams/health-promotion/enhanced-wellbeing/eighth-global-conference

63. Rudolph L, Caplan J, Ben-Moshe K, Dillon L. *Health in All Policies: A Guide for State and Local Governments.* The Public Health Institute; 2013. http://www.phi.org/uploads/files/Health_in_All_Policies-A_Guide_for_State_and_Local_Governments.pdf

64. World Health Organization. *The Innov8 Approach for Reviewing National Health Programmes to Leave No One Behind: Technical Handbook.* Author; 2016. https://www.who.int/publications/i/item/9789241511391

65. Wernham A, Teutsch SM. Health in all policies for big cities. *J Public Health Manag Pract.* 2015;*21*(suppl 1):S56-S65. doi:10.1097/PHH.0000000000000130

66. Central Intelligence Agency. *The World Factbook: maternal mortality ratio.* https://www.cia.gov/the-world-factbook/field/maternal-mortality-ratio/

67. Central Intelligence Agency. *The World Factbook: infant mortality rate.* https://www.cia.gov/the-world-factbook/field/infant-mortality-rate/

68. Central Intelligence Agency. *The World Factbook: life expectancy at birth.* https://www.cia.gov/the-world-factbook/field/life-expectancy-at-birth/

69. The National Institute of Diabetes and Digestive and Kidney Diseases. *Overweight & obesity statistics.* https://www.niddk.nih.gov/health-information/health-statistics/overweight-obesity

70. Tolbert J, Drake P, Damico A. *Key facts about the uninsured population.* Published December 19, 2022. https://www.kff.org/uninsured/fact-sheet/key-facts-about-the-uninsured-population

71. National Research Council (US), Institute of Medicine (US). Public health and medical care systems. In: Woolf SH, Aron L, eds. *U.S. Health in International Perspective: Shorter Lives, Poorer Health.* National Academies Press; 2013:106-137. https://www.ncbi.nlm.nih.gov/books/NBK154484/#ch4.s18

72. Wallace LS. A view of health care around the world. *Ann Fam Med.* 2013;*11*(1):84. doi:10.1370/afm.1484

73. World Health Organization. *Universal health coverage (UHC).* Published January 24, 2019. https://www.who.int/news-room/fact-sheets/detail/universal-health-coverage-(uhc)

74. Kolata G. *Death rates rising for middle-aged white Americans, study finds. The New York Times.* November 2, 2015. https://www.nytimes.com/2015/11/03/health/death-rates-rising-for-middle-aged-white-americans-study-finds.html

75. Kara J. *Who is dying in Connecticut's opioid overdose crisis?* Trend CT. https://overdose.trendct.org/story/who

76. Rudd RA, Aleshire N, Zibbell JE, Gladden RM. Increases in drug and opioid overdose deaths—United States, 2000–2014. *MMWR Morb Mortal Wkly Rep.* 2016;*64*(50-51):1378-1382. doi:10.15585/mmwr.mm6450a3

77. Centers for Disease Control and Prevention. *U.S. overdose deaths in 2021 increased half as much as in 2020—but are still up 15%.* Published May 11, 2022. https://www.cdc.gov/nchs/pressroom/nchs_press_releases/2022/202205.htm

78. Singhal A, Tien Y-Y, Hsia RY. Racial-ethnic disparities in opioid prescriptions at emergency department visits for conditions commonly associated with prescription drug abuse. *PLoS One.* 2016;*11*(8):e0159224. doi:10.1371/journal.pone.0159224

79. Chang H-Y, Daubresse M, Kruszewski SP, Alexander GC. Prevalence and treatment of pain in EDs in the United States, 2000 to 2010. *Am J Emerg Med.* 2014;32(5):421-431. doi:10.1016/j.ajem.2014.01.015

80. Daubresse M, Chang H-Y, Yu Y, et al. Ambulatory diagnosis and treatment of nonmalignant pain in the United States, 2000–2010. *Med Care.* 2013;51(10):870-878. doi:10.1097/MLR.0b013e3182a95d86

81. Centers for Disease Control and Prevention. *Understanding drug overdoses and deaths.* https://www.cdc.gov/drugoverdose/epidemic/index.html

82. International Narcotics Control Board. *Report of the International Narcotics Control Board for 2008.* United Nations; 2009. https://www.incb.org/documents/Publications/AnnualReports/AR2008/AR_08_English.pdf

83. Fields HL. The doctor's dilemma: opiate analgesics and chronic pain. *Neuron.* 2011;69(4):591-594. doi:10.1016/j.neuron.2011.02.001

84. Swedlow A, Ireland J, Johnson G. *Prescribing Patterns of Schedule II Opioids in California Workers' Compensation.* California Workers' Compensation Institute; 2011. https://www.cwci.org/document.php?file=1438.pdf

85. Gounder C. *Who is responsible for the pain-pill epidemic? The New Yorker.* November 8, 2013. https://www.newyorker.com/business/currency/who-is-responsible-for-the-pain-pill-epidemic

86. Addictions.com. *The role of pharmaceutical companies in the opioid epidemic.* Updated May 13, 2019. https://www.addictions.com/opiate/the-role-of-pharmaceutical-companies-in-the-opioid-epidemic

87. Ethics Unwrapped. *Oxycontin & the Opioid Epidemic.* https://ethicsunwrapped.utexas.edu/video/oxycontin-the-opioid-epidemic#:~:text=In%201996%2C%20in%20its%20first,Purdue%20is%20the%20Sackler%20family

88. Centers for Disease Control and Prevention. *CDC guideline for prescribing opioids for chronic pain.* Updated April 17, 2019. https://www.cdc.gov/drugoverdose/pdf/Guidelines_At-A-Glance-508.pdf

89. U.S. Department of Health and Human Services. *National opioids crisis: help and resources.* https://www.hhs.gov/opioids

90. Goodnough A, Tavernise S. *Opioid prescriptions drop for first time in two decades. New York Times.* May 20, 2016. https://www.nytimes.com/2016/05/21/health/opioid-prescriptions-drop-for-first-time-in-two-decades.html

91. Rudd RA, Seth P, David F, Scholl L. Increases in drug and opioid-involved overdose deaths—United States, 2010–2015. *MMWR Morb Mortal Wkly Rep.* 2016;65(5051):1445-1452. doi:10.15585/mmwr.mm655051e1

92. Gloucester Police Department. Gloucester Police Department Volunteer ANGEL Program. https://gloucesterpd.com/wp-content/uploads/sites/17/2015/05/Gloucester-Angel-Program.pdf

93. Becker D. *Gloucester Police Mark 1 Year Since Launch Of 'Angel Program' To Combat Opioid Crisis. WBUR.* June 2, 2016. https://www.wbur.org/morningedition/2016/06/02/gloucester-police-angel-program-anniversary

94. Schiff DM, Drainoni M-L, Bair-Merritt M, et al. A police-led addiction treatment referral program in Massachusetts. *N Engl J Med.* 2016;375(25):2502-2503. doi:10.1056/NEJMc1611640

95. Marcelo P. *Researchers: Gloucester's Angel Program helped nearly 400 drug addicts. CBS Boston.* Published December 21, 2016. https://boston.cbslocal.com/2016/12/21/gloucester-police-angel-program-helped-400-drug-addicts

INDEX

Note: An *f* after a page number indicates a figure. A *t* indicates a table.